Classics in Psychiatry

Psychological Healing

A Historical and Clinical Study

Pierre [Marie-Felix] Janet

Volume I

ARNO PRESS

A New York Times Company

New York • 1976

Editorial Supervision: EVE NELSON

——◆——

Reprint Edition 1976 by Arno Press Inc.

Reprinted from a copy in
  The University of Illinois Library

CLASSICS IN PSYCHIATRY
ISBN for complete set: 0-405-07410-7
See last pages of this volume for titles.

Manufactured in the United States of America

——◆——

Library of Congress Cataloging in Publication Data

Janet, Pierre, 1859-1947.
  Psychological healing.

  (Classics in psychiatry)
  Translation of Les médications psychologiques.
  Reprint of the 1925 ed. published by Macmillan,
New York.
  Bibliography: p.
  1. Psychotherapy. I. Title. II. Series.
[DNLM: WM420 J33me 1925a]
RC480.J3613 1975   616.8'914   75-16710
ISBN 0-405-07437-9

PSYCHOLOGICAL
HEALING   I

Psychological Healing

A Historical and Clinical Study

By

Pierre Janet

Member of the Institute
Professor of Psychology at the College of France

Translated from the French by
Eden and Cedar Paul

IN TWO VOLUMES—VOL. I

NEW YORK
THE MACMILLAN COMPANY
1925

TO

Dr. JEAN NAGEOTTE

PROFESSOR OF COMPARATIVE HISTOLOGY

AT THE COLLEGE OF FRANCE

PHYSICIAN TO THE SALPÊTRIÈRE

Table of Contents

VOLUME ONE

PART II

UTILISATION OF THE PATIENT'S AUTOMATISM

PART III

PSYCHOLOGICAL ECONOMIES

INTRODUCTION

In the autumn sessions of 1904 and 1906, at the Lowell Institute in Boston, Massachusetts, I gave a series of lectures upon The Chief Methods of Psychotherapeutics. Some of these lectures were repeated at Liége, Belgium, during the exhibition of 1905, and also at Baltimore, Maryland, in March 1906. In 1907, I lectured at the College of France upon The Psychological Concepts underlying Psychotherapeutic Methods. The present work is a reproduction of these courses of lectures.

During the years mentioned, and subsequently, the treatment of various diseases by psychological methods, the more or less definite use of psychotherapeutics, was arousing general interest. Shortly before, the revival of hypnotism had been received with widespread enthusiasm. " The mind," said Bernheim twenty years earlier, " is not a negligible quantity. There is such a thing as psychobiology. There is also such a thing as psychotherapy. This is a powerful lever, and one which the human intelligence and medical therapeutists must turn to full account." [1] There were many doctors willing to endorse what Myers said in 1893: "Nascitur ars nova medendi. We now propose to heal the patient's tissue, not through the stomach nor through the blood, but through the brain. . . . At each step we touch the ill more intimately ; we call more directly upon the patient's own inward forces to effect the needed change." [2]

It is true that hypnotism and suggestion underwent a period of decadence after the struggle with the school of Charcot. Nevertheless, mental therapeutics continued to exist under a different name. People spoke of treatment by reasoning and by persuasion. At the beginning of the present century, there was in all lands and all tongues, and especially in English-speaking countries, an enormous output of litera-

[1] Bernheim, La suggestion, 1886, p. 48.
[2] Proceedings of the Society for Psychical Research, 1893, p. 207.

ture concerning these new methods for the relief of suffering humanity.

To take one example only, in the United States, psychotherapeutic chairs were established. Morton Prince lectured on psychotherapy at Tufts College Medical School in Boston ; lectures were delivered upon all aspects of the subject ; periodicals, such as the " Journal of Abnormal Psychology," were devoted to their study ; numerous books on psychotherapeutics were published. William B. Parker issued a huge work in three quarto volumes entitled *Psychotherapy, a Course of Reading in Sound Psychology, Sound Medicine, and Sound Religion.* This appeared in New York in 1908 and 1909, professors of neurology and psychiatry, philosophers, psychologists, and divines belonging to various creeds, being the collaborators. The American Therapeutic Society, at its annual meeting held at New Haven, Connecticut, in 1909, had a long discussion concerning these new therapeutic methods. The debates were incorporated in a remarkable volume entitled *Psychotherapeutics, a Symposium,* published at Boston, Mass., in 1910. It was obvious that the scientific world and university teaching had been greatly influenced by the various movements issuing from the study of animal magnetism, the study of hypnotism, and the study of Christian Science inaugurated by Mrs. Eddy. In these circumstances, my lectures on psychotherapeutics delivered at Boston in 1904 and at the College of France in 1907 played their part in an interesting movement, and were perhaps able to discuss certain problems from a rather individual point of view. That is why I prepared them for the press, so that they were ready for publication at the outbreak of the war.

The war, of course, interfered with my plans for immediate publication. To-day it might seem that such studies occupy a less important place. But the decline, I think, is apparent merely. The movement which developed so powerfully in all lands will soon resume its course. These historical studies, which display the leading part played by French philosophers and medical practitioners in the development of so promising a science, these therapeutic studies for whose practical application there is unfortunately only too much need thanks to the neuropathic disorders engendered by the war, still retain their interest.

My general study of psychotherapeutics comprises three groups of studies. The first of these, as we have just seen, mainly consists of a historical investigation into theories and practices which have played a great part in the development of psychotherapeutics, and which are worthy of a place in the history of medicine and the history of psychology. The first studies of this kind bear upon miraculous, religious, and philosophical methods of treatment. Among these, we are entitled to include animal magnetism, for although this method had certain claims to be regarded as scientific, its main inspiration was drawn from an undue fondness for systematisation and from a love for the marvellous. For a long time I have been collecting facts relating to the history of animal magnetism, but it will suffice to epitomise the most important of these. I think it is difficult to understand the evolution of medical and psychological ideas, whether in America or in France, unless we start from the concepts of animal magnetism, whose place in the history of this development seems to me extremely important. Next we have to consider Mrs. Eddy's Christian Science, little known in France, although in America it has initiated a notable movement of ideas. Christian Science is a link between animal magnetism and some of the most modern methods of treatment by moralisation. What are known in the United States as the Emmanuel movement and the New Thought movement are offshoots of Christian Science, and lead us in turn to various interesting methods of the treatment of neuroses. Although the history of hypnotism has often been written at considerable length, I have found it necessary to give that history a place once more in my discussion of the development of psychotherapeutics. Besides, the later phases of this history, those subsequent to the struggle between the Salpêtrière School and the Nancy School, have hardly been studied as yet, although they are rather important.

Part One and Part Two are mainly concerned with such historical studies of the opening phases of psychotherapeutics. We then pass to consider more recent methods. The treatment of nervous disorders by rest has come very much to the front during recent decades, due especially to the teaching of Weir Mitchell of Philadelphia. It has aroused a good deal of controversy, for the doctors who treat disease by moralisation are inclined to make light of the fatigue of which neuropaths complain. Treatment by isolation in special institutions underwent an extension after the regime of asylums had been reformed owing to the efforts of Philippe Pinel in France and those of William Tuke in England. In this connexion there arise for consideration all the problems that concern the social influence exercised by human beings on one another. In the history alike of medical science and of psychology, a place has to be given to the doctrines which developed first of all in Austria and subsequently in the United States under the name of psychoanalysis. These doctrines, which are especially connected with the name of Sigmund Freud, originated out of the studies made by French investigators concerning traumatic memories. Despite much exaggeration and distortion, psychoanalysis has unquestionably done a great deal to promote interest in psychiatric researches and has initiated a notable movement of ideas. My book, therefore, contains a lengthy chapter on psychoanalysis, one which amplifies the report upon this subject which I presented to the International Congress of Medicine held in London in 1913. Nothing must be ignored in the history of medical science, for many things are reborn which may have seemed dead and buried. The queer methods of metallotherapeutics (æsthesiogenism) are the starting-point for an understanding of the methods of treatment by various excitations, the methods which have been recently revived. They lead us, moreover, to the remarkable procedures of the latest American schools of psychotherapeutics, although at first sight the resemblance is not obvious. We have not to do here solely with the history of medicine. I am confident that these studies will lead to a blossoming of the psychological sciences, and that my account of such developments is a contribution to the history of psychology and philosophy as well as to the history of medical science.

The second group of studies may be regarded as a collection of psychological investigations anent various concepts indispensable to the psychotherapeutist. The concepts in question are continually recurring in books on psychotherapeutics, and yet they are seldom accurately defined. It is obvious that a whole treatise on psychology would be required for the full analysis of the phenomena and the ideas underlying such terms as suggestion, hypnotism, mental disinfection, rest, isolation, the awakening of sensibility, excitation, etc. Still, we shall find it possible to dismiss certain hazy and inexact interpretations of a kind which have often facilitated the reproduction of the same facts under new names. In the case of some of the before-mentioned terms we shall be able to provide, if not definitions, at least explanations that will introduce a certain amount of clarity into our studies. I have laid especial stress upon some concepts which I regard as peculiarly valuable in medical psychology : the notions of psychological strength and weakness ; the notions of psychological tension and depression ; and the influences which act upon the former or the latter. In Chapter Ten, that dealing with treatment by isolation, I have done my best to throw light on the important problem of the fatigue which human beings produce in one another, the expenditure demanded by social relationships, the impoverishing action exercised by antipathetic individuals. When discussing treatment by excitation, I have been mainly concerned with the inverse problem, that of the stimulant influence of social life, that of enrichment by guidance, that of the advantages derivable from association with sympathetic individuals. Few people realise how numerous are the moral problems opened up by the simplest psychiatric studies ; few realise what a wealth of interesting details is furnished even by the most superficial study of mental disorder.

That is why the before-mentioned researches have been supplemented by a considerable number of clinical observations bearing upon the various psychoneuroses known by the names of neurasthenia, hysteria, psychasthenia, cyclothymia, and dementia præcox. If we disregard anatomical or etiological considerations concerning which little is as yet known, and if we confine ourselves to a descriptive treatment of symptoms and to the field of psychological analysis, all these troubles can be presented as different grades of a mental depression which reduces the energy or the tension of mental activity. For more than thirty years, with a collector's zeal, I have been accumulating records of such cases, and my notebooks now contain more than 3,500 of them. Many of the patients have been under observation for years, some for as long as fifteen or twenty years. I have thus been enabled to study neuroses from a special point of view, that of their evolution. It has been possible to note the modifications undergone by the disease as life advanced, and to study the influences affecting these modifications favourably or unfavourably. In most of the patients I have, for long periods, made use of, now one, now another, of the psychotherapeutic methods whose history and rationale are studied in the present work. By keeping the patient under observation for months or years after such courses of treatment, I have been enabled to ascertain the immediate and the remote effects of the various therapeutic procedures, and to secure a sort of experimental verification of their value. Herein will be found important supplementary illustrations to our study of psychotherapeutics.

Unfortunately, considerations of space have made it impossible, in most cases, to give even a brief account of these numerous medical and psychological observations. Only in instances of peculiar interest could I summarise the individual history of my patients. In general, I have had to content myself with allusions to coordinated clinical phenomena, derived from the observation of a number of like cases of illness and giving expression to a mental and moral state common to all the members of the group ; I have had to be satisfied with statistical statements showing the number of persons affected by particular circumstances or relieved by this or that remedial measure. Though I have done my utmost to abridge the analyses, such observations occupy a considerable space, especially in Part Three of the work. Such a bulking of the material is unavoidable in studies of this character, for nothing but a detailed description of psychological phenomena will enable the reader to understand and reflect upon the interpretations. The development of the psychological sciences is still at a stage in which clinical observations and descriptions of characteristic types are more useful than systematised theories.

The main divisions of my book correspond to an advance which may I think be noted in the succession of psychotherapeutic methods. The earlier treatments of this character were general and vague ; the healer was satisfied with exercising some sort of *moral action* upon the patient. Subsequently, psychotherapeutics, as I shall endeavour to show, became more specialised ; it now appealed to latent mechanisms, to preexistent tendencies ; it acted by *utilisation of the patient's automatism.* A still more advanced method was that of those who were concerned to study the expenditure requisite for human activity, and to prescribe rest and isolation, thus organising an *economy* of the forces of the mind. Finally, psychotherapeutists of a still more adventurous type, have aimed at supplementing the inadequate forces by happy speculations, by new *acquisitions.* Thus Part One discusses the search for mental and moral action, and Part Two deals with the utilisation of the patient's automatism. Part Three is devoted to treatment by psychological economies ; to the various forms of treatment by rest, by isolation, and by psychological disinfection. Part Four is a study of the psychological acquisitions which have been sought with the aid of various psychophysiological methods of treatment, with the aid of different forms of excitation and with that of moral guidance.

Since the death of Professor Raymond in 1910, my psychological laboratory, which was originally organised in connexion with the Salpêtrière clinic, has been partly transferred to the clinic of my friend and colleague Dr. Jean Nageotte, Professor at the College of France and Physician to the Salpêtrière, whom I take this opportunity of thanking. Although, unfortunately, my own studies of pathological psychology fall far short in respect of accuracy and scientific truth of Nageotte's admirable researches concerning the histology of the nervous system and that of connective tissue, they have been inspired by the same ardour for knowledge and by a like sincerity. I am glad, therefore, to be able to dedicate this book to my friend.

PART ONE

SEARCH FOR MENTAL AND MORAL ACTION

CHAPTER ONE

MIRACULOUS HEALINGS

FROM time to time it has been the fashion to laugh at miracles and to deny that they occur. This is absurd, for we are surrounded by miracles ; our existence is a perpetual miracle ; every science has begun by the study of miracles. The miraculous enters into a huge category of phenomena which conflict with scientific determinism. I refer to phenomena which cannot be accurately predicted, and above all to those which cannot be made to occur unfailingly by causing a prior determinant to take place. When such phenomena are quite indifferent to us, we call them chance happenings ; when they are hurtful to us, we describe them as fate ; and when these undetermined phenomena are agreeable to us, we speak of them as miracles. If I am told that some unknown person has won the first prize in a lottery, I say that he has done so by chance ; but if I am myself the winner, I talk of a miracle, or of providential intervention.

But in most miracles there is another element. The undetermined happening is not merely one which interests us, but one we endeavour to make happen, one for whose happening we pave the way. Man always plays his part in the production of miracles. Almost always there is a magician or a priest at work ; there are ceremonies and sacred rites ; there is effort on the part of the person who will profit by the miracle. Sad experience teaches us, however, that all this preparation will not suffice to ensure the regular happening of the desired event. Ceremonial, however carefully practised, has not the same effect upon the production of a miracle as the application of heat has in making water boil. Man does not succeed in becoming a complete producer ; he is aware that he does not act alone, but is merely a collaborator with powerful forces which are, unfortunately, capricious. In this respect, a miracle resembles a work of art, which is certainly produced by man, but cannot be produced by all men, or even by the same man in all conditions. The work of art, like the miracle, results from man's collaboration with a mysterious and capricious inspiration.

Since these things are so, it is natural that the cure of disease should be, in especial, the domain of miracle. Cure is often uncertain, inexplicable by our limited science, impossible to foresee and produce at will. On the other hand, it is never indifferent to us, for man ardently seeks relief from his ailments, and will make immense sacrifices for this end. But even in provinces of medicine where we have made considerable progress, cure has still to be achieved by medical *art*; it is not surprising, therefore, that in provinces where our knowledge is less assured, cure should remain a matter of miracle.

1. Religious Miracles.

The first miraculous cures were regarded by most primitive folk as religious phenomena, for the mysterious forces which came to the aid of man's inadequate activities were conceived by them in the form of gods. These divine beings, fashioned after the image of the human mind, were supposed to behave in an extremely irregular and unpredictable manner, under the stimulus of motives which were often beyond our ken. This explained the capricious character of miracles.

At the outset it is probable that religious methods of treatment were applied to all diseases without exception. Before long, however, science began to develop, so that men became able to treat with almost unfailing success a certain number of unfortunate happenings whose nature was especially plain and intelligible. Treatment in these cases advanced a stage beyond miracle to become a work of art. Quite early, the gods lost interest in the treatment of dislocations and fractures, and handed over these elementary matters to the surgeons. But there still remained a huge multiplicity of diseases for whose relief the aid of the gods had to be invoked. Thus in ancient days there were two distinct practices of medicine. One of these was official and human, for here the results of treatment were explicable, and could be obtained with sufficient certainty to be regarded as the outcome of human science. The other medicine was religious, more or less secret in character, applied to the cure of comparatively hidden and obscure illnesses. A description of many of these religious practices and of numerous antique miracles will be found in the writings of Salverte,[1] Bouché-Leclercq,[2] and Paul Girard.[3]

One of the most interesting among such descriptions is that of the Asclepieion (Temple of Aesculapius) at Epidaurus. The description has been made famous by Charcot in his article entitled *La foi qui guérit*,[4] an article containing a comparison between ancient miracles and those which occur in our own days.

Within the sanctuary was a statue which was supposed to have miraculous healing powers. Around this statue and in other parts of the temple stood acolytes of all kinds, and priests to whom various duties were assigned. Some had to carry or to lead the patients. Others were doctors whose duty it was to ascertain the nature of the ailment when the sufferer arrived, and to decide whether there had been a cure when he departed. Some, again, were intercessors whose business it was to act as the patient's proxy, and to invoke the god's aid in his behalf. Some were interpreters who had to explain the treatment ordered by the god and to supervise its application. Others, finally, were concerned only with the financial side of the matter, and took charge of the gifts made by grateful patients.

The sufferers arrived in crowds from the most distant parts after long and arduous travel. On arrival, hoping to predispose the god in their favour, they laid valuable offerings at the entry to the temple and plunged into the cleansing waters of the fountain. After these preliminaries they were admitted to the porch, and had to pass one or more nights there. Not until after this period of probation, spent in public prayers and in listening to eloquent exhortations, was the sick man at length allowed access to the interior of the temple, where he was given advice in the form of oracles or prophetic dreams. Inscriptions record details of remarkable cures. " A blind soldier, Valerius Aper, having consulted

---

[1] Des sciences occultes, essai sur la magie, les prodiges et les miracles, 1856.
[2] Histoire de la divination, vol. iii, p. 298. [3] L'Asclepieion, 1881.
[4] " Archives de Neurologie," 1893, vol. i, p. 74 ; " La Revue Hebdoma-daire," December 3, 1892.

the oracle, was told to mix the blood of a white cock with honey in order to make an ointment with which he was to rub his eyes for three days. He recovered his sight and gave thanks to the god before the multitude. . . . A consumptive, Lucius, took ashes from the altar, steeped them in wine, and rubbed his chest with the mixture. He was instantly cured, and all the onlookers mingled in his rejoicings."

Those who had been cured in the temple of Aesculapius decorated the walls with votive inscriptions which were to preserve the memory of the miracle and were at the same time to make famous the name of him on whom it had been worked. The before-mentioned Valerius Aper is still trumpeted for having been cured, as if he had done some heroic deed. Grateful patients used also to attach to the walls small objects fashioned of more or less valuable material to represent the part of the body which had been healed. Thus in the ancient sanctuaries of Egypt, Greece, and Rome, we find arms, legs, necks, and breasts, made of common stone or of marble, of silver or of gold. It is a matter for regret that these images so seldom reproduce the exact malformations of the diseased limb. Still, Paul Richer has been able to publish the description of a votive offering which accurately reproduces the position of a foot in a state of hysterical contracture.

In the Middle Ages, although the name of the god had changed, the mode of treatment by miracle remained exactly the same. There were the same pilgrimages, the same ceremonies in front of the temples, the same fees, the same votive offerings. In some cases the miracle may be ascribed to a sacred statue and in others to a healing spring. Sometimes the essential role is played by a fragment of the true cross, or by one of the bones of a saint. Every church had its speciality, and in like manner the saints were often specialists. St. Marcoul cured scrofula ; St. Clair, diseases of the eye ; St. Fiacre, piles ; St. Ouen, deafness ; St. Roch, plague ; St. Petronella, fevers ; St. Mein, various skin troubles ; St. Cloud, boils ; and so on.

By the simple authority of their names, by the mere influence of their words, pious personages would sometimes exercise remarkable powers of cure, and they themselves could find no better explanation than that these cures were miracles, were the outcome of divine intervention. The

Reverend Curtis Manning Geer has published an interesting study of the miracles wrought by three of these notabilities : Eligius, Bishop of Noyon, 640–655 ; St. Malachi ; and Bernard of Clairvaux, 1146–1147. Geer tells us that Eligius once saw a man " contracted in all the limbs." The bishop exhorted the sufferer to have faith in Christ and in St. Denis, and to promise to have faith in God for the future. Then Eligius prayed over the sick man, took him by the hand, and said : " In the name of Jesus Christ, arise and stand upon your feet." Instantly, the sick man stood up, the contractures having passed away.[1]

In other instances, the individual through whose instrumentality the miracle was performed was a thaumaturge in virtue of his exalted function. Thus, the kings of France and the kings of England were believed to have the power of curing scrofula by the laying on of hands—" touching for the king's evil." Various studies have been published concerning the strange ceremonies associated with this practice. I may refer to a remarkable one by Edouard Brissaud on the king's evil[2] ; the writings of Cabanès and Landouzy, who describe the picturesque incidents which occurred when the king of France was touching for scrofula ; Helme's study ; and the work of Rondelet, who reproduces an old account written by Thomas Plattner of Basle in 1599. In France, the ceremony was discontinued in the reign of Louis XVI ; and the attempt of Charles X to revive it was unsuccessful. " Faith had been lost," writes Landouzy ; " touching for the king's evil is now nothing more than a historical memory, the reflexion of vanished beliefs, prejudices, and customs."[3]

But miracles had not ceased, and they were still needed. Very remarkable miracles were worked at or about the year 1736 in the Saint Médard cemetery at the tomb of Deacon Pâris. A valuable book, that of Carré de Montgeron, preserves their record. It is remarkable to find that those who write

[1] Psychotherapy, a Course of Reading in Sound Psychology, Sound Medicine, and Sound Religion, edited by W. B. Parker, 3 vols, New York, 1909, III, i, 65, and III, ii, 56, Curtis Manning Geer, Healing in the Middle Ages.— In this and subsequent references to Parker's Psychotherapy, the large Roman numeral denotes the volume, the small Roman numeral the part, and the Arabic numeral the page.

[2] Le mal du roi, " Journal du Magnétisme," viii, 493.

[3] Landouzy, Le toucher des écrouelles, l'hôspital Saint Marcoul, le mal du roi.

histories of the Lourdes miracles refer with contempt to Carré de Montgeron.[1] The reason may be that the latter's book was used by Charcot as a text when he was searching for a rational explanation of certain miracles. Notwithstanding the scorn of the Lourdes historiographers, Montgeron's account of the illness of the Demoiselle Coirin, who suffered from paralysis of the legs and ulcer of the breast, and his description of the cases of the Demoiselle Fourcroy and Marie-Anne Couronneau, affected with paralyses and contractures, are excellent medical observations. They may also serve as proofs of the reality of certain miraculous cures.

If miracles have not ceased to-day, this is simply because medical science has not yet advanced to a stage at which miracles will become needless. They do, in fact, still happen in all lands. Percival Lowell's book, *Occult Japan, or the Way of the Gods*, published in 1895, shows us that in Japan in our own days there occur miraculous cures precisely similar to those described in the literature of ancient Egypt and classical Greece. Similar miracles still take place in France. Various curative pilgrimages have been noted in our land. The holy blood of Fécamp, whose registers I have myself studied, has had remarkable successes ; for a long time the shrine of Our Lady of Salette has attracted crowds of pilgrims.

But the fame of these healing shrines has been eclipsed by that of the miraculous spring at Lourdes. The study of the Lourdes miracles is extremely interesting both from the psychological and from the medical point of view. Numerous books and articles on this topic have been published. I may refer, among others, to Lasserre's *Les épisodes miraculeux de Lourdes*, 1883 ; Boissarie's *Les grandes guérisons de Lourdes*, 1900 ; the admirable paper by the two Myers, *Mind Cure, Faith Cure, and the Miracles of Lourdes*, 1893 ; Georges Bertrin's, *Lourdes, apparitions et guérisons*, 1905 ; Mangin, *Les guérisons de Lourdes*, " Annales des Sciences Psychiques," December 1907. These writings give detailed accounts of the legends surrounding this movement of popular faith, the legends which have furnished the healing spring with the requisite prestige. They tell us of the huge crowds which have since 1868 flocked to the wonder-working church, and they depict the impressive ceremonies designed to act on the minds

[1] See Bibliography.

of those who come to be cured. They relate the most remarkable miracles, and the writers' desire to be accurate and truthful is obvious. One of the best accounts of the Lourdes miracles is that of Bertrin, but I should like to refer, in addition, to a very interesting book by Maria Longworth Storer, *The Story of a Miracle at Lourdes*, published at New York in 1908. This describes the case of a young woman who was twenty-seven years of age when she came to Lourdes. Eight years earlier, she had had an attack of typhoid, and thenceforward had suffered for years from abdominal pains which were ascribed to chronic appendicitis. When she was twenty-three, an operation was performed, with unsatisfactory results. The abdominal pains continued, abscesses occurred in the scar of the operation wound; there was pain and stiffness in the muscles of the back, so that the patient was bedridden, and had for a long time to wear Bonnet's apparatus. Three fæcal fistulas formed near the crest of the ilium. For two and a half years she suffered from retention of urine, so that the catheter had to be used, and throughout this time the urine contained pus. The transport of this patient to Lourdes was a difficult and painful matter, but within a few days after her first immersion in the piscina, a cure had been effected. Such occurrences are frequent at Lourdes, and we of the twentieth century are certainly entitled to congratulate ourselves upon the contemporary occurrence of miraculous cures which are hardly, if at all, less remarkable than those which took place at the temple of Aesculapius many centuries before Christ.

2. MAGICAL HEALINGS.

Cures effected under religious auspices are not the only ones entitled to be termed miraculous. The essential characteristic of a miracle is that man should ardently desire the occurrence of a certain phenomenon, but should not be sufficiently well informed as to the conditions that determine it, and should therefore be unable to bring it to pass without fail. Tentatively, he may try certain methods, knowing all the time that they are inadequate, and that for a successful issue there must be collaboration on the part of capricious forces. These forces, whose aid man invokes in so haphazard a fashion, were in the first instance gods. Subsequently, thanks to an evolution akin to that of which Comte speaks in formulating his Law of the Three States, they became natural forces, but forces of an extremely mysterious character, whose laws of action were unknown, so that there was a persistent analogy with divine caprice. Some recent authors have maintained that an appeal to a vague power of this kind was made antecedently to the origin of the idea of divine intervention.[1] The problem of the relationships between magic and religion is most interesting, but for our present purposes the only important point is that magicians, like priests, are not in a position to predict with confidence the results of their intervention. The magician has no reason to be surprised at failure, for he knows that failure is very likely ; all that he has when he begins operations is a certain measure of confidence and hope. This attitude of mind is closely akin to that characteristic of the priest who is preparing for the occurrence of a religious miracle. We must not draw too sharp a distinction between faith and doubt. Between these extremes, there are many intermediate sentiments which play a considerable part in all religions and in all systems of magic.

Many magical methods of treatment are still in close touch with religion ; they are based upon ancient and half-forgotten pacts with a god or a demon. The sympathetic powders and the celestial plasters of the Rosicrucians healed wounds, cured ulcers, and stopped bleeding. There are still extant talismans which were hung round the necks of patients by Apollonius of Tyana, and, in more recent days, by Paracelsus. We know that the word Abracadabra was a cure for tertian fever ; that the words Max, Pax, et Adimax, were a sovereign remedy for hydrophobia ; and so on.

In the case of other remedies of this kind we catch a glimpse of the idea that unknown chemical, physical, or physiological forces are at work. This accounts for the high repute of anise, red coral, the viper broth of which Madame de Sévigné speaks, orvietan, bezoar, theriac, powdered stag's horn, powdered crab's eye, etc. A medieval physician advised that a sow should be tied up close to the patient's bed ; a still

[1] Hubert and Mauss, Esquisse d'une théorie générale de la magie, "Année Sociologique," 1902-3.

more effective remedy was to put a litter of puppies into his bed. Here are some of these strange prescriptions : " To remove eye pain, take a wolf's right eye and pick it to pieces, and bind it to the suffering eye." . . . " For swollen eyes, take a live crab, pull his eyes out, and put him alive again into the water, and put the eyes upon the neck of the man who hath need. He will soon be well." . . . " For him that may not speak well, give him to drink hound's tongue." [1] To cure hysterical attacks : " It is a good thing to have ready glowing charcoal, and thereon to throw birds' feathers, especially partridge feathers, and old shoes, or bones, and pieces of woollen cloth, or pieces of fur, or asafoetida, and such stinking things. Let the patient inhale the smoke through mouth and nose." [2]

James Graham, a quack doctor who had studied medicine at Edinburgh and came to London towards the close of the eighteenth century, established there a Temple of Health with the special object of curing sterility. If the divine balsam which was his first prescription proved ineffective, he had recourse to an " electrical throne " and a " celestial bed." This bed was in a huge room, and was supported on six transparent pillars ; it had a purple satin coverlet. In the next room was a metal cylinder, which was supposed to act as conductor of the celestial and vivifying fire ; and oriental perfumes were also brought to the bed through glass tubes. Thus, the bed was filled with celestial and electric fire issuing from magnetic vapours. The cost of a night's lodging was only £50.[3]

It would be easy to enumerate thousands of similar methods of treatment, all of which had a passing vogue.

3. ANIMAL MAGNETISM.

One of the methods of treatment which at the outset closely resembled the magical methods considered in the last section deserves special attention. I refer to animal magnetism, which seems to me to have played an intermediate role between

---

[1] Parker, op. cit., III, i, 68 (Curtis Manning Geer, Healing in the Middle Ages).

[2] Chirurgie de Franco de Turriers, see Bibliography, Franco.

[3] Demangeon, De l'imagination considérée dans ses effets sur l' homme et sur es animaux, etc., 1829, p. 129.

magical methods of treatment and scientific psychotherapeutics. Moreover, the studies to which it gave rise paved the way for the analyses of pathological psychology, and gave a peculiar turn to much of our psychological science. Some day, full justice will be done to these hardy pioneers on whom so much contempt has been poured. Lengthy histories of all their doing will then be written. Here I can do no more than briefly indicate their place in the evolution of psychotherapeutics.

Mesmer [1] is regarded as the founder of animal magnetism, and mesmerism is an alternative name for the doctrine, but he is perhaps the least interesting of these writers. He is in line with the series of therapeutists before his day, those who effected miraculous cures by an appeal to mysterious forces ; he was clever enough to speak of forces whose nature was still little known, but which were beginning to attract attention—such forces as magnetism, electricity, and nervous energy, whose activity seemed real enough to the comparatively uneducated. It was easy to believe that these forces might act upon the human organism and might affect our health. Goclenius, van Helmont, Robert Fludd (1574–1637), and Winding (known also as Vindingius, 1673), had already pointed this out. The Scottish physician William Maxwell was the first to assemble into a definite body of doctrines the utterances of the ancients concerning the curative influence of magnetism.[2] He regarded all diseases as an outcome of the withdrawal of a vital fluid from our organs, and he believed that a proper balance could be reestablished by simply restoring the requisite amount of magnetic force. Substantially, Mesmer's propositions are an almost complete reproduction of Maxwell's aphorisms.

Mesmer was born in 1734, at the village of Iznang near Radolfszell, in Baden, on the Lake of Constance. Already in 1766, he attracted attention by the publication of a remarkable medical thesis in which he discussed the influence of the planets on the human body.[3] " This action," he wrote, " is exerted through the instrumentality of a universal fluid, a

---

[1] Good summaries of the early history of animal magnetism will be found in the following books : Ricard, Traité du magnétisme, 1841 ; Baragnon, Étude du magnétisme animal, 1853, p. 348 ; Noizet, Mémoire sur le somnambulisme, 1854 ; Schneider, L'hypnotisme, Paris, 1894.
[2] See Bibliography, Maxwell.   [3] De planetarum influxu.

kind of impalpable and invisible gas in which all bodies are immersed." Since this fluid had many " attractive properties " resembling those of the magnet, and since on the other hand its action was mainly exercised upon living beings, he termed it " the fluid of animal magnetism." His theory was that the human will was competent to set this fluid at work ; to withdraw it from one point and concentrate it at another ; and to produce very remarkable effects upon living creatures. Man, like a magnet, is divided in two from above down ; the left side contains poles opposite to those of the right side. Disease is merely a disorder of the harmonious distribution of these fluids. The proper treatment is to reestablish harmony by the application of magnetism.

Mesmer had little success either in Germany or in Switzerland. In 1778 he removed to Paris, at a date when the wonders worked at the Saint Médard cemetery had predisposed people to believe in mysterious forces. In association with a physician named Deslon, he founded a clinic at which he treated all kinds of diseases. Mesmer used an elaborate apparatus, and his practice was attended with a ceremonial similar to that employed at miraculous shrines. The patients were ushered into a hall of which all the windows were thickly curtained, so that darkness prevailed. The air was filled with plaintive strains from a pianoforte. In the middle of the room was a large oaken tub, Mesmer's famous " baquet." This was filled with a mixture of water, iron filings, and powdered glass. It had a lid pierced with holes, and coming up through the holes were jointed iron rods. The patients, upon whom absolute silence was enjoined, linked hands and applied the rods to the ailing spot. Mesmer, the great magnetiser, now appeared, wearing a silken robe of a pale lilac colour, and holding in his hand a long iron wand. He passed slowly through the ranks, fixing his eyes upon the patients, passing his hand over their bodies or touching them with his iron wand.

Many of the patients were unable to notice much result. Baron de Holbach and the literary critic La Harpe declared that they could feel absolutely nothing. But some of the patients coughed, spat, felt as if insects were running over their skin. Some, finally, especially young women, would fall down and go into convulsions, so that the hall certainly deserved the name of the "Hell of Convulsions." This convulsive state, attended by hiccough, outbursts of laughter, and sometimes delirium, constituted what was known as "the crisis," and was supposed to be most salutary. After two or three sittings of the kind, many persons declared that they had been cured of the most multiform disorders.

To begin with, Mesmer's success was remarkable. When he spoke of leaving France, splendid offers were made to induce him to remain. Those who attended his courses were pledged to secrecy. They founded a Society of Harmony which had branches in various provincial towns, such as Strasburg, Lyons, and Bordeaux. A Society of Magnetism was even founded in San Domingo. The grand master of the Sovereign Order of the Knights of Malta adopted the discovery with enthusiasm, and all the knights of the Order undertook to cure by magnetism.

Unfortunately, certain official bodies, the Academy of Medicine and the Academy of Sciences, intervened. Two commissions of enquiry sat. The first of these issued an indecisive report. The second, among whose members were Lavoisier, de Jussieu, and Bailly, was definitely unfavourable to Mesmer's claims, deciding that the phenomena included nothing which could not be explained by imitation and imagination, and that in the long run the effects of the treatment could not fail to be unwholesome. Although de Jussieu added a note of a more favourable tenour, these reports did Mesmer a good deal of harm. Fashion, fickle as usual, turned against him, and a few witticisms brought about his final ruin. One of his patients died at the very time when a letter of gratitude from this patient was being published. "Monsieur Court de Gébelin," wrote one of the papers, "has just died, cured by animal magnetism." A piece was staged ridiculing the doctors of the new school; and a few humorous songs finished their discomfiture. In his mortification, Mesmer shook the dust of France off his feet. When, subsequently, he wished to return, his place had been filled; magnetism had undergone changes, and had entered a new phase.

The second period of animal magnetism began towards 1786 or 1787, with the publication of the works of the Marquis de Puységur and Dr. Petetin of Lyons; though it was not until 1813, when the first writings of Deleuze were published, that this phase attained its climax. The new departure was initiated by some remarkable observations made by Puységur on his Buzancy estate, where, following Mesmer's example, he magnetised all the patients who came for relief. Applying the method one day to a young shepherd named Victor, he tried to induce the salutary crisis. But the youth, instead of exhibiting the familiar contortions, passed into a quiet sleep. There was, however, something very strange about this sleep. For a time nothing could awaken Victor, who was unaffected either by noises or by shakings. Then, after a while, he spontaneously got up without waking, though he walked, talked, and went about his avocations with considerably more intelligence than he was in the habit of displaying in his ordinary waking life. In this sleepwalking condition, he obeyed all Puységur's orders, for the marquis seemed to be able to modify Victor's ideas and sentiments at will. When Victor finally woke up, he felt very well, but seemed to have completely forgotten all that had just happened. Such were the primary characteristics of the condition to which Puységur gave the name of *somnambulism*, by analogy with natural somnambulism, with which people were already familiar.

Mesmer's defenders declared that the same phenomenon had occurred round the famous tub. This was probably true, for somnambulism is common in neuropaths who have been subjected to fatigue or emotion. But the occurrence of a phenomenon is not the same thing as its discovery ; those who are present when it happens must notice it, describe it, and, above all, understand its importance. Such a study of artificially induced somnambulism was certainly the work of Puységur, Petetin, and Deleuze.[1]

This form of somnambulism, which was accompanied by a certain degree of intellectual exaltation and by a marvellous agility, seemed extremely interesting to the before-mentioned authors. They believed that the mind of the somnambulist had been profoundly modified. The strange appearance of the person who spoke while asleep, and who, after awakening, could not remember what he had said, made them believe

[1] Puységur, Rapport des cures opérées à Baïonne par le magnétisme animal, 1784 ; Petetin, Mémoire sur la découverte des phénomènes que présentent la catalepsie et le somnambulisme, 1787 ; Deleuze, Histoire du magnétisme animal, 2 vols., 1813.

that a quasi-miraculous transformation had taken place. A form of thought so different from the normal must be all-powerful. Such thought must surely be free from the limitations imposed by the harsh necessities of our senses and by the laws of time and space. The somnambulist reminded the observer of the inspired prophets, and of the pythonesses (the priestesses of the temple of Apollo at Delphi). Surely those whose mode of thought had been transformed, those who could see with their eyes shut and act while asleep, must also be able to see through obstacles, to see at any distance, to know the past and the future. The discovery that the mode of thought was transformed, and the recognition of the strange character of the transformation, aroused wonder in the minds of persons who were novices in the study of pathological psychology, and led them to the idea of somnambulist *lucidity*.

This was a revelation; artificial somnambulism was regarded with overpowering interest, and it monopolised attention. How magnificent, how divine, to transform a human mind in this way, to render a man capable of seeing, understanding, and knowing everything! What splendid services such a mind might render! At any cost, the means of producing this mental transformation must be studied; the observers must learn how to make use of the wonderful instruments they had created; they must strive to render the somnambulists more " lucid " than ever. Such was the aim eagerly sought for half a century by a number of able investigators. To that end, they devoted a vast amount of intelligence and patience. The animal magnetism of the French school is the outcome of their search for this philosopher's stone, the " ultra-lucid somnambulist."

The general principles adopted by these investigators during the second period differed little from those taught by Mesmer in earlier days. The question at issue was always the transformation of a human being by the action of a mysterious fluid resembling electricity and magnetism. It is true that the magnetisers no longer talked about the stars, and that they were less inclined to trouble themselves concerning the universal fluid. The fluid they wished to turn to account was somewhat less pretentious, and more human. " The magnetic fluid," said Deleuze, " is an emanation from ourselves

guided by the will; . . . he who magnetises for curative
purposes is aiding with his own life the failing life of the
sufferer." The fluid was invisible to ordinary persons, but
somnambulists, who can see everything, saw it exuding from
the magnetiser's hands and eyes. To some it appeared white,
whilst others saw it as red or yellow or blue. No general
agreement as to colour could be secured, but it was certain
that the magnetiser could bottle it, and that if carried to a
distance in bottles it continued to have an effect. These
were minor details; the essential point was still the supposed
existence of a mysterious agent which people were trying to
use without knowing what it was, and in whose power to
work wonders they had faith rather than scientific conviction.
It was in practical matters that the new magnetism differed
notably from the old. The magnetisers were mainly concerned with the production of lucid somnambulists. Here
they were confronted with a remarkable problem, one whose
difficulty and interest are equally conspicuous. The question
was, how to produce, experimentally and at the desired
moment, an extensive psychological modification; and how
to restore the subject to the normal state without much
trouble and at an opportune time. The modification must
not be brought about by administering any substance capable
of producing intoxication; it must be secured through the
instrumentality of an invisible fluid, by non-material action,
without violence of any kind, and without administering a
poison. Those who are hardy enough to attempt the solution
of such a problem must perforce study the mental condition
of their subjects, that they may be enabled to recognise the
somnambulist modification whenever it occurs. They will
have to take careful note of the subject's sayings and doings;
to ascertain his character, his memories, his sensations. The
magnetisers will form the habit of keeping a written record
of all that can be observed during the sittings; they will note
down the subject's most trifling observations, together with
everything said in his presence. I have studied the work of a
very interesting magnetiser, Dr. Perrier of Caen, and am
greatly indebted to his son for sending me the manuscripts containing the notes made by Dr. Perrier during
attempts to magnetise patients. They are extremely careful and detailed medical observations. Above all, they

are psychological observations made upon persons studied in isolation.

The magnetisers were likewise constrained to search for every possible way of transforming the mental condition, and this led them to study the role of emotion, attention, and fatigue. They knew that the subject did not become " lucid " if he was unable to concentrate, and they were continually calling him to order. They learned that the somnambulist quickly grew tired, and that the sittings must not be indefinitely prolonged. Those who were persistently engaged in the study of somnambulism and its variations had to interest themselves in all the nervous and mental phenomena (many of them morbid) which are akin to somnambulism. The magnetisers were the first to gain a familiar acquaintance with neuropathic disorders and the various forms of nervous crisis. During half a century they were engaged in studies which became the foundation of modern psychology.

Furthermore, those who were passing whole days in contact with their subjects, and who were taking so much pains to understand the working of the subjects' minds, necessarily became interested in them as individuals. It was no longer a question of a physical operation upon an unknown person ; it had become a question of sympathetic penetration into a mind. " Desire your patient's welfare," wrote Deleuze. " Do not allow yourself to be turned aside from your enterprise, and you will necessarily convey to him the impetus and the impression of the sentiment which animates your own mind. . . . The first requisite for those who wish to magnetise is will ; the second is the confidence which the magnetiser has in his own powers ; the third is kindly interest and a wish to do good." Teste, again, tells us : " It is essential to regulate the physical and moral life of the subject." It was natural that psychotherapeutics should issue from animal magnetism.

The magnetisers did not forget that the primary aim of their method had been the cure of disease ; they continued attempts at treatment side by side with their psychological studies. There were two different modes of treatment. The first I have to describe was simpler than the other, and less interesting. The patient was brought to a somnambulist who, in a condition of marvellous lucidity, was able to see the lesions deeply placed in the sufferer's body and to indicate the desirable remedies. " This patient's stomach is full of pimples. . . . I see a ball of hair blocking the bowel. . . . Your chest is all grazed inside, and you must not sing for several days ; it looks as if it had been scraped with a knife, and your lungs are full of dust." [1] The remedies are sometimes peculiar. One of Perrier's somnambulists was fond of prescribing that the chest should be ironed with a hot smoothing iron ; another would frequently order a powder made from the callosities of a horse's legs—the strangeness of these remedies made them all the more effective. Dr. Clapier reported that in two months he had been able to effect more than sixty perfect cures, thanks to the advice of his somnambulist. " Indeed, I have nothing to do with the cure, for I have merely carried out the somnambulist's prescriptions." [2] What admirable modesty !

This was nothing more than the speedy and commonplace treatment of comparatively uninteresting patients. The essential aim of the magnetiser's treatment was always to exercise a directly transformative action on the patient, who was thus to become an ultra-lucid somnambulist. All the psychological and neurological studies previously mentioned were made upon patients who, in pursuit of health, were trying to become somnambulists. With this end in view, they would modify their whole course of life, visiting the magnetiser daily or every other day, and devoting many hours to the sittings. They adopted a new system of physical and moral hygiene, and sedulously watched their own metamorphosis, studying the modifications in sensation and memory. In fine, they collaborated with the magnetiser both in their own cure and in the making of the splendid discoveries which were to transform the human race.

These psychological and therapeutic studies aroused almost incredible enthusiasm. Towards 1840, animal magnetism underwent a blossoming which must not be forgotten by those who wish to understand subsequent and analogous but less extensive surges of enthusiasm. The number of investigators devoted to such studies between 1813 and 1850 was very large. It would be a mistake to imagine that these magnetisers

---

[1] " Journal du Magnétisme," vol. i, p. 76 ; " Hermès," 1826, p. 40.
[2] " Hermès," 1826, p. 216.

were all simpletons or quacks. Many of them were persons
of high distinction ; doctors, naturalists, and philosophers.
I do not count among them such men as Bertrand, Ordinaire,
and Faria ; nor those who styled themselves "animists."
These belong to a different group of investigators, and we
shall have to consider them among the forerunners of hypnotism. I am thinking only of the magnetisers properly so
called, of those whose direct aim was to bring about a transformation of the nervous system that would determine the
onset of lucid somnambulism. Among them are a great
many names which should not be forgotten, such as those of
the physician Deleuze and the philosopher Bouillet, who were
collaborators with the celebrated physicist Ampère. Among
noted doctors and physiologists who were magnetisers, the
following may be mentioned : de Lausanne, Chardel, Dupau,
Ricard, Aubin Gauthier, Henin of Cuvillers, Charpignon,
Teste, Chambard, Lafontaine, Morin, Olivier, Dupotet de
Sennevoy, Perrier of Caen, Charles Despine. Magnetic
societies were founded all over the place. There were several
in Paris. In the provinces there were : the Magnetic Society
of Rennes ; the Troyes Athenæum of Mesmerology (1847) ;
the Magnetic Society of Caen ; the Magnetic Society of
Rheims, in which town a magnetic congress was held in 1845 ;
and others. A branch society was even formed at New
Orleans. Numerous periodicals were issued by these magnetic
societies, among which the following may be enumerated :
" Archives du Magnétisme Animale " (1820–1823) ; Deleuze's
journal which ran to four volumes (1826–1829) ; " Hermès "
(1826) ; " Le Propagateur du Magnétisme Animal " (1828) ;
Ricard's " Journal du Magnétisme Animal" (1839) ; " Annales
du Magnétisme," 8 vols. (1814–1826) ; " La Bibliothèque du
Magnetisme " by a member of the Society of Magnetism ;
" Le Révélateur " (1837–1838) ; Dupotet de Sennevoy issued
" Le Journal du Magnétisme " (1847) ; " The Zoist, a journal
of Cerebral Physiology and Mesmerism," 13 vols. (London
1844–1856). As for books dealing with the subject, they are
too numerous to find mention here.

These societies were extremely active ; they issued
periodicals, distributed prizes, and founded a Magnetic Order.
The general public was inclined to be derisive, but was nevertheless passionately interested. The clergy were, for the most

part, favourably disposed towards magnetism, and suggestions
were made in the press that the new science should be taught
to nursing sisters. Lacordaire preached sermons about magnetism, saying that it was the last effulgence of the power
Adam possessed before the expulsion from the Garden of
Eden, and that the prophets were the first to rediscover it.
Hospitals for magnetic treatment were founded in London
and Calcutta. The fourth page of the newspapers, the one
now devoted to the trumpeting of quack medicines, was
full of puffs of somnambulists, described as " lucid," " very
lucid," or " ultra-lucid," according to the fees demanded.
Magnetism made a great deal of noise in the world. On
May 23, 1850, there was a splendid celebration of Mesmer's
birthday : impressive cards of invitation ; rewards of merit ;
a concert ; a banquet, with interminable toasts ; and songs
specially written for the occasion. Here is one of the refrains :

> Ce sont les nerfs, ce sont les nerfs,
> Qui font mouvoir tout l'univers,
> C'est par les nerfs, oui par les nerfs
> Que nous possédons l'univers.

Magnetism even invaded the platform and the stage. In
1850, Adolphe Didier gave magnetic performances resembling
those given by Donato at a later date. The program was
alluring : A Feast of Wonders, Magnetic Séance by the
renowned somnambulist Adolphe Didier, New Demonstrations
of Sight with the Eyes blindfolded, The Transmission of
Thought, Voyages into Space, Ecstatic Poses. In the regular
drama, magnetism became the pivot of the play, like Scapin
of old. *La croix de Saint Jacques* in five acts and six tableaux
was staged at the Gaieté Theatre. All I have been able to
learn about it is that among the characters were three young
women who were continually being magnetised. In the lucid
state they discovered one another's secrets, and thus unravelled
a complicated intrigue which could never have been unravelled
without this aid. In his famous play *Urbain Grandier*,
Alexandre Dumas shows that the best way of getting into a
convent is to magnetise the portress, the mother superior, and
all the nuns you meet.[1]
   The downfall of magnetism was largely due to the extrava-

[1] " Journal du Magnétisme," 1849–1850, passim.

gances of its adepts ; and, just as in the case of mesmerism,
the adverse decisions of learned bodies helped the decline.
A first commission considered magnetism as early as 1831.
Husson's report, though very critical of clairvoyance and
lucidity, was not strongly adverse on the whole. He wrote :
" It is impossible, I will not say to withhold belief from, but
at any rate to restrain astonishment, at what occurred during
this séance." The Academy was much surprised by the
tenor of this report. In view of the increasingly obvious
inconsistencies, and owing to the dissatisfaction of its members
with Husson's report, a second commission was appointed in
1840 to examine two somnambulists presented by Dr. Berna.
This report, edited by Dubois of Amiens, was extremely
critical. All the phenomena were discountenanced ; even the
occurrence of anæsthesia was denied ; the manifestations were
regarded as the outcome of ingenious mystification. This was
manifestly an exaggerated view. Berna entered a protest,
and was supported by several members of the Academy. The
quarrels that broke out concerning Burdin's proposal that a
prize should be offered to persons who could read with the
eyes blindfolded, and the ludicrous discussions that arose in
connexion with the bandage used to blindfold Mademoiselle
Pigeaire, helped to make the study of magnetism absurd.
Thenceforward, animal magnetism was tabu to the scientific
world. Its practice lingered on in obscurity for another
twenty years, but to an increasing extent it fell a prey to
quackery, and gradually sank into oblivion. The errors, the
exaggerations, the extravagances, and, above all, the utter
confusion that prevailed in these studies, had hidden the kernel
of truth.

The students of magnetism erred in two ways ; they were
unduly ambitious alike from the scientific and from the
practical point of view. In the realm of science, they tried
to inaugurate all in a moment an entire physiology of the
nervous system. As concerns practice, although their notions
as to the changes of an unknown nature they could produce
in the human mind were still extremely vague, they wished
to apply these notions forthwith, for the disclosure of all the
secrets of the world and of the future, and for the relief of
every kind of suffering. They had to pay for their immoderate
ambition. Their work and their personality were subjected

to the last extremity of ridicule, and the whole topic fell into hopeless disrepute. It is difficult to realise how strong the animus against studies of this character became. A doctor who avowed an interest in magnetism risked his whole career. Men of great distinction and high station were afraid to admit that they were engaged in the study of somnambulism. Morel of Rouen, the famous alienist, never admitted quite openly that he magnetised some of his patients. I have at my disposal a very remarkable account of a distinguished medical practitioner in a country town, who was all his life a great magnetiser but sedulously concealed the fact. Under the public eye, and as an ordinary citizen, he lived in the town. He would start forth early in the morning, a botanist's collecting box slung over his shoulder, ostensibly to gather herbs in the countryside. In actual fact, he made his way to a neighbouring village, where he had secretly established a cottage hospital for nervous diseases. The inmates were poor women, somnambulists, under orders to live in retirement. They were to remain asleep and motionless during his absence. Upon these inmates he conducted interminable researches. Some day, I hope to tell this remarkable story at greater length, for the account of the arbitrary seclusions will read like a novel.

During this period, a number of remarkable studies on magnetism were published, but none of them could overcome the indifference and distrust of the scientific world.

Animal magnetism has left a few traces. The problems which the magnetisers brought prematurely to the front continue to interest certain investigators. In magnetic and psychic congresses people still speak of nervous force, of the influence of one person's nervous system upon that of another, of the fluids and the polarity of the human body. But these studies are repugnant to the majority of scientists, the general view being that such researches are fruitless. The public no longer has faith in the assertions of the magnetisers; no one seriously believes them to have occult forces at their command. The scepticism of their patients has deprived the would-be healers of most of their curative power.

But the reader must not suppose that methods of treatment based on the utilisation of mysterious remedies have quite lost their vogue. It is extremely probable that part, at least, of the admitted efficacy of electrical treatment, treatment by radium, and even serum treatment, may be the outcome of kindred psychological phenomena. Consider, for instance, what is known as osteopathy, a therapeutic method widely celebrated in the United States. The mechanism of the method resembles that of treatment by animal magnetism. An account of this remarkable medical method will be found in the writings of E. R. Booth,[1] G. D. Hulett,[2] D. L. Tracker,[3] and in the " Massachusetts Journal of Osteopathy." [4] This new method of universal cure was founded by Dr. Andrew Taylor Still of Baldwin, Kansas, in 1874. The first school of osteopathy was established at Kirksville, Missouri, in 1892. " Osteopathy is the treatment of all diseases by the removal of their cause through an anatomical readjustment. . . . The disease is due to a trifling anatomical defect which gives rise to pressure upon or obstructs the course of the nerves or bloodvessels supplying the affected part. It is more scientific to remove the cause with the fingers, rather than to treat the effects merely, to treat symptoms by the administration of drugs." The dislocation regarded as a primary cause of all diseases is supposed to be a slight luxation of one or more vertebræ, seeing that the least displacement of the spinal column must modify the circulation and must affect the condition of the spinal marrow and the nerves. The localisation of the disease depends upon the part of the spinal cord affected. If the displacement is in the neck, then the eye, the ear, or the nose will suffer ; if it is in the upper part of the back, there will be trouble in the heart or the lungs ; if it is lower down in the back, abdominal disorders will ensue. The proper treatment can be deduced from these principles ; it will consist of deep massage, a sort of kneading of the muscles along the spine. This is the only treatment used by the practitioners of the osteopathic school, and it is applied by them in all diseases.

However strange it may seem, the treatment has had a great vogue. According to a recent issue of the " Journal of Osteopathy," there are more than 3500 osteopathic practitioners in the United States. Numerous books and periodicals

[1] History of Osteopathy and Twentieth Century Medical Practice.
[2] Principles of Osteopathy.   [3] Ibid.
[4] R. K. Smith, " Massachusetts Journal of Osteopathy," November and December 1905.

are devoted to a description of the successes of the method;
persons who have been cured by osteopathy and whose
gratitude makes them enthusiastic advocates of the system
are to be met everywhere. Whatever the cause of these cures
or apparent cures, it is improbable that the massage of the
spinal column has much to do with the matter. We may
presume that here, likewise, forces are at work of which both
the patient and the osteopath are unaware. The prestige of
anatomical science plays its part, just as the prestige of
astronomy functioned in Mesmer's practice, and just as the
prestige of the physical science of electricity functioned in
magnetic treatment. Despite the claim of osteopathy to be
scientific, we have to do with one of those methods of treatment which belong to the realm of magic. Its success shows
that magic still plays a part in medicine.

4. VALUE OF MIRACULOUS METHODS OF TREATMENT.

It is only too easy to make fun of stories of miraculous
cure. Not merely are sceptics prone to use this weapon of
ridicule, but the faithful do the same thing. The devotees
of a religion are strongly inclined to attack kindred super-
stitions. Nothing will persuade the adepts of Lourdes that
the miracles worked at the shrine of Aesculapius were genuine.
Who could induce the admirers of animal magnetism to take
a serious view of such miracles as those of Lourdes? Each
one attacks his neighbour, and is quite unaware that his criticisms rebound upon himself.

Manifestly, the chief difficulty of such studies does not lie
in the interpretation of the miraculous phenomena, but in
their accurate record. We need not follow Bertrin in his
unending discussions as to whether the rapidity of a cure is a
sign of miracle; or as to whether, when the Blessed Virgin
effects a cure, she should or should not leave a scar.[1] What
we really want to know is very simple, but at the same time
extraordinarily difficult. We want to know what actually
happened. But our knowledge of the facts is derived from
the witnesses, and every one knows that the reports of witnesses
are untrustworthy. The experimental studies of Binet,
Claparède, and Le Bon have shown how rarely the witnesses

[1] Bertrin, op. cit., pp. 173 et seq.

of an event can describe it accurately, even when they have
to do with simple phenomena which are not of a kind to
arouse emotional reactions. What, then, are we to think of
these accounts of happenings difficult to appreciate, of these
diagnoses of chronic diseases, of these stories of temporary
or permanent cures, these reports made by enthusiasts under
stress of emotion, influenced by the fear of death, by an eager
wish for the cure of themselves or their dear ones, crazed by
religious or by political passion ? " The untrustworthiness of
testimony is especially conspicuous," writes Le Bon, " when
we have to do with religious or political happenings. That
explains the stories of miracles and apparitions with which
the books are packed. During ten centuries, thousands of
persons saw the devil, and if the unanimous testimony of a
vast number of observers could be regarded as proving anything, we should be entitled to assert that no one's existence
is more certainly proved than that of the devil. . . . As far
as testimony is concerned, it is the good faith of witnesses
that is dangerous, and not their bad faith."

A possible rejoinder would be that those who have first-
hand knowledge of the facts must surely know better than any
armchair critic. One of the defenders of Lourdes thinks he
can convince us by showing that a certain diagnosis was made
by a hundred doctors in council. But, for our part, we know
that observation and diagnosis become more difficult, and
that their accuracy is more open to question, as soon as two
or three doctors are gathered together. A careful examination
by one skilled observer will have more weight with us than
that of a council. Besides, we shall continue to think that
the title of doctor affords no guarantee against ignorance or
human passion. Nor does this title abrogate the old logical
rule that the criticism of testimony must be rigorous in proportion to the manifest incredibility of the phenomena
testified.

I have often been asked : " Why don't you undertake
such a criticism yourself ? Why don't you yourself verify
the miracles of Lourdes, seeing that the account of these
miracles has interested you so much ? " The questioner
perhaps hardly realises how much time and labour would be
needed to pierce the mists of imposture, to smoothe down
ruffled sensibilities, to check the testimony of each individual

witness. He does not realise how much bitterness would be aroused by the attempt to gain a clear notion of the motives which induced the experts to sign such certificates. Great pains would be expended to secure a minimal result. It is easy to understand why so many conscientious observers have abandoned the attempt in disgust, and are content to accept the conclusion of Paul Dubois of Berne : " In these pilgrimages, the recorders are in a peculiar mental state. Lourdes is not far from Tarascon ! . . . The student returns with an oppressive feeling that he has been in a world of superstition." [1]

Nevertheless, it seems to me that such an attitude is most unfortunate. Collections of observations concerning miracles are not scientific works, and should not be criticised in the same manner as collections of medical observations. It is extremely difficult to appreciate the worth of each individual fact, and yet there emerges a general impression of the truth of the whole. There are instances in which the calculus of probabilities can establish quasi-certitude as regards a collection of facts, although it cannot justify a definite affirmation concerning any one of the facts taken alone. Speaking generally, I believe that cures take place at Lourdes. I believe, too, that there were numerous cures when the faith in animal magnetism was at its height. Many circumstances contribute to produce this general impression, the most notable being precisely the success of the pilgrimages or the magical practices. Bertrin has good reason for recording the number of trains that enter Lourdes every day, for insisting upon the number of the bishops and the pilgrims, and, more than all, for dwelling upon the vast figures totalled by the subscriptions and freewill offerings. Such data have far more convincing force than Bertrin's medical observations. The really remarkable success of magnetism for half a century ; the numbers of patients whose cases are recorded by Mauduit, Guéritant, Cloquet, Deleuze, Aubin Gauthier, Pigeaire, Lafontaine, etc.— these facts prove the reality of magnetic action during the period in question. There is no smoke without fire, and recourse to religious and magical methods of treatment would not have continued for centuries if these methods had been utterly devoid of value. Scientific medicine (or medicine

[1] Les psychonévroses et leur traitement moral, 1904, p. 247.

which is nearly scientific) has perfected some of the methods of religious or of magical medicine, and has made the application of these methods more trustworthy; but scientific medicine would never have been born unless the methods of religious and magical medicine had already justified the confidence of mankind by their proved efficacy.

Let me add that we regular practitioners all have opportunities from time to time of observing some of these cures that bear the stamp of the miraculous. Even at the Salpêtrière, patients have been cured by having the Blessed Sacrament held over their heads.[1] Paul Dubois, whose attitude towards Lourdes is so critical, records the history of a patient "whose neck and jaws had been rigidly fixed for years, who had been fruitlessly treated by a number of famous physicians and surgeons, but who was promptly cured in the piscina of Lourdes."[2] I have myself been able to cure a great many patients by methods resembling those of magnetism. The cures wrought by thaumaturges follow the same laws as the cures effected by regular medical practitioners, and this entitles us to believe in the reality of the former. Charcot insisted on this point when he was studying the cures at the tomb of Deacon Pâris; I have referred to the same thing in connexion with a case recorded among the cures wrought by the Precious Blood of Fécamp; more recently, Mangin has made a similar remark regarding some of the Lourdes miracles.[3] As concerns the reality of these miracles, we may adopt the conclusion drawn by the two Myers. They considered that stories of "mediumistic marvels" and "alleged miracles of healing" could be grouped in three classes. The first group comprised cases entirely devoid of evidential value. The second was made up of cases which could be paralleled by phenomena due to ordinary causes (including fraud). In the third class was a small residue of cases not obviously liable to these fatal objections, and therefore demanding further study.[4]

We have, then, to admit the reality of miraculous cures. Man desires them, and seeks them with the aid of special methods; but he attains the wished-for end so rarely, and the sequence is so irregular, that he cannot ascribe absolute

[1] Cf. Régnard, Les maladies épidémiques de l'esprit, etc., 1887, p. 109.
[2] Op. cit., p. 440.
[3] "Annales des Sciences Psychiques," December 1907.
[4] Proceedings of the Society for Psychical Research, 1893, p. 165.

efficacy to the methods he employs. Consequently, he is forced to believe that unknown forces, capricious and mysterious, play their part. Still, such cures are common enough to have been subjected, like other phenomena of the same character, to observation and discussion.

Charcot, in his remarkable study of *The Faith Cure*, was one of the first to point out, with regard to miraculous cures, that they continually recur under closely similar conditions. His account of Faith Healing made its appearance in English in the London " New Review " (issue for January 1893), the French original being simultaneously published in the " Archives de Neurologie," vol. xxv, pp. 72 et seq. No matter, said Charcot, whether the miracles we study are ancient or modern, we almost always note the same surroundings : a fine mountain country, a sacred spring, the dark cave which the ancients used to describe as the earth's mouth, the wonder-working statue. " Among the servitors of the temple are the doctor-priests who are charged with noting and aiding the cures—that is to say, the Medical Board which the shrines of to-day never fail to maintain if they are of sufficient importance."

In this connexion, Charcot makes an amusing observation. He has learned that in Poitou there are certain old women whose profession is to act as intercessors at the tomb of Saint Radegonde on behalf of those who, although believers in the faith cure, either cannot or will not come to the shrine in person. Precisely similar intercessors were found in classical days at the temple of Aesculapius. The preparatory stages of the miracle have always been the same. The patient is one who has come from a distance, and has had an arduous journey. The local residents are not good subjects for these miraculous cures—which accounts for the remarkable fact that there are still sick people in and near Lourdes! The patient is not allowed to dispense with preliminaries. He must not straightway touch the relic or drink the healing waters of the sacred spring. There is a probationary period, a propitiatory novena. There are long waits at the gateway of the temple during which the sufferer listens to sermons and repeats prayers. Above all, during these periods of probation, the sick hear a great deal about miraculous cures, and have an opportunity of looking at the numberless votive offerings. In a word, their entry into the temple is a slow one, and their minds are prepared by a special incubation. If the miracle is wrought, the patient must then return public thanks to the deity, and must decorate the temple with material evidence of gratitude. All these things happen to-day at Lourdes just as they used to happen of old at the temple of Aesculapius. The same remark applies to animal magnetism. In the solemn sittings round Mesmer's " baquet," in the occult practices around the clairvoyante who spoke in a trance, in the initiatory rites and hermetic instructions, we recognise the same preparation of the patient under a somewhat different form.

This community of practice throughout the ages and in such widely separated countries is highly significant. We learn from it that miracle is less arbitrary, less free, than we had fancied ; we learn that even a miracle is subject to immutable laws. The god who works miracles does not cure any chance comer, nor cure in a haphazard fashion. You will find it useless, at one of these sanctuaries, to ask that the god or the wonder-working fluid shall restore an amputated limb or remove the scar of a wound. You will be given good reasons. The adepts will tell you that the god likes the traces of the miracles to persist ; and so on. At long last you will be told that you must not be importunate, and that the god is not interested in that particular kind of surgery. On the other hand, there is no end to the number of cures of disorders of sensation and movement. In many such cases, a cure can be confidently expected. A miracle, in fact, is no more arbitrary than lightning, which the ancients likewise believed to be the work of the gods. We must learn, says Charcot, to understand the determination of these new phenomena, these natural phenomena which occur everywhere. We must study the science of miracles so that we may be able to reproduce them at will. Day by day, he adds, the domain of the supernatural is being restricted, thanks to the extension of the domain of science. One of the most notable among scientific victories over the mysteries of the universe will be achieved when we have tamed, have domesticated, the therapeutic miracle.

Having thus realised the determinism of miracles, science can make a further step forward. We are beginning to understand that we have to do with a particular kind of determinism,

that which regulates mental phenomena. The ancients were
on their way to recognise this. Galen wrote : " We have
proof at the temple of Aesculapius that many serious illnesses
can be cured solely by the shock administered to the mind."
To-day we have a fair amount of evidence in support of
this supposition. First of all, the majority of the patients
cured under such conditions are neuropaths. That is to say,
they are persons whose illness is to a preponderating extent
due to mental causation. Selecting a year haphazard, I have
studied the cures that took place at Lourdes. Among these
I found 110 cases of considerable interest. Without trying
to eliminate the errors and frauds which must have modified
a good many of these case-histories and have rendered it
more difficult to ascertain their real nature, I have been able
to decide that 92 out of the 110 were cures of neuropathic
disorders. When we study the reports of cures by animal
magnetism, we find an even larger proportion of neuropathic
cases. The magnetisers frankly admit the fact. Aubin
Gauthier,[1] Rostan,[2] Morel, Prosper Despine,[3] Georget, and
others, were aware that the magnetic influence was chiefly
exerted upon neuropaths. The conditions which have come
to be recognised as desirable preliminaries to the miracle—a
long pilgrimage to the shrine, tedious waiting, tales of wonder,
religious exaltation, public sittings, the emotion induced by
the marvellous and the terrible—are all familiar causes of mental
perturbation. Of late years, the study of one specific psychological phenomenon, suggestion, has shown that in certain
cases it is possible, by purely psychological methods, to induce
phenomena closely akin to those observed in instances of
miraculous cure. The general conclusion has been drawn
that we must look into the domain of psychology if we wish
to throw light on the determinism of miracles and to learn
the means of producing like effects by a regular causal sequence.
Some authors, advocates of a purely religious interpretation
of miracles, protest against these deductions, although their
protests have little force. They demur to the description of
the Lourdes patients as neuropaths for the most part ; and
they even exhibit a certain amount of hostility towards those
patients who are undeniably neuropaths, regarding the cure

of these as a matter of little interest. A strange mistake, this! Nothing is more difficult than to cure a confirmed neuropath, and Lourdes would deserve all its reputation and more if it were preeminent for the cure of neuropaths alone. Very little medical knowledge is requisite to show that, among the patients cured at Lourdes, most even of those whose illnesses are classed under some other head, are really neuropaths in whom the nervous character of the disorder has been masked.

Other discussions of the subject have turned, as a rule, upon the unhappy word "suggestion." The objectors have endeavoured to show that some of the cures spoken of as miraculous cannot be explained by suggestion, so that such cures do not belong to the realm of psychological phenomena. The arguments used are sometimes remarkable. Bertrin, in particular, seems to have a very hazy notion of suggestion. It is, he writes, "a well-known force; . . . we quite understand what it can do, and we understand even better what it cannot do." [1] But science is far from making any such claim. The International Society of Medical Psychology and Psychotherapy, when meeting at Brussels in 1910, devoted itself to the study of the nature of suggestion, but was unable to arrive at definite conclusions upon all points. As for Bertrin, some of his opinions concerning suggestion are very remarkable : " To induce suggestion there must be a clear, categorical, authoritative affirmation. Hope has no influence in psychotherapy [!]. . . . Suggestion does not occur when the would-be suggester begs instead of ordering." [2] Doubtless some suggestions have an imperative character, but it is no less certain that well-marked suggestion can be effected without anything like an order ; in fact, suggestion by insinuation is often far more potent. It is really surprising that anyone so incompetent as Bertrin should venture to undertake such studies.

Still, a detailed discussion of suggestion would be superfluous here, seeing that I am perfectly willing to admit that some of the phenomena of miraculous cures are not explicable by suggestion. This admission does not invalidate the con-

---

[1] Op. cit., p. 298.
[2] Op. cit., pp. 185 and 189.—On this point, consult Marcel Mangin in " Annales des Sciences Psychiques," December 1907.

clusion that we have to do with psychological phenomena ; for it would be strange, and even absurd, to limit the field of psychology to suggestion more or less perfectly understood. The psychological phenomena which occur in connexion with such treatments are extremely numerous, and about some of them we know very little. There can be no doubt that religious faith must play a great part, or faith in science ; though the faith may be in pseudo-religion or pseudo-science, with all their content of exaggerated hopes and potent tendencies. Nevertheless, we may admit that " patients are cured who had no hope of cure, blind unbelievers who spoke evil of religion and were none the less cured ; and there have been others who have been cured after returning home, when they had ceased to expect a cure." [1]   This merely proves that religious faith is not the only factor ; the instinctive respect for wealth and power has made it possible for kings to cure illness just as well as priests. The journey, fatigue, the strangeness of the environment, a new physical and moral hygiene, emotional shocks of all kinds, the effect of public opinion exercised in virtue of the reputation of the remedy, the powerful and little understood influence of the crowd—all these things combine to work on the patients' minds. Zola puts the matter very well in his description of Lourdes : " Autosuggestion, emotional perturbation due to long expectation, the excitement of the journey, prayers, hymns, increasing exaltation ; above all, the breath of healing, the unknown force exhaled by the crowd during the acute crisis of faith." [2]

Among all these influences, I should like to emphasise one which I regard as important, though little known, and one which we shall meet again in the sequel.   I refer to the nervous and mental excitation produced in an individual by the part he is made to play.   We are only just beginning to understand that many diseases, physical as well as mental, are due to the depression of nervous energy, and that this depression is maintained by troubles of every kind, and by inaction.   How many prople fall sick because they have nothing of interest to do ; because their life is commonplace, dull, and monotonous ; because they have no hope, no ambition, no aim ; because no one is interested in them, and because they see no prospect of arousing anyone's interest.   Take a person of this

[1] Bertrin, op. cit., p. 185.   [2] Lourdes, p. 199.

type and make him understand that the Blessed Virgin is going to work a miracle in his favour, that the all-powerful divine being has chosen him from among thousands to grant him a special favour which no one will be able to overlook, that he will become the living proof of the truth of religion and will promote the eternal salvation of an impious century. Take a woman who is hopelessly bored, who has no interest in life and no part to play in it, and make her understand that she is going to become an ultra-lucid somnambulist, one whose thought can transcend the limits of time and space, one who can amaze her fellow human beings and overwhelm them with benefactions ; make her understand that she is to become the collaborator with a person of quite exceptional gifts, to whom she will give her time, her life, and some of her affection, so that, thanks to her, he may be able to write a wonderful book which will save humanity. Is it not plain that such persons will be morally and physically transformed, and that the transformation is fully explicable without having recourse to the power of the gods or the action of a mysterious fluid ? Such are some of the psychological influences concerned in the working of miracles. Probably there are many others which still elude analysis.

We have thus been led to surmise that psychological phenomena play a notable part in miraculous cures, and we have realised that miracles still constitute to-day one of the most elementary among psychotherapeutic methods. But we must not forget that these psychological influences operate in an extremely vague and confused way. They are ignored, not only by the patient, but also by the operator, who believes himself to be utilising forces of a very different character. We have to do with unwitting psychotherapeutics. For this reason, however real the psychotherapeutic action, its range is greatly restricted. I have tried to show that miraculous methods of treatment are sometimes successful, but I hope that none of my readers will dispute the assertion that more often they fail. The persons who have made a pilgrimage to wonder-working springs, who have besought the aid of the gods in accordance with the prescribed ritual, who have swallowed theriacs, or have been magnetised, without deriving any benefit by these procedures, may be counted by millions. The failures greatly outnumber the cures.

Furthermore, we have discovered no indication of any method by which we can learn whether one individual has better chances than another of being cured by a miracle. The operators will not allow of any distinction between the diseases with which they have to deal. They claim that they can cure anything, everything. Diagnosis counts for naught, and the sufferer's chances will not be improved by making him suit his conduct to particular circumstances. Do we ask that the patient's moral predispositions shall be taken into account ? We are told that faith is of no moment, that it cannot determine the choice of Providence, and that frequently unbelievers are given a preference. We are not to consider the sufferer's suggestibility, for it is wrong to invoke psychological influences. In a word, there is no clue to guide us through the maze ; we are to play blind hookey ; we are to buy tickets in a lottery where the prizes are few and far between.

'Twould not be so bad if the game had no other drawbacks ; but the cost of the journey, the upkeep of the priest who lives upon the shrine, the magician's fees, empty the patient's pockets. Can we say that such methods of treatment never induce serious fatigue or other troubles ? Among all the patients I have known to visit these abodes of miracle (some were sent by myself), one or two have returned better than they were before they set forth, and the improvement has lasted several months ; the others have come back worse than when they started, more hopeless than ever. The time spent upon these fruitless endeavours has often been long, so that the disease has gained ground when it might have been more successfully treated in some other way. As long as the only available medicine was the medicine of miracle, men may have been well advised to risk the remnants of their health by taking tickets in this lottery. But to-day, surely, they might find something better to do.

CHAPTER TWO

PHILOSOPHICAL METHODS OF TREATMENT

THE evolution thanks to which scientific psychotherapeutics is destined to arise out of miraculous methods of treatment has been a slow one and has already passed through several stages. One of the most interesting of these stages is represented by the remarkable practices which for some decades have had a great vogue in the United States under various names, such as Mind Cure, Faith Cure, Divine Healing, Mental Healing, and, above all, Christian Science. The last-named school or church has played a considerable part. It has shown the importance of mental or moral treatment, and has been the starting-point of the extensive development such methods have undergone in America. Furthermore, it has brought into the limelight a conception of the role of thought in disease and health which has made it possible to interpret the effects of earlier miracles and to out-do them. Finally, the life of Mrs. Eddy, the founder of the sect, was an extraordinary one, and the details of her career are of great interest to students both of psychology and of psychotherapeutics. The history of Christian Science is little known in France, and I shall, therefore, describe it at considerable length. A great many works on Christian Science have been published, especially in Britain and the United States. The following may be mentioned : Frances Lord, *Christian Science Healing,* London, 1888 ; Buckley, *Faith Healing, Christian Science, and kindred Phenomena,* London, 1892 ; Schofield, *Faith Healing,* London, 1892 ; Myers, *Mind Cure, Faith Cure, and the Miracles of Lourdes,* Proceedings S.P.R., 1893, p. 160 ; E. R. Knowles, *The True Christian Science,* Providence ; J. A. Dresser, *The true History of Mental Science,* Boston, 1887 ; Albert Moll, *Christian Science, Medicine, and Occultism* ; Riley, *The personal Sources of Christian Science,* " Psychological Review," November 1903 ; Mark Twain, *Christian Science,* New York and London, 1907 ; Milmine, *The Life of Mary Baker G. Eddy and the History of Christian Science*, New York and London, 1909. The last-named work contains a good deal of adverse criticism, and records numerous biographical details which do not always redound to the honour of the founder of the new faith. An official reply was, therefore, issued in 1908 (Georgine Milmine's book was originally published as a serial in " MacClure's Magazine " during the year 1907), *The Life of Mary Baker Eddy*, by Sibyl Wilbur, Concord Publishing Co., New York. I may also refer to a French study, a university thesis by Emmanuel Philippon, *La médication mentale dans la doctrine de la Christian Science* ; also to an adverse criticism by an English medical man, Stephen Paget, *The Case against Christian Science*, London, 1909. I shall myself have space for no more than a summary of historical details concerning the cult and its founder, my information being drawn from several of the works just enumerated, and especially from Milmine's biography.

1. EARLY HISTORY OF MRS. MARY BAKER GLOVER PATTERSON EDDY.

" The woman who was in due time to become the prophet of a widespread religion, one of the richest and beyond question the most powerful woman in the United States of America, was born at a little farm in the township of Bow, not far from Concord, New Hampshire, on July 16, 1821." Her ancestors had been New England farmers for five generations. Her parents were extremely religious, and not conspicuous for enlightenment.

Some of the hereditary influences are worth noting. Her father, Mark Baker, was a harsh and energetic man, narrowly religious, and with a domineering character which was reproduced in various members of the family. Mary was the youngest child, and is described as being pretty and graceful. " Her nose was gently aquiline. She had a rather long and pointed chin ; the lines of her mouth betokened firmness ; her forehead was both high and broad ; she had fine eyes, and these were to play a great part in her career." Every one spoiled her, and she knew how to keep all the villagers at her beck and call. She seldom went to school, and had little power of application. The fact was that from early childhood she was perpetually ailing, being subject to severe nervous disorders. Convulsive seizures were frequent. She would fall suddenly to the ground, grinding her teeth, rolling about, struggling, and uttering cries of alarm ; sometimes she would have hallucinations, or would pass into a state of general contracture, or would be motionless for hours in a faint. Since doubts concerning the existence of hysteria were not yet fashionable, the local doctor, Ladd by name, when hastily summoned to the girl whose condition was supposed to be desperate, would reassure her parents by telling them that there was nothing much the matter—only an attack of hysteria.

At the age of twenty-two she married George Washington Glover, a friend of her brother's, and removed with him to Charleston, South Carolina. Glover died shortly afterwards of yellow fever, leaving her in a state of destitution. Her son was born posthumously. Her mother was dead, her father had married again, and she had to take refuge with one of her sisters. Her nervous troubles were aggravated by this distressing situation. The attacks became more violent than ever, alternating with long periods of lethargy which were broken from time to time by fugues[1] or by the onset of somnambulist delirium. She would be in bed, apparently moribund, and a moment later she would have vanished, and would have to be pursued all over the countryside. She was cared for with the utmost devotion, for she was always able to get her own way. Her poverty did not make her humble, but the reverse, and she made claims upon her hosts as if it had been a great honour to grant her an asylum. During this period she became affected with a strange fancy to which her housemates patiently submitted ; she had to be rocked in a cradle like a child, for nothing else could assuage her crises and soothe her delirium. At first she had tried having a swing in her bedroom, but subsequently she used an enormous cradle well lined with pillows. At one end of this was an extension seat for the person who rocked the cradle, by rocking himself as in a rocking chair. Her nephew would perform the duty of swinging her in the swing for hour after hour, and sometimes

---

[1] Janet uses the term "fugue" in its derivative sense to denote a "flight," an impulsive flight from the customary environment, as a symptom of neurosis. —E. & C. P.

other boys of the village would earn a few cents by coming to " swing Mrs. Glover."

After a while she married again, the second husband being an itinerant dentist and homeopath, Patterson by name. We read of his fetching from his wife's previous home the huge cradle in which Mrs. Patterson had to be rocked to sleep. The second marriage was an unhappy one. Then came the civil war, and Patterson was a prisoner in the south for two years. His wife sued for a divorce, and, being successful in the suit, resumed the name of Glover.

She now lived for a time with her sister Mrs. Tilton, and proved, as before, at once attractive and intolerable. Her beauty increased with the years. She took a great deal of pains with her appearance, spoke mincingly, and ransacked the dictionary for unusual and grandiloquent words. In her somnambulist crises she was clairvoyant, and would help people to find lost or stolen articles. Once she tried to locate the body of a drowned person. On another occasion she disclosed the hiding-place of Captain Kidd's treasures—but the treasure was not there! She was fascinated by the rise of spiritualism, and, like the Fox sisters, she could hear spirit rappings in the walls. All this made her extremely interesting, but her domineering ways and extravagant claims were, in the end, too much for Mrs. Tilton, and she had to seek refuge elsewhere.

We cannot follow our heroine through all the peregrinations of the next few years, her wanderings from house to house in search of a means of livelihood. The reader must turn to Milmine's book for a full account of the misadventures when she was staying with the Carters and with the Websters, for these throw a strong light upon Mrs. Eddy's character. She had wormed her way into the household of a superstitious elderly lady, declaring that the spitits had told her that this was to be her home. Here she acted as medium, the two women communing with the spirits together, and undertaking the important work of " a revision of the Bible by the spirits." The hostess' family were not best pleased at this invasion, but found it difficult to get rid of the unwelcome guest. After heroic struggles, the husband and the son-in-law had to carry the medium's luggage into the street and to slam the door in her face. These were hard trials for a woman who was both

proud and overbearing. But she was undaunted, and sought
hospitality elsewhere. Finding favour with her new hosts, she
immediately began to establish her tyranny over the whole
household.

One point must be emphasised, and that is the increasing
gravity of her morbid symptoms. The convulsive seizures
and the somnambulism continued ; the hallucinations now
began to trouble her in the waking state ; visceral disorders
were superadded. She suffered from pain and spasm in the
stomach, refused food, and became extremely weak. To
aggravate her misfortunes, she slipped on the frozen curbstone
one winter day and was stunned by her fall. It was natural
that in a hysterical patient this accident should be followed by
contracture of the lower limbs, and soon by complete paralysis.
It is difficult to understand why her doctors, who had hitherto
fully grasped the functional nature of all her disorders, should
now have begun to talk of an incurable affection of the spine !
The sufferer had recourse in vain to all kinds of treatment,
both allopathic and homeopathic. For several years she was
bedridden, despairing of cure.

In 1862, when Mrs. Glover was forty years of age, something
occurred to give her mind an entirely new turn. To help my
readers to understand what happened, I must introduce to
them a new person of the drama, Quimby by name, " Doctor "
by courtesy, a magnetiser or healer.[1] In the previous chapter
I pointed out that the study of animal magnetism, originating
in France, had been eagerly adopted in the United States of
America, and that as early as 1835 a magnetic society had been
established at New Orleans. American magnetisers had
published works of considerable interest.[2] About 1840, a
French magnetiser, Charles Poyen, visited the State of Maine.
He gave lectures at Portland and Belfast, published a book on
the power of the mind, and exhibited somnambulists at public
sittings. One of his audience, a watchmaker by trade, was
filled with enthusiasm, and felt that he likewise possessed

---

[1] Concerning Quimby, consult Evans, The Mental Cure, 1869 ; Mental
Medicine, 1872 ; Myers, op. cit., p. 175 ; Goddard, " American Journal of
Psychology," vol. x (1899), p. 447 ; A. G. Dresser, The Philosophy of P. P.
Quimby, Boston, 1895 ; H. W. Dresser, The Quimby Manuscripts, Werner
Laurie, London, 1922.

[2] See, for instance, the references in the Bibliography under Grimes and
Dods respectively.

magnetic powers. This was Phineas Parkhurst Quimby, born at New Lebanon in New Hampshire, of working-class parentage and himself a working man, but of an inventive turn of mind and a good observer. Discovering a favourable subject for experiment, a lad of seventeen named Lucius Burkmar, he exhibited the youth in a series of public sittings. Quimby's success was rapid. Reviled by some, he was extolled by others, became the talk of the newspapers, and was much sought after by sick persons desirous that an ultra-lucid somnambulist should disclose what was going on inside them.

It was now that Quimby began to make interesting observations upon the mental attitude of his patients and upon the effect of the remedies prescribed by Burkmar. One day the somnambulist prescribed an expensive remedy, though the patient was very poor. When Quimby pointed out this difficulty, Burkmar promptly modified his prescription, ordering the use of an inexpensive drug, and one whose known physiological effect was the very opposite of that of the costly remedy. But the cheap medicine did the patient just as much good as the other could have done. Quimby drew the inference that the consultation of the somnambulist served merely to produce in the patient a confident hope of cure, and the further inference that the medicament really counted for nothing. Dismissing Burkmar, he ceased to practise magnetism in the ordinary sense of that term, and devoted himself to the elaboration of his own conception of " Mind Cure," working first at Belfast, and in 1859 removing to Portland. He was an energetic man with an attractive personality, and a keen student of mental phenomena. He speedily acquired much influence over his patients, and aroused general enthusiasm. It was currently said of him that he had " solved the enigma of life " ; that he " made the blind to see and the deaf to hear." People came from great distances to consult him.

This was the person to whom, in her despair, Mrs. Glover now turned. After negotiations which lasted for a considerable time (for she was so poverty-stricken that she had to ask to be treated almost gratuitously), she came to Portland in 1862. From the very first interviews, physician and patient were charmed with one another. To Quimby this handsome woman, this confirmed neuropath, seemed an admirable subject for his studies. Mrs. Glover, on the other hand, felt for the first time that she had aroused some one's serious interest, and this is always a revelation to a hysterical patient. Hitherto, as Georgine Milmine tells us, she had herself had no absorbing interest. Her life had been most unhappy, full of disappointment and failure. Neither of her marriages had been happy. Maternity had not softened her, nor brought her consolations. Wrapped in a mantle of egoism, she had thought of nothing but her own unending ailments. "Quimby's idea gave her her opportunity, and the vehemence with which she seized upon it attests the emptiness and the hunger of her earlier years " (Milmine, *Life*, etc., p. 57).

As a result, the paralysis and the imaginary disease of the spinal cord were cured in a few days ; and, to do credit to her doctor, Mrs. Glover briskly climbed the staircase of 182 steps at the Town Hall. This cure was at a later date regarded as the wonderful revelation of Christian Science. There was no longer any thought of illness, and Mrs, Glover had now no room in her mind for anything but Dr. Quimby. She wrote him enthusiastic and extravagantly worded letters ; she composed love sonnets addressed to him ; in 1864 she came back to see him at Portland, and stayed three months in the town ; her mind was wholly occupied with the thoughts and the philosophical labours of her physician and master. Now Quimby, from 1859 onwards, had been penning manuscript volumes, which in time numbered a dozen or more. These were the first drafts of books on religion, the interpretation of the Scriptures, spiritualism, disease, clairvoyance, happiness, wisdom, and even on science and on music. None of them had been finished ; none of them had been published. Mrs. Glover, who spent all her afternoons with Quimby, imagined herself to be helping him in his work. She pattered all he said about science, errors, and faith ; and, like him, she discussed mesmerism and spiritualism. She even tried to cure patients by Quimby's methods, but could make little progress with a certain Miss Jarvis. In collaboration with a Mrs. Crosby, she dipped into spiritualism once more, calling up the spirit of her dead brother, Albert Baker, incarnating it, assuming the deceased Albert's voice, and so on. She was thus leading an active and busy life, and fancied she had now found her true vocation as Quimby's secretary and collaborator. But the poor woman seemed to have been born under an evil star, so that disaster continually dogged her footsteps. Quimby, who had cured so many others, was a physician who could not heal himself. Becoming affected with an abdominal tumour, he died rather suddenly on January 16, 1866.

Though still extremely poor, Mrs. Glover met this new stroke of ill-fortune with a faith and an enthusiasm which were worth more to her than wealth. For some years she resumed her life of wandering from house to house, but her whole outlook was different from of old. She was no longer a paralysed invalid continually suffering from convulsions or delirium ; she had become an energetic and ambitious woman, bent on fulfilling her mission. Some of Quimby's manuscripts were already in her possession, and she succeeded in laying her hands upon others. Her fancy was to edit them, for she believed that her true vocation would be to diffuse this precious doctrine throughout the world. She copied them again and again, adding interpretations from the Bible and weird commentaries of her own. This unlettered woman, who was unable to pen a grammatical sentence and did not understand the first elements of punctuation, undertook to write a book. Wherever she went, she made a parade of her treasures, her manuscripts, and continually spoke of the new revelation which was to make an end of all diseases. From time to time she gave advice to sick people, sometimes paying for her lodging in this way. What she said was hard to understand, and was seldom understood. Nevertheless, her lordly ways, her good looks, the strangeness of her garments, her highly figurative speech, her interest in the mysterious, her claim that she had a great mission—all these, while arousing a certain amount of ridicule, combined to make her a well-known figure throughout the smaller towns in the neighbourhood of Boston.

We now come to a very remarkable fact. This woman who was continually talking of mental medicine and of moral methods of treatment, was never able to become a successful practitioner, a successful exponent of her own doctrines. She was a failure as a healer. She did not know how to talk to her patients, or how to guide them, and her first attempts were absurd. Having the wit to realise her own awkwardness, she decided to remain in the background; she would teach Quimby's theory, but would leave practice to others. She was fortunate enough to convert Richard Kennedy, a young man of twenty-one, who agreed to practise under her direction. There was considerable difficulty in installing the clinic at Lynn, Mass.; but once this had been effected, Kennedy had a fair number of patients, so that at the end of the first month it was possible to cover expenses. The young healer was intelligent and amiable; he inspired confidence, effected some cures, and continued to attract patients. For Mrs. Glover, this signified the end of poverty. Her circumstances became comparatively easy, and she was no longer exposed to humiliations. It might have been thought that she would have been grateful.

In actual fact this unwonted prosperity enabled her to give freer expression to her dictatorial and jealous temperament. She began to order Kennedy about, and to humiliate him in various ways, notably when others were present. Grudging him his successes, she would not bear to leave him alone with his patients, especially when they were women. There were repeated quarrels. Again and again she accused Kennedy of robbing her, and of trying to kill her by transferring to her mentally all the ills of which he had relieved his patients. At this date, Mrs. Glover began to suffer from an obsession which was to play a great part throughout the remainder of her life. She had learned from Quimby that animal magnetism was useless, that it could not possibly benefit patients, that it could only do harm. She now came to believe that anything which she fancied might menace her powers was "malicious mesmerism" or "malicious animal magnetism." Kennedy was the first culprit to be charged with practising malicious magnetism. For a time he displayed all the patience of an affectionate son, but at length he found that life with Mrs. Glover was impossible, and in 1872 he declared his intention to break off their association. Mrs. Glover had a severe hysterical attack, but she retained enough self-command to insist upon her partner's paying her a forfeit of six thousand dollars—the profits began to roll in! Kennedy opened a new office in Lynn, and had a reasonable measure of success, but he no longer took his teacher's doctrines very seriously.

Mrs. Glover, retaining a few pupils whom Kennedy had

found for her, continued to give a quasi-medical instruction. Each pupil had to pay a premium of one hundred dollars, and to promise a high percentage of all prospective earnings as a healer. These students were attracted by the hope of gaining marvellous powers at small expenditure both of time and money. The most remarkable among Mrs. Glover's pupils during this period (1875–1879) was Daniel Harrison Spofford. He had a fair number of patients, and was soon able to keep his instructress in funds. He also undertook to revise the manuscripts at which she was continually working, and which she now presented as entirely of her own composition, poor Dr. Quimby being forgotten. Spofford found that the manuscripts were utterly incomprehensible, and he had to rewrite them as best he could. This was the first editing of the famous book *Science and Health*, which was issued at the cost of enthusiastic pupils (for Mrs. Glover shared only in the profits). The first edition, a poor looking volume, appeared in 1875, and attracted little attention. At this time, Spofford introduced a new pupil, Asa Gilbert Eddy, who was to assist Mrs. Glover in her work. She soon displayed a preference for the new comer. At length, despite jealousies and rivalries, she married him in January 1877, thus taking the name by which she has become most widely known.

Unfortunately, Mrs. Eddy soon began to feel about Spofford much the same as she had felt about Kennedy. She considered him too popular among the students and the patients. She did not think him sufficiently docile. Just as she had done with Kennedy, she ordered him about and humiliated him. " I am wisdom," she said ; " this revelation is mine, not yours." She accused him of " immorality, adultery against the faith." When treating his patients, Spofford, she said, thought about her, thus robbing her of her strength in order to pass it on to the sick. At length she accused him, just as she had accused Kennedy, " the young Nero," of practising malicious magnetism. Spofford was apostrophised (1875) in the following terms : " thou criminal mental marauder, that would blot out the sunshine of earth, that would sever friends, destroy virtue, put out truth, and murder in secret the innocent, befouling thy trade with the trophies of thy guilt. . . ."

This time, Mrs. Eddy's onslaughts upon her partner were

to take a more serious form. Turning to account the complaints of one of the patients, she accused Spofford of wizardry and tried to revive in the Boston of 1879 the witch-hunting trials of Salem in 1692. This absurd legal action was, of course, ineffective. But Mrs. Eddy continued to spend all her time in the Boston law-courts, bringing suits against her pupils for arrears of fees, charging them with disclosing her secrets, and the like. Enraged at her failure to convict Spofford as a wizard, she became more and more troubled in her mind, and her nights were spent in attacks of delirium during which she railed against her enemy. At length she organised a conspiracy against Spofford, paying a large sum to a bravo who was to lure Spofford into an ambush and put the offender to death. The upshot was a public scandal, and a trial at which Mrs. Eddy and her husband were sentenced to a fine. These incidents did not improve the standing of Mrs. Eddy's school. Many of the pupils were growing weary of malicious magnetism and of these incessant quarrels and law-suits. Enthusiasm waned, and there were backsliders. For a year, Mrs. Eddy continued the struggle, trying to quell the revolt ; but in the end she felt that the Lynn school must be closed. Her third husband died in 1882 ; and she quitted Lynn, accompanied only by half a dozen of the faithful, but fully determined to make a fresh start elsewhere. She was then sixty-one years of age.

2. DEVELOPMENT OF CHRISTIAN SCIENCE.

Mrs. Eddy was endowed with self-confidence and indomitable energy ; having failed in an attempt upon a narrow platform, she decided that her new endeavour should be on a more extensive scale. Removing her school to the great city of Boston, she opened her course in the drawing-room of a lady friend, with whom she hastened to quarrel. In order to attract public attention, with the aid of a man named Buswell she founded a small monthly, containing eight octavo pages and entitled the " Journal of Christian Science." The few pupils who had remained faithful to her clubbed together to defray expenses, for of course none of the cost was to be borne by Mrs. Eddy. " Although her subscription-list was small, Mrs. Eddy knew what to do with her " Journal."

Copies found their way to remote villages in Missouri and Arkansas, to lonely places in Nebraska and Colorado, where people had much time for reflection, little excitement, and a great need to believe in miracles. . . . Lonely and discouraged people brooded over these editorials, which promised happiness to sorrow and success to failure." [1]

The journal published prophecies; it contained reports of wonderful cures; and it was full of declamatory writing anent malicious mesmerism, which was made to account for all the failures. Simultaneously, *Science and Health* was revised by the Rev. James Henry Wiggin, who endeavoured to put the book into comparatively intelligible English (the work has been retouched again and again, by about thirty persons in all); and the second edition was now published. Several other books were issued in 1888: *Unity of Good; Christian Healing; People's Idea of God; Christian Science, No and Yes; Mind Healing, an Historical Sketch;* etc.

The Boston school was officially established in 1883, and became a valuable source of revenue. Each course of lectures lasted three weeks, and was given to fifty students at a time. The primary course was followed by a normal course, by one of "metaphysical obstetrics," and by a course of theology; the fees for the whole series were $800 per head. There was an abundance of pupils, so that the lectures had to be given over and over again. Ere long, branch institutions began to spring up, preparatory courses being given in California, Nebraska, and Colorado; at New York, Chicago, Denver, and a dozen lesser towns.

Patients likewise abounded. The journal was packed with the reports of cures. "Absent treatment" was now inaugurated, and this was extremely profitable, for the fee was $500, and all that was requisite was to think about the patient and thus ensure the restoration of health. Mrs. Eddy's activities were manifold and amazing. She was continually lecturing and giving public addresses; she was never content unless she was being talked about; and she encouraged every one to shower gifts on her. Her financial success enabled her to take a fine house in Commonwealth Avenue, and the "Journal of Christian Science" gave an impassioned description of the founder's sumptuous mode of life.

[1] Milmine, op. cit., pp. 313–314.

It must not be supposed that difficulties were at an end. Fresh troubles occurred from day to day, so that at times the movement was involved in serious danger. For instance, Mrs. Corner, a sometime student of the course of "metaphysical obstetrics," was attending her own daughter's confinement when the latter died of hæmorrhage. A charge of malapraxis was brought, and there was a newspaper campaign against these obstetric students of Mrs. Eddy's "who knew no more about obstetrics than the babes they helped into the world." In the end, Mrs. Corner was acquitted. Mrs. Eddy had not stirred a finger in her defence. She was content to repudiate the pupil as incapable, and this had a very bad effect on public opinion.

In 1883, Julius A. Dresser, an old patient of Quimby's, who had known Mrs. Eddy when she, likewise, had been under Quimby's care for nervous trouble, came to Boston, and was astonished to learn the part she was playing. He told all he knew concerning the relationships between Mrs. Eddy and Quimby, publishing the grateful letters and poems formerly addressed by her to the healer. The documents were in sharp conflict with what Mrs. Eddy was now saying about her miraculous cure and her revelation.[1]

Infuriated by this, Mrs. Eddy declared that the letters and sonnets quoted by Dresser had been written under the influence of Quimby's malicious magnetism, and she endeavoured to heap opprobrium on the memory of the man whom she had once so ardently admired. Attention being thus directed to Quimby, there were some who wished to study that healer's teachings. They turned for information to the writings of Warren Felt Evans,[2] and to some of Mrs. Eddy's pupils it seemed that Quimby's teaching was far more rational than hers. This was the origin of a schism ; it led, not without difficulties, to the foundation of the New Thought movement. A student who believed himself to be numbered among the faithful endeavoured to publish a book which was to clarify some of Mrs. Eddy's teachings, but this also involved the risk of establishing heresies.

---

[1] See letter to the Boston "Post," February 24, 1883 ; also Dresser's book The true History of mental Science, Boston, 1887, new edition, 1899.
[2] The mental Cure, 1869 ; Mental Medicine, 1872 ; Soul and Body, 1875 ; The divine Law of Cure, 1881 ; The primitive Mind Cure, 1885 ; Esoteric Christianity, 1886.

The founder of Christian Science stood four-square to all the winds that blew. She issued draconian rules forbidding her pupils to read a single line of a work on mental treatment which was not signed by her name; and forbidding them to publish any commentary upon or any translation of her own writings. This was in accordance with the traditional methods of threatened religions, which protect themselves by putting unorthodox works on an expurgatory index. Mrs. Eddy turned the method to good account. Thanks to her energy, her pride, and her invincible self-confidence, she overcame all obstacles, and in the end was able to achieve apotheosis.

Having escaped the danger of a really serious schism, the woman of seventy secured additional pupils, was able to get Christian Science puffed on all hands, founded churches in town after town, and soon became omnipotent. In 1888 there was a triumphal demonstration in Chicago : " Mrs. Eddy had to receive more than 3,000 persons. People jostled one another in the attempt to touch her ; fragments were torn from her dress as relics ; paralytics were healed by touching the hem of her vesture ; a mother who failed to get near her held high her babe to look on their helper." The faithful spoke of this as the Pentecostal Manifestation.

The members of the Christian Science cult, united to form a sort of congregation and governed by a committee, had built a church in Boston. Mrs. Eddy was not wholly satisfied, for two reasons ; the building was not imposing enough for her taste ; and it was not her absolute property. After a good deal of clever manœuvring, she was able to arrive at her goal. An appeal having been issued to all the faithful, in 1894 the foundation stone of Mrs. Eddy's cathedral was laid. This Mother Church of Boston was not to be a local church, but was to be the head of all the other churches. Mrs. Eddy was " pastor emeritus." She ruled with the aid of a quasi-imaginary board of directors " on which Mrs. Eddy and God comprised a majority." The building, costly though it was, was speedily finished, and the dedicatory service was held on January 5, 1895. The original Mother Church now forms the front of an entirely new building dedicated in 1906. The old church is still called the Mother Church ; while the new structure, although many times larger than the old, is termed the

Annex. Built of marble and granite, the church is an imposing edifice which can seat two thousand persons. It has for the use of its pastor a Mother Room finished in rare woods, marble, and onyx, and gold, the furniture being supplied by the children of the Christian Scientists organised into a society known as the Busy Bees. When Mrs. Eddy came to Boston for the opening ceremony, thirty thousand persons were waiting at the entrance to the temple. Five successive services had to be held to satisfy a portion of this vast public; and a great number of the faithful, admitted a dozen at a time, defiled through the Mother Room reverentially as if going to receive the Blessed Sacrament.

After this solemn hour, Mrs. Eddy made few public appearances. Withdrawing to her Concord estate, " and living there in an isolation like that of the Grand Lama, she presided over her own beatification, nay, divinisation." Ardent disciples hold that Christian Science is the offspring of a communion of Mrs. Eddy with God, just as Jesus was the offspring of the communion between the Blessed Virgin and the Holy Ghost : " the outcome of this second immaculate conception is a book and not a man because our century is more spiritual than that of Christ." In the ceremonies at the cathedral, a man reads verses of the Gospels ; and a lady dressed as for a great occasion, and representing Mrs. Eddy, responds by reading verses from *Science and Health*, which always refute the verses from the Gospels, for " the feminine idea of God is far more elevated than the masculine idea, and Jesus was no more than the masculine representative of the spiritual idea." These tangled phrases are still somewhat hesitant, but soon Mrs. Eddy would have been deified without qualification.

Unfortunately, she died at Boston on December 4, 1910, succumbing to an attack of pneumonia at the age of eighty-nine years. Her disciples kept the death as quiet as possible, for in their religion there is no death, and the word must not be spoken. Mrs. Eddy had simply entered a new phase of existence, where her individual labours would continue, and where she could still progress. The Christian Scientists have no funeral rites, and all the services have gone on exactly as if the founder were still alive. She did not die ; " she passed out of the flesh." There was some talk about Mrs. Augusta E. Stetson, First Reader of the New York church, becoming

chief priestess of the Christian Scientists, but this lady declared
that Mrs. Eddy could have no successor.

At the time of writing, the Boston congregation numbers
nearly 50,000 members, and there are 668 Christian Science
churches in the United States. These churches are served by
1,336 ministers, and have 85,096 communicants; there are
innumerable healers all over the Union. Branches of the cult
exist in various other lands: Italy, France, Great Britain,
Canada, British Columbia, Germany, Norway, Sweden,
Hindustan, China, South Africa, Australia, etc. The British
branch would seem to be the most important of these. It
first developed under the guidance of Dr. Schofield, and was
subsequently influenced by Countess Dunmore, but it does not
seem to have shown conspicuous originality.[1]

3. " SCIENCE AND HEALTH."

We must now study the nature of the doctrines and
methods which have had so amazing a success. The Scientists
are never weary of telling us that the whole body of teaching
is to be found in the famous book first published at Boston
in 1875, and subsequently re-issued in more than 180 editions.
Mrs. Eddy recommends her own volume with an abundant
measure of self-satisfaction : " My book on Christian Science
is absolute truth. . . . It is the soul of divine philosophy, and
there is no other philosophy. . . . It is not the search for
wisdom, but wisdom itself. . . . When God speaks, I listen."
Let us turn, then, to *Science and Health*. My own copy of the
176th edition is a small octavo volume sombrely bound in
black, tooled in gold on the cover with a cross and a crown
encircled by the words : " Heal the sick, raise the dead,
cleanse the lepers, cast out demons." The full title is *Science
and Health with the key to the Scriptures*. The work begins
with maxims from the Gospels, and with quotations from
Shakespeare, one of which at least is extremely apt : " There
is nothing either good or bad, but thinking makes it so." An
enthusiastic preface tells us that the time for thinkers has
come, and that truth is knocking at the portal of humanity ;

[1] The statements in the text regarding the death of Mrs. Eddy and the
numerical strength and diffusion of the Christian Science movement are
taken from an article some one was good enough to send me from Boston,
in a number of the " Sun " dated December 5, 1910.

it shows us that a great discovery was made in 1866, one thanks to which we can simultaneously heal both disease and sin. The opening chapter on Prayer does not lack eloquence. It insists that silent prayer rather than vocalised prayer, prayer conjoined with a fervent wish to know and do the will of God, enables us to make our way to truth, and has a beneficial influence on disease, giving the mind more power over the body through a blind faith in God.

The book is divided into three unequal parts. The first of these, the longest and the most important, discusses in haphazard order various philosophical and historical topics : Atonement and Eucharist ; Marriage ; Christian Science versus Spiritualism ; Animal Magnetism Unmasked ; Science, Theology, Medicine ; Footsteps of Truth ; Science of Being— such are the titles of the principal chapters. Part two is entitled the " Key to the Scriptures," and is an attempt to interpret certain biblical texts. Part three, " Fruitage," is a single chapter, containing records of the more remarkable among the cures wrought by Christian Science.

Science and Health is difficult reading, especially for a foreigner.[1] Not only is there an entire lack of order in the composition, but the author's style is a very remarkable one. A Frenchman must speak diffidently here, but at any rate the use of biblical terms, archaisms, and numerous fantastic and far-fetched expressions peculiar to Mrs. Eddy, combine to make her writing, in many cases, almost incomprehensible. It seems to me that English critics are well advised in what they say about the matter. One of them writes : " We need a glossary to understand this book. In it, the word ' bridegroom ' means ' spiritual understanding ' ; the word ' death ' means ' illusion ' ; the word ' mother ' means ' God ' ; and so on." In these circumstances, the comprehension of Mrs. Eddy's philosophical ideas would be a difficult matter if *Science and Health* had any new or complicated notions to present. Fortunately,

[1] There are now official French and German translations, the translation in each case being published side by side with the English text. In the preface to the German edition Mrs. Eddy declares that for a long time she was opposed to the idea of a translation, " which could not adequately express her revelation of Truth in its primitive strength and purity." All the versions are paged alike, and the lines of each page are numbered in the margin. Thus any word (except the words of relation) can be readily found, as far as the English original is concerned, by the use of Conant's Complete Concordance, compiled from the 1910 Edition of Science and Health as finally revised by its Author, Stewart, Boston, 1916.—E. and C. P.

however, the book contains nothing more than a few simple
and familiar thoughts reiterated in season and out of season,
and interspersed amid a profusion of metaphors. The extraction of these thoughts to summarise them is an easy task.

For our purposes, little need be said concerning the interpretations of the Bible. They are of an extraordinary
character, and are often amusing. One of Mrs. Eddy's
favourite methods is to transform the texts she quotes with
the aid of simple word-plays. Where they do not lend themselves to such a transformation, and the plain meaning is
repugnant to her, she speaks of copyist's errors. These
devices enable her to show that Holy Writ is merely a preparation for her own book. " Divide the name Adam into
two syllables, and it reads *a dam*, or obstruction. This
suggests the thought of something fluid, of mortal mind in
solution " (338 : 14) [1]. . . . Jesus " took no drugs to allay
inflammation. He did not depend upon food or pure air to
resuscitate wasted energies. He did not require the skill of
a surgeon to heal the torn palms and bind up the wounded side
and lacerated feet " (44 : 13). " Our Master fully and finally
demonstrated divine Science in his victory over death and the
grave " (45 : 6).—Such interpretations are significant, for they
give Christian Science a religious character, and link it on to
Christianity. In other respects they do not concern us.

The greater part of *Science and Health* is devoted to the
affirmation of a philosophy that is crudely and aggressively
idealistic and spiritualistic (in the philosophical sense of the
term). I say " affirmation," for Mrs. Eddy, though she talks
of " science," never troubles herself with explanation or proof ;
she does not seem to imagine that there can be anything
beyond affirmation, and, once more, affirmation. Her philosophy may be summed up in three basic maxims :

" God is All-in-all " (113 : 16).
" God is good. Good is Mind " (113 : 17).
" God, Spirit, being all, nothing is matter " (113 : 18).

Mrs. Eddy sagely remarks that these fundamental propositions can be reversed without disturbing the sense, thus

---

[1] The large figures denote the page in Science and Health. The small
figures denote the line at which the foregoing quotation begins.

"showing mathematically their exact relation to Truth" (113 : 13). This is one of the rare occasions on which she deigns to talk of proof, and certainly that sort of proof is easy. In a word, everything is spiritual, and the spirit of the universe is God "who is its divine immortal principle" (554 : 3). "Life, Truth, and Love constitute the triune Person called God,—that is, the triply divine Principle, Love" (331 : 26). "Father-Mother is the name for Deity, which indicates his tender relationship to His spiritual creation" (332 : 4). The name of God can be substituted by various synonyms relating to his functions, such as divine principle, life, truth, love, soul, mind or spirit. Finally, it should be mentioned that Mrs. Eddy, who terms her philosophy Christian Science, does actually allot a certain place in that philosophy to Christianity. She believes in Jesus Christ, the Son of God ; she believes in the Holy Spirit (359 : 9) ; she accepts the idea that sin is expiated by Jesus' incarnation, crucifixion, and resurrection. But she rarely mentions these dogmas, and makes no attempt to associate them with her idealist system.

Life is a manifestation of God : "Spirit is God, and man is His image and likeness" (468 : 13). "The spiritual man's consciousness and individuality are reflections of God. They are the emanations of Him who is Life, Truth, and Love. Immortal man is not and never was material, but always spiritual and eternal" (336 : 14).

The negative side of this philosophy comes next, being more important and more fully developed than the positive side. Mrs. Eddy abhors the concept of matter, and declares again and again that matter does not exist. She does not try to explain it or to transform it, but is consistently radical, and simply suppresses it. Such is the meaning of her third basic principle, God, Spirit, being all, nothing is matter. "Cain very naturally concluded that if life was in the body, and man gave it, man had the right to take it away. This incident shows that the belief of life in matter was 'a murderer from the beginning'" (89 : 27). "Matter is nothing beyond an image in mortal mind" (116 : 18).

A great many other concepts share the fate of matter. For instance, evil, sin, poverty, disease, and death are equally displeasing to our reformer, and are incontinently suppressed. Here we have a fourth fundamental principle : "Life, God, omnipotent good, deny death, evil, sin, disease.—Disease, sin, evil, death, deny good, omnipotent God, Life " (113 : 19). " Nothing is real and eternal,—nothing is Spirit,—but God and His idea. Evil has no reality. It is neither person, place, nor thing, but is simply a belief, an illusion of material sense " (71 : 1). " When will the error of believing that there is life in matter, and that sin, sickness, and death are creations of God, be unmasked ? " (205 : 7).

The pity of it is that such denials do not suffice. Why is it that people continue to believe in the existence of matter, in the reality of pain and death ? Here, likewise, the answer is simple. They do so because of an absurd error, a fundamental illusion which leads the human intelligence astray. Mrs. Eddy terms the illusion " mortal mind." This vague phrase, whose inadequacy she recognises (114 : 12), signifies for her all possible errors. It is the flesh opposed to the spirit ; it is " the human mind and evil in contradistinction to the divine Mind, or Truth and good " (114 : 4). " What is termed matter, being unintelligent, cannot say, ' I suffer, I die, I am sick, or I am well.' It is the so-called mortal mind which voices this and appears to itself to make good its claim. To mortal sense, sin and suffering are real, but immortal sense includes no evil or pestilence " (210 : 25). " You say a boil is painful; but that is impossible, for matter without mind is not painful. The boil simply manifests, through inflammation and swelling, a belief in pain, and this belief is called a boil. . . . The fact that pain cannot exist where there is no mortal mind to feel it is a proof that this so-called mind makes its own pain—that is, its own *belief* in pain. . . . We have smallpox because others have it ; but mortal mind, not matter, contains and carries the infection " (153 : 16). " Death will be found at length to be a mortal dream, which comes in darkness and disappears with the light " (42 : 6).

It is easy to infer the nature of the physiological and medical theories that arise out of such conceptions. " Physical science (so-called) is human knowledge,—a law of mortal mind, a blind belief " (124 : 3). " The act of describing disease— its symptoms, locality, and fatality—is not scientific. Warning people against death is an error that tends to frighten into death those who are ignorant of Life as God " (79 : 1). The truth is much simpler : the body does not exist, and therefore has no part to play. " To understand that Mind is infinite, not bounded by corporeality, not dependent upon the ear and eye for sound or sight nor upon the muscles and bones for locomotion, is a step towards the Mind-science by which we discern man's nature and existence " (84 : 19). There is no death, and illnesses are non-existent ; the body and its organs have nothing to do with life. " Discard all notions about lungs, tubercles, inherited consumption, or disease arising from any circumstance " (425 : 32). " Inflammation, tubercles, hæmorrhage, and decomposition are beliefs, images of mortal thought superimposed upon the body ; . . . they are not the truth of man ; they should be treated as error and put out of thought. Then these ills will disappear " (425 : 9).

Unfortunately, obstinate people continue to talk of disease and pain. How is this possible ? It is all the outcome of illusion, of the false beliefs of mortal mind. " Matter cannot be inflamed. Inflammation is fear " (414 : 32). " The cause of all so-called disease is mental, a mortal fear, a mistaken belief or conviction of the necessity and power of ill-health ; also the fear that Mind is helpless to defend the life of man and incompetent to control it. Without this ignorant human belief, any circumstance is of itself powerless to produce suffering " (377 : 26). " A man was made to believe that he occupied a bed where a cholera patient had died. Immediately the symptoms of this disease appeared, and the man died. The fact was, that he had not caught the cholera by material contact, because no cholera patient had been in that bed. If a child is exposed to contagion or infection, the mother is frightened and says, ' My child will be sick.' The law of mortal mind and her own fears govern her child more than the child's mind governs itself, and they produce the very results which might have been prevented through the opposite understanding. Then it is believed that exposure to contagion wrought the mischief " (154 : 10). In like manner, if a child has worms or any trouble, the invariable cause is that its elders have the idea of the illness in their minds.

Obvious and crude objections surge instantly into our minds, but Mrs. Eddy forthwith sweeps them away. " If a dose of poison is swallowed through mistake, and the patient dies even though physician and patient are expecting favourable results, does human belief, you ask, cause this death ? Even so, and as directly as if the poison had been intentionally taken. In such cases, a few persons believe the potion swallowed by the patient to be harmless, but the vast majority of mankind, although they know nothing of this particular case and this special person, believe the arsenic, the strychnine, or whatever the drug used, to be poisonous, for it is set down as a poison by mortal mind. Consequently, the result is controlled by the majority of opinions, not by the infinitesimal minority of opinions in the sick-chamber " (177 : 25). It may be contended that our horses and kine do not think about their lungs. But the answer to such an objector is easy. The domesticated animals are controlled by the thoughts of their human masters. We have corrupted the horses and the kine, and have made them acquainted with pneumonia and colic.

4. PHILOSOPHICAL THERAPEUTICS.

Under these conditions, therapeutics becomes a very simple matter. Diagnosis is superfluous. Here is a patient, and that suffices. The healer's behaviour does not vary from case to case, for the same treatment applies to all diseases. Mrs. Eddy frequently emphasises her contention that Christian Science methods must not be restricted to the relief of nervous disorders, but must be applied indiscriminately for the cure of every kind of disease. " Should all cases of organic disease be treated by a regular practitioner, and the Christian Scientist try truth only in cases of hysteria, hypochondria, and hallucination ? One disease is no more real than another. All disease is the result of education, and disease can carry its effects no farther than mortal mind maps out the way. . . . Decided types of acute disease are quite as ready to yield to Truth as the less distinct type and chronic form of disease " (176 : 21).

Christian Science therapeutics is essentially negative. First and foremost, it absolutely forbids the use of any of the surgical or medical methods discovered by human science ; they are all equally futile and equally absurd. The pupils of the " Metaphysical College," being utterly ignorant of anatomy and physiology at the outset of the curriculum, received not a word of instruction concerning these subjects, nor yet con-

cerning pharmacy or hygiene ; they were no more to be taught
how to tie a cut artery than how to take the patient's temperature. Especially to be avoided was any practice which seemed
to smack of animal magnetism. " The author's own observations of the workings of animal magnetism convince her that
it is not a remedial agent, and that its effects upon those who
practice it, and upon their subjects who do not resist it, lead
to moral and to physical death " (101 : 21). Finally, all
hygienic precautions are to be disregarded : Dyspeptics can
eat and drink whatever they like, for God has given man
dominion, not only over the fish of the sea but likewise over
the poison which is in his stomach. We must not trouble
about fatigue, or periods of repose ; and we should not even be
greatly concerned about cleanliness. " The daily ablutions of
an infant are no more natural nor necessary than would be the
process of taking a fish out of water every day and covering it
with dirt in order to make it thrive more vigorously in its own
element. . . . Water is not the natural habitat of humanity.
I insist on bodily cleanliness within and without. I am not
patient of a speck of dirt ; but in caring for an infant one need
not wash his little body all over each day in order to keep it
sweet as the new-blown flower " (413 : 12).

A second feature of this negative therapeutics is yet more
important. We must absolutely discard the mental precautions which we are accustomed to take against disease.
We must overcome our perpetual fear of illness, must master
the disquietude with which we become affected when we have
the most trifling sensations of disorder. " That mother is not
a Christian Scientist, and her affections need better guidance,
who says to her child : ' You look sick,' ' You look tired,'
' You need rest,' or ' You need medicine.' Such a mother
runs to her little one, who thinks she has hurt her face by
falling on the carpet, and says, moaning more childishly than
her child : ' Mamma knows you are hurt.' The better and
more successful method for any mother to adopt is to say :
' Oh, never mind ! You're not hurt, so don't think you are.'
Presently the child forgets all about the accident, and is at
play " (154 : 24). We may say that the struggle against the
dread of disease is the most essential part of Christian Science.
Mrs. Eddy is never weary of repeating : " We should master
fear, instead of cultivating it " (197 : 16). " The doctor's

mind reaches that of his patient. The doctor should suppress his fear of disease, else his belief in its reality and fatality will harm his patients even more than his calomel and his morphine " (197 : 30). " Always begin your treatment by allaying the fear of patients. Silently reassure them as to their exemption from disease and danger. Watch the result of this simple rule of Christian Science, and you will find that it alleviates the symptoms of every disease. If you succeed in wholly removing the fear, your patient is healed " (411 : 27). Further, it is just as important to suppress the fear of disease in the doctor's mind as in the patient's. " A patient's belief is more or less moulded and formed by his doctor's belief in the case, even though the doctor says nothing to support his theory. His thoughts and his patient's commingle, and the stronger thoughts rule the weaker. Hence the importance that doctors be Christian Scientists " (198 : 23).

Nay more, if patient and doctor are to be fully reassured, the very belief in illness must be suppressed. " Would a mother say to her child, who is frightened at imaginary ghosts and sick in consequence of the fear : ' I know that ghosts are real. They exist and are to be feared ; but you must not be afraid of them ' ? " (352 : 12). " Palsy is a belief that matter governs mortals, and can paralyse the body, making certain portions of it motionless. Destroy this belief, show mortal mind that muscles have no power to be lost, for Mind is supreme, and you cure the palsy " (375 : 21). " Spead the truth to every form of error. Tumours, ulcers, tubercles, inflammation, pain, deformed joints, are waking dream-shadows, dark images of mortal thought, which flee before the light of Truth " (418 : 28).

Let us replace all these absurd and futile medical methods of treatment, all these false fears and beliefs, by potent and salutary beliefs. Let us replace them by the conviction " that Mind governs the body, not partially but wholly " (111 : 28). The system based upon this conviction " has proved itself, whenever scientifically employed, to be the most effective curative agent in medical practice " (111 : 32). " If Mind is foremost and superior, let us rely upon Mind " (114 : 3). It is in order to achieve this result, in order to permeate the minds of our patients with these truths, that we have to expound to them the whole of Mrs. Eddy's metaphysical system, to convince them that mind is all and that matter is nothing. This system derives its curative power from the suppression of the idea that disease really exists.

The Christian Scientist must be encouraging and sympathetic. " The physician who lacks sympathy for his fellow-being is deficient in human affection, and we have the apostolic warrant for asking : ' He that loveth not his brother whom he hath seen, how can he love God whom he hath not seen ? ' " (366 : 12). The American psychologist Goddard tells us that the whole system has always to be expounded with professions of a disinterested zeal for the good of others, with immense self-confidence, and (it must be avowed) with declamations that remind us rather too obviously of the trumpets of the Salvation Army.[1]

Mark Twain, in his book Christian Science,[2] gives an admirable account, both lively and amusing, of this metaphysical therapeutics in its actual working, in its indiscriminate application to all possible diseases. There is, manifestly, an element of caricature in his description, but it is substantially just. In the opening pages the hero tells us how he had a fall when mountaineering, " and broke some arms and legs and one thing or another. By good luck," he goes on, " I was found by some peasants who had lost an ass, and they carried me to the nearest habitation." A lady practitioner of Christian Science is called to his bedside, and comes rather tardily, preferring when first summoned, late at night, to deal with the case for a few hours by " absent treatment." Making no attempt to examine the injuries, she harshly reproves the sufferer for the groans forced from him by pain. Here are some extracts from the ensuing conversation :

" You should never allow yourself to speak of how you feel, nor permit others to ask you how you are feeling ; you should never concede that you are ill, nor permit others to talk about disease or pain or death or similar non-existences in your presence. Such talk only encourages the mind to continue its empty imaginings." Just at that point the Stubenmädchen trod on the cat's tail, and the cat let fly a frenzy of cat-profanity. I asked, with caution :

[1] The Effects of Mind on Body, as evidenced by Faith Cures, " American Journal of Psychology," 1899, vol. x, pp. 430 et seq.
[2] Harper, New York and London, 1907.

" Is a cat's opinion about pain valuable ? "

" A cat has no opinion : opinions proceed from mind only ; the lower animals, being eternally perishable, have not been granted mind ; without mind, opinion is impossible.

" She merely imagined she felt a pain, for imagining is an effect of mind ; without mind, there is no imagination. A cat has no imagination."

" Then she had a *real* pain ? "

" I have already told you there is no such thing as real pain."

" It is strange and interesting. I do wonder what was the matter with the cat."

" Peace ! The cat feels nothing. Your empty and foolish imaginings are profanation and blasphemy, and can do you an injury. It is wiser and better and holier to recognise and confess that there is no such thing as disease or pain or death."

" I am full of imaginary tortures," I said, " but I do not think I could be any more uncomfortable if they were real ones. What must I do to get rid of them ? "

" There is no occasion to get rid of them, since they do not exist. They are illusions propagated by matter, and matter has no existence ; there is no such thing as matter."

" But if there is no such thing as matter, how can matter propagate things ? "

In her compassion she almost smiled [the lady has been described as having a resolute and austere countenance]. She would have smiled if there were any such thing as a smile.

" It is quite simple," she said ; " the fundamental propositions of Christian Science explain it, and they are summarised in the four following self-evident propositions : 1. God is All-in-all. 2. God is Good. Good is mind. 3. God, Spirit, being all, nothing is matter. 4. Life, God, omnipotent good, deny death, evil, sin, disease. There—now you see."

The patient, dumbfounded, ends by repeating the formulas after the Christian Scientist, and murmuring " Wonderful ! "

Finally, the lady brings " an itemised bill for a crate of broken bones mended in two hundred and thirty-four places— one dollar per fracture.

" Nothing exists but Mind ? "

" Nothing," she answered. " All else is substanceless, all else is imaginary."

Thereupon, says the writer, "I gave her an imaginary cheque, and now she is suing me for substantial dollars. It looks inconsistent."

There is obviously a great deal of truth in this humorous narrative, for neither the Scientist healers nor their unfortunate patients understand a word of what they are saying. Both the physicians and the sick do nothing but murmur empty phrases concerning God, mind, matter, sin, disease, health, harmony, the denial of error, and so on. Still, we must never forget that these empty phrases have built churches, and have relieved millions of sufferers. In "Fruitage," the concluding chapter of *Science and Health*, we find an account of eighty notable cures, together with letters from grateful patients and a record of acts of thanksgiving. The "Journal" is continually publishing documents of the same description. The cures run through the whole gamut of diseases : migraine, constipation, alcoholism, eczema, cataract, mania, epilepsy, valvular disease of the heart, cancer, consumption. There are even cases of "mental surgery"; broken bones, dislocated joints, and (dislocated) spinal vertebræ have been cured by Christian Science treatment (402 : 6). Nor do the cures take place only in cases of disease in the ordinary sense of the term ; moral disorders, likewise, can be radically suppressed, vice and sin overcome. "If sickness and sin are illusions, the awakening from this mortal dream or illusion, will bring us into health, holiness, and immortality" (240 : 4). No previous metaphysical system has produced such marvellous results. Although, theoretically considered, Mrs. Eddy's doctrines may seem to be nothing more than those of a trite and very illogical idealism, the practical results of Christian Science are unrivalled, and give the philosophy the stamp of originality.

It seems proper to associate with Christian Science methods which may differ in appearance but are founded on the same principle. The advocates of these methods may try to differentiate themselves from Mrs. Eddy's school, and may even actively oppose it, but they are really imitators of Christian Science, and hope to profit by its success. One of the most interesting of such developments is the American school of metaphysics led by Leander Edmund Whipple, author of *The*

Philosophy of mental Healing, 1893, and *Practical Health*, 1907. Here we are told that health is the natural inference from a metaphysical principle that discloses the true relationship between man and the universe. Whipple also maintains, just like Mrs. Eddy, that disease is the outcome of our false ideas. He tells us that if there are microbes in a rabbit's blood, it is because man thinks there are ; and he adds that if we were to suggest to the guinea-pig not to think so much about Koch's bacillus, the animal would not become tuberculous. A remarkable point about this school is that its course of studies embraces a whole system of philosophical branches like those taught in our higher schools. The students learn : 1, general philosophy, 15 lessons ; 2, symbology, 12 lessons ; 3, ethics, 16 lessons ; 4, mentality, 16 lessons ; 5, science, 16 lessons ; 6, the normal course of metaphysical treatment, 12 lessons. There are also 24 lessons for oral practical instruction. This complete course of philosophy may be interesting, but it is hard to understand how the whole curriculum can be regarded as medical training, and as supplying an adequate introduction to the practice of medicine. The trail of Mrs. Eddy is over it all.

In the same connexion I shall mention a certain Antoine the Healer, who has recently attained considerable notoriety at Jemeppe near Liége, and also in northern France. He is the author of an extraordinary little book entitled *Le couronnement de la révélation d'Antoine le Guérisseur, l'oréole de la conscience* (1907–1909). He issues a " Revue Mensuelle de l'Enseignement du Nouveau Spiritualisme," and here we read that " there is only one remedy for the cure of mankind." This remedy is " the denial of illness and pain, the denial of evil, a non-existent entity." No doubt, the theoretical side of Antoine's system is very simple, and his practice resembles that of ordinary miraculous cures, but we certainly find in his writings, here and there, a good many expressions that recall the phraseology of Christian Science. We are perhaps entitled to assume that Christian Science has had an influence, more or less indirect, upon Antoine. In any case, a detailed and separate account of these minor metaphysical or spiritualist schools is needless. The brief remarks I am about to make concerning Christian Science will apply equally well, mutatis mutandis, to the imitations.

5. VALUE OF PHILOSOPHICAL THERAPEUTICS.

If we wish to understand and appreciate the remarkable movement of ideas comprising Christian Science and the metaphysical methods of therapeutics, we can do so from three different outlooks. First of all, we have to study the fundamental notions underlying these doctrines; we have to ascertain their true origin. Secondly, we shall try to discover the reasons for their success, the determinants of this vast movement of popular credence. Thirdly, and lastly, we shall grasp the importance of these doctrines from a practical standpoint when we compare Christian Science and its congeners with the miraculous methods of healing described in the opening chapter.

Christian Science borrows part of its name from that of a noted religion, and it assumes the semblance of a religion, but we should err if we were to classify it as a religion. Various writers on the subject emphasise this fact, and it has especially been brought into relief by Mark Twain. In the literature of Christian Science we find nothing which makes us think of the fear or the love or the adoration felt for a superhuman power ; there is no trace of the sentiment of mystery, or of the humility appropriate to those who realise the impotence of man when faced by the problems of existence. Nor is there any sign of a real affection for poor humanity ; charity has no place in Christian Science. Mark Twain writes : " I have hunted, hunted, and hunted, by correspondence and otherwise, and have not yet got upon the track of a farthing that the Trust [i.e. organised Christian Science] has spent upon any worthy object. . . . To the question, ' Does any of the money go to charities ? ' the answer from an authoritative source was : ' No, not in the sense usually conveyed by this word.' " [1]

Such religious formulas as are scattered through *Science and Health* are of minor importance, having been borrowed either from the dominant religion or from local superstition. Woodbridge Riley [2] traces the influence exercised by the Shakers, and points to the formulas plagiarised from the teaching of the prophetess Ann Lee. Fundamentally, there is no true religion in Christian Science ; there is nothing but a religious staging.

[1] Christian Science, pp. 75 and 77.
[2] " Psychological Review," November 1903, p. 606.

Some critics think they draw nearer to the truth by regarding Christian Science as a system of philosophy, and above all as a system of idealist philosophy. To me it seems quite erroneous to ascribe much importance to this element of idealist philosophy, or to suppose that such a philosophy has occupied a prominent position in the thought of Mrs. Eddy and her disciples. Their idealism is incoherent and illogical, packed with absurd contradictions in every line. Those who are continually asserting that matter is an illusion, are in fact continually talking about matter, and are really asserting the existence and importance of matter. The illusion and its multiform manifestations still require explanation. The appearance, we are told, is a product of the " mortal mind." Maybe. But what is this " mortal mind " which replaces matter, to raise in its turn exactly the same problems ? Whence comes it, and how does it engender the illusion of matter ? Mrs. Eddy has but one answer : " Mortal mind has no origin and no action, for it does not exist." But if mortal mind, too, be non-existent, how can it explain anything ? We always come back to the practical question : If matter does not exist, how and why do you behave as if it did exist ? Mark Twain says that from first to last Christian Science has recognised only one thing as real, the dollar ! But if matter be unreal, why should a Christian Scientist expect to be paid in real dollars ? As C. G. Pease observes, one who avows that there is no such thing as matter, and in the same breath offers us a chair, is simply lying. Mrs. Eddy pays no heed to these obvious objections, and never attempts a systematic exposition of her teaching. We ourselves, as critics, extract the principles of this idealist system, and formulate them in philosophical terminology for the convenience of summary statement. In actual fact, no exposition of the system has ever been attempted by its adepts ; the philosophy is dispersed amid a thousand and one heterogeneous things. Like the religious formulas, the philosophy appears to be superadded to a building of which it does not constitute anything more than a trifling part.

We must not forget that Christian Science is, preeminently, a medical method, a therapeutic system ; and that the author of *Science and Health* was always and exclusively preoccupied with the problem of treatment. Now, the basic idea of Christian Science treatment is the idea that what the patient thinks about his own illness exercises an all-powerful influence upon the course of the disease. If the sufferer abandons hope, the disease is aggravated ; if he has a confident expectation of cure, his cure becomes a much easier matter. This familiar and trivial observation, disproportionately magnified, makes up the whole of Mrs. Eddy's inspiration. The patient must be made to feel contempt for his disease ; must be convinced that his disease is neither dangerous nor important ; that the disease is nothing, and that he himself, the patient, is great, a superior being, able to conquer this contemptible malady. No one has discerned more accurately than William James the essential characteristic of Christian Science. In his book *The Varieties of religious Experience*, he shows that the kernel of the doctrine is the sentiment of optimism, trust in one's self and in the universe. " The leaders in this faith had an intuitive belief in the all-saving power of healthy-minded altitudes as such, in the conquering efficacy of courage, hope, and trust, and a correlative contempt for doubt, fear, worry, and all nervously precautionary states of mind [pp. 94–95]. . . . This system is wholly and exclusively compacted of optimism. ' Pessimism leads to weakness. Optimism leads to power ' " [p. 107].

Mrs. Eddy's system seems to me designed merely to give this fundamental idea a sort of logical foundation, and to cultivate this feeling of self-confidence and of contempt for illness. It is to rob illness of its apparent power that the Christian Scientists protest against the tyranny of the flesh ; that they deny the existence of pain, fatigue, and physical lesions ; that they seek to suppress the body by proclaiming it to be an insignificant illusion. It is to strengthen the patient's self-confidence that he is raised to the rank of a pure spirit, eternal, all-powerful, immune to suffering and death. The result of this teaching is the emergence of an idealist system ; but the author is utterly indifferent to philosophy, and the appearance of such a system in her writings is a great surprise to herself. Religion is likewise mingled with the brew ; for so much talk of spirit, of the immortal soul, necessarily calls up religious ideas. All the better, for the religious sentiments thus accidentally evoked will endow the doctrine with fresh strength. The lack of coherence in the exposition matters little, seeing that it is not Mrs. Eddy's aim to construct a philosophical or religious system. Enough that the idea of marvellous power has been implanted in the patient's mind, enough that his soul should have learned to soar at an altitude far above bodily troubles.

What was the origin of this basic idea? A number of painstaking studies have supplied the answer to this question.[1] The notion derives from Quimby, who cured Mrs. Eddy of hysterical paraplegia in 1862, explaining his method to the patient, and entrusting her with his manuscripts. In Quimby's writings we can find all that is essential in the utterances of Mrs. Eddy, but garnished with fewer declamations. As we have already seen, the sometime watchmaker, turned magnetiser, came by degrees to renounce all kinds of medical treatment, magnetism not excepted. In the later part of his career, he trusted wholly in the spoken word, and in the instructions he gave to his patients. "I give no drugs," he wrote as early as 1859. "I simply sit down by the patient, I explain to him the truth about himself and things, explain to him that which he believes to be his disease, and my explanation is the whole of my treatment. If I succeed in correcting his errors, I change the fundamental state of his system, and reestablish in him truth and health ; truth comprises all my treatment. . . . When I used to mesmerise the subject, he would prescribe for himself a few simples which did him neither harm nor good, and sometimes he would get better. This led me to believe, at that time, that certain medicines cured in certain cases if the patient prescribed them for himself. But through a great many mistakes, and the prescription of a great many useless drugs, I was led to reexamine the question, and came in the end to the position I now hold : the cure does not depend upon any drug, but simply upon the patient's belief in the doctor or the medium. Now I confine myself to the denial of the truth of disease ; I insist that it is an error, just like the other baseless tales which are handed down from generation to generation, to become a part of the life of the nations." That

[1] See, in especial, the following : Goddard, " American Journal of Psychology," 1899, p. 447 ; Julius A. Dresser, The true History of mental Science, new edition, Boston, 1899 ; Woodbridge Riley, The personal Sources of Christian Science, " Psychological Review," November 1903 ; Milmine, The Life of Mary Baker G. Eddy, 1909.

he might be justified in denying the existence of the disease, Quimby insisted upon the superiority of mind, and upon the non-reality of all that is inferior and material, thus developing a hazy idealist system closely resembling the one we have been studying in the works of his pupil Mrs. Eddy. In 1863, Quimby was already calling his system Christian Science. At this date, too, he was making use of the formulas which were subsequently to comprise the foundations of Mrs. Eddy's *Science and Health* : " Error is sickness, truth is health " ; " error is matter, truth is God " ; " God is right, error is wrong " ; and so on.

During the first years after her cure, and even after Quimby's death in 1866, Mrs. Eddy did full justice to her forerunner. She continued to declare that her only aim was to spread the knowledge of Quimby's teachings, and photographs of her letters to this effect will be found in Milmine's *Life*. Content to sing Quimby's glories, she declared that he did not mesmerise, but healed the sick after the same manner as Christ ; and she even composed a poem on the subject. It was towards 1872 that she began to suppress Quimby. At first her story was that she was merely going to write a preface to her master's book. After a time, she was going to incorporate the preface in the text, and to write a book that would be partly Quimby's work. Finally, coming to the conclusion that her own interpretation excelled the interpretation to be found in the Quimby manuscripts, she declared that the book she published in 1875 was entirely her own work. This was nine years after Quimby's death, and she now claimed that *Science and Health* had been foretold in the Gospel according to St. John. It was the fruit of divine inspiration, for the Holy Ghost had descended upon her. The date alleged for this revelation varies, being sometimes given as 1844, sometimes as 1853, and sometimes as 1864. Now when referring to Quimby she was beginning to accuse him of every possible crime, and especially of " malicious magnetism." If there was anything meritorious in Quimby's writings, it was only what she herself had taught him. As for the letters to Quimby, which on the face of it were certainly compromising, her explanation was that they had been written under Quimby's mesmeric influence.

These protests are childish. The best that can be said in Mrs. Eddy's excuse is that, like so many hysterics, she was unable to transform her wishes into honest beliefs. Students of the history of psychotherapeutics know as a fact that Quimby was the real founder of the remarkable doctrine which underlies Christian Science. Those who like to understand the affiliation of ideas will find it interesting to recall that Quimby was a pupil of the French magnetiser Charles Poyen, and that Poyen had been the introducer of Deleuze's teachings into the United States. Further traces of animal magnetism will be found in Christian Science, as for instance in the theory of unconsciousness, that of a rapport between healer and patient, that of the power of the will, of the communication of thoughts, of the diagnosis at a distance which is implicit in absent treatment.[1] Mrs. Eddy's invectives against magnetism need not be taken seriously. We are witnessing the quarrels of brothers who have fallen out. The fact of real interest is that, in the United States, Christian Science was born of animal magnetism, just as in France hypnotism had the same parentage. Mrs. Eddy's personal contribution to the strange edifice of Christian Science concerned matters of practical organisation. It was thanks to her that the little consulting room of the obscure Dr. Quimby grew into the huge Mother Church of Boston. I think her work can be best described as the financial exploitation of Quimby's idea. What she achieved in this field is sufficiently remarkable.

The marvellous success of the exploitation is what now remains to be explained. Why did Christian Science undergo so vast a development in the United States? Many explanations have been offered, and some of them are worth considering. It is certainly true that Mrs. Eddy's native country and time were peculiarly favourable to the spread of mystical and somewhat superstitious doctrines. The Shakers had had considerable influence, and there was a flourishing Shaker colony at East Canterbury, not far from Tilton, New Hampshire, where Mrs. Eddy passed many of her early years. Miraculous cures were common at this epoch. John Alexander Dowie, born in Edinburgh in the year 1848, the inventor of divine healing and the founder of Zion City on the west shore of Lake Michigan, much resembled earlier miraculous healers.

[1] Cf. Riley, op. cit., p. 607; also, Mental Healing in America, Comptes rendus du Congrès de Genève, 1909, p. 772.

So did the Rev. A. B. Simpson of New York City. Inspired healers, such as Schrader, and Bradley Newell, toured the villages. The most famous specimen of this type, Francis Schlatter, believed himself to be Christ. He wore an appropriate garment, and copied the traditional postures of Jesus, giving himself out to be an envoy from God, and charged by his divine father to heal the ills of suffering humanity. The public mind was thus prepared for such a revelation as that of Christian Science, and was not likely to find Mrs. Eddy's words and ways unduly startling.

While Christian Science could furnish satisfaction for certain mystical trends, it had likewise an eminently practical character, well adapted to please persons of an ambitious and active type and those whose main concern was with material success. It is not a religion for weaklings and repiners. Health, strength, and courage are demanded of all the adherents. Illness, pain, and weakness do not exist; this is quite simple; and since they do not exist we must ignore them. No burial services are held in Christian Science churches, for death is an illusion, and must be neither recognised nor made the object of ceremonial observance. Poverty, too, is non-existent. Consequently, the churches are fine places; the ceremonial is sumptuous; everything is done upon a large scale and in costly fashion; charitable practices have no place in the new religion. Besides, Christian Science promises the faithful wealth as well as health. Both Mark Twain and Georgine Milmine lay especial stress upon this aspect of the cult. *Science and Health* repudiates government, civilisation, and science; but no doubt is ever breathed concerning the importance of business. Christian Science has a message of joy for all; it exalts health, vanity, and material prosperity, as lofty virtues. They are manifestations of union with God. Far from despising riches, this religion makes much of them, and continually insists upon the worth of life and upon its security; in these respects it is the very opposite of the old religions. It thus ministers to the sense of satisfaction and wellbeing characteristic of the prosperous classes in the United States. To this strong appeal to certain typically " American " traits, Christian Science is obviously indebted for much of its success.

It was a practical characteristic of this kind which enabled

Mrs. Eddy to attract a swarm of pupils and to become the centre of so vast a circle of devout healers. The laws regulating medical practice in the United States are laxer than those of most European countries. In America, all sorts of medical schools, varying much in value, are able to grant the title of Doctor of Medicine, and the public must form its own judgment as to the worth of the diploma issued by this or that school. Mrs. Eddy could promise a lucrative practice to those who graduated at her college, and all that was needed was the undertaking of a brief and vague course of metaphysical study. Thus healers could be readily recruited from all classes of the population. The practitioners of Christian Science are ex-schoolmasters ; sometime dressmakers, tailors, or musicians ; they are housewives, or young married women with a good deal of spare time. Milmine (op. cit., pp. 366–369) tells us of the delight of a captain in the mercantile marine when he learned that in three weeks he could become a wonderful doctor—at a cost, it is true, of several hundred dollars. This prospect was an irresistible attraction to a crowd of poor wretches who had their living to make. Mrs. Eddy was not likely to lack disciples as soon as the success of her school was assured.

But the initial success still remains to be explained. The reasons hitherto adduced are, I think, inadequate. They have been no more than contributory causes. It seems to me that the main factor of the success was the character of the founder ; her determination, perhaps we should say her genius. All the historians of the movement have been greatly struck by the organisation of the school, and by the discipline which Mrs. Eddy established among her staff of healers. Mark Twain writes (op. cit., p. 230) : " If she has overlooked a single power, however minute, I cannot discover it. If she has found one, large or small, which she has not seized and made her own, there is no record of it, no trace of it. In her foragings and depredations she usually puts forward the Mother Church—a lay figure—and hides behind it. Whereas, she is in manifest reality the Mother Church herself. It has an impressive array of officials, and committees, and Boards of Direction, of Education, of Lectureship, and so on—geldings, every one, shadows, spectres, apparitions, wax-figures : she is supreme over them all, she can abolish them when she will : blow them out as she would a candle. She is herself the Mother Church."

Medical practitioners are well acquainted with this lust for wielding authority, this jealous desire to hold despotic sway. They know how it becomes a monomania in certain neuropaths. Ordinarily, however, the impulse cannot get beyond the stage of being an unsatisfied passion which, precisely because it is never satisfied, is one of the factors of the delusion of persecution. The remarkable feature of Mrs. Eddy's career was that she was actually able to establish the domination of which she dreamed. All her associates were marvellously docile. The young folk who attended her lectures, cut loose from their families and sank their own individualities. They sacrificed everything for Mrs. Eddy, sacrificed their fortune and their dearest affections ; they submitted to the harshest treatment ; and they could not shake off the shackles even when they were no longer in personal contact with the founder.

What was the foundation of Mrs. Eddy's charm, of her power of domineering over her associates ? She had had almost no education. To judge from her writings, whose only merit is to be found in the ideas taken from others, her intelligence was a poor one. She never manifested any generous feeling, and seems never to have had a strong affection for any one. Her only child, the posthumous son of her first husband, Glover, played no part in her life ; she handed him over to others' care when he was quite young, and took no interest in him thenceforward. In fact, her life was always guided by the dictates of a narrow selfishness. It seems to me that all her strength, all her seductive power, depended upon her imperturbable will. When she was practically destitute, when she was exposed to the most distressing humiliations, after the revolts among her pupils who thrice shattered her life's work, when she was more than sixty years of age—still she would never admit defeat. She was endowed throughout with an amazing and inflexible pride, with an absolutely indestructible self-confidence. These are master qualities ; and, in conjunction with a practical intelligence, they explain the successes of great men of business and of conquerors. " Mrs. Eddy was born with a far-seeing business eye . . . and with a large appetite for power." . . . If she had been " second-assistant cook in a bankrupt boarding house," writes Mark Twain, " I know the rest of it, I know what would have happened. She would have owned the boarding house within six months ; . . . in two years she would own all the boarding houses in the town, . . . in twenty all the hotels in America." [1]

We cannot but be surprised, none the less, to find such will power and such tenacity of purpose in a woman who had been subject to hysterical paroxysms and hysterical paralysis until she was over fifty years of age. We must suppose that her will was unable to develop its full potency until after the revelation from Quimby. Then only did the goal become manifest to her, then only did she conceive the guiding thought of her life. Thenceforward she was able to get the better of her neurosis and to prove that she possessed an indomitable will. Students of psychotherapeutics can learn more from the story of Mrs. Eddy's life than from the lady's writings.

We are now in a position to understand how it was that the financial exploitation of Quimby's therapeutical principle came to be so profitable. But we still have to ask what the principle was worth in itself, and whether it was as valuable to the patients as to those who made money out of it. Here we touch upon a thornier problem, one concerning which accurate statements are far from easy. Certainly, the distressing realities of illness and death are not shuffled out of the world by the simple denial of their existence. Those who refuse to see real evils are behaving like the ostrich which buries its head in the sand in order to avoid the sight of danger. Such a method is of dubious utility, for it can hardly protect us from danger, and may intensify evils which a little wisdom would have enabled us to avoid. Whatever the defects of traditional medicine, there are things which it can do, and can do very well. Certain troubles can be relieved far better by a simple operation, or by the use of such a drug as mercury, than by the wisest psychology in the world. Sufferers from disorders of these kinds are exposed to great danger by those who try to cure them by moral exhortations. American regular practitioners are never weary of drawing attention to cases in which Christian Scientists have allowed patients to die of blood-poisoning without opening abscesses or having recourse to the most elementary antiseptic procedure ; cases

[1] Op. cit., pp. 263-264.

where peritonitis has been caused by the neglect of dietetic precautions in typhoid patients; and cases where infection has run riot in schools because Christian Scientists have refused to enforce isolation. But we must not dwell too much upon such considerations when we encounter phenomena which appear to belong to a new order. If the facts speak for themselves, we must bow to them. Are the facts overwhelming? Goddard remarks that the curative power of the new medical method must certainly be small, seeing that, in the regions where Christian Science has the greatest vogue, far from there having been a decline in the death-rate from the most prevalent diseases, there has rather been an increase. We cannot rest content with a general observation of this kind. The method must be judged by particular instances, by a study of the records of particular cases.

There is no lack of material for such a study. We are overwhelmed by a positive deluge of amazing records. All possible diseases, all imaginable illnesses, have been satisfactorily cured after a few conversations. Persons who have been bedridden for thirty years and have been declared incurable by distinguished specialists, arise and forthwith begin to dance about the room. There are records in plenty; more than enough, it would seem, to convince the most sceptical. Why, then, does doubt persist?

The reason is that the editing of the reports is not such as to inspire confidence. They are obviously written by amateur physicians, who have had no training in medical observation, or in practical observation of any kind. Some of the case-notes are irresistibly comical. Here, for instance, is one quoted by Milmine : " A four-year-old horse had overeaten itself and had a bad fit of indigestion. She said to it : ' You are God's horse, perfect, like all God's work. Being God's work, you cannot eat too much ; you cannot have colic ; material nourishment cannot fight against the activity and the freedom of spiritual nourishment.'—Before the treatment the poor beast was hanging its head, and its breathing was shallow and rapid ; but an hour later it was all right again." Not all the records are so quaint as this, but for the most part we read of poor wretches who have suffered manifold ills for years, have lost the use of all their senses, whose internal organs have been displaced but who recover perfectly " because everything goes

back into its place." In this connexion the Myers write:
" We cannot but remember the case of Maria Jolly, advertised
in every newspaper in the days of our youth, where ' thirty
years of indescribable agony ' were cured at once by the use
of ' Revalenta Arabica,' which turned out to be the flour of
lentils." [1]

The Myers made a little experiment to show how incapable
these good healers were of accurately recording what they had
seen. In a list of marvellous cures they found one described
as complete cure of a congenital deformity of the right foot,
and cure of subsequent maldevelopment of the right leg. Such
a cure should have been easy to check. Unfortunately, the
published report of the cure, while giving remarkable details
concerning the specially made and expensive cork-soled shoes
and the specially cut trousers which the patient had had to
wear, quite failed (by an oversight, doubtless) to mention the
facts that would have been of real use to the scientific student.
There was not a word about the actual position of the bones,
the joints, the muscles, the actual condition of the reflexes, the
amount of atrophy, the electrical reactions, and so on. The
Myers wrote to the person who had recorded the case, asking
for a few additional details, this being the usual practice when
a doctor has published an interesting report and a colleague
has an appetite for further information. The answer in this
instance was an extraordinary one, and the Myers have
published it.[2]

As might have been expected, the miraculously healed
patient made no attempt to furnish the requisite details, and
probably did not understand what his correspondent was
driving at. His reply was reprobatory in tone. There was
only one way, he said, of learning how to understand such
reports. The correspondents were referred to the example of
the prophet Jonah. They must come out of the darkness of
the whale's belly. " If Mr. Myers and those with whom he is
associated will open their minds to the truth that there is no
life, substance, or intelligence in matter, . . . if they will
come out of their material beliefs, they will learn more in one
day than they can otherwise learn in an age." They must
" do as Jonah did, i.e. come out of their belief of life, substance,

[1] Proceedings of the Society for Psychical Research, vol. ix (1893–4),
p. 174. [2] Op. cit., p. 173.

and intelligence in matter." The poor Myers, who could not follow Jonah's example, had to abandon the hope of learning what had been the actual condition of the patient's muscles before and after the cure. There was no possibility, therefore, of passing a scientific judgment upon this case.

Alas, whenever we try to begin the scientific study of the cures effected by Christian Scientists, we are faced by the same difficulty. We are concerned with popular diagnoses, made by the patients upon the strength of their own sensations, and dictated to the healer. The healer will be better pleased with the diagnosis in proportion as the name given to the disease sounds more formidable, so that the honour of the cure may be greater. But the reader of the report has no clue to what the words really mean. Furthermore, as many critics have shown, such observations are often full of contradictions. Doctors and patients have frequently had occasion to protest against the publication of spurious cures. Those who have been treated unsuccessfully for many years (despite their ardent faith) have been numbered among the "cured." Taking all these facts into consideration, the reader will understand that it is very difficult to form a reasoned opinion concerning Christian Science, despite the wealth of case histories the Scientists have published.

All the same, a blank negative would be just as unreasonable as enthusiastic admiration. By no means all the records are so absurd as those I have quoted. Some of them have a strong air of probability, and we have no right to reject them in the mass. I have myself known persons in whom the practice of Christian Science seems to have brought about the undeniable relief of neuropathic troubles. I have known drunkards who have really given up drinking; morphinists who have been cured of their addiction without having been subjected to isolation treatment; sufferers from depression in whom the crises of depression have been arrested. It is quite possible that the same cures might have been effected by other means. But the actual fact is that they were effected by Christian Science. There is one point in particular that must be placed to the credit of such idealist interviews. I refer to their effect upon chimerical dreads, upon the exaggerated precautions which so many people adopt in the hope of preserving their health. "It is the anxiety and fretting about colds, and fevers, and draughts, and getting our feet wet, and about forbidden food eaten in terror of indigestion, that brings on the cold and the fever and the indigestion and most of our other ailments ; and so, if Christian Science can banish that anxiety from the world I think it can reduce the world's disease and pain about four-fifths." [1]

To sum up, and to repeat what I have already said concerning miracles, such a success as Christian Science has had (a far more considerable success than that of Lourdes), would be unintelligible unless Mrs. Eddy's methods of treatment exercised some sort of beneficial influence. With all due reservations made, I am confident that Christian Science contains some useful ideas, and that official psychotherapy must turn them to good account.

The general upshot of the foregoing remarks is that the metaphysical therapeutics of Quimby, Mrs. Eddy, and their successors, has a close resemblance to miraculous therapeutics. We have the same uniformity of treatment for all kinds of diseases, the same vagueness of diagnosis, the same ignorance of the specific factors concerned in bringing about the observed changes. The analogy is manifest. The later therapeutic method is obviously derived from the earlier. This is plainly shown by the religious character which Christian Science continues to preserve.

But we should be unjust were we to ignore the differences between the two methods of treatment, were we to be blind to the advance which has been made in passing from one to the other. In miraculous healing, both operator and patient are working together in the dark. They know that they have to do with a great force which may be turned to useful account, but they are ignorant of its origin or its nature. That is why they ascribe it vaguely to Apollo or the Blessed Virgin. The practitioners who undertake metaphysical treatment have advanced a stage ; they have made the great discovery that the mysterious force is in the human mind. No longer do they appeal to an entirely occult and external power ; they know that they must appeal to a power that lies within us, to the power of thought. This idea that human thought is potent even against the maladies of the body, began to germinate during the study of animal magnetism ; but it

[1] Mark Twain, op. cit., p. 55.

blossomed for the first time in the full light of day when Christian Science was born. This merit must be frankly recognised.

When it became necessary to define the healing power of thought, to say what it consisted of, to explain how we could distinguish potent and efficacious thoughts from those which had no such efficacy, these first healers developed an idea which, according to our present lights, seems both strange and perilous. They imagined that the effective thought was true thought ; that thought was potent in proportion to its truth, and above all in proportion to its objective and metaphysical truth. Thus they were led to suppose that, in order to cure himself, the patient must know the essence of things, and must understand the principle of the world. For the thought had to be true ; the further it made its way into reality, the more potent it would be. Such, I believe, was the starting-point of these remarkable courses of philosophy undergoing transformation into courses of medicine, and of these idealist systems applied to the cure of indigestion.

The illusion, strange though it may seem, was very natural. In former days, thought was mainly known under the form of intelligence, as the faculty of knowledge ; its chief power was regarded as the knowledge of truth, and of absolute truth. On the other hand, truth, though one of man's thoughts, was also supposed to be an external reality ; it was a loosely defined entity, simultaneously subjective and objective. For thinkers who set out from the notion of miracle and of mysterious powers external to man, and passed thence to the study of human thought, the notion of truth, metaphysical truth, was an intermediate stage easy to conceive. Everywhere metaphysics preceded science, and metaphysical methods of treatment have paved the way for psychological methods of treatment.

The absurdities in which metaphysical methods of treatment have culminated, disclose the inadequacy of these first attempts to replace the old dependence on miracle. I do not think it likely that Mark Twain's forecast will be realised ; I do not believe that Christian Science is destined to spread throughout the United States, and ere long to seize the reins of government. The doctrine is unlikely to survive its illustrious founder for many years. During her own lifetime, this domineering high priestess was able to forbid thought and argument, and could maintain union among the faithful. Henceforward it will be difficult to impose the uniform acceptance of dogmas that are so absurd ; discussion and the spread of heresy will soon bring about the dissolution of the creed. Moreover, Christian Science has to encounter increasing hostility from without. At first the doctors were taken aback, but now they are organising crusades. At the last neurological congress, Lloyd Tuckey declared that the new sect had become a public danger.[1] Prosecutions for criminal neglect are becoming more frequent. In England a mother has been punished for having allowed her daughter to die of pneumonia without seeking qualified medical aid.[2] In an address to the Congregational Union at Sheffield, Stephen Paget declared that Christian Science is red with the blood of its victims.[3] Deprived of their leader, the unhappy Scientists will not be able to offer effective resistance. But, more than all, the dissolution of the cult will be promoted by the development of a genuine psychological therapeutics. When true psychotherapeutics replaces Christian Science, it will be incumbent on its practitioners to remember what they owe to the forerunner.

[1] Comptes rendus du Congrès de Neurologie d'Amsterdam, 1907, p. 869.
[2] " Daily News," October 15, 1909.
[3] The Case Against Christian Science, p. 27.

CHAPTER THREE

MEDICAL MORALISATION

Now that we have studied the remarkable religious and medical movement especially prevalent in the United States and known by the name of Christian Science, it will be interesting to discover whether any analogous system of instruction has originated in Europe. Some authors describe the Lourdes miracles as akin to Christian Science. The comparison seems to me inapt, for in mental healing there is an element which plays no part in the Lourdes miracles, namely the idea of a mental and moral determinism which plays a part in these cures. Others have compared the American movement with the French development of hypnotism, but this comparison also seems ill-advised, for hypnotism is a far more definite method both psychologically and clinically. Hypnotism presupposes comparatively precise observation and diagnosis, and is thus a marked advance upon Christian Science.

In my opinion, we can find on this side of the Atlantic a movement more closely resembling Christian Science than either of the two before-mentioned. It has not had a very wide vogue, but is important none the less. I refer to a method of treatment based on moral influence, one that has been practised with fair success in a number of Swiss sanatoria. It has also been adopted by a good many medical practitioners in the United States.

This method appeals to man's intelligence, to his reason, to his moral and religious sentiments, relying on these influences to bring about the restoration of health. It is an old method, as I have shown in the Introduction. Still, if we think of widespread practice rather than of theory, it will be proper to regard Paul Dubois of Berne, a famous Swiss doctor, as the pioneer of this therapeutic method. To his writings I shall turn when expounding the principles of treatment by medical moralisation. Then we shall have to consider the modifications introduced by some of Dubois' successors, and to discuss the value of these.

I. PAUL DUBOIS OF BERNE AND HIS METHOD.

Dubois' personal history is not so remarkable as that of Mrs. Eddy, and need not concern us. It will be enough to enumerate the studies which decided the bent of his life's work. At quite an early stage of his medical career, his interest was concentrated upon nervous disorders. At first he treated them by electrical methods, but soon found the practice wearisome. " I found the occupation of moving an electrode to and fro over the patient's body an irksome one. Sometimes I would interrupt the electrical treatment in order to talk to the sufferer, and I soon came to realise that a kindly word or a little philosophical advice did far more good than half an hour's faradisation ; I found encouraging conversation to be the only efficient weapon." During his study of these moral methods of treatment, he devoted some time to hypnotism, which was then fashionable as the only psychological method of treatment, and he worked under Bernheim at Nancy. But with hypnotism, too, he was dissatisfied. Quite wrongly (in my opinion) he regarded hypnotic suggestion as an unscrupulous way of abusing the patient's credulity. No doubt the invalid could be cured in this way, but only by being humbugged. To Dubois the thought of deception was intolerable and humiliating. He decided to fight disease more frankly, in the full light of day, and simply by reasoning and moralisation.

Such was the spirit in which he taught psychotherapeutics at the University of Berne, and in which he treated a large number of patients in his sanatorium. His leading ideas concerning the treatment of disease by transforming the patient's moral state, and reports of a few out of a large number of successful cases, will be found in the most important of his books, *Les psychonévroses et leur traitement moral*, 1904. The reader may also consult *L'éducation de soi-même*, 1909 ; the interesting articles contributed by Dubois to Parker's great compendium of psychotherapeutics, and entitled, *The Method of Persuasion* (II, iii, 5 ; II, iv, 22 ; III, i, 33 ; III, ii, 31) ;

and various other articles, notably *La pathogénie des états neurasthéniques* (Rapport au dixième Congrès de Médecine, Geneva, September 1908).

The first thing we note in these studies is a negative characteristic, a strong inclination to eliminate many things to which most medical practitioners attach considerable importance. For instance, it is plain that Dubois does not trouble himself to study symptoms closely, or to make an exact diagnosis. I should wrong him if I were to imply that he is as utterly indifferent to diagnosis as were Quimby and Mrs. Eddy ; he does not propose to apply his method to all diseases indifferently, but limits it to psychoneuroses (p. 19) [1] ; this is a manifest advance. But, first of all, these psychoneuroses are vaguely defined, the term being used to include all illnesses wherein mind is a dominant factor in causation ; and, secondly, Dubois makes no attempt to distinguish among what he terms psychoneuroses. " It is a futile endeavour when we try to give to hysteria the characteristics of a morbid entity, or to separate it artificially from neurasthenia, with which it is almost invariably combined. Among these patients, too, we often encounter manifest symptoms of hypochondria and melancholia " (p. 210). Dubois has no interest in the problems which have been one of my own chief concerns for a great many years ; he pays no attention to the interpretation of neuropathic symptoms, to their hierarchy, their pathogenesis. His " neuropaths " are merely patients whose mind is troubled in one way or another. What does it concern the doctor to understand the exact nature of the disease ? His business is to cure. Nothing but treatment is of real interest.

Dubois is no less rigid and restrictive in his choice of methods of treatment. The various surgical procedures now so much in fashion for the relief of abdominal troubles and for the cure of maladies of the sense organs, seem to him too highly esteemed and often harmful. " In certain specialities, would it not be better to operate and cauterise and curette rather less frequently, and to recognise that morbid autosuggestions have an enormous influence even in the case of diseases that seem to be local " (p. 113). He has no use for hydrotherapy (which has certainly been much abused) ; and he stigmatises as

---

[1] The parenthetical page-references are to the 1904 edition of Les psychonévroses et leur traitement moral.

quackery, massage, hypodermic injections, and treatment by organic extracts (p. 23 ; also Parker's *Psychotherapy*, II, iv, 33). " After having seen nothing but microbes everywhere, we now dream only of internal secretions, and have strayed into the fantastic domain of organotherapy " (p. 8). " We must make an end of all this, and must march against the disease unarmed, without medicaments ; thus we shall give the patient confidence that there is no danger, and this is of great importance " (p. 487). " Our only weapon must be encouraging conversation " (p. 301). We are, therefore, limited to moral methods of treatment, but some even of these are to be excluded. I need hardly say that miraculous treatments, like those of Lourdes, are ridiculed (p. 247). But Dubois' harshest criticism is directed against hypnotism and suggestion. " Rational psychotherapeutics has no need of this sort of preparatory narcosis termed hypnotism, no need of this hypersuggestibility which is itself suggested. It is above all upon suggestion, as understood by his former master Bernheim, that Dubois delivers such furious onslaughts. Nowhere does he tell us in set terms what he means by suggestion, but it must be something dreadful, for he overwhelms it with invectives. " I reflected on the nature of suggestion, resolved to abandon it, not because I doubted its efficacy, but because I found it artificial. My respect for honesty in all lines of thought restrained me from using subterfuges, however prompt and complete their results might be. . . . The operator who makes use of suggestion . . . views only the final favourable result and gives no thought to the more or less irrational character of the means used." We go too far if we simply lay a hand upon the patient's forehead, for this verges upon a physical therapeutic method.[1] In like manner, Mrs. Eddy was infuriated if any of her pupils ventured to lay a hand upon a patient's forehead, for this, she said, was malicious magnetism. But let us return to Dubois. " Our aim must not be to make the patient stupidly suggestible, but to restore to him his power of self-mastery " (p. 131.) If, sometimes, for unexplained reasons, Dubois makes up his mind to employ suggestion (for instance, in the treatment of nocturnal incontinence of urine), he is bitterly ashamed, and blushes at his own behaviour (p. 380). He is no less strongly adverse to the exercise of authority than to

[1] Parker, op. cit., II, iv, 23–25.

the use of suggestion. He finds himself compelled to exercise authority on occasions, as when he has to do with a young woman who refuses food ; but he is greatly distressed by this lapse, and would if he could avoid exercising any kind of influence acting on the patient exclusively through emotional channels.

When the methods to which Dubois objects have been eliminated, what remains ? The patient is first of all sent to the Lausanne sanatorium, where isolation from the domestic environment can be secured. For a week he is kept in bed, upon a pure milk diet (8 pints in the 24 hours) ; then he gets up and resumes an ordinary diet (pp. 310 and 315). These, however, are unimportant accessories (p. 489). The essential factor is an intimate daily conversation, which does far more for the patient than douches or chloral. The real doctor does far more good by his words than by the prescriptions he writes. He should be content with sitting down beside his patient, and with working a cure by moralising conversation (p. 27). There is a remarkable analogy between these phrases and those of Quimby.

What is the aim of such conversations ? " Their primary aim must always be reason and truth. . . . We cannot communicate an idea to the patient unless we ourselves accept it in its entirety. . . . Above all, we have to respect the patient and his mental faculties " (p. 27). But what is the truth which we have to communicate to the patient ? We have to make him understand the truth about his illness ; we must explain to him the theory of his illness. This is important, for when the patient comes to consult a doctor his mind is filled with false notions about his troubles. He has two fundamental ideas concerning his malady. First of all he believes that he is affected with a lesion of some kind, with a disorder which is the outcome of organic changes ; and that he is subject to the consequences of this lesion, and is powerless to overcome them by an act of will. In the second place, he believes these lesions to be incurable.[1] By means of a prolonged and painstaking discussion, we must convince him of his error ; we must persuade him that there is no real lesion in his stomach, his intestine, or his brain. There

[1] Parker, op. cit., II, iv, 30 ; III, i, 33.

are a great many nervous disorders in which the patient falsely imagines himself to be suffering from heart disease, meningitis, brain tumour, tubercular peritonitis—when, in reality, the disease has no organic basis whatever (p. 117).

The troubles of which the patient is aware are purely functional; in themselves, they are neither serious nor important; this becomes plain to the patient as soon as he has been enlightened concerning their true nature and their origin. "Don't take your palpitations seriously; they are due to your persistent uneasiness, and are not dangerous. . . . The variations in the frequency and tension of your pulse, and even the occasional intermittence, are due to emotional stress " (p. 360). " The gastric and intestinal troubles to which nervous patients are subject have no serious consequences ; they are due to the influence which ideas exercise upon the viscera. There is nothing so prone to upset the stomach as gloomy thoughts. Barras showed this clearly as long ago as 1820 in his treatise *Les gastralgies et les entéralgies ou maladies nerveuses de l'estomac et des intestins.*" The chief cause of enterocolitis is a defective mental representation, the fixation of thought upon the intestine. The insomnia from which so many of our patients suffer, dependent upon chronic uneasiness, is of no consequence, and we should pay no attention to it. A few sleepless nights are a trifling matter. Let the patient adopt towards sleep an attitude of indifference which can be expressed by the phrase : " If I sleep, all the better ; if I don't sleep, no matter " (p. 400). Disorders of sensation are not worthy of a moment's notice. " Sensation can be annulled by distracting the attention, or by inhibitive autosuggestion ; it can be intensified by attention ; it can be created de novo by mental representation " (p. 155). Convulsive seizures are merely the exaggerated expression of moral uneasiness ; paralysis and paresis are equally unimportant. " You are paralysed ? What are you talking about ? You are merely suffering from nervous fatigue, which is natural enough after all the troubles you have been through. Don't worry about it, you'll be better to-morrow " (p. 449). " The obstacles that stop you are not in your nervous system but in your imagination. . . . You think that you cannot pass water ; the failure of the urinary function depends upon undue attention " (pp. 376 and 379). Above all we should be careful to avoid talking of pain or distressing sensations. " The human machine is so complicated, that hardly a day can pass without our becoming aware that there is something a little out of gear. One day, it is a gastric uneasiness ; another, a vague pain somewhere ; another, an attack of palpitation ; another, a fleeting neuralgia. Have more confidence in you health. Dismiss these petty ailments with a smile."

But surely the mental and moral disorders from which the patients suffer are more serious ? Not a bit of it. They are all quite wrong to complain of emotional upsets. " The things that trouble them are not the graver misfortunes of life, but little matters, trifling vexations, pinpricks. A little philosophy, easily learned, will restore the mental balance " (p. 111). Among such mental troubles must be numbered a feeling of which nervous patients are always complaining, the feeling of fatigue. Here is one who feels utterly exhausted after he has walked twenty paces. If he tries to force himself to go any farther, all sorts of distressing symptoms ensue. Another suffers from a like fatigue in social life ; he cannot endure company for more than a few minutes at a time. Another has no power of sustained mental work, and if he begins to read he is forced to lay aside the book after turning over a few pages. In many of these patients, the sense organs are quickly wearied ; close visual attention is impossible to them for more than a few seconds. Such facts are familiar, and I believe them to be of essential importance. But how does Dubois interpret them ? How does he explain them to his patients ? Quite simply ! They are false feelings of fatigue ; their origin is purely mental ; they are belief that one is tired, nothing more. " We all know what it is to grow tired, and healthy persons are aware that a brief spell of rest will remove the sensation of fatigue ; but the neurasthenic takes fright, is distressed to note his weariness, and perpetuates it by excess of attention " (p. 118). This problem of the feeling of exhaustion from which neuropaths suffer is, in my view, an exceedingly complicated one, and almost the whole of the ninth chapter of the present work is devoted to its consideration. Dubois thinks otherwise, and for him the matter is amazingly simple. Equally simple are all the other troubles of thought. " Innumerable are the neurotics who are seized with headache as soon as they see a heating apparatus ; who feel faint when there are cut flowers in the room; who feel chilly even in summer weather; who put on gloves before they will lift a cup of milk " (p. 157). " In all neuroses, the salient factor is the effect of mental representations. It is ideation which originates or maintains these functional disorders " (p. 18).

We shall understand our patients better when we realise that under the influence of erroneous ideas they have adopted a number of bad mental habits. They pay undue attention to certain sensations which exist in all of us, but which healthy people disregard; " vague impressions aroused by the sexual instincts, sensations of fatigue, trifling pains in the stomach." It has become a habit with them to expect a phenomenon, to foresee it, to look out for it. " We expect palpitations (p. 364) . . . nervous cough (p. 369). . . . Expectant attention, chronic uneasiness, transforms an idea into an action, though the person concerned is unaware of what is going on " (p. 439). Superadd habitual emotional trends, such as fear, anger, waywardness, sulkiness, and you will understand how extremely complicated disorders may develop under the influence of a few erroneous ideas. At bottom, the only real thing in such illnesses consists of the false ideas upon which they depend. Dubois' patients, like Mrs. Eddy's, are simply " in error."

These are the truths which you must hammer into your patient's head. To achieve this, your main resource will be your attitude towards the various symptoms of which he complains. You will not take the symptoms seriously; you will not treat them at all. " You must give up sounding the stomach, test meals, chemical examination of the gastric secretions. You must ignore hysterical aphonia and hysterical anaesthesia. . . . I no longer pay any attention to paralysed limbs, and I have given up testing sensibility with a pin. I declare straightway that these disorders no longer exist " (pp. 209 and 373). Furthermore, we must discuss every aspect of the question. " Logical persuasion is a true enchanter's wand " (p.109). " Discuss matters with your patient in the frame of mind of a barrister convinced of the justice of his plea, as one who knows how to present and multiply arguments, as one who can hammer the truth into the patient's head " (p. 272). " The doctor must destroy all the scaffolding of fears and false theories ; he must take by storm the mental mechanism whereby the patient has manufactured so many false notions " (p. 164). " He must never be weary of saying : ' Don't think about your troubles ; act as if they did not exist ; dismiss these petty ailments with a smile ' " (p. 436).

While carrying on this medical and psychological discussion, the doctor must arouse the idea of health in his patient's mind. It may seem strange to speak of seeking health to a person when we have just been proving to him that he has no illness. Still, we may go so far as Mrs. Eddy, may agree that there is an illusion of illness, and that the illusion has to be cured. " Impress upon the patient the fixed idea that he will get well ; maintain the fixity of this idea until the cure is complete ; arouse conviction by reasoning that grows ever more cogent " (p. 273). The neurotic is on the high road towards health as soon as he is convinced that he will get well ; he is cured when he believes himself to be cured " (p. 245). To reach this goal, we must point out the little things that will enable him to secure a partial improvement. In this connexion Dubois gives some practical advice concerning the best way of overcoming constipation in neuropaths (p. 344), this being one of the rare disorders which he condescends to treat by concrete measures. " We must optimistically insist upon all the progress that has been made, and may even exaggerate a little to encourage the patient " (p. 289). Thus the idea of health will enter his mind, replacing the idea of disease due to incurable lesions. This idea of health, realising itself, will bring about a complete transformation.

Relapses may be speedy and frequent. The patients will not be able to keep the idea of health persistently before their minds. Other thoughts will intrude, and we must be on our guard against such an intrusion. Here we come to the core of the method. The neuropath's absurd notions must be replaced by sublime philosophical thoughts. The patient must be made to understand the importance of thought, the power of his own mind, the superiority of mind over body. " You must be ready to discuss predestination, free-will, responsibility, natural religion, etc. ; for the patient will speedily involve you in philosophical discussions, and you must have ideas upon the topic " (p. 40). It is the doctor's supreme duty to insist upon the power and the freedom of the will. " If you are determined by your inimical tendencies, you are also the slave of your beneficent impulses, your good sensibilities, your clear notions of the true, the good, and the beautiful. A plain view of the goal should be enough to ensure your marching straight forward " (p. 57).

The essential point, in fact, is to gain moral ideas competent to guide our life, to regulate our conduct towards ourselves and others. Morale is indispensable to these patients. Unaided, this " can bring about a profound change in their mentality. You must reeducate their reason, must make them understand how dangerous it is to think too much of themselves.

" Show the patient by examples carefully chosen from your own experience as a man and a doctor, the immense value of moral courage, and the existence of a natural tendency towards the perfectionment of our moral personality " (p. 40). " What we need in life is not will . . . but intelligence. Above all, let us cultivate this moral intelligence which enables us to distinguish between good and evil, and to throw light on the path bordered by pitfalls along which we have to walk through life." [1] " Forget your stomach and your bowels ; bear your discomforts cheerfully ; and make it your ambition to lead a bold and active life " (p. 336). " We must live with an imperturbable confidence in our own powers of resistance. We must acquire good habits, and yet have no fear of discarding them on occasion. We must take an interest in everything, develop all our powers, continually improve our moral state. We must desire good health, . . . and must know how to throw all our discomforts into the waste-ailment basket " (pp. 499 and 541). " The doctor's consulting room must become a psychotherapeutic dispensary, not one at which prescriptions to be made up by the chemist are written, but a place in which the doctor impresses upon the patient's understanding all the wisdom of the stoics, all the maxims of the serene but not frigid reason, which can alone make good the defects of our inborn or acquired mentality." [2]

The best way of forgetting ourselves is to devote a little more thought to others ; the best way of winning happiness for ourselves is to seek the happiness of others. " There is one form of egoism which cannot be too highly extolled. I mean altruism, which is only a perfected egoism." [3] " Solace

[1] L'éducation de soi-même, p. 72. [2] Ibid., p. 201. [3] Ibid., p. 101.

those who suffer, instead of regaling them with the spectacle of your own folly. Duty, however arduous, ought to be done joyously." [1] This little volume upon the education of self contains some admirable pages upon tolerance, forbearance, moderation, sympathy, kindness. I cannot but think that these excellent sermons written for sick folk might be even more useful to those in good health. If Dubois could succeed in inculcating such exalted rules of conduct, he would certainly have good reason for his assertion that " people are wrong in speaking of degeneration, for the upward progress of mankind is continuous " (p. 239).

The foregoing exposition may have led the reader to think that Dubois' moral therapeutics is solely addressed to the intelligence, and that its only appeal is to cold reasoning. Such is the complaint of Dejerine, who believes that he has made a new departure in Dubois' therapeutic method by supplementing it with the influence of a few sentiments. I regard Dejerine's criticism as unjust. Dubois stresses the importance of reasoning because he thinks that it is urgently necessary for the patient to arrive at a certain measure of self-understanding; but he is continually appealing to all the sentiments as well. The doctor must arouse the patient's confidence, and must even arouse the latter's pride by making him understand how much that is beautiful and good can be found within himself (p. 289). " Try to discover his best qualities. Make him understand that he is intelligent. Awaken his religious sentiments, and turn them to good account " (p. 285). " The doctor must himself enjoy a sense of mental euphoria, and must be competent to inspire optimistic feelings " (p. 106). He must be able to acquire something more than the patient's confidence ; he must win friendship, and if he is to do this, he must make the patient feel that he is inspired with a real sympathy and affection towards the latter.

" If we wish to modify the state of mind of one who has fallen, it will not suffice to tell him that we know there were extenuating circumstances, or to show him a forced sympathy ; we must love him like a brother, must enfold him in our arms with a profound feeling of our common weakness " (p. 242). " In these conversations we must show our patient that our sympathy for him is so keen and so all-embracing, that he

[1] L'éducation de soi-même, p. 110.

would really be very ungrateful not to get well " (p. 264). Dubois has good reason for insisting more than once that in his method of treatment he " makes the strings of all the moral sentiments and of the reason vibrate in unison " (p. 264).

2. OTHER MORALISING METHODS OF TREATMENT.

Dubois' writings furnish the fullest and most typical account (typical even in its exaggerations) of the psychotherapeutic method which works by the moralisation of the patient, and that is why my summary has been made in the form of quotations from this author. But my readers must not imagine that Dubois has a monopoly of the idea, which is simultaneously medical and moral. Closely similar methods of treatment were advocated almost simultaneously in various quarters, and it will be interesting to compare these different expressions of the same fundamental thought.

In Germany several authors, and in especial Strümpell, Oppenheim, and Jolly, began a good while ago to insist upon the influence of psychological phenomena upon the genesis of nervous disorders. They went on to declare that psychological phenomena could also become factors promoting the cure of such troubles, and that this must be turned to good account. In 1906, Hermann Oppenheim of Berlin published a selection of letters written by him to patients, Englished by Alexander Bruce under the title *Letters on Psychotherapeutics*. These letters contain excellent practical indications concerning the best way of exerting a moral influence. Buttersack, of Berlin, insisted in 1903 on the value of the doctor's moral influence, acutely analysing the operation of psychical factors, and emphasising the great importance of an optimistic philosophy. In 1905, Auguste Forel of Zurich published a work entitled *Hygiene der Nerven und des Geistes im gesunden und kranken Zustande* ; and in 1906, *L'âme et le système nerveux, hygiène et pathologie*. Here Forel gives advice concerning the mental training of children. He wants it to become more concrete, but his leading recommendation is that there should be an education of the sentiments. " We must impress upon the child feelings of contempt and horror for all that is bad and false, for lying, and for the selfishness that exploits others." [1]

[1] *L'âme et le système nerveux*, p. 279.

He maintains that " repining and fruitless despair on account of lost good are rooted in the narrowness and in the egoism of our love sentiment, which is so apt to be concentrated upon certain specially selected objects. . . . Let us always direct our steps towards a humanist ideal that is lofty, great, and wide, and let us never look backwards " (p. 311). An important element in cerebral hygiene is " to pay as little attention as possible to functional nervous troubles, whatever their nature, that we may avoid magnifying them through habit. Painful affections can be greatly mitigated if we distract our attention from them by work, so that we may perhaps get rid of them altogether " (p. 312). " The odd moments which are available even for those who are very busy can be used for the promotion of a harmonious mental balance, by setting the mind to work as vigorously as possible in new fields " (p. 313). " Those who desire their old age to be happy should never renounce their optimism ; secondly, they should never waste their time in brooding over the past and mourning over the death of those dear to them ; thirdly, they should continue at work down to the day of their death, in order to keep their brains elastic " (p. 318). We find here the same inspiration as that which animates the writings of Dubois. Health and happiness are to be secured by a hygiene of the mind, by the cultivation of the intellect, and by the exercise of moral virtues. But Forel applies these principles less crudely, and his therapeutic method is not so exclusive as that of Dubois. The systems of thought are akin, but Forel's inspiration is independent.

Certain French writers, however, have been the direct disciples of the Bernese professor, and merely reproduce his teachings word for word, or with trifling modifications. Dejerine, who had worked under Dubois at Berne, undertook to make the latter's method known in France, and to apply it practically. In 1904 he wrote a preface for Dubois' *Les psychonévroses et leur traitement moral*, from which I quote the following passage : " The leading, perhaps the unique, role in the treatment of psychoneuroses must be assigned to what I should like to call psychical pedagogy, meaning by this the reeducation of the reason. Dubois is the first to have based his whole system of treatment upon this guiding idea." Writing in the " Journal de Médecine " on March 12, 1910,

Dejerine made an eloquent declaration of spiritualist faith, and expounded Dubois' ideas anent treatment by persuasion. " To cure nervous troubles, which always issue from the affective life, we must fight the deceptive and sterile systems of monism, fatalism, scepticism, and determinism ; we must encourage the use of reason, must overcome the patient's obsessions, and must help him to reconstruct his mentality. Every one ought to set before his higher faculties an ideal which will enable him to find in himself a support during the trials of daily life. We must keep before the patient's mind, ideas of the beautiful, the just, and the noble ; we must insist upon the feeling of satisfaction which follows upon the fulfilment of duty ; must develop the notions of solidarity and charity ; must not forget that the brain should always be guided by the heart. Such will be the true medicine of the future."

Dejerine has made an interesting attempt to realise in hospital practice the moralising method of treatment which he had learned to admire at Berne. He uses the method in his practice at the Salpêtrière. The remarkable ward for patients undergoing curative moralisation is described in Manto's thesis for the degree of doctor of medicine. A yet fuller account will be found in the work by Camus and Pagniez entitled *Isolement et psychothérapie*, published in 1904. In this ward, a women's ward, the patients are kept in bed, each bed being surrounded by curtains. They may neither receive nor write letters, nor have any visitors until there has been a great improvement in their health. The only people they may speak to are the visiting physician, the house physician, and the ward sister. The ordinary nurses may not go near the patient's bed without the sister's orders, and they must not speak to the patient. Unless there is a special indication to the contrary, the patient is put on a pure milk diet for some time after admission. During the early phases of the treatment she is not allowed to read either newspapers or books. Every morning and every evening the visiting physician or the house physician holds a psychotherapeutic séance at each bedside. The writers tell us that complete isolation should be enforced for at least four weeks, but they add that there is not much advantage in continuing it for more than three or four months.[1]

There are two reasons for the rigidity of this isolation.

[1] Isolement et psychothérapie, pp. 101–107.

The first aim is to withdraw the patient from the influence of the other patients, which might be unwholesome. The second is to subject the patient more fully to the moral influence of the doctor who practises the moralising treatment in his morning and evening visits. What is this treatment? What does the therapeutist do at the patient's bedside? We can gather no fresh information on this matter from *Isolement et psychothérapie*. The ideas and the phraseology are identical with those of Dubois. As before, drug treatment and surgical treatment are forbidden. As before, there are somewhat rhetorical attacks upon suggestion, "in which the subject obeys without criticisms, without reflection, without reasoning or judging, and without having either to accept or to check what is said" (p. 26). Persuasion must take the place of suggestion. "What is requisite is a dialogue in which the doctor tries to turn the patient's thoughts away from the illness, to encourage him, to give him hope, to change his state of mind, to make him understand the possibility of getting better and the importance of collaborating in his own cure." For the guidance of the treatment, the authors declare more explicitly than Dubois that science, study of any kind, is utterly useless. This therapeutic method "no longer demands of the doctor that he should be a sort of priest of an esoteric science. He is merely to be an honest man in the exalted sense given to this term in the seventeenth century, and one well informed concerning all that can be done by the language of the reason addressed to a trusting patient" (p. 82). This is not the place for a discussion of a recent work by Dejerine and Gauckler, *Les manifestations fonctionnelles des psychonévroses et leur traitement par la psychothérapie*. Although this book is of the same character as the foregoing, it contains certain comparatively precise notions which entitle it to a place among studies relating to educational methods of treatment.

Some other French writers, though rather slowly, have followed Dejerine's example in the attempt to make simple moralisation an exclusive method for the treatment of neurotic patients. Even Bernheim, to whom we are indebted for his admirable studies upon suggestion, and whose only mistake was his contention that suggestion was everything, now prefers to say that suggestion is nothing and that he has never aimed at anything beyond persuasion. Dubois is outraged by such a change of front. He reproaches Bernheim " with trying to purify [!] his psychic influence, to make it more rational,"[1] with wanting also to fly the psychotherapeutic flag—as if Bernheim had no right to do anything of the kind. This is a quarrel about words, and about words which neither of the two disputants has troubled to define. In 1898, Paul Emile Lévy was still making use of a simulacrum of hypnotism which seemed innocent enough ; he was merely asking the patient to keep the eyes closed during the famous moralising conversation. Dubois waxes indignant about this : " There is still too much artifice in M. Lévy's method. . . . We recognise in him a pupil of M. Bernheim."[2] Camus and Pagniez likewise grow eloquent when they denounce this crime.[3] Since then, Lévy has made praiseworthy efforts to mend his ways. Influenced by the prevailing fashion, he now tells us that hypnotism has fallen into disfavour " because it is regarded as a special nervous condition." He, too, wants the patient to participate in the work of cure, which is, of course, to be " rational." The patient must learn to discipline himself morally and physically. In a word, the whole of Lévy's therapeutic system depends upon " rational education and re-education."[4]

The same tendency can be traced readily enough in the medical literature of other lands ; but we shall find nothing, in this connexion, that differs notably from the teaching we have just been discussing. Suffice it, therefore, to mention : Canfield (of Bristol, U.S.A.), *Practical Considerations in the Treatment of Neurasthenia*, a series of articles in the " Boston Medical and Surgical Journal," 1907 ; and articles by J. Antonio Agrelo and Bravo y Moreno which appeared in the " Archivos de Psiquiatria de M. J. Ingegnieros," during the year 1908, under the respective captions, *Psicoterapia y reeducacion psiquica* and *Notas de psicoterapia*.

We must return to the United States for the study of

[1] Les psychonévroses, p. 25.   [2] Ibid., p. 485.
[3] Isolement et psychothérapie, p. 57.
[4] Lévy, L'education rationnelle de la volonté, son emploi thérapeutique, p. 19 ; La cure définitive de la neurasthénie par la reéducation, " Archives Générales de la Médecene," February 6, 1906 ; Traitement psychique de l'hystérie, " Presse Médicale," April 29, 1903.

a more original and more interesting development of the method of moralisation. This remarkable movement now links itself on to Dubois' teaching, but to understand its true affiliations we must retrace our steps a little. Mrs. Eddy, when she insisted that any other moral treatment than her own was evil and dangerous, was merely trying to monopolise an idea that is general property.[1] She succeeded fairly well, for " to-day thousands of persons believe that they owe their health and their happiness to a healing power revealed by God to Mrs. Eddy, and, by Mrs. Eddy, to the human race." Nevertheless, the principle of psychotherapeutics had an independent existence and several of Quimby's disciples preserved and developed the latter's teaching without towing in Mrs. Eddy's wake. Several years before the appearance of the first edition of *Science and Health*, Warren Felt Evans was already saying that disease originates in a false belief, and that it can be cured by changing this belief (*The mental Cure*, 1869 ; *Mental Medicine*, 1872). Julius A. Dresser developed the same ideas in *The True History of mental Science*, 1887 ; and Henry Wood in *New Thought Simplified*, 1903. These writings gave birth to the New Thought movement and its numerous varieties. The idea underlying them all is that a stronger mind can aid a weaker mind to overcome bad ways of thinking. Plato said long ago (the phrase is chosen as the motto for Parker's *Psychotherapy*) : " This is the great error of our day in the treatment of the human body, that physicians separate the soul from the body." New Thought teaching was much more reasonable than that of Christian Science. Its exponents did not merely admit the reality of the body ; but, going further, they agreed that the body was as important in its own place as the mind. The body must be regulated, and turned to good account ; its existence must not be denied. These teachings left room for rational hygiene and for indispensable surgical procedures. Provisionally, the use of a few drugs might be tolerated. Of course such physical measures were mere accessories. The essential feature of New Thought treatment was, and is, nothing more than moral exhortation.

Among the exponents of the method, some of the bolder spirits hold views very like those of Mrs. Eddy. That was

[1] Woodbridge Riley, Mental Healing in America, " American Journal of Insanity," January 1910.

why, in the last chapter, I mentioned Leander Edmund Whipple among the imitators of Christian Science. But others, such as P. M. Heubner, R. J. Ebbard, X. Lamotte Sage, William Walker Atkinson, and V. Turnbull, hold well-defined and practical ideas. It seems to me expedient, however, to distinguish the methods of these authors from Dubois' rational persuasion or general moralisation, and to study them later, in the chapter on Treatment by Excitation. The whole of the New Thought movement, deriving from Quimby's treatment, is an interesting one.

Of late years this form of psychotherapeutics has had a great vogue in the United States, thanks to an alliance between medicine and the church.[1] " Mrs. Eddy has awakened clergyman and doctor from inertia and dogmatic sleep." The amazing development of Christian Science alarmed the churches by robbing them of their flocks, and touched the pockets of the regular medical practitioners by taking away their patients. The fear of the common enemy brought about an unexpected alliance.

In October 1906, Elwood Worcester and Samuel McComb, rectors of the Emmanuel Episcopal Church of Boston, in collaboration with certain medical practitioners, founded the Emmanuel Church Health Class for the treatment of nervous disorders. This Emmanuel Movement must not be confused with the doings of the Society of Emmanuel founded in London during October 1905, for the last-named body works upon entirely different principles, and its practice belongs rather to the domain of miraculous methods of treatment.[2] The original feature of the Boston Emmanuel Movement is that the treatment of the sick by priests in temples has for the first time ceased to be conducted upon a footing of hostility towards treatment conducted by regular medical practitioners. The Emmanuel Movement takes the form of an association of clergymen and doctors. This characteristic is plainly indicated in the rules, drawn up by a committee which included four doctors among its members. These rules were published in the " Boston Transcript " on January 28, 1909. [Retranslated from the French.] " No one can be treated without a pre-

---

[1] Cf. Goddard, " American Journal of Psychology," 1898, p. 449 ; Max Eastman, The new Art of Healing, " The Atlantic Monthly," 1908, i, p. 645
[2] Cf. Parker's Psychotherapy, I, ii, 88, The Society of Emmanuel.

liminary examination by the family doctor, whose report
must be appended to that of the minister of religion. . . .
A patient who has no medical adviser must consult one and
must be under medical guidance before he can receive instruction at the Emmanuel Church. The only patients acceptable
for treatment at the Emmanuel Church are those suffering
from maladies arising out of the abuse of alcoholic stimulants,
or from hysterical, neurasthenic, or other neuroses." [1] Speaking generally, the Boston doctors supported the Emmanuel
Movement. Not only were they willing to examine the
patients who applied for treatment to the clergy, but they even
sent on some of their own patients to the church. Some of
them took part in the discussions at the religious gatherings.
J. J. Putnam, a specialist in nervous diseases and a professor
in Harvard University, delivered from the pulpit lectures
designed to give the sick advice that should be simultaneously
medical and moral.

A movement thus supported could hardly fail to spread.
From the Emmanuel Church at Boston it spread to churches
in Chicago, Rochester, Cambridge, Northampton, Waltham,
Newark, Detroit, Buffalo, Brooklyn, Jersey City, etc. Soon,
courses of lectures on medical moralisation were being given
in Philadelphia ; then in two leading churches of New York ;
then in Portland. Crossing the seas, the movement made its
way to Japan, South Africa, and Australia. It was not confined to Episcopal churches. Treatment by these methods
and under like auspices was carried on in Baptist, Unitarian,
and Presbyterian churches. It was tacitly approved by the
Roman Catholics, even though it may not have been practised
in Catholic churches.[2]

Parker's *Psychotherapy*, published at New York in 1908–
1909, as " a course of reading in sound psychology, sound
medicine, and sound religion," is a symposium, both churchmen and doctors being numbered among the contributors.
The book gives literary expression to the moralising enterprise
jointly undertaken by doctors and the clergy. Among the
articles written from the religious standpoint, there are several
historical studies dealing with spiritual methods of treatment in the days of classical antiquity and as described in the

[1] Cf. Richard C. Cabot, The American Type of Psychotherapy, in Parker's
Psychotherapy, I, i, 5.   [2] Parker's Psychotherapy, I, i, 15.

New Testament. There are also accounts of the development of the Emmanuel Classes in various parishes. The Rev. Herbert M. Hopkins dilates upon the changes wrought in certain small parishes. He assures us that the whole spirit of the congregation was modified ; there was less touchiness and a notable increase in cheerfulness. The Rev. Charles A. Place and the Rev. Lyman P. Powell described their treatment of the sick every evening in the church, recounting their attempts to free their patients' minds from grief and to bring calm to troubled spirits. They think that this new development will be helpful to the church and will give it a new life. Among the medical contributions to Parker's *Psychotherapy*, three may be specially mentioned : articles by Dubois, containing an exposition of the teachings with which we are already familiar ; J. J. Putnam's noteworthy studies in medical philosophy ; and Richard C. Cabot's researches, which are of a more practical order. Another symposium to be mentioned in this connexion is that by Morton Prince and others, entitled *Psychotherapeutics* (1910). A particularly interesting contribution to this volume is the article by E. W. Taylor, *Simple Explanation and Reeducation as a therapeutic Method.*

In these various writings we can study the characteristic features of the therapeutic method we are now considering. First of all we may note a persistent endeavour to avoid the exaggerations and the narrowness which make Christian Science absurd. Respect for scientific medicine is continually proclaimed. Nothing must be done without medical approval. In all the towns where the movement flourishes, the collaboration of the local medical practitioners is invited. " The sick body is also real. As Kant declares, a dream which all men dream together and which they cannot help dreaming, is no longer a dream but a reality. The Emmanuel Church must not reject what is good in medicine." [1] The treatment must be eclectic. It must have room for all the doctrines " which aim at relieving the sick by mental, moral, or spiritual methods ; it must work in harmony with all those who study nervous diseases or psychology, and must embrace within its unity all psychological methods of treatment." It is necessary to include educational science as well as psychology within the scope of

[1] Samuel McComb, " Boston Weekly Transcript," February 1907.

our studies, for pedagogy has a marked bearing on therapeutics. Cabot refers in this connexion to William James' little book *Talks to Teachers on Psychology and to Students on some of Life's Ideals*, and to the same author's studies concerning the formation of habits, for the doctor's task is in many cases to bring about the replacement of bad habits by good ones.[1] Attention may also be drawn to the fact that the Emmanuel Movement is interested in social studies, in researches concerning criminal tendencies, idleness, vagabondage, work shyness and the like. The captains of industry and the leaders of sports are invited to collaborate, no less than army officers.[2] I think that in all the points I have been enumerating, this psychotherapeutic method differs a little from Dubois' system of moralisation. It is more catholic in its scope, relying more than Dubois relies upon ordinary medical methods and on psychology.

The main differences will be found in the principles and in the general theories, for as far as practice is concerned the new method closely resembles the one expounded in Dubois' book. We have the same " conversations with the patient " in which a vigorous attempt is made to explain everything fully.[3] Lewellys F. Barker puts the matter very well when he says : " We must give plenty of time to each patient, and must win his confidence. We shall do little good by bluntly saying to him : ' There is nothing the matter with you ; get on with your work.' "[4] In these conversations, the disease must always be carefully explained to the patient, and we must cure him of the idea that he is the victim of some uncanny influence.

In order to dispel the patient's absurd and hypochondriacal notions, we are to fill his mind with grand and noble thoughts, and are to work for his moral uplifting. No one has more aptly insisted upon the practical importance of such lofty ideas than J. J. Putnam, who has dealt with the matter both in his lectures at the Lowell Institute (1906), and in his contributions to Parker's *Psychotheraphy*. "Hitch your wagon to a

---

[1] Parker's Psychotherapy, II, i, 27.
[2] Cf. Cabot, Whose Business is Psychotherapy ?, Parker's Psychotherapy, III, iv, 5.
[3] F. K. Hallock, The Methods of Education and Simple Conversation in Psychotherapy, Parker's Psychotherapy, II, iv, 5.
[4] Barker, On the psychic Treatment of some of the functional Neuroses, 1906, p. 8.

star," said Emerson. "Those who know how to do this can free themselves from many of the maladies of body and mind. . . . The important thing is that we should be able to take interest in a great many things, and that we should know how to feel enthusiasm. . . . Every one ought to have a philosophy. . . . Most people are inclined to regard philosophy and metaphysics as unpractical and unprofitable studies. In reality they form a splendid road along which the intelligent can travel into the world of beauty, order, and reality." Consider, too, Hallock's saying : " We must fully realise the value of optimism, and must never forget that pessimism is but another name for fear."

The patient cannot make his way into these "templa serena " all in a moment. We must help him along the road. " We must help a man to rise when he has fallen and is disheartened. . . . We must be at hand in all the great crises of his life. We must not let him brood over disagreeables or over aches and pains ; nor must we let him concentrate his attention unduly upon personal matters, friendships, love affairs, household concerns." These thoughts, which continually recur throughout the three large tomes of Parker's *Psychotherapy*, are certainly much like the ideas of Dubois, and the various authors are quite ready to quote Dubois' authority.

But a special characteristic of this American school is that religious exercises play so large a part in the medical treatment. "Weekly services, religious meetings, prayers, the singing of hymns ; these are of great value." . . . "The highest form of the religious act is to pray, no longer for God's gifts, but for his presence itself. And this very prayer is a potent force in transforming the inner man." [1] William James had already insisted upon the view that religious faith provided the best treatment for nervous disorders. He said that the religious minded expected their church to play the first part in curing them ; and that religious faith could not only cure nervous disorders, but could put an end to selfishness and avert domestic tragedies. Thus the American schools of psychological healing, supplementing medical and psychological studies in the strict sense of the term by religious

[1] The Rev. Dickinson S. Miller, What Religion has to do with Psychotherapy, Parker's Psychotherapy, I, iii, 42.

practices, have amplified the notion of the treatment of disease by moralisation. That is what gives these schools their special place in the history of psychotherapeutics.

3. PRINCIPLES UNDERLYING THERAPEUTIC MORALISATION.

These different attempts in the line of moral therapeutics must be regarded with respect and sympathy. The pioneers of the movement have considerable scientific and moral endowments ; they have undertaken a very difficult task in a disinterested spirit, and animated by a profound conviction ; and they have effected a notable advance in psychotherapeutics. Still, for the very sake of the studies to which they have devoted themselves, criticism is essential. We shall first examine the principles on which this therapeutic method appears to be based, and then consider the practical results that have been achieved.

We have seen how psychotherapeutics gradually emerged, as it were, out of the analysis and interpretation of miracles. The Christian Scientists were already well aware of the essential character of the mysterious force which the primitive miraculous healers and their patients used all unwitting. Dubois and those of his school are still better acquainted than the Christian Scientists with the moral character of this force, and they impress an understanding of its nature on their patients. Whereas Mrs. Eddy's patients do not understand a word of her metaphysics, and conceive that a miraculous power is at work, those of Dubois cannot make the same mistake, for their doctor gives them a clear explanation of the forces he is setting in motion.

The advance in the interpretation of miracles is shown, first of all, in the choice of patients. Mrs. Eddy applied her treatment to all comers, making absolutely no distinction between one case and another. This uniformity of application is one of the most obvious flaws of Christian Science. The exponents of medical moralisation have achieved a better analysis of the effect of miraculous methods of treatment. Studying what happened at wonder-working shrines, and in the practice of animal magnetisers, they noticed that certain classes of patients were cured more readily than others. Observation showed that it was futile to bring to the shrine the kind of patients in whose cure the god had no interest. Since the forces at the disposal of the medical moralisers were akin to those which effect miraculous cures, they must be applied to favourable subjects; Mrs. Eddy's " metaphysical obstetrics " must be rejected, and no attempt must be made to treat fractures by moralisation. The concept of the neuroses and of the psychoneuroses seems to furnish an accurate definition of the category of diseases suitable for medical moralisation, and herein we can see a notable advance in psychotherapeutics.

A further advance is shown in the choice of the ideas which are to have a curative influence. Mrs. Eddy, in her search for a potent thought, found it necessary to appeal to the thought of truth, being guided here by the traditional association between knowledge and power, between a true doctrine and a fruitful doctrine. She imagined that the mere knowledge of metaphysical truth, thought concerning the essence of things, would suffice to cure all our petty ills. The moraliser's conception of the effective thought is simultaneously wider and more precise. The potent thought is not merely a true thought; it is also a good thought, moral weal being super-added to truth. We discern here a sort of confident optimism. A man who knows the truth and a man who acts morally is a perfect man; he cannot be a weakling or an invalid. More-over, the moraliser's notion of truth is far more precise than Mrs. Eddy's. He no longer speaks of metaphysical or scientific truth left undefined; he is concerned with a particular truth which has a definite bearing on the cure of the disease. The patient need only know the truth about the functions of his body, about the origin and mechanism of the troubles from which he is actually suffering. We all know that the patient's own idea concerning his illness has a considerable influence on its course; it will therefore be well that he should know the true meaning of his symptoms. This especially applies to neuropathic symptoms determined by thought, and commonly regarded as much less serious than symptoms arising out of organic lesions. The part played by moral ideas has also become far more definite. The main desire of the medical moraliser is to make his patient perform real actions, lofty and noble actions which will require attention and effort, thus developing will power and moral energy. There is, therefore, far more clarity and simplicity about the teaching of Dubois and his school. Treatment by the general moralisation of the patient presents itself as the last stage of the evolution which began with the analysis of miracles. It is easy to understand why medical moralisation has had a considerable vogue, and why in many countries it is still regarded as the best way of treating neuroses.

Nevertheless, this method, especially as expounded by Dubois, has been sharply criticised, as, for instance, by de Fleury, J. Bonjour [1] of Lausanne, and Sollier.[2] The last-named writes vivaciously on the topic : " The light now comes to us from Switzerland. Hitherto the essentials of the treatment of nervous diseases in Switzerland have consisted of altitude, which we know to have a bad influence ; fresh air, which can be had anywhere ; the view of blue lakes, white peaks, and green pastures, with a Kursaal close at hand; elaborate baths and sometimes douches in a hotel masquerading as a sanatorium. Now there have been added macaroni and nouilles, which can only be had to perfection in Lausanne, and philosophical discourses which are a specialty of Berne and to which the patient listens while lying in bed and swilling milk. But there are peevish folk who declare that they can do better for themselves without so long a journey."

The critics reproach the moralisers with ignoring the history of medicine, and with " discovering " old-world therapeutic methods ; they are unwilling to make any distinction between medical moralisation, miraculous healing, and Christian Science. There is no more than partial truth in such reproaches. While it is true that Dubois does not pay enough attention to historical developments, Camus and Pagniez have published valuable studies concerning the origin of psychotherapeutics. Moreover, Parker's *Psychotherapy* contains a number of noteworthy historical articles. As I have just been showing, therapeutic moralisation is distinguished in many ways both from miraculous healing and from the practice of Mrs. Eddy.

Graver criticisms must now be considered. A good many writers accuse the moralisers of ignoring, not merely medical history, but medical science. The moralisers, say these critics,

---

[1] Psychothérapie et Hypnotisme, " Revue de l'Hypnotisme," June 1906, p. 357.   [2] " Archives des Conférences de l'Internat," 1905, p. 5.

have a contempt for diagnosis, and their reports of cures cannot
be checked because there is no means of ascertaining the real
nature of the malady, or of learning what treatment was actually
employed. There is a good deal of truth in these allegations,
for the moralisers certainly lack precision upon the two points
in question.

We have seen that Dubois does not propose, like Mrs. Eddy,
to treat all comers. He selects what he regards as suitable
cases. But which cases does he choose, and what are the
grounds of choice? He tells us that he treats neuropaths,
for in their troubles psychological phenomena are a notable
determining factor. The answer does not help us. Since
man is a thinking being, psychological phenomena play their
part in almost all diseases, if it be only in the form of pain,
anxiety, or despair ; and it would be absurd to deny the importance of such phenomena in illness of every kind. In
Parker's *Psychotherapy* there is an interesting essay on the
part played by psychological phenomena in the development
of pulmonary tuberculosis, and the author recommends the
moralisation of consumptives. On the other hand, it is obvious
that mental disorders are the diseases in whose evolution psychological phenomena play the most notable part, and Dubois
does not propose to treat these by his method. In a recent
work of my own I have tried to show that the vagueness and
the worthlessness of the definition that neuroses are diseases
determined by psychological phenomena.[1]

In actual fact, the moralisers make very little use of the
foregoing definition, and their choice of patients is determined
for the most part by two purely negative characteristics. For
them, neuropaths are persons who have no organic lesions and
are free from mental disorder. Apart from the customary
defects of negative definitions, this definition is based upon
two vague and practically unintelligible concepts. I have
myself declared more than once that I am unable to understand what people mean when they speak of illnesses without lesions.[2] Just as there can be no normal functioning
without a transient organic change, and just as there cannot
be a good habit without a more or less durable modification
of the organism, so there cannot be disease without a change
in the organs, that is to say without a lesion. Our science

[1] Les névroses, 1909, p. 378.   [2] Ibid., p. 377.

may not enable us to detect this lesion to-day ; perhaps we shall be able to detect it to-morrow. This matters little. We may hope that the lesions are fugitive. But many of the diseases we term organic are likewise transient. The lesions of the nasal mucous membrane that accompany a cold in the head are transient, but we do not for that reason regard a cold as a neurosis. Nay more, this exclusion of diseases in which there are organic lesions involves the rejection of a very large number of illnesses in which psychotherapeutics might be advantageous. Let me instance chorea, migraine, and epilepsy, all of which are often classed among the neuroses. Nowadays, epilepsy is in very truth the " morbus sacer," for no one dares touch it. If a tenth part of the time and trouble devoted to the study of hysteria had been applied to the understanding of this strange malady, extremely important physiological and psychological discoveries would probably have been made. But epilepsy is suspected to be due to organic lesions, whereas hysteria is regarded as a purely " functional " disease. This has been enough to make medical psychologists fight shy of epilepsy, and to make the medical moralisers refuse to have anything to do with sufferers from this disease. " It is useless to concern ourselves about the epileptic," writes Dubois, " for he perpetually relapses into the fatalism of his morbid self-centredness."[1] So arbitrary a limitation of the field of psychotherapeutics is very remarkable. The day will assuredly dawn when there will be no more talk, in season and out of season, of the absence of lesions in the neuroses, for the phrase has neither meaning nor interest.

The neuropaths, as moralisers understand this term, are, then, the only patients for whom moralising treatment is suitable. But the cases selected for treatment are distinguished by a second negative characteristic. The patients have mental troubles, indeed, but they must be free from mental disorder as the alienist defines it. This radical distinction between neuropaths and the insane is not peculiar to the laity, for it is often made by medical practitioners. Not long ago, Dejerine published a remarkable lecture in which he claimed the whole galaxy of neuropathic patients for the neurological specialists, leaving the alienists out in the cold. Their only

[1] Les psychonévroses, p. 17.

concern was with raging maniacs. Ballet has good reason for making fun of this claim.

It certainly seems rather remarkable to withhold the advantage of psychotherapeutics from the very patients who need it most, from the very patients for whom treatment determined by psychological considerations would seem to be most appropriate. But, in my opinion, the whole controversy is subordinate to the decision of a more important problem. What is the true significance of such words as lunatic, mad, and insane ? These are not medical or scientific terms ; they are popular terms, and may even be said to smack of the police court. A lunatic is an individual who is a danger to others or to himself, and is not legally responsible for his actions. This definition is not based upon the sufferer's intrinsic characters, or upon this or that definite change in his psychophysiological functions, but upon an extrinsic character arising out of the situation of the patient. It is impossible to contend that in this or that trouble defined by medical science the patient is always harmless, while in this or that other he is always dangerous to himself or others. Certain melancholics, general paralytics, and dements are quite harmless, and ought not to be spoken of as lunatics in the legal sense of the term ; certain psychasthenics with uncontrollable impulses are dangerous, and must be classified as insane. The danger to be apprehended from a patient depends far more upon his social surroundings than upon the nature of his psychological troubles. If he is rich, if he does not need to work for his living, if he is surrounded by careful watchers, if he lives in the country, if his environment is uncomplicated, he may have very serious mental disorder without being a danger to himself or any one else, and his doctor may euphemistically describe him as a " neurasthenic." If he is poor, if he is a wage earner, if he lives unguarded and in a large town, if his position is one that presents delicate or complicated issues, the very same mental disorders, at the same level of intensity, will make him dangerous, and his doctor will have no choice but to have him certified as a lunatic and put under restraint. Now this is a practical distinction, a matter which concerns public order, but has no bearing upon the outlooks of scientific medicine. The diagnosis is just the same in either case. The prognosis is unaffected, except in so far as the patients put under restraint are apt to get well sooner than those allowed to remain at large. Since these things are so, what right have we to use the word " non-insane " to distinguish the neuropaths in whom psychotherapeutic methods can be applied with a fair prospect of success, while we refuse to practise psychotherapy upon those to whom the qualifying term " non-insane " seems inapplicable ? I cannot but feel that Dubois' use of the word lunatic, and similar expressions, is arbitrary. For him, a patient whom he is unable to cure is insane ; and that's that ! In Dejerine's psychotherapeutic wards, a patient who is bored to death behind the curtains which shut him off from the world, who proves intractable, and who tactlessly continues to insist that he is not cured, will also be christened " insane." Very simple, and very practical ! In this way the doctor is enabled to draw up admirable statistics of cures, but from the diagnostician's point of view it is difficult to take such distinctions seriously.

The conception of psychoneuroses, when it is based solely on these two negative characters, is hopelessly vague. The patients in whom moralising treatment is applied are chosen almost haphazard, After the choice, there is no accurate classification of the cases. Doctors who have to deal with organic disease do their best to make a prompt and accurate individual diagnosis, believing that successful treatment depends upon successful diagnosis. But the moralisers make no attempt to analyse with precision each pathological instance. They make no distinction between different symptoms, or between different neuroses. With almost incredible light-heartedness, all the cases are lumped together. " All the neuropaths are classed among psychoneurotics, the latter word being simply an additional epithet. Hypochondria, melancholia, hysteria, and neurasthenia are considered to be practically identical. Dubois' patients are suffering simultaneously from three or four diseases, unspecified." [1] This confusion is quite comprehensible, and there is no reason for an accurate analysis of the cases, for the treatment is always the same, whatever the patient's symptoms may be.

But when we consider more closely these methods of treatment which seem at first sight more definite and more logical

[1] Bonjour, " Revue de l'Hypnotisme," 1906, p. 330.

than Mrs. Eddy's system, we shall soon realise that they are
not very intelligible after all, and not very rational despite
their parade of rationality. I will say nothing about the
crude rejection of surgical operations and of drugs ; this is
obviously no more than an overstatement of the case, no more
than a question of degree and of circumstance. Besides, the
Emmanuel School in the United States is less intolerant
than Dubois in this respect. The heedless attacks on hypnotism
and suggestion need not be considered at this stage. Enough,
now, to deal with the essence of these methods. Both
with Dubois and with all the American practitioners of the
same school, the main idea is to instruct the patients and to
moralise them. The invalid is to be taught the philosophical
truth about the universe, and the medical truth about his own
illness ; his character is to be uplifted ; he is to be taught
how to behave finely, energetically, and nobly.

A splendid idea, but is the treatment really medical, and
shall we find that it will suffice to cure disease ? In former
days, few would have disputed the contention, for these ideas
derive from the exceedingly old conviction that illness is the
outcome of sin and error. In earlier phases of civilisation,
disease was regarded as a moral malady, because it rendered
the sufferer useless to society and dangerous by being a centre
of contagion. The invalid was knocked on the head or driven
out of the community. The notion is deep rooted and
persistent, and we still find it difficult to free ourselves from
a sentiment of repulsion for hateful diseases. Nevertheless, as
time passed, a gentler mood prevailed. The sick were looked
upon as blameworthy to a moderate degree only, like those
who make mistakes through inattention or because they lack
education. Illness has become a form of error. This idea
dominates Christian Science. When the founder of the faith
died of the bronchopneumonia to which very old persons often
succumb, the Scientist newspapers wrote with perfect seriousness
that Mrs. Eddy " has been ten days in error." Dubois would
seem to have remained at the same level of mental development, for he is continually talking about error, and he treats
his patients as if they were simply in a state of sin and error.

I shall not stop to discuss this juxtaposition of illness with
sin. Our present notions concerning responsibility and liberty
(ideas underlying our conception of moral action) forbid us

to confound a disease with a fault. Even when the illness follows the commission of a sin, we regard the sequence as accidental. If a man becomes infected with syphilis, this is not because he has misconducted himself, but because he has been unlucky in the choice of partner. A friend of his who misconducts himself in precisely the same way will escape infection—obviously because he has been more fortunate in his choice.

The idea of " error " is a vaguer one than that of " sin," for the word error connotes the thought of a more or less mechanical intellectual operation for which we are not responsible, though it also connotes the thought of an act of will and attention. You are not entitled to say I am in error unless you consider that I might have thought differently ; unless you are prepared to assert that I might have arrived at a different conviction by more careful attention in the opening phases of my reasoning, and that I shall be able to modify this conviction by talking matters over with you. It is an abuse of terms when we say that an idiot or a dement makes a mistake. By an illusion, we are putting ourselves in his place, for we know that if we had acted as he has done we should have been in error. But as regards diseases, do we still contend that they are simply the outcome of intellectual voluntary actions, or that they are due to a lack of attention which might have been remedied by the power of the will ? As far as organic disease is concerned, such a belief belongs to the past ; and we may leave to Mrs. Eddy the proud privilege of being in error when she is dying of bronchopneumonia. But when we have to do with maladies about which we still know little, with the neuroses in which psychological symptoms make their appearance, we are instinctively inclined to be influenced by the old tradition. We still venture to say that a woman affected with hysterical paraplegia is mistaken when she believes herself to be paralysed, seeing that we know her motor functions to be in perfect order. In more enlightened days than our own, this will be regarded as a misstatement no less gross than the misstatement about Mrs. Eddy's bronchopneumonia. What is paralysed in the hysterical patient is a real constituent of the motor function, the personal and conscious element of that function ; and the patient is not mistaken, is not " in error," when she declares that she cannot move her legs. Errors and faults may have been committed at the outset of the illness, but different mechanisms have got to work since then. To-day, the patient's medical adviser has no right to say that he is confronted solely with an error.

If there were really an error, it would not be necessary to treat the patient medically, and psychotherapy would be useless. I have missed my way, you point out the right road, and that is an end to the matter. Your function is to instruct, to advise. You do not " treat " me. A man falls sick because he sleeps with doors and windows shut in a room heated by a stove which draws badly. The doctor explains what is amiss, and the patient answers : " All right, I'll let the stove go out and will open the window." Is that psychotherapeutic medication ? A girl cuts down her food unduly, believing that this will be good for her health. If she is merely making a mistake, it will be enough to explain to her that a person of her stature needs more calories. She will modify her diet accordingly, and will have no need to visit Dubois' sanatorium. Your rejoinder is obvious. " She will not believe you ; or even if she does believe you in the main, she has not the will power that will enable her to follow your advice." I am well aware of the fact. This is the crux. She is incapable of understanding certain things, and incapable of willing to act on her knowledge when she has understood. That is her malady ; not an error, but something quite different. The proper treatment consists of something more than a mere physiological demonstration, something more than good advice ; the demonstration and the advice have to be given in a particular way, which is not Dubois' way. The essence of the treatment lies in the way the advice is given, and here we are in a very different domain from that of the pure and simple inculcation of the truth.

Having recalled these elementary ideas, we are now in a position to understand better what elements of exaggeration and irrationality there are in the principles of moralisation. Dubois, after putting the patient into a sanatorium and after enforcing a pure milk diet for a week (this dietetic regimen being certainly a concession to the familiar methods of disintoxication), tries in his conversations to explain to the invalid the medical truth concerning the illness. But why ? Are we sure that the patient cannot get well without knowing the truth about the mechanism of the disease from which he is suffering? Surely there is no lack of persons who have recovered from measles or typhoid without understanding anything at all about the matter! " But it is different in the case of mental troubles, for in these the patient's ideas about the illness affects the course of the illness." The generalisation is absolutely unsound. A highly skilled pyschiatrist may become affected with mental depression or with fixed ideas. He will not recover more speedily than one who is ignorant of the mechanism of these disorders. Many sufferers from melancholia have got perfectly well after two or three months without any understanding of the nature of their mental trouble. " At any rate you must admit that patients are reassured as soon as they know that their troubles are purely moral, and that they have no organic lesions; this knowledge cannot fail to help them." It is far from certain that reasoning of this sort will reassure the patient. A great many patients are terrified at the idea that they have mental disorders, and would much rather feel convinced that the root of their troubles is physical. Besides, the proof of moral causation may be far to seek.

Here, in fact, we encounter the cardinal difficulty of moralisation. The doctor wants to cure his patients by teaching them the truth about their illness—but what is the truth? Quimby used to tell his patients : " The truth is my system." With Mrs. Eddy the phrase ran : " The truth is health." Dubois concludes his explanations of neurasthenia by saying to the patient : " The truth is what I tell you." Yet it seems most improbable that these three truths are precisely the same. They have, indeed, a common element, the claim to cure; but treatment will become a difficult matter if we must first of all be in possession of indisputable and definitive proof. Dubois asserts that the exhaustion from which psychasthenics suffer depends wholly upon " the idea of fatigue," and that there is no real underlying exhaustion. I venture to doubt. Dubois convinces a young woman suffering from paralysis that the sole cause of her trouble is an idea. I know that it is the fashion to-day to contend that a hysterical woman is ill because she has a fancy to be ill, or because her doctor has put the fancy into her mind. Such pathology is extremely simple, but is it a true statement of the matter ? A good many people share my doubts. I could multiply the instances. There is not a single one of Dubois' psychological explanations which is not open to objection ; not one which a well-informed patient could not contradict.

The truth you are serving up to the patient is hypothetical and fugitive. Perhaps you will convince him in the long run, for he is ignorant, and a doctor can make his patients swallow anything ; but you have no right to say that you are curing by administering the truth. Monsieur Dubois you are deceiving your patient, and I am outraged, just as you were outraged at my use of suggestion. Dubois will answer that he may be mistaken, but that he says nothing which he does not believe to be the truth ; he is perfectly sincere, and that is the essential point. It may be essential if we are mainly concerned with Dubois' moral integrity. Is it essential if we are mainly concerned with the patient's interest ? What does the absolute sincèrity of the doctor matter to the patient, save in the most exceptional cases ? If the doctor is an ignoramus, he may be as sincere as you please, but he is not the doctor for me. I would rather put myself in the hands of one who will tell me what will do me good. That is why I am far from convinced of the rationality of this incessant explanation, in all cases ; of this perpetual presentation of a medical hypothesis to our patients.

Moreover, Dubois and his congeners are not satisfied with inculcating what they allege to be medical truth. They are eager to expound more important truths ; they give the patient lectures on general philosophy, teach him a whole system. They talk of freedom of the will, which seems to me a very obscure topic. Human freedom, they tell the patient, is a particular kind of determinism. Freedom is determinism by ideas, a rational determinism, in contra-distinction to mechanical determinism. The lofty notions of the True, the Beautiful, and the Good, play a great part in human life ; they guide our will, and in thus guiding it they emancipate it from the tyranny of the passions and advance it to a higher degree of perfectionment, which consists of disinterested and noble activity ; and so on, and so on. We all know this philosophy. There is a strain of Leibnitz in it, with a dash of Victor Cousin ; and it has been admirably expounded by Paul Janet. It is the philosophy which presided over our childhood, which we passed on to others for years ; and it still reigns supreme in manuals for students of moral philosophy. Far be it from me to decry it. I am convinced that in due time justice will be done to Paul Janet for his excellent presentation of it. But do all these medical philosophers really believe it to be ultimate truth, or even the philosophical truth of our own day ? Why should this philosophy, which already is beginning to have a musty flavour, suffice to give calm and happiness to all minds ? Long ago, in glorious verse, Lucretius expounded Epicurus' materialism as the supreme consolation for those who were uneasy in mind and sore at heart. One philosophy after another has made a similar claim, and why should this particular one be chosen as a panacea ? Why should you disturb the religious convictions of one patient or the contented materialism of another ? Are you quite certain that your approved manual will give him more faith and hope ?

To continue ; the moralisers tell us that convictions count for nothing without actions. What we need to reform is the patient's behaviour as a whole. The patient must be taught how to lead a worthy life, by inculcating a sort of stoicism mitigated by Christian charity. His will must be transformed. " Suggestion has, it is true, certain limited effects, and can dispel morbid symptoms. But it cannot make the subject perform Actions in the full sense of the term, actions in which his whole physical and moral being takes part. It cannot regulate a life, a form, a character. . . . Persuasion, on the other hand, making its appeal to the higher mental functions, can have such an effect." [1] This profound change in morality will indirectly lead to the relief of all the troubles ; for obviously when the will has attained so lofty a level, no more weaknesses can be tolerated. The cure will be complete, for, by transforming the individual we shall have rendered the existence of the disease impossible.

All this is magnificent from the theoretical outlook ; but when I turn to practice, doubts arise. I do not dispute that it would be an excellent thing to transform a timid idler into a bold worker, an egoist into an altruist ; I do not deny that such a transformation ought to have an excellent effect upon

[1] Camus et Pagniez, op. cit., p. 176.

the morbid symptoms. But such a transformation cannot always be brought about ; and fortunately, it is not always indispensable. Is it what the patient wants of us when he comes to us complaining of neuralgia, sleeplessness, or stomachache ? We are only doctors. Have we time to play the moraliser's part, and are we competent ? Most of our patients are poor devils whose morale is below par ; and who, if they are to become heroes and saints, must be given another kind of life, another occupation, a new environment, better luck in money matters. Above all, in most cases, their shoulders must be freed from the burden of heredity. Of course the doctor must help them in all these ways, as far as may be ; but he must not expect the impossible of his patients, and he must relieve their immediate distresses before asking them to undertake costly reforms. Even if the patient should remain a weakling, incapable of doing " Actions in the full sense of the term," he will thank us for curing his limp or his sick stomach. If, later, he has to reform himself and to become a hero, he will do this all the easier because he no longer limps or vomits. If you ask too much, you may repel your patient and get no results at all. I once had a confidential talk with a young woman who had passed some time in the Berne sanatorium, and who, strange to tell, came away without having been cured. Her report of the conversations, I may say the disputes, between herself and the physician was amusing. " ' Mademoiselle,' said the doctor to me, ' all your nervous troubles, all your sufferings, are the outcome of your bad disposition. What you need most of all is a change of heart ; you must turn it, like an omelette in a frying pan.'—' There is nothing I should like better,' I answered. ' But it is not my fault that I do not know how to turn myself. You must turn my omelette for me.'—Since the doctor did not manage to do this, I came away just as ill as I had been when I first went to the sanatorium."

One of my own hospital patients was a hysterical street walker from the poorer quarter of Paris. She was addicted to drink, and was in a very bad way indeed. After a quarrel and an assault, she became affected with hysterical contracture of the shoulder, so that she was unable to move the right arm. The trouble was cured in half an hour by massage and suggestion, and she returned to her customary occupation.

Three years later I heard that there had been no relapse. No doubt I was very much to blame. I ought not to have paid any attention to the contracture, which would have disappeared in due course thanks to the general advance of the patient's freedom of will. My part should have been to achieve the moral reform of this sinner, teach her how to Act, and how to give her life an exalted and noble aim. Of course I might put in a plea or two for the defence ; might say that the conversion would probably have been a long job, that time pressed, that other patients were awaiting their turn, that it was not my trade to be a moral reformer, that I was loath to let the contracture drag on ; but I will not dwell on these considerations. I know that the moralisers will pronounce an anathema on me, but I hope that some of my medical colleagues will absolve me.

The foregoing remarks apply to the other methods of moralising treatment as well as to Dubois' practice, but the Emmanuel Movement in the United States has peculiar characteristics which demand a special examination. The founders of this therapeutic organisation have thought well to associate clergymen with doctors in the treatment of nervous diseases ; or, to put the matter more accurately, having had the neurosis diagnosed by a medical practitioner, they consign the patient to a clergyman for treatment. Their view is that moral influence will be reinforced by religious influence, and that this will facilitate the cure ; they also hold that the prestige of religion will be augmented by its therapeutic renown. Very pretty theories these, at first sight, and yet I have never been able to free myself from a sense of uneasiness. I could not but wonder at the ostensibly unanimous approval of the Boston doctors. But I have recently had the advantage of reading a remarkable protest, voiced by Münsterberg (of Boston) in his *Psychotherapy*, published in 1909. I am in full accord with the arguments expounded in the twelfth chapter of that work, entitled " Psychotherapy and the Church." In especial I would refer the reader to p. 319.

The collaboration between medicine and the church is a relic of the ancient superstition according to which the neuropath is " in error," is blameworthy. The practitioners of the Emmanuel Movement call in the doctor to begin with, just for safety, to give the treatment a scientific aspect, to make sure that the patient is suffering from a neurosis and not (let us say) a brain tumour. Then the patient is taken out of the hands of a doctor who would treat him medically, and entrusted to the care of a priest who instructs and corrects him. To me this seems most undesirable, whether from the medical or from the religious outlook. The treatment of disease is not simply a matter of preliminary diagnosis; it demands the continued study of symptoms, and of the changes they undergo. To say once for all that the illness is not an organic trouble but a neurosis, does not suffice. We want to know the nature of the neurosis, the form it exhibits at this moment or that, the part played by antecedent tendencies, the influence of various happenings in the life of the patient; and these factors must be subjected to persistent medical observation and interpretation. Continually we have to intervene, not by sermons, but by therapeutic action, whether material or moral.

Religious emotion, to which the champions of the Emmanuel Movement appeal, is indubitably a potent remedy : but it is so at certain moments and not always, in certain cases but not in all. Besides the dosage must be carefully regulated, for it belongs to " that category of medicines of which five grains will cure while fifty grains will kill." The priest plays his natural part when he tries to promote religious influences to the uttermost; we cannot ask him to restrict the amount of faith he inspires in his patients, or to be niggard in the dosage of religious sentiment. It is likely enough, therefore, that, in many instances, a craze of over-scrupulousness or some mystical frenzy will be superadded to the primary neurosis. If the priest suspects such complications to be imminent, and if, in his therapeutic zeal, he wishes to safeguard the patient from these dangers attendant upon religious ecstasy, he will have to abandon his proper functions as priest and to seek for other methods of treatment. He will then become an irregular practitioner of medicine, and this is a most undesirable development.

In their first enthusiasm, the adepts of the Emmanuel Movement believed that it was destined to breathe new life into the churches. This seems to me unlikely. "Among primitive folk, the priests were also magicians and doctors;

among the Australian blacks the koonkies,[1] and among the Siberian tribes the shamans, are healers to this day." " In every niche of the Catholic churches in all Europe there are kneeling before the burning candles those who pray for nothing but their health." [2] Is it really advantageous to religion that it should retrace its steps in this way, and should encourage such proceedings ? Are we to regard it as the true role of modern religion to become a remedy for disorders of the stomach and imaginary visceral pains ? The advocates of the method may agree that it is not an exalted one, but they will contend that at any rate it will promote religious faith. There is a misunderstanding in the contention. When the doctor invokes the aid of religious faith for the cure of a neurosis, his outlook on the religious sentiment is purely psychological : he thinks that faith may cure the illness, but he does not care a rap whether the faith be in Jupiter, Odin, or Jehovah ; and when he sends the patient to a temple, he does not (as doctor) himself believe in the power of the god in whose honour the temple was built. Is it proper that a priest should adopt a similar outlook ; should try to achieve a cure by arousing the patient's religious sentiment, without himself attributing to the god any effective share in the cure ? If, as will be natural enough, the priest believes that his god has a share in the cure quite apart from the purely human influence of the religious sentiment, why should he restrict himself to the treatment of neuroses, and why should he not try to work a real miracle such as the cure of a cancer ? The doctor who forbids him to do this is robbing the priest of his truly religious function, and is discrediting religion. The doctor and the priest join hands in the work without understanding one another ; each is humbugging the other, and I do not think that true religion will gain much by the comedy.

I fancy it would be better, would be both more dignified and more useful, if each were to keep within his own sphere, and if doctor and priest were to render one another reciprocal service. When the doctor thinks that religious instruction is indicated, let him send the patient to the priest, who can speak of religion as a priest without intruding into the domain of medicine. When the doctor thinks that enough religious instruction has been given, and that more might become

---

[1] Münsterberg, op. cit., p. 320.   [2] Ibid., p. 327.

dangerous, he can withdraw his patient. The priest will not have to bother about dosage, or to nip faith in the bud. If the religious instruction fails to cure the patient, neither the priest nor the religion can be blamed for this, seeing that the doctor is responsible. It is on these terms that I have myself often invoked the aid of Catholic priests or Protestant pastors. I have always been able to congratulate myself on their collaboration, and they have never had to regret the assumption of a false role. I must admit that I am not hopeful about the future of an intimate association between medicine and religion. I am inclined to put more trust in the old French proverb : " A chacun son métier et les malades seront bien gardés." [1]

I am extremely sorry to have been constrained to utter these words of criticism. Treatment by moralisation is a notable medical achievement ; the method will form part of the permanent foundations of the psychological therapeutics of a coming day ; but it was essential to show that its principles and teachings are still far too vague and ill defined.

4. PRACTICAL VALUE OF MORALISING METHODS OF TREATMENT.

I do not lay much stress upon my theoretical criticism of the medical and philosophical principles underlying treatment by medical moralisation. The essential problem lies elsewhere. The only question of real importance to the practising physician is this : Does the method in question give, in general, good results ?

At the first glance this question may seem an easy one to answer. The phenomena occur in the open. We no longer have to do with such rudimentary diagnoses as those of the Christian Scientists. If we ask Dubois to give us fuller particulars about one of the cases he reports, he is not likely to begin a discourse about Jonah in the whale's belly. Some of those who practise medical moralisation publish statistics which seem instructive. Thus Dr. Worcester writes : " One hundred and seventy-eight cases were treated in an American church between March and November 1907. In fifty-five of these, the result was vague, or was not reported ; in forty-eight, no good effect was noted ; seventy-five of the patients

[1] Let every one stick to his own trade and the sick will be well cared for.

were cured or greatly improved." Dejerine reports in 1910 :
" Among neurasthenics, putting aside those suffering from
algias (whose treatment is difficult), we get 100 per cent. of
cures. Relapse is rare, being noted only in 5 per cent. of the
cases." These statements seem plain and precise, so there
ought to be no difficulty in forming an opinion as to the value
of the method.

Unfortunately, real precision is lacking. I do not think
that trustworthy statistics can be drawn up ; I do not think
that we can place any reliance whatever upon the statistics
that have been published. Neither the total number of
patients treated nor the number of cures has a genuine significance. As regards the total number of patients, this would
only be a valuable datum if, while including all the patients
presenting themselves for treatment, we could be certain that
the diseases from which they were suffering belonged to a
scientifically defined category, and that the patients were not
arbitrarily chosen. Now, we are concerned with psychoneurotics, that is to say with patients in whom the nature of
the illness has not been strictly defined. As we have just seen,
this " psychoneurosis " is for Dubois and his followers a
vague concept. The patients are selected in accordance with
negative characteristics ; they are such as appear to be free
from organic lesions ; they must not be epileptics ; they
must not be lunatics. We can include or exclude whatever
we please when we have to do with a group thus vaguely
defined. In some of the clinics, when a patient who, to begin
with, was labelled neurasthenic, does not get better or fails
to listen patiently to the sermons, he is relabelled " lunatic,"
and his case no longer enters into the statistics. Furthermore,
as Sollier justly remarks, " the choice is not made only by the
doctor. The patients, likewise, have a say in the matter.
Those who voluntarily submit to a regime of isolation and
philosophical discussions must be favourably predisposed to
the treatment." [1] Substantially we may take it that the total
of patients in such statistics includes only the patients who
have been relieved or cured. That is why some of the moralisers
confidently announce 100 per cent. of cures.

Turning now to consider the cures, I may be a hardened
sceptic—but I am sceptical. Many of these patients declare

[1] Sollier, op. cit., pp. 11 and 15.

themselves cured because the sanatorium treatment is costly, and they do not want to go on paying for it ; because they are weary of the isolation, and want to regain their liberty ; because they have had enough of the doctor, or because they want to please him ; or simply because they have so great a desire to be cured that in the end they believe that they have been cured. Dubois will tell us that the last criticism counts for nothing ; that a neuropath who believes that he is cured is in fact cured, seeing that neurosis is only the idea of disease. People are fond of repeating such phrases, but in truth there are neuropaths who are not cured though they believe themselves cured. The members of the patient's family know the true state of affairs, and will say : " He thinks he is cured, but he is just as intolerable as before ; perhaps the way in which he makes himself intolerable is rather different, that is all." I know a woman who is very ill when she ceases to be aware of her fatigue and of her morbid state ; she is on the mend when she realises that she has been very bad and that she is still ailing. Let me add that when we are dealing with such patients we must never be in a hurry to decide that they are cured. We must wait for a time which is always rather long, though it varies in different cases, if we are to avoid being misled by one of the fluctuations that are so frequent in neu-rotics. In many instances there will be " relapses " which are in reality nothing more than an evolution of the primary disease.

You must be on your guard, likewise, against including among your cures the patients who are really cured, but in whom the cure has taken place because the time was ripe, quite independently of your moralising treatment. Nowadays, far too much play is certainly made with the concept of the " manic-depressive psychosis." It is none the less true that certain depressive states caused by fatigue or emotion seem to have a definite duration, after the lapse of which they undergo a spontaneous and inevitable cure. The lucky practitioner is the one who has been consulted shortly before the end of the crisis, but he will make a mistake if he allows such instances to swell his record of cures. In a word, the percentage of cures is difficult to ascertain, seeing that the " cure " is no less ill-defined than the " disease." Each author interprets cures as pleases him best, and will have a smaller or larger percentage according as he is modest or the reverse. In such circumstances, is it possible to draw accurate conclusions from these statistics ?

Happily, in these studies concerning the effects of moralisation we find something more than pretentious statistics ; we often find admirable medical and psychological observations. For the most part, medical science is still in the stage of individual observations, and the remark applies above all to psychiatry. A good description of a pathological type that has been well understood is worth more than a great many arbitrary theories and classifications. Both in Europe and in the United States the authors previously quoted have analysed numerous neuropathic troubles, and have shown clearly enough how these troubles can be modified by moral methods of treatment. Sollier (whose criticisms are in this respect pushed too far) maintains that the cures occur only in minor ailments, " in slight cases of hysterical anorexia, in overworked neurasthenics, in persons suffering from a moderate degree of phobia." I do not agree with this author. We can never foretell the gravity of a commencing neurosis ; and these careful observations disclose definite symptoms identical with those we have all seen in grave cases. If the neurosis runs a favourable course, we are often entitled to suppose that it has been mitigated by moralisation. Those interested will do well to study some of Dubois' observations in patients suffering from depression, astasia-abasia, contractures, various algias, phobias, obsessions, hypochondria—patients who seem to have gradually undergone a real transformation. The case recorded by Dubois on p. 448 seems all the more striking to me because I am so well acquainted with patients of this type, persons who are continually obsessed with the idea of fatigue, and agonised at the thought of the most trifling movement. I do not interpret these cases as Dubois interprets them ; but, like him, I have often tried to stir such patients into activity, and I know how difficult it is to do so. Dubois' results, therefore, seem to me remarkable.[1] Many similar cases are to be found in the writings of Dubois' French disciples, and in the works published in the United States by those who have taken part in the Emmanuel Movement. Though I criticise their theories, I value the

[1] Cf. Dubois, Un cas de phobie guéri par la psychothérapie, Société Suisse de Neurologie, Berne, March 1909.

practical results they have secured in many difficult cases. There can be no doubt that the skilful use of moralisation has saved a large number of patients from incurable disease and from mental alienation.

If we want to convince ourselves of the value of this method, we can look nearer home, and can reconsider the cases that have come under our personal observation. We shall then find that, intentionally or otherwise, we have often made use of this method of moralisation in the treatment of our own patients. We shall find that psychotherapeutists, when more definite treatment fails, make a practice of talking to the patient, of reassuring him by showing him that his illness is less serious than he had fancied and is not incurable, of encouraging him to seek distraction and to resume a more active life. We shall find that in a great many instances this treatment has had excellent results, better results than could be secured in any other way.

I find in my own case-books notes concerning seven young men (their ages ranged from nineteen to twenty-eight) whose troubles can certainly be classed as belonging to the same type. After undue fatigue, or after some serious disappointment, they suffered from a sense of fatigue and from a strong disinclination to work ; they became affected with a mania for fastidious accuracy, or with a questioning spirit which complicated all their activities, slowing these down and rendering them yet more difficult ; they suffered from an inhibition of attention and from intellectual incapacity ; they were affected with tics of various kinds, such as a swallowing tic, and even aerophagia ; they suffered from minor phobias, and more or less aggravated obsessions. For reasons which differed from case to case I was unable in these patients to make use of more definite methods of treatment, and I confined myself to sermonising, to educational discourses, to the guidance of their reading. The results were most gratifying, and the patients were cured in a few weeks.—In a different group we may class cases of tics and spasms of a more definite kind. A woman of fifty-three, greatly distressed by the behaviour of her children, was suffering from depression, attended by spasms of the abdominal muscles, and a tic which must be described as a sort of half-developed sob. She was fully cured in three months by a course of conversations which had a calmative influence from the first.

The cases of Len., a woman of thirty-eight, and of Lye., a man of thirty-seven, were extremely remarkable, for they both suffered from oesophageal spasm, which is apt to be a very obstinate disorder. In one of these patients we used the radioscope to watch the antics of a cachet containing bismuth, which moved up and down the oesophagus without being able to make its way into the stomach. Len., had always been fussy about her throat. She had a fine voice and had hoped to become a professional singer ; she was always examining her larynx, and running after some new method of treatment. At the age of thirty she failed in an examination when success would have secured her a good post. After this disappointment she began to have difficulty in swallowing. Soon the dysphagia became intractable, and she had to be fed by means of an oesophageal tube. In this patient, explanations concerning the nature of her malady, moral exhortations, and guidance towards another career in which success came easily, brought speedy relief to a trouble which had seemed grave. The man's case was very similar. Some good advice and the ability to resume his work as schoolmaster were enough to cure a spasm which had lasted for several years.

I could quote numerous examples of algias and of phobias in which a perfect cure has resulted from exclusive treatment by moralisation.—Loe., a man of forty-five, was suffering from depression, the dread of permanent paralysis, claustrophobia, dread of society, fear of crowds, vertigo, aprosexia, and a feeling of inability to understand anything. He was completely cured by moral guidance during a period of four months.— Bab., a woman of forty-five, with phobias relating to digestion, ambulation, and sleep, was cured in like manner by treatment for five months. Rox., a woman of twenty-two, terrified by a burglary in her house, had become so timid that she was unable to walk in the streets. There was a remarkable exception to this inability ; she was able to go out into the streets when she was menstruating, though not at other times—this is a matter to which we shall have to return in the chapter on treatment by excitation. Except when menstruating, she had not left the house for two years. She was treated by moralising conversations like those described by Dubois and his disciples. Repeated every other day for two months, they sufficed to dispel her terrors. To quote the patient's own words : " I wanted to talk frankly about my illness, and this has cured me quickly by restoring my self-confidence."

Paul, a man of thirty, after suffering from all kinds of phobias, was monopolised by a very remarkable one. He had a terror of towns. He could go about freely in the country, but nothing would induce him to visit Paris. Conversation with him about these strange psychological phenomena, simple advice, a few exhortations ; these measures speedily enabled him to get the better of the phobia, so that he could come to consult me in Paris without any of the troubles he had so greatly dreaded. Before this, he had not set foot in the city for ten years.

I shall mention here only one case, among many, of obsessions properly so called. Bal., a woman of thirty-five, was so much tormented by the fear of death, and by the obsession of the world to come, that she was unable to continue her work as schoolmistress. She spent all her time groaning about the sad lot of elderly women for whom death was near at hand, and she was being reduced to poverty. My first concern was to persuade her to resume her work, and this speedily brought about a marked improvement of morale. A few explanations were then sufficient to overcome the crisis.— I could multiply examples indefinitely, but shall be content with the foregoing. All doctors who have interested themselves in such methods of treatment can furnish plenty of instances from their personal experience. If they will study their case-books in this light, they will, like me, come to the conclusion that they have often made use of the method of moralisation, and they will realise that the cures obtained by this method are often extremely remarkable.

The reader may wonder how it is that such remarkable cures can be obtained by therapeutic methods which, as I have shown, are so vague and so little based on reason. I do not think there is any contradiction. Dubois and the other moralisers, when expounding their system of treatment, attempt to interpret the facts they observe and to account for the obvious results ; and they state their theory of the cures that ensue. Now, the facts are sound ; but the theory is unsound, or at any rate incomplete. Their explanation is that the cures are the outcome of their reasoning. In some of the cases, the reasoning may be one of the factors of the cure ; but it is certainly not the sole factor of these cures, nor even the chief determinant.

Let us enumerate the other psychological phenomena that have played a part, potent influences every one. First of all, there has been in many instances a journey to Switzerland ; change of air and scene. Often the patient's mood, though he is going to consult a qualified medical practitioner, is that of one who visits a distant shrine in search of a miraculous cure. I have been told that the inhabitants of Pau are never cured at Lourdes ; I fancy that those who live in Berne will not be the most favourable subjects for psychotherapeutics. Additional factors in many of the cases are isolation, rest in bed, and discipline. R. C. Cabot points out that Dubois puts all his patients on a pure milk diet, and adds that this practice is not so absurd as it might seem. Most of the patients have been very irregular in their habits, and the rationing with milk every two hours is already a rigorous discipline.[1] Other moral influences are superadded. There are threats, for instance, and even punishment. Substantially, the patients are in solitary confinement, and are given to understand that the duration of their imprisonment depends on their own behaviour. When the treatment is most rigorously applied, the bed is curtained off, and the patient is denied even a book, denied all occupation, until there has been a real or apparent change for the better. I am not criticising the details of the method ; I merely point out that there is a good deal at work here besides pure reasoning, many influences besides those of logic. Some of the procedures are simply educative. For instance, the patient must monotonously repeat certain things at fixed hours of the day. His powers of attention are trained by making him listen to a daily lesson in philosophy. Various stimuli are applied, the patient being assured that he is regarded as an intelligent being, as one whose sole guide is reason. Dubois especially recommends us to magnify the invalid's good qualities, to flatter the patient's self-esteem. We have also to take into account the influence of example. The doctor is one whose character is firm and whose convictions are solid. How can these persons who have never believed in anything fail to be impressed by their contact with a man who is so absolutely certain of the truth of Leibnitz' philosophy ?

[1] Parker, op. cit., II, ii, 27.

There is yet another influence at work (horresco referens !) ; the influence of suggestion. It is extremely difficult to prevent the interaction of automatic phenomena. The personality or the words of the physician cannot fail to influence the patient's mind in this way. Even Dubois admits the fact (p. 108) : " No doubt our moral influence upon our neighbour is not always rational. The weaker his mentality, the more readily will he be guided by our injunctions. We are fully entitled to turn this circumstance to account if our aim is to effect a cure or to bring solace." Again (p. 101) : " The doctor succeeds because he is a stranger, because the patient regards him as a person equipped with moral authority, because he knows how to act by persuasion." Bonjour, who has noted the part played by suggestion in Dubois' practice, makes a pungent criticism : " This incessant blowing of one's own trumpet, this reiteration to the patient that one can cure everything, is it perfectly moral, does it not verge on sophistry ? " [1] Without being so harsh as this, I should like to point out that Dubois certainly has no right to abuse those who understand the indispensable part played by suggestion, and who deliberately make use of the influence.

Medical moralisation, then, is not, as many of its advocates would have us believe, purely rational. It appeals to all sorts of influences besides those of the reason ; to the sentiments, to the passions, to the patient's automatism. It would fain turn to account a medley of psychological influences, simply because they are psychological ; for those who practise the method have recognised in a general fashion the power of thought. In this connexion I may recall the history of theriac, a medicament which played a great part in the Middle Ages. It was a universal remedy, one suitable for every possible disorder, for this electuary contained scores of drugs, all the active substances known at the time. The patient was made to swallow the composite remedy in the hope that one of the ingredients, at least, would touch the spot. The therapeutic method we have just been studying may be regarded as a sort of psychological theriac. " Medical moralisation " huddles all the phenomena of thought together pell-mell ; it appeals to all the mental operations in every patient, whatever the nature of the disease,

[1] Op. cit., p. 330.

the hope being that each patient will discover in the amalgam the element that suits him best.

Therein lies the great merit of medical moralisation. Those who practise it have thoroughly recognised the therapeutic power of thought. Without waiting to solve all the scientific problems involved in the distinction between psychological phenomena, they have brought this power into the limelight far more effectively than ever before. It is hardly possible, as yet, to be less summary than they have been. Our diagnosis of psychological troubles is rudimentary ; our knowledge of essential psychological phenomena is minimal. We may try to write a precise psychological prescription, we may believe that we are acting by suggestion or by psychomotor education or by mental stimulation ; but we do not fully understand what we succeed in doing. The result achieved depends upon numerous phenomena to which we have made a quite unintentional appeal. More often than we are aware, we have slipped back into the simple method of moralisation, which is to-day the most common and most practical form of psychotherapeutics.

Does this suffice ? Are we never to get beyond this stage ? Obviously, we must try to advance, for the lack of precision in diagnosis and treatment entails many drawbacks. Such general and confused methods of treatment have their advantages ; but they have all the defects of theriac, a remedy which has disappeared from the pharmacopoeia. No doubt successes can be obtained by the method of moralisation, but it is impossible to foresee or guide them, so that we can never tell whether we shall be able to produce a similar result in another patient. For example, a few pages back I recorded the cure of oesophageal spasm in two of my patients simply by moralising conversation. Shall I be able to apply the same treatment with confidence in all cases of the kind ? Unfortunately not, for in six other cases of oesophageal spasm, of exactly the same type to outward seeming, this treatment did no good whatever. I do not know why the treatment was so successful in two of the cases, and why it failed in the other six. I cannot tell whether it will do good in a new case, and I have to apply it haphazard. That is always the trouble with moralisation. We cannot advance by reasoning from case to case ; we cannot profit by experience. We hope for a run of good luck, but if we have a series of failures we console ourselves by blaming it on the patients. We say they were not sane enough for the treatment.

Since in our own practices we cannot be sure of being able to do the same thing twice over, there is scant justification for advising others to use the method we are so doubtful about ourselves. Some writers have no illusions on this point, for they declare that the moralising method of treatment cannot really be taught to pupils. Since your success depends upon a number of unknown factors, and perhaps upon many factors that are purely personal (your stature, your beard maybe, or the tone of your voice), you are not in a position to teach your pupils how to succeed by following your example. You will explain to them your theories concerning moralisation, that is to say the most insignificant part of your system, and the most fallacious. If they subsequently attempt to apply your teaching—exaggerating certain elements of it, while suppressing the essentials which you have not imparted, and whose existence has remained beyond their ken—they will merely expose themselves to ridicule, and will bring discredit upon your methods.

Psychotherapy by moralisation contains the germ of a medicine of the mind, just as the medieval theriac contained the germ of modern methods of drug treatment. A long time will elapse, and a great deal of hard work will have to be done, before this germ will develop into a method of treatment that will be at once precise, practical, and capable of being taught.

PART TWO

UTILISATION OF THE PATIENT'S AUTOMATISM

CHAPTER FOUR

HISTORY OF SUGGESTION AND HYPNOTISM

" It is really rather late to talk about hypnotism and suggestion," some of my readers will say. Treatment by hypnotism
and suggestion, which was all the rage for a dozen years or so,
fell into a decline. There came a period in which no one
remembered the palmy days of hypnotism ; in which no one
recalled the enthusiasm of twenty years earlier, when hypnotism
cured everything. It has been my tendency, my misfortune
perhaps, to have a fondness for moderation, and to dislike the
absurd exaggerations of extremists. That is why, twenty years
ago, I exposed myself to contempt by saying that hypnotic
suggestion was not everything ; and that is why, to-day, I
run the risk of making people laugh at me by saying that
hypnotism counts for something after all. The contempt and
the laughter leave my withers unwrung. Moderation is the
best aid to the discovery of truth. If my book be ignored
to-day, it will be read to-morrow, when there will have been a
new turn of fashion's wheel, bringing back treatment by
hypnotic suggestion just as it will bring back our grandmothers'
hats. The study interests me, for the methods of treatment
of which I am now going to speak differ in many respects from
the generalised methods we have hitherto been studying. I
regard them as the type, as the starting-point, as the more
special and more accurately defined methods of psychological
healing which are ultimately destined to dispute the field with
the psychological theriacs.

1. First Studies concerning Suggestion and Hypnotism.

Attention is first drawn to a particular force by its exceptional manifestations. Not until then do people begin to
acquire knowledge about the everyday phenomena that result
from the working of this force. For ages observations had
been made concerning certain individuals in whom strange

modifications of behaviour took place in relationship with certain ideas which seemed to exercise a remarkable effect. Charms and amulets, wishing-rings and forgetting-rings, spells whereby an enemy could be rendered sexually impotent or unable to void his urine (" nouer l'aiguillette," " cheville-ment," etc.), conjurations with waxen images pierced with pins and melted before the fire, powders of sympathy and unguents of the soul, even exorcism—these were not mysterious to every one. In the Middle Ages there were already persons competent to understand the rationale of such activities, and able to turn their knowledge to good account.[1]

In the seventeenth century, Malebranche was a pioneer in the work of associating these strange phenomena with familiar happenings. The third part of the second book of the famous treatise *De la recherche de la vérité* is entitled " La communication contagieuse des imaginations fortes," and shows a remarkable knowledge of these phenomena. The author explains very well how " passionate persons arouse passion in us, and make upon our imagination impressions resembling those with which these persons are affected. . . . Visionaries, by excess of folly, go so far as to believe that they see before their eyes absent objects of which we speak to them." Malebranche records a remarkable instance, reported by a friend of his : " An old gentleman that lived with one of my sisters became sick, a young maid held the candle whilst he was blooded in the foot : but as she saw the surgeon strike in the lancet, she was seized with such an apprehension as to feel three or four days afterwards such a piercing pain in the same part of her foot as forced her to keep her bed all that time " (Book II, Chapter vii, Section 2 : T. Taylor's transla-tion). I wish there were space to quote in full this author's admirable explanation of the origin of beliefs relating to the Sabbath. The theory of these phenomena is expounded by Malebranche in a most interesting way : " Among these per-sons," he writes, "an idea fills the mind so exclusively that they can pay no attention to any other thing than that represented by these particular images." Towards the close of the

---

[1] Cf. Dom Calmet, abbot of Senones, Les apparitions des esprits et sur les vampires ou les revenants de Hongrie, de Moravie, etc., 1751, vol. i, p. 214 ; E. Portalié, L'hypnotisme au moyen âge, Avicenne, Richard de Middletown, " Études des Péres de la Cie. de Jésus," March and April 1892, pp. 481 and 577 ; Régnard, op. cit., p. 51.

eighteenth century and the beginning of the nineteenth, various authors described phenomena of the same nature, and showed how they could be explained in the light of the general laws of thought. I may refer especially to Maine de Biran, *Oeuvres inédites*, vol. iii, p. 485 ; also to de Beauchène, *De l'influence des affections de l'âme dans les maladies nerveuses des femmes* (1781) ; and to Demangeon, *L'imagination considérée dans ses effets directs sur l'homme et les animaux*, 1829.

It must, however, be recognised that this study was suddenly transformed, and received a fresh impetus, when the time came for the study, from the same outlook, of the phenomena of somnambulism induced by animal magnetism. Here were remarkable happenings whose salient character could not fail to arouse attention ; and they were phenomena which could be reproduced at will under varying conditions. The study of these phenomena, which were at a later date to be called " suggestions," was the foundation of experimental psychology.

In 1784, the members of the governmental commission appointed to study Mesmer's doings, was already able to report : " All the subjects were, to an amazing extent, under the influence of the magnetiser ; though they might seem to be asleep, his voice, or a look or sign from him, would arouse them. We cannot fail to recognise in these invariable effects a great power at work upon the patients, controlling them, a force which seems to be at the disposal of the magnetiser." Puységur writes in even plainer terms regarding his somnambulists : " When it seemed to me that these ideas were having a disagreeable influence upon the subject, I called a halt, and tried to instil more cheerful thoughts ; nor did I find this a difficult matter. . . . Then the subject became quite happy, imagining himself to be winning a prize, dancing at a party, and so on. . . . I encouraged these ideas in him, and I made him move about freely in his chair." [1]

Attention having been drawn to these phenomena, various observers began to take note of the modifications of behaviour which can be very readily produced in somnambulists by the simple measure of modifying their thoughts through the influence of the spoken word. Bertrand, in his *Traité du somnam-*

---

[1] Lettres de Puységur, May 8, 1784.—See also Gauthier, op. cit., vol. ii, p. 251.

bulisme (1823), describes the movements and the actions which
a word can induce in somnambulists, and speaks of the hallucinations which can be aroused in their minds. This observer
was likewise one of the first to describe what may be called
negative suggestions. " The will," he writes (p. 256), " can
prevent their seeing some one who is in the room." Again
(p. 288) the will " can make them forget something which they
know perfectly well." He lays especial stress on suggestions
whose performance is postponed—what we now call posthypnotic suggestions. These are not acted upon until after the
subject has been reawakened. He shows, too, that a like
phenomenon may be observed in connexion with spontaneous
frenzies. " The ecstatics of Saint Médard foretold in the crisis
that they would fast when it was over, and then they could not
help doing this." [1]

Deleuze's writings (1813 and 1825) are well known. He gives
remarkable instances of the kind just described, speaking of
suggested anaesthesias and amnesias, and of various other
kinds of posthypnotic suggestions. " You will return home
at such and such an hour ; you will not go to the theatre this
evening ; you will wear this or that article of clothing ; you
will find no difficulty in taking your medicine ; you will drink
no wine, or no coffee ; you will no longer heed this or that
concern ; you will cease to be afraid of something which now
troubles you ; you will forget this, that, or the other. The
somnambulist will have a natural urge to do what he has been
told ; he will remember the instruction without being aware
that he is merely remembering ; he will feel drawn towards
what you have advised him, and will be repelled by what you
have forbidden him." [2] In 1825, Abbé Faria, in a remarkable
book which, I am glad to say, has just been reprinted, published
studies of the same character. These are not so original as is
commonly supposed, seeing that the phenomena described by
Faria had been previously recorded both by Bertrand and
by Deleuze. Delatour's articles in " Hermès " are likewise of
interest in this connexion.

For some years after this, animal magnetism was under a
cloud, but at length we find renewed accounts of such

[1] Cf. Teste, Manuel pratique de magnétisme animal, p. 133 (English
translation, p. 100) ; Gauthier, op. cit., vol. ii, p. 259.
[2] Deleuze. Instruction pratique sur le magnétisme animal, 1825, p. 118.

phenomena in the writings of Charles Despine (1840), Teste (1840), and Charpignon (1842 to 1848). The last-named published interesting researches concerning the duration of suggested hallucinations,[1] and concerning the physiological changes which can be induced by suggestion. He writes (op. cit., pp. 364 and 365) : " We may also find that an imaginary pain [one induced by suggestion] will be attended by local physical symptoms ; or that an imaginary blister will redden the skin where it is supposed to be situated." All these experiments were reproduced in public by Dupotet, and were described in his lectures (1849). Dupotet signalises the importance of the medico-legal problem, to which Charpignon had already referred ; he likewise points out that, under the influence of suggestion, a prolonged dream may occupy the mind of the subject, attended by actions as well as by hallucinations. One of the most remarkable instances given by this author is that of a dream that there has been a metamorphosis of personality.[2] To the same epoch belong the remarkable studies made by Perrier of Caen (1849-1854).[3] This investigator paid special attention to induced hallucinations and contractures. Thus, as early as the middle of the nineteenth century there were being studied in somnambulists the contractures which develop with comparative ease when the skin is touched or the muscles are lightly struck. We shall see, subsequently, that this fact is of some historical significance.

Generally speaking, scant justice is done to many of these authors. J. P. Durand (called " Durand de Gros ") waxes indignant at the way in which, a few years ago, those who were studying suggestion believed themselves to be making pioneer experiments when they were merely repeating those that had been made long before. He adds : " All that our modern contemporary suggesters can offer in the way of observation and experiment, was furnished, with a wealth of detail, in an American treatise, of which the first edition was published in 1851. I refer to *The Philosophy of Electrical Psychology*, by John Bovee Dods." [4] Other writers are prone to refer to James Braid of Manchester, whose first publications on the

---

[1] Physiologie, médecine et métaphysique du magnétisme, Paris, 1848, pp. 81-82.
[2] Cf. " Journal du Magnétisme," vol. viii (1849), pp. 396, 589, 593
[3] Unpublished. Studied by the author of the present work in MS notes. See below, p. 190. [4] See Bibliography

subject date from 1841, as the most notable forerunner in the fields of hypnotism and suggestion. In " Brain," Part LXXIII (Spring, 1896), will be found an excellent account of Braid's work, with a list of his writings, by J. Milne Bramwell ; but this author inclines to overestimate Braid's importance. It is probable that Braid was the introducer of the term " suggestion," but (dismissing theoretical questions for the moment) Braid's works contain no essentially new facts. All the phenomena observed by him had already been admirably described in the writings of Puységur, Bertrand, Deleuze, and Charpignon. It is, indeed, very interesting to note that the fundamental facts were ascertained at a very early stage, and that no important discoveries were made in the sequel.

Has a more notable advance been made in the interpretation of the facts ?   A purely mechanical interpretation, one which absolutely denies the mental character of the phenomena, was not favoured at the outset of the researches ; but it found expression later in the books of Heidenhain, Prosper Despine, and MacKendrick of Glasgow.   In an article in the " Nineteenth Century " (January, 1896), Ernest Hart, the editor of the " British Medical Journal," presented the same outlook.   In one of the early chapters of my book *L'automatisme psychologique*, I discuss the mechanical interpretation.   Milne Bramwell puts forward identical arguments in a critique of Hart.[1] As a matter of fact, there is not much to be said in favour of these premature attempts to furnish a mechanical explanation, and the early observers were well aware that they had to do with psychological phenomena.   But Puységur and Deleuze believed that they were dealing with psychological phenomena of a wholly abnormal character, peculiar to the state of induced somnambulism.   Since they believed magnetism to be the essential factor in the production of somnambulism, it followed, in their view, that all the abnormal phenomena were dependent on magnetism.

The theory of suggestion is based upon a very different conception.   Its real founder was Alexandre Bertrand.   Educated at the Ecole Politechnique, qualifying as a medical practitioner, and subsequently becoming a member of the scientific editorial staff of the " Globe " and the " Temps," Bertrand took a lively interest in the phenomena of animal

[1] Proceedings of the Society for Psychical Research, 1896, p. 212.

magnetism, and believed he had found a satisfactory clue to lead him through this labyrinth. His idea was that the facts could be explained, on scientific and determinist lines, by an adequate study of the mental condition of the subjects, and the morbid or artificially induced modifications exhibited by these. He was assisted by one of the most notable among the doctors who devoted themselves to such studies, Charles Despine, who sent Bertrand all his own notes upon somnambulism and catalepsy.[1] Bertrand's intention was to publish a sort of encyclopaedia, in six volumes, upon the phenomena of pathological psychology ; the volume actually published, a posthumous work, is no more than an introduction. In this work, Bertrand develops the general view that the psychological phenomena observed during the magnetic state are not exceptional phenomena, but are normal, or are at least phenomena which can be observed under various other conditions. Artificial somnambulism, said Bertrand, serves merely to render conspicuous and to amplify phenomena dependent upon the working of the general laws of imagination, expectant attention, and desire. If normal psychology could give a satisfactory explanation of these phenomena, the same explanation would be applicable to all that was witnessed in somnambulist patients, however strange it might appear at first sight.

To the same period belongs the work of General Noizet, a friend of Bertrand, and likewise educated at the Ecole Politechnique. Noizet became acquainted with Abbé Faria's teaching, and passed it on to Bertrand. His book, *Mémoire sur le somnambulisme et le magnétisme animal*, was not published until 1854, but it had been drafted in 1820 as a memorial to the Royal Academy of Berlin, and contained in essentials, at that early date, the ideas subsequently expounded by Bertrand. The fundamental psychological law which is at work here is, says Noizet, the law in accordance with which every idea tends to become an action ; the suggested action is performed because the idea of the action has made its way into the subject's consciousness. The author does not seem to have asked himself why the working of this law is not constantly manifest in the normal state, seeing that it is so rigorously applicable in the case of suggestions. Nevertheless, Noizet's

[1] Cf. in this connexion, the preface to Charles Despine's book, De l'emploi du magnétisme animal, etc., p. xliv.

book is of great importance from the historical outlook, for, if 1 mistake not, this author's theories form a link between the teaching of Bertrand and that which was to emanate much later from the Nancy School.

Braid, in 1842, likewise declared that the phenomena of suggestion were nothing more than special instances of familiar psychological facts ; but he was more inclined to dwell upon one of the peculiar characteristics of these phenomena, the monoideism of which Bertrand and Noizet had already spoken. It seemed to Braid that the easy passage of the idea into action, the essential feature of suggestion, was determined by an excess of attention. Braid, therefore, was one of the originators of the theory that suggestion is to be explained by an excess of attention—a theory which, as we shall see, has of late been revived and developed by Münsterberg.[1]

Joseph Pierre Durand of Gros, in his remarkable works, *Electrodynamisme vital* (1855) and *Cours de braidisme, ou hypnotisme nerveux* (1860), also insists upon the fact that there is something peculiar and specific about suggestion. He points out that the disposition to receive suggestions is not universal, and that its intensity is not constant in any individual. In addition to the "ideoplastic" phenomena of suggestion, we must, says Durand, study the state of suggestibility, the "hypotaxic state" into which the subjects are thrown by various influences. The other writings of this epoch are more concerned with medical and therapeutic outlooks, and pay little heed to the psychological study of the phenomena. Still, I regard Mesnet's work as important.[2] He gives a long description of a man who had crises of spontaneous somnambulism after an injury to the head. In these crises the patient performed various actions which seemed to be determined solely by the sight of objects or by contact with them. If he had a roll of paper in his hand, he would unroll it and begin to sing ; if he was holding a stick, he would go through his musketry drill ; if he saw a bright gem, he would try to steal it. We learn from these observations, says Mesnet, that the influence of an operator issuing orders is not indispensable, and that inert objects which are not offered to the subject by another person

---

[1] Cf. Milne Bramwell, "Brain," 1896, p. 10 ; Hypnotism, its History, Practice, and Theory, 1903
[2] "Union Médicale," 1874, No. 87.

can serve as the starting point of suggestions. Like phenomena were noted by Moreau de Tours when studying the effects of hashish.[1] Lights and other objects in the room could change the trend of the subject's dreams, and even modify his actions. —All these researches paved the way for the psychological study of suggestion, and already effected considerable advances along the road.

Observers wanted to turn these phenomena to account before they had really begun to understand them. Their first application was in the interpretation and production of the somnambulist state, in connexion with which they had first come to light. Somnambulism was still regarded as essential to their occurrence.

In the earliest days of animal magnetism, there began a famous quarrel, that between the " fluidists " and the " animists." Its progress can be followed in all the journals of the period, and especially in the " Journal du Magnétisme " (vol. ix, pp. 114, 119, 525, 590, etc.). The fluidists, without troubling much about details, thought that the changes in the subject's state must be regarded as due to the physical effect of a fluid emanating from the magnetiser. The animists ridiculed this unwarranted assumption, and declared that everything depended upon the changes induced in the subject's mental state. The magnetiser's action was a mental or moral one. The subject's thoughts were modified, and all the rest was an outcome of this modification. Already, there was manifest the essential distinction between magnetism and hypnotism. These two disciplines bear upon the same phenomenon, namely upon artificially induced hypnotism ; but the typical feature of the hypnotic theory is the scientific attitude towards the phenomena under consideration. The dominant desire of the hypnotic school was to dismiss the wonderful, occult, and miraculous elements in which the magnetisers took delight. Furthermore, the hypnotic school endeavoured to explain the happenings by psychological laws instead of appealing to physical or physiological forces.

If this formulation of the differences between the two schools be accepted, we must recognise that hypnotism began with Bertrand in the early twenties of the nineteenth century.

[1] De haschisch et de l'aliénation mentale, 1845.

He was the first to say in plain words that artificial somnambulism could be explained as being due solely to the working
of the subject's imagination.   The somnambulist went to sleep
because he thought about going to sleep, and awoke because
he thought about waking.   To Faria belongs the merit of
turning this idea to practical account, for he was the first to
induce somnambulism in his subjects simply by saying to them :
" I wish you to go to sleep."   Next in the series must be
mentioned the work of General Noizet, who laid stress upon a
kindred but risky theory, that induced somnambulism was
analogous to natural sleep.   In the same connexion I may
refer to Heidenhain's book (1880), and to some remarkable
letters contributed by Ordinaire to the " Journal du Magnétisme " (1850, pp. 120–207).

Braid's book, *Neurypnology* (1843) deserves mention, in
my opinion, only after the foregoing.   It is known that Braid
reached his idea in the course of an attempt to reproduce the
experiments of the magnetiser Lafontaine.   He was able to
induce sleep, or somnambulism, in his subjects by making
them fix their gaze upon the glass stopper of a water-bottle.
He thus dispensed with all thought of utilising the activity
of the " nervous fluid " of which Lafontaine had spoken,
but he set another physiological phenomenon to work, to wit,
the fatigue caused by fixation of attention.   His investigations
were thus upon a different plane from those of Bertrand and
Faria.   This might have been made the starting-point of
interesting researches anent the part played by fatigue in the
determination of these phenomena, but Braid did not follow
up that line of investigation.   He wandered off into an attempt
to apply to the study of somnambulism Gall's theories of
phrenology and cranioscopy, and he believed that he was able
to stimulate this or that moral faculty by rubbing the suitable
" bump " in the patient's head.   Still, as Bramwell shows,
Braid did not stray long in such perilous paths.   His main
interest was the study of suggestions and the part played by
these in the induction of artificial sleep.   His ideas were thus
in line with those of the French pioneers of hypnotism.

These studies of hypnotic sleep were still embryonic.   Only
one character had as yet been adequately analysed, the disposition to mental inertia and the disposition to suggestibility.
Nevertheless, one important fact had been brought to light.   It

had been shown that the mental state of certain subjects could be modified either by suggestion or by methods which induced fatigue.

At that date, moreover, the majority of such studies were primarily aimed at achieving therapeutic results, the theoretical interest being subordinate ; suggestion and hypnotism had hardly been born when they were applied to the treatment of patients. As long ago as 1780, Deslon had written : " If M. Mesmer had no other secret than that he has been able to make the imagination exert an effective influence upon the health, would he not still be a wonder worker ? If treatment by the use of the imagination is the best treatment, why do we not make use of it ? " [1] A number of investigators were on the look out for facts proving the influence of imagination on health—in some cases facts showing that ideas could cause disease, and in other cases facts showing that ideas could cure disease. Hecquet quoted the instance of a man " who, seeing some one hanging by the heels to a carriage which was dragging him along, was seized by so intense an emotion that he instantly felt a sharp pain in the heel, and limped for the rest of his life." [2] William Charles Ellis (*A Treatise on the Nature, Symptoms, Causes, and Treatment of Insanity*, 1838) records the case of a woman who fancied that she had been infected with syphilis, and who was cured by bread pills. She was told that they were mercurial pills, and they induced well-marked salivation. J. H. Bennett, Carpenter, and David Brewster record similar facts. There is good ground, therefore, for applying this treatment to all diseases in which the imagination appears to play a notable part.

To begin with, at any rate, the hypnotists were less ambitious and more cautious than the magnetisers. They did not claim that they were able to cure all diseases, and the case-histories they published show that they were mainly concerned with the treatment of nervous disorders. Bertrand speaks of curing ecstatics and somnambulists. In 1862, Charpignon is studying " the part which moral medication plays in the treatment of nervous diseases." The cures reported by Braid are, above all, cases of contracture ; he tells of " a contraction of the neck towards the left shoulder, dating from

[1] Observations sur le magnétisme animal.
[2] " Journal du Magnétisme," vol. viii, p. 488.

six months back, cured in two sittings," and speaks of relieving pains and disorders of sensibility ; he has great hopes of relieving deafness (but does not seem to exercise sufficient care to distinguish between functional and organic deafness). Charles Despine speaks of the use of hypnotism in education. He uses the method, above all, in the treatment of hysterical patients, and records some remarkable cures. I shall not dwell here on the case of Estelle, the one discussed at such length, for I think that the treatment of this patient was on lines that transcended the limits of suggestion and hypnotism in the strict sense of those terms. (The matter will be considered more fully in Chapter Thirteen, § 1.) Lasègue pointed out that " sleep [hypnosis] is the most potent modifier of the nervous system, for it wards off hysteria, arrests chorea, and induces epilepsy." [1] Morel, in his *Traité des maladies mentales* (1860), already recommended hypnotism for the treatment of hysteria, and Georget declared that he had secured good results by hypnotising insane patients.

Hitherto I have made no mention of Liébeault's book, for I consider it of little interest as far as the theory of suggestion is concerned. It reproduces, almost without modifications, the substance of Noizet's teaching. That is why I suspect that Noizet's influence may be traced here—for Noizet was Bertrand's pupil. He lived for a long time at Metz, and may have been one of the intellectual fathers of the Nancy School founded by Liébeault. But from the therapeutic outlook the importance of the latter's work must on no account be underestimated. Liébeault was a man of generous disposition, and exercised great moral influence over a very large number of patients. He was convinced that thought affects health profoundly. He was continually declaring that moral representations, whether during sleep [hypnosis] or during the waking state, could exercise great power over the organism, and he showed that dreams could modify physical states.[2] Moreover, he did not confine himself to the treatment of nervous disorders, for he believed that suggested ideas could do good in organic diseases as well as functional, and could work as antidotes to poisons. He considered that by suggestion he was able to cure anaemia,

---

[1] Lasègue, Études médicales, vol. i, p. 207.
[2] Liébeault, Le sommeil et les états morals au point de vue de l'action du moral sur le physique, 1866, p. 157 ; " Revue de l'hypnotisme," vol. i, p. 145.

intermittent fever, pulmonary tuberculosis, disorders of menstruation, dental troubles, neuralgia, and migraine. Among the disciples of Bertrand who were prompt to turn to therapeutic account these psychological phenomena that were still so little understood, Liébeault was the most convinced and the most enthusiastic. Demarquay and Teulon in an interesting little book (1860),[1] Trousseau, Mesnet (1866), Michéa, Macario, and Baillif (1868), record numerous attempts in the same direction.

Most of the other writers on this subject were less ambitious, and confined their attention to some specific problem in treatment. To ensure the success of hypnotism, and to turn it promptly to practical account, the main endeavour was to induce by this means anaesthesia for surgical operations. Récamier (1821), Cloquet (1829), Oudet (1837), Ribaud, Broca, Follin, Guérineau, Vulpian, and in England Topham (1842), Elliotson (1843), and, in especial, Esdaile, performed surgical operations under anaesthesia induced by hypnotic sleep and by suggestion. Many of these were major operations, including even amputation at the hip-joint. But in 1846 came the discovery of anaesthesia by the inhalation of ether, and in 1847 that of anaesthesia by the inhalation of chloroform. These methods being much easier and more trustworthy, an unfortunate result was that the use of hypnotism for surgical purposes fell into abeyance, and the whole study of induced sleep was neglected. A few books, like the little volume by Demarquay and Teulon (1860), were subsequent to this date, but by 1865 suggestion and hypnotism seemed as dead as animal magnetism.

2. Rebirth of Hypnotism. The Salpêtrière School

For nearly twenty years, hypnotism was contemptuously abandoned to charlatans. A few healers still used it secretly ; and from time to time there were also public demonstrations with hypnotised subjects, the hypnosis being in many cases fictitious. Donato, a Belgian, Alberti, an Italian, Hansen, a Dane, and Montus, a Frenchman, travelled from town to town, demonstrating to amazed audiences the postures and jerky movements of persons under the influence of suggestion.[2]

---

[1] Recherches sur l'hypnotisme ou sommeil nerveux, etc
[2] Cf. " Revue de l'Hypnotisme," vol. i, p. 347

Men of science no longer dared to study hypnotism. Animal magnetism had an evil reputation, and hypnotism was classed in the same category. The study of the topic involved great difficulties, and it was easy to say that scientific investigation was rendered impossible by the perpetual risk of fraud. It was taken for granted that all the mistakes had been due to the bad faith of the subjects of hypnosis, had been due to simulation. An attempt was made to evade this difficulty by studying hypnotic sleep in the lower animals. But the work of Kircher, Czermak, Heubel (1877), Preyer (1878), Beard (1881), and Danilewski (1889), was not very successful. In actual fact, the phenomena studied by these investigators were for the most part manifestations of fear rather than of real hypnosis,[1] and no advance could be made until the study of hypnotism in human beings was resumed.

Charles Richet was one of the first to make headway against the prejudice which ascribed all hypnotic phenomena to fraud. In a series of studies published between 1875 and 1883 in the "Journal d'Anatomie et de Physiologie," and in Ribot's "Revue Philosophique,"[2] he showed again and again that the theory of incessant fraud was an extremely improbable one. After the judgment of the Academy in 1840, and after the report of Dubois of Amiens (supra, p. 40), it had been declared that the advocates of induced sleep had better make up their minds whether they were to be regarded as dupes or accomplices. Richet showed that a scientist could study these problems without being either the one or the other. Have we any right to accuse of trickery and dishonesty all the people who have been thrown into a state of artificial sleep ? "Am I to suppose," said Richet, "that, by an amazing run of ill luck, all my associates, my relatives, and my friends, are in league to deceive me, and to make me commit gross errors ? " The difficulty the critics had to face was that there were so many somnambulist subjects. It was a legitimate hypothesis that one or two persons, here and there, might like to play this little comedy ; but how could there be hundreds and thousands of them ? There was no motive ; no obvious advantage to be gained by such trickery. Besides, the simulation of induced

[1] Cf. Bramwell, Proceedings of the Society for Psychical Research, 1896, p. 214.
[2] The studies are summarised in Richet's book L'homme et l'intelligence, 1884.

sleep would often demand much knowledge as well as a good deal of heroism, for the subjects in whom somnambulism was induced were always found to exhibit the same phenomena, and they could not have known these in advance.—The last contention is the weakest, for Richet only described, as characteristic of the somnambulist state, familiar psychological phenomena, the most interesting of which was the amnesia that followed the somnambulism. On the whole, the phenomena were ill defined, and could certainly have been reproduced by subjects who had had very little instruction.

Besides studying this problem of simulation, Richet undertook a valuable investigation into the psychology of induced somnambulism. He described all the phenomena of suggestion, emphasising the point that suggestions could be induced by attitudes, movements, and gestures. The kinaesthetic sensations which played the part of suggestions might be fortuitous, and quite independent of the experimenter. In a person under the influence of hashish, a spasm in the neck might become the starting-point of a complicated dream.[1] Suggested dreams, said Richet, can develop through the association of ideas, and can bring about an entire change of personality. (Here we are back at the transformation by suggestion spoken of by Perrier and by Dupotet.) Richet also emphasised the importance of a psychological notion whose value we recognise to-day, namely, that the idea which is to be transformed into a suggestion must be isolated in the mind.

Richet was a pioneer among those who have studied hypnotism from a point of view which seems to me of quite exceptional interest ; among those who have studied induced somnambulism without any preconceived ideas, and animated by the desire to effect a psychological analysis of all the phenomena of this state. Thus Richet must be regarded as the founder of a psychological school of hypnotism to which we shall return in the sequel. For a time, however, this trend was eclipsed by the development of two other schools, which were really much less interesting although they made a good deal more noise in the world.

The first of these two schools was the one led by Charcot at the Salpêtrière. A specialist in nervous diseases, Charcot

[1] Ricket, " Revue Philosophique," 1884, vol. i, p. 471.

was well aware that, alike from the medical and from the philosophical point of view, there was much to be learned from the study of the phenomena of induced somnambulism, which had been clamouring for recognition for more than a century, but had again and again been rejected without examination by the exponents of official science. When entering this dangerous field, he wished to guard against the risk of fraud, and to adopt a method of investigation which should be above criticism from the scientific point of view. He had recently achieved notable successes through the analysis of the symptoms of persons suffering from diseases of the spinal cord, and it seemed to him that the best way would be to make use of the same methods in the study of hypnotic states. Beyond question he was aware that strange and important psychological phenomena were factors in these states ; he was familiar with the working of suggestion, and did not hesitate to make use of it in case of need. But he was never weary of repeating that these psychological phenomena were of a very complicated kind ; that their study was a delicate matter ; and that all the mistakes of the magnetisers had been due to faulty methods, and their unfortunate way of beginning the study of a problem at the most complicated end. For his part, he would be guided by Descartes' rule, and would begin by the study of simple facts, of those in which scientific investigation is easiest. Before studying psychological intricacies, the involved happenings in the mind of a person in an abnormal state, we must first of all ascertain the precise characteristics of this abnormal state, and must learn how to recognise it by definite signs which cannot be counterfeited. For Charcot, a neurologist accustomed to the examination of patients suffering from locomotor ataxia or from lateral sclerosis, the definite symptoms which could not be counterfeited were changes in the condition of the muscles, variations in the reflexes, and modifications of sensation. If the condition of the nervous system had undergone any real alteration, it ought to be possible to detect definite changes of the before-mentioned kind. Thus it was that Charcot, in his endeavour to work out a strictly scientific method, devoted himself to a study of the movements and reflexes of the subjects brought to him by some of his pupils, and declared by these pupils to be in a condition of hypnosis.

Among the collaborators of the early days, among those

who joined with Charcot in the practice of " major hypnotism," there are well-known names, such as those of Bourneville, Brissaud, Chambard, and Paul Richer. Others of the group are less well known, but two, at least, must be mentioned, for I think they played an important part. I refer to Ruault ; and to Londe, the director of the photographic laboratory.

These pupils, familiar with their master's wishes, brought Charcot various patients, and in especial three young women (Witt., Bar., and Gl.), who displayed abnormal muscular reactions during the hypnotic state. In this state there was manifest a certain amount of muscular and nervous hyperexcitability. When a group of muscles, or the nerves supplying this group, were stimulated by a slight blow or by massage, vigorous muscular contractions would ensue, and would persist in the form of obstinate contractures until in some way, as by a stimulation of the opposing muscles, they could be checked. The contractures occurred in accordance with well-known anatomical laws. Stimulation of the median, the ulnar, or the musculospiral nerve would induce a contracture of the muscles supplied by the respective nerves, so that the hand assumed a characteristic position which the study of organic nervous lesions had already made familiar. Once initiated, the contracture spread in accordance with Pflüger's laws. From the left thenar eminence, it would pass to the whole of the left hand, the left arm, and the left shoulder ; thence to the right shoulder and down to the right hand ; finally, in certain instances, the left leg and then the right leg would become affected.[1] Sometimes catalepsy ensued. If one of the subject's limbs was raised by the experimenter, it would retain the position for an indefinite period without any sign of fatigue becoming apparent, and without the possibility of detecting even by graphic methods the respiratory changes which a tiring attitude will rapidly induce in normal subjects. In some of the experiments, stimulation of the muscles would give rise to paralysis, whereas previously the same stimulation had brought about contracture. Finally, in a group of studies initiated by Ruault, there occurred contractures brought about by gentle

---

[1] Charcot and Paul Richer, Contribution à l'étude de l'hypnotisme chez les hystériques, du phénomène de l'hyperexcitabilité neuro-musculaire, " Archives de Neurologie," 1881, ii, p. 32 ; Charcot, Oeuvres, ix, p. 305 ; Chambard, " Encéphale," vol. i, p. 241 ; Charcot and Brissaud, Oeuvres, ix, p. 383 ; Paul Richer, La grande hystérie, second edition, 1885, p. 537.

stimulation of the surface of the skin. These appeared to depend upon an exaggerated sensitiveness of the cutaneous reflexes, just as the contractures previously studied had appeared to be the outcome of an exaggerated sensitiveness of the deep reflexes.

All these phenomena could be successfully linked to Charcot's earlier studies. They could be examined with the guidance of the same anatomical ideas. The same method and the same instruments could be used. The same little hammer could be employed for testing the reflexes. As of old, demonstrations could be made by the chief to an admiring circle of pupils. It was still possible to seek upon the bared limb of a subject the place where a blow with the hammer would most readily induce a well-marked contracture, and one plainly visible to all beholders. To Charcot, this was irresistible. He declared that the study of such phenomena could be conducted by a perfectly sound method; that the method sufficed to exclude the possibility of fraud, which had invalidated the old experiments upon somnambulists; and that it was in the light of the data acquired by this method that a critical review of all the recorded phenomena of animal magnetism must be undertaken.

An exact classification of the phenomena was now begun. According as the various reactions were differently combined, three well-marked states could be distinguished, being known respectively as lethargy, catalepsy, and somnambulism. In " lethargy," which was induced by closing the subject's eyes or in some other way, there were all the appearances of profound slumber. The subject could hear nothing, and was irresponsive to stimuli, except that the before-mentioned neuromuscular hyperexcitability was present. If, now, his eyes were suddenly opened by the experimenter, the subject passed into the state of " catalepsy," in which the limbs retained any position imposed on them by the experimenter, for the previous hyperexcitability had given place to a disposition towards paralysis. By various procedures, and in especial by friction of the vertex, the subject could now be thrown into the " somnambulist " state. He could then hear and speak. Now he manifested a readiness to accept suggestion, and displayed various other psychological phenomena which were not, for the moment, to be studied. What especially interested Charcot and his pupils was that in the somnambulist state there were manifest new forms of contracture, induced this time by the superficial stimulation of the skin. Taken as a whole, these three states comprised " major hypnotism," which was entirely distinct from " minor hypnotism." The latter was the condition in which psychological phenomena were observed. Its study was a more hazardous affair, and must be postponed for a time.[1]

For the moment, these investigators were content to study all the varieties of the before-mentioned phenomena, and to examine the conditions under which they occurred. They discovered one very remarkable phenomenon, whose occurrence accentuated yet further the analogy between the study of major hypnotism and that of organic diseases of the nervous system. I refer to the existence of " états dimidiés," in which some particular phenomenon (such as a disposition to deep or super-ficial contractures, to catalepsy, etc.) existed on one side only of the body. When this happened, a notable experiment could be performed. By the application of a suitable stimulus, and especially by moving a large magnet towards the affected limbs, the characteristic symptoms could be displaced to the other side of the body. This was spoken of as " transference," and its study at the Salpêtrière was extremely interesting, for a link was thus established between the old theories of animal magnetism and another study, equally strange and equally fallen into disrepute, that of metallotherapy. The founders of metallotherapy, Burq and Dumontpallier, had already noted the phenomenon of transference, but had not been able to persuade others to admit its reality. Now transference re-appeared, and received the same official imprimatur as induced somnambulism.

Finally, the important fact emerged that all these phenomena occurred in female patients suffering from a peculiar disturbance of the nervous system. In a word, all the patients in whom the phenomena were studied by Charcot and his associates were hysterical women. The investigators drew the inference that the phenomena, while certainly induced by special causes, could not be induced in subjects of any other kind. The symptoms were not present in all hysterics ; but all the hysterics in whom the symptoms of " major hypnotism "

[1] Charcot and Babinski, Oeuvres, ix, pp. 505–530 ; Paul Richer, Études cliniques sur l'hystéro-epilepsie, ou grande hystérie.

could be induced, were sufferers from grave forms of hysteria.

Such were the leading ideas of a paper read by Charcot at the Academy of Sciences on February 13, 1882, describing the various nervous states induced by hypnotism in hysterical patients. It must not be forgotten that the Academy had already thrice condemned all researches into animal magnetism, and that it was a signal exploit to make this learned assembly listen to a lengthy description of kindred phenomena. Charcot was able to achieve this, not only thanks to his high standing in the scientific world, but also because of the method he had employed, for he was able to show that he had been constantly on his guard against simulation, and had taken the most elaborate steps to verify the anatomical types of the contractures. An additional point in his favour was the general trend of his paper, which presented the phenomena described as nothing more than the symptoms of a special disease. The members of the Academy in general, like Charcot himself, believed that this study was in a field remote from animal magnetism, and was the final condemnation of the latter. That is why the Academy showed a sympathetic interest in a study which was to put an end to the dispute which had raged so long round the topic of animal magnetism—a dispute concerning which a good many members of the Academy had uneasy consciences.

Charcot's success had very important results. It seemed as if he had broken down a dam behind which a vast head of water had been accumulating. No matter that the topic had to be considered under a new name. The study of animal magnetism was no longer prohibited, now that discussion of it had been revived at the Academy of Sciences. No longer need people hide what they had long been studying in secret. What a splendid subject for theses, and for magazine articles ! Since the observers of old days, discredited by having been called magnetisers, were dead and forgotten, what harm could there be in grubbing up their whilom observations, which could be published as new discoveries. Here was an inexhaustible mine ! Everywhere, " hypnosis redivivus," as Hack Tuke called it in 1881, gave rise to numberless books and articles. An enumeration of the authors of these would include the names of most of the neurologists of that day, both in France and in other lands, for there were few who failed to be influenced at this epoch by the teaching which emanated from the Salpêtrière. It will suffice to mention a few of the leading authorities. As early as 1880, when Charcot's studies and lectures were beginning to become widely known, appeared the writings of Bourneville and Régnard, Berger, Cohn, Preyer, Chambard, Tamburini, and Seppili. In 1881, Paul Richer, in his excellent book *La grande hystérie*, described and pictured the various phases of hypnotism as enumerated by Charcot. From the beginning of 1882 we find that all the reviews (not medical reviews only, but those devoted to philosophical and even literary topics), and the proceedings of all the learned societies, are full of articles on major hypnotism. Among the writers, I shall mention only Brown-Séquard, Tamburini, Seppili, Ladame, Vizioli, Pitres, Descourtis, Dumontpallier, and Leblois. Coming to 1883, we note contributions to the discussion from the pens of Paul Richer, Luys, Barth, Babinski, Brissaud, Legrand du Saulle, and Emile Yung (of Geneva). In 1884 there were writings by Pitres, Bérillon, Bottey, Mocquin, Féré, Gilles de la Tourette, Tageret, and Paul Magnin. To the following years belong the works of Brémaud, Azam, Morselli, Lombroso, Bianchi, Sommer, Dujour, Paul Janet, etc. Special reviews were founded, such as Bérillon's " Revue de l'Hypnotisme," the " Revue des Sciences Hypnotiques," and the " Zeitschrift für Hypnotismus."

These numerous observers were not concerned merely to describe the physiological phenomena of hypnotism and to study the strange manifestations of the hypnotic state. Many of them were now beginning to apply hypnotic methods to the practical treatment of disease, and a number of observers recorded that major hypnotism was therapeutically useful, especially in the treatment of neuroses. To Charcot, these practical applications seemed premature. He would have preferred that the phenomena and the methods should have been more exhaustively studied before being turned to therapeutic account. In this respect he showed a certain simplicity of mind, for patients want to be cured, and doctors are not willing to wait indefinitely at the stage of observation. Besides, difficulties were about to thicken, and Charcot was not to be allowed to finish his work in the leisurely and logical fashion of which he had dreamed.

3. THE NANCY SCHOOL.

In 1884 appeared the manifesto of a rival school. This was a slim volume of 110 pages, simply and brightly written, extremely readable. The author, Hyppolyte Bernheim, a professor at Nancy University, published a summary account of the researches in which he had been engaged for several years. He had worked quite independently of Paris, and gave his readers to understand that his outlook was very different from that of the Parisian school. He begins his book by saying : " I owe my knowledge of the method I use to M. Liébeault, a Nancy medical practitioner." We already know of Liébeault's book, and how it originated out of the teachings of Noizet, Bertrand, and Faria. We are concerned, then, with a revival of the " animist " conception, of the theory that the phenomena of magnetism are explicable psychologically, and above all by the power of ideas.

Bernheim, in fact, approaches the question from an outlook that differs utterly from Charcot's. He does not waste time considering the problem of fraud, or the need for taking precautions against it. There is but one cautious allusion to this matter : " No doubt we may occasionally have to do with persons who are deliberate humbugs, or who simulate through complaisance. . . . Here, as always, experience will soon teach the observer how to discriminate, and to ascertain whether the influence is a real one." [1]   I agree with Bernheim. We cannot persist indefinitely at the stage of investigation, on the ground that we believe that the pathological or physiological phenomena we are studying may sometimes be imitated by practical jokers. We have to take risks, for the problem of fraud is not one of general interest, but concerns us only in particular cases. In earlier days, however, a different view prevailed, and public opinion inhibited research in these fields because fraud was possible. Not until the publication of Charles Richet's studies and the official endorsement of Charcot's teaching, was it possible to overcome these prejudices ; and Bernheim's book would have been ignored had not Richet and Charcot already flung themselves into the breach. The fact should not be forgotten. Bernheim himself does not

[1] La suggestion, p. 43.

wholly ignore it, for he makes his acknowledgments when referring to the works of these two authorities (p. 81).

Being unconcerned with the problem of fraud, Bernheim does not trouble himself to describe in detail the character-istics of the condition into which his subjects pass ; he is content to record the methods employed to induce the state, and the results achieved. Having reassured the patient by explaining that there is no question of producing anything more than a simple sleep which may occur in any one under the same conditions, Bernheim comes to the point as follows : " I say to the patient : ' Look at me fixedly, and think only about going to sleep. You will feel your eyelids grow heavy, and your eyes will become tired. Your eyelids are flickering, your eyes are watering, your vision is becoming confused. Your lids have closed, you cannot open your eyes. You no longer feel anything ; your hands are motionless ; you see nothing more ; you are going to sleep.' I add in a somewhat commanding tone : ' Sleep. ' In many cases, this word turns the scale ; the patient's eyes close ; he goes to sleep " (p. 5).

When the subject has gone to sleep, or seems to be asleep, the operator goes on talking to him, and by word or sign conveys the idea of certain actions or the idea of certain sights. In the one case, the subject then performs the action that is spoken of ; in the other case, he behaves as if he were really witnessing the sight which has just been described. In this way a suggested catalepsy can be induced ; the subject's limbs then remain fixed in any position that is imposed on them, but this only happens when the subject understands that it is to happen : in like manner we can induce the performance of various movements, gestures, dances, etc., or can induce all kinds of hallucinations : these are " positive suggestions." Conversely, if we introduce into the subject's mind the idea that he cannot act, that he does not feel or does not see, then a real paralysis will ensue, or the subject will behave as if he could not see a certain thing or could not hear a certain person speak : these are " negative suggestions," or, to use Bernheim's own term, " negative hallucinations." Such effects can be induced during the period of sleep, or they may be postponed until a stated moment : " I suggest to Cl. while he is asleep that, when he wakes up, he will see M. S. (a colleague who is in the room) with his face shaved on one side only, and with a huge silver nose. When the subject awakens, and he catches sight of my colleague, he bursts out laughing, and says : ' I suppose you've done it for a wager, shaving your face like that on one side ! And what an extraordinary nose ! I suppose you've paid a visit to the Invalides ? ' Another time, in a hospital ward, I suggest to him that when he awakens he will see in every bed a large dog instead of the patient who is really there. When he wakes up he is amazed to find himself in a dog hospital " (p. 24). These are " posthypnotic suggestions," and they can be varied indefinitely. Hypnotism, says Bernheim, is nothing more than a multiform combination of suggestions of different categories.

These suggestive phenomena are (says Bernheim) easy to understand ; they are only an exaggeration of phenomena of frequent occurrence in us all. A great many actions are performed by us directly the idea of performing them enters the mind : the movements of facial expression, for instance ; beating time to music ; keeping step ; imitative coughing or yawning ; and the like. All these actions result from a natural inclination towards obedience, imitation, and belief ; they are adequately explained when we recall the existence of " natural credivity."

In some persons, and under certain conditions, these natural faculties undergo a marked development. There is then " a peculiar aptitude for the transformation of any idea that is received, for the transition to action . . . and this transition occurs so rapidly that there is no time for the intervention of intellectual control " (p. 85). *Suggestion* turns these tendencies to account ; " it *consists of the influence exercised by an idea that has been suggested, and has been accepted by the brain* " (p. 73).

Sometimes, continues Bernheim, we shall do well to bring about a temporary enhancement of this natural suggestibility. By suggestion itself we can induce psychological states, such as somnolence or sleep, in which there is increased suggestibility. *The hypnotic state is nothing more than such a sleep brought about by suggestion.* We must not imagine that this condition can only be induced in exceptional individuals, that neuropaths are alone susceptible. No doubt impressionability varies from person to person. Some are predisposed to passive obedience by education or occupation; but "experience shows that the great majority of persons can be readily inclined towards it" (p. 6). Merely by instilling the idea of sleep, we actually cause various grades of sleep attended by suggestibility of differing degrees of intensity. These range from slight somnolence, in which the subject believes himself to be wide awake but is nevertheless unable to open the eyes at will, up to profound somnambulism in which the most complicated suggestions are instantly and accurately carried into effect without the subject's having (after waking) any memory of what has happened. Such are the exceedingly simple phenomena which Bernheim sets forth in his little book; pointing out, in conclusion, that a knowledge of them is likely to lead to important practical results.

In subsequent years these studies were continued and further developed by Bernheim and his fellow-workers, among whom the most noteworthy were Beaunis, professor of physiology at Nancy, and Liégeois, professor of jurisprudence in the same university. The researches undertaken during this period may be studied in the following publications: Beaunis' book, *Du somnambulisme provoqué* (1886); various articles by Liégeois, and in especial a memorial addressed to the Academy of Moral Sciences in 1884, entitled *De la suggestion hypnotique dans ses rapports avec le droit civil et le droit criminel;* above all, the second edition of Bernheim's book, which appeared in the year 1886.

These writings contain some interesting psychological studies—I may mention, in especial, Beaunis' examination of the memory of the carrying out of suggestions—but psychology is not the main concern of these authors. Their aim being to make a practical use of the power of suggestion, their chief endeavour is to demonstrate that power, and to ascertain its utmost limits. Especially they want to learn whether suggestion is capable of determining abnormal physiological phenomena which cannot be induced by the unaided action of the will; this would facilitate quite a number of practical applications, and would be a great safeguard against fraud. That is why Bernheim and his collaborators were so prompt in devoting their attention to *experiments in the production of blisters by suggestion.* As early as 1848, Charpignon declared that the skin could be reddened by imaginary blisters. In 1860, de Mirville asserted that phrases could thus be written in blood-red letters on the subject's arm—a contention concerning which a measure of scepticism may be permitted. Charcot, before Bernheim, had described the appearance of pemphigoid vesicles on a hysterical woman's arms after the suggestion of an imaginary burn. Bernheim, working in conjunction with Focachon, under fairly rigorous conditions, was able in a number of instances to obtain well-marked blisters by suggestion (pp. 77 and 83). Various other investigators worked along the same lines. During the years 1883 to 1885, Dumontpallier presented to the Academy of Medicine a series of observations upon the vasomotor action of suggestion. He reported that when a bland dressing, described as a blister, was applied to the leg, a rise in surface temperature amounting to 3° or 4° could subsequently be detected. Many others studied like phenomena, and in this connexion I may menion, the names of Pitres, Mabille, Ramadier, Bourru, Burot, Fontan, and Ségard. Good summaries of these investigations will be found in the writings of Bérillon [1] and Myers.[2] I do not think that they justify definite conclusions, but they contain a larger measure of truth than most people imagine.

The problem of criminal suggestion is an important subdepartment of the general field of suggestion. Is mere suggestion competent to make any one perform criminal actions which are out of keeping with his character and opposed to his interests ? The members of the Academic commission which reported on animal magnetism in 1787 (supra, p. 32) had already mooted this question. One of them asked Deslon whether magnetised subjects could be incited to crime ; the answer was in the affirmative. The question was subsequently discussed by Joseph Pierre Durand, by Bellanger (1854), by Brierre de Boismont (1855), Macario (1857), and Charpignon (1858). In 1860, the last-named published a work entitled *Les rapports du magnétisme avec la jurisprudence et la médicine légale.* In 1883, Bernheim returned to the question, and recorded the experiments which had led him to form an opinion : " Wishing to ascertain how far the power of suggestion could go, I one day staged a little drama for this

[1] Bérillon, " Revue de l'Hypnotisme," December 1887, p. 183.
[2] Proceedings of the Society for Psychical Research, vol. vii (1891–2), p. 337.

subject. I showed him an imaginary person standing in front of the door, and said this person had insulted him ; I then gave him a paper-knife, telling him it was a dagger, and ordering him to stab the offender. He leapt forward and stabbed fiercely at the door, and then stood rigid, wild-eyed, and trembling violently " (p. 34). At a later stage, this subject, one of the spectators having been transformed by suggestion into a magistrate, accused himself of the crime, but made no mention of the fact that its commission had been suggested to him. In the same connexion, Bernheim reproduces a note made by Prosper Despine in 1865, concerning a tramp who had taken advantage of a girl after throwing her into a strange condition which was supposed to have been a hypnotic trance. These possibilities of suggestion were, said Bernheim, most important and extremely dangerous.

Liégeois' memorial on the same question is even more complete. In a lengthy series of experiments, all perfectly successful, he suggested to hypnotised subjects a number of splendid crimes, which were savagely performed with wooden daggers and cardboard pistols. They could be made to perjure themselves, bearing false witness before some one promoted to the magistracy for the occasion. They could be made to sign cheques of fabulous value payable to Liégeois, and to give incredibly vast donations to this, that and the other. Obviously, all this showed the possibility of serious danger to the public. " To summarise this teaching," wrote Binet and Féré, " it was held that it would be possible to take any one haphazard, put him to sleep in a few seconds, in any odd corner, and send him to commit any imaginable crime." [1] Many authors whose names are mentioned by Liégeois, in an article in the " Revue Philosophique " (1892, vol i, p. 256), shared his view that these experiments were of great importance, and that the possibility of criminal suggestions was a grave menace to the public. " There are more than 10,000 persons in Paris to whom any sort of crime could be suggested by a word." Legislative reforms must instantly be undertaken to defend society against these dangers. Before being tried, every accused person ought to be hypnotised in order to ascertain whether the crime had been performed under the influence of suggestion.

[1] Le magnétisme animal, 1887, p. 273.

This interest in the problem of criminal suggestions was displayed by a good many of the writers who grouped themselves round Bernheim, but even more characteristic of this group was the desire to turn the influence of suggestion to immediate practical account for therapeutic purposes. The main reason why the second edition of Bernheim's book was so much larger than the first was, that it contained a great many reports of cures. Bernheim reminds us that in 1872 and 1873 Charcot had drawn attention to the miracles of St. Louis, and to the cure of cases of paralysis thanks to pilgrimages to the tomb of St. Denis after the mortal remains of Louis IX had been buried at that shrine. He quotes and discusses carefully chosen instances from among the recorded miracles at Lourdes, cures of paralysis, of imaginary hip-joint disease (p. 215), of amaurosis, of paraplegia (p. 217) ; and he expounds in this connexion the principles of suggestive therapeutics. " It is a physiological law that sleep [hypnosis] induces in the brain a psychical state in which the imagination accepts and recognises as real the impressions which are received by it. The role of hypnotic psychotherapeutics is, by hypnotism, to lead to the appearance of this peculiar psychical state, and to turn to account, in order to cure or to relieve, this artificially enhanced suggestibility " (p. 218). " Suggestion attacks the disease in one of its elements. The suppression of this morbid element has a happy influence upon the whole pathological apparatus, all of whose elements are reciprocally subordinated one to another " (p. 410). " Functional restoration leads to organic restoration " (p. 410). Furthermore, there are no dangers attendant upon the use of this valuable remedy ; or, if any troubles should arise owing to its employment, these can readily be cured by the use of suggestion, which is facilitated by the hypnotic state.

Bernheim goes on to record a number of his successes. He speaks of instant or speedy cures in hysterical disorders analogous to those treated in the same way by the practitioners of Charcot's school : restoration of cutaneous sensibility and of the visual functions by the use of a pretended magnet (pp. 285, 291, and 299) ; restoration of the power of walking in hysterical hemiplegia (pp. 293 and 305) ; cure of hysteroid crises by somnambulism (p. 302) ; cure of hysterical aphonia (pp. 212, 309, and 358). He passes on to relate the cure of various other neuropathic symptoms which, for reasons that are not given, he does not wish to term hysterical: gastric troubles (p. 317); loss of appetite, depression of spirits (p. 327); pains of various kinds (pp. 319, 320, and 325); tremors and choreic movements (pp. 332, 335, and 346); writer's cramp (p. 349); fixed ideas, sleepwalking (pp. 328 and 357). The pains and other troubles attendant on rheumatism are relieved in like manner. Finally, suggestion can do a great deal of good, even if it cannot cure, in serious disorders dependent upon unmistakable organic lesions of the central nervous system; for instance, in insular sclerosis (p. 235), locomotor ataxia (p. 275), and cerebral haemorrhage (pp. 267 and 272). " In a great many such cases, the functional disorder persists after the subsidence of the cause or the organic lesion which has given rise to them. . . . Certain pains are perpetuated after the lesion that first induced them has ceased to exist. . . . Thanks to this dynamogenic stimulation, the influence emanating from the brain is able to make its way once more to the motor nerve cells, and the reestablishment of conductivity leads to a restoration of function. . . . The possibility of impressing upon the joint the movements essential to its integrity, leads to a renewal of the suppleness of the fibro-serous tissues, gives rise to a fresh lubrication of the joint surfaces with synovial secretion, activates the capillary circulation, and by these means relieves or cures the joint trouble " (p. 410). To sum up: " Muscular pains, the ' painful points ' of consumptive patients, hysterical anaesthesia, the lightning pains of ataxics (sometimes), certain dynamic contractures resulting from organic affections of the nerve centres, certain movements which persist after an attack of chorea, nocturnal incontinence in children—will often disappear as if by magic thanks to a single suggestion or to quite a small number of suggestions " (p. 226).

This therapeutic method was received with enthusiasm and widely practised. The doctors of all lands began to publish reports of similar cases. I may mention, among these, the interesting work by Delboeuf, *De l'origine des effets curatifs de l'hypnotisme*, which appeared in the year 1887. As the starting-point of his argument Delboeuf refers to a burn due to suggestion, in which " the idea of the suffering has given rise to the disease " ; and he asks whether the absence of pain would not prevent the development of the disease.   In a remarkable series of experiments made upon persons who were good enough to submit to them, he cauterised both arms.   One of the burns was rendered insensitive by suggestion, the other being left painful.   He believed himself able to detect that the healing of the burn was far more rapid in the arm that had been rendered insensitive.   " Pain is the chief cause of disease " (p. 22) ; and it is upon pain that hypnotic suggestion has an especially powerful influence.

I may also refer to the investigations of Auguste Voisin concerning the use of suggestive therapeutics in mental disorders.[1]   His first observations related to four cases of hysterical delirium and to two cases of melancholic delirium with refusal of food.   He contended that the insane could be hypnotised even when suffering from delirium, and that their state could be completely modified by suggestions.

Interesting though these studies are, they do not suffice to give this group of workers a definite unity or a well-marked originality.   What characterised and integrated the members of the Nancy School was, as so often happens, the need for forming a united front against a common enemy.   Before all, the Nancy School was composed of those who were adversaries of the school of Charcot.

4. STRUGGLE BETWEEN THE TWO SCHOOLS.

In the first edition of his book, Bernheim wrote with studious moderation.   He quoted Charcot's experiments approvingly, and described them as " memorable."   His only criticism took the form of a statement, that, as far as he himself was concerned, when he was careful not to lead the subject to expect that contractions of the muscles would follow the application of pressure to the nerve supplying them—the musculospiral, the ulnar, or the facial nerve, as the case might be,—no such contractions ensued (p. 14).   He pointed out that suggestion might cause phenomena resembling those attributed to the magnet ; but he did not deny the activity of the magnet, and, indeed, was led by his own observations to regard that activity as important (p. 50).   Finally, while insisting that all the phenomena of hypnotism and suggestion could be induced in

[1] " Annales Médico-Psychologiques," 1884, vol. ii, pp. 150 and 285 ; 1886, p. 238.

normal persons, he was more disposed to speak of experiments made upon hysterics, and his most characteristic facts were derived from the study of such patients (pp. 4, 21, 25, 27, 40, and 48). At this date, then, there was no strong divergence between the outlooks of Charcot and Bernheim.

A few years later, Bernheim had become more aggressive. In the interim, Charcot's pupils, pushing their master's method to an extreme, had begun to publish more and more extraordinary observations. They described medicines that acted at a distance ; they cured patients by making these sit back-to-back with hysterics, and by then transferring the maladies to the hysterics through the influence of a magnet ; and so on. On the other hand, they attacked Bernheim's writings as unscientific, on the ground that Bernheim did not recognise Charcot's three states of major hypnotism. Liégeois' memorial to the Academy of the Moral Sciences concerning criminal suggestions had been criticised by Paul Janet, and criticised in a manner which left a good deal to be desired. Janet did not deal with essentials, but censured Liégeois for lack of precision, for having failed to watch for and describe in his subjects the positive signs of hypnosis standardised by the investigators of the Salpêtrière School. There was obviously good warrant for Bernheim's intervention.

In an article on the role of fear (1886), and, even more emphatically, in the second edition of his book on suggestion (1886), Bernheim made a definite attack on Charcot's teaching : " If, in our researches, we failed to take as our starting-point the three phases of hysterical hypnotism described by Charcot, this was because we were unable, by our own observations, to confirm their existence. We could not detect either neuromuscular hyperexcitability or exaggeration of the reflexes. . . . In all the states, the subject understands the operator perfectly well, and can be awakened by a word " (p. 93). " We were unable to ascertain that the action of opening or closing the subject's eyes, or friction of the vertex, modified the phenomena in any way ; or that in subjects who were not disposed to manifest certain phenomena under the sole influence of suggestion, such phenomena could be induced by any of the physical stimuli just mentioned " (p. 94). " Conversely, all the phenomena can be readily obtained when they are described in the subject's presence, and when the idea of them is allowed to permeate his

mind. Not only can all the classical effects of the magnet
be induced in this way, but the same thing applies to all the
varieties of transference. I say : ' I am going to move the
magnet, and when I do so there will be a transference from the
arm to the leg.' A minute later, the arm falls and the leg rises.
Without saying any more to the subject, I next move the
magnet back to the leg ; thereupon there is a fresh transference
from the leg to the arm. If, without disclosing the fact to the
subject, I substitute for the magnet a knife, a pencil, a bottle,
a piece of paper, or nothing at all—still the phenomena are
witnessed " (p. 98).

What inference should be drawn ? Sometimes Bernheim
hesitates : " I do not try to explain by suggestion the facts
recorded by other investigators ; all I say is that I have not
myself been able to produce the phenomena without suggestion " (p. 195). " If I am mistaken, if these phenomena
can occur as primary manifestations, in the entire absence of
suggestion, then it must be admitted that major hypnotism
is exceedingly rare. Binet and Féré tell us that during a
decade there have been only a dozen such cases at the
Salpêtrière. A dozen such cases among thousands upon thousands in which the phenomena have not been noted—does
this afford sufficient foundation for the theory of hypnosis ? "
(p. 95). Usually, however, his criticism is more direct. He
says that the Salpêtrière investigators were wrong in believing
themselves to have eliminated suggestion by dealing with
subjects in the state termed " lethargy," for in that state
the subject could hear perfectly well, though Charcot and his
associates thought otherwise. " Why should I conceal the
impression produced in my mind by the examination of a young
woman who had been in the Salpêtrière, and in whom all the
three states could be observed ? It seemed to me that she had
been subjected to a specialised training ; that, thanks to
unconscious suggestion, she was imitating the phenomena
exhibited in her presence by other somnambulists of the same
school ; that she had been drilled to reproduce, imitatively,
certain reflex phenomena in a typical order ; that she was not
a natural hypnotic, but *was suffering from a suggestive hysterical
neurosis* " (p. 95). By degrees, Bernheim became more
downright in his assertions. In an article remarkable for
clarity of style, published in the " Temps " on January 29,

1891, he concluded as follows : " The Nancy investigators draw the inference that all the phenomena witnessed at the Salpêtrière—the three phases, the neuromuscular hyperexcitability characteristic of the period of lethargy, the special form of contracture that is induced during what is styled somnambulism, transference under the influence of magnets—are non-existent when the experiments are made under conditions wherein suggestion can play no part. In other words, the subjects only manifest these phenomena when they know that such manifestations are expected of them ; when they have witnessed similar manifestations in others, or have heard talk of them ; in a word, when the idea of the phenomena has been introduced into their minds by suggestion. The hypnotism of the Salpêtrière is an artificial product, the outcome of training."

On another point Bernheim has become ever more insistent with the passing of the years. While he recognises that a predisposition to hypnotic states is well marked among hysterics, and that a mere trifle will suffice to induce somnambulism in such persons (p. 197), Bernheim reiterates that hypnosis is not a mere variety of hysteria, and is not a morbid state grafted upon the neuropathic temperament ; it is a physiological condition, with as good a title to that name as normal sleep ; it is, perhaps, a derivative of normal sleep, and it can be produced in the great majority of normal persons (p. 202). Statistics are unanswerable here. Of 1,000 persons whom Liébeault attempted to hypnotise in the year 1880, only 27 proved refractory. Every one of the others was more or less influenced. Substantially, this means that during that year Liébeault hypnotised all comers. Compare this with the results obtained at the Salpêtrière. There, in a decade, Charcot came across only a dozen cases of hypnotism. These numerical differences underline the contrast between the two schools. There were all the grounds for a formidable conflict.

Battle had been joined. Though their position had become untenable, Charcot's lieutenants continued to fight valiantly as long as their chief was still alive. The Salpêtrière was stoutly defended, and vigorous counter-attacks were delivered by Cullerre, Binet and Féré, Gilles de la Tourette, and Blocq (1889). One of the most interesting of such counter-attacks was an article by Babinski, which appeared in the " Gazette Hebdomadaire," in July 1891. The author showed how vague were the the psychological notions of the Nancy School, and how the Nancy investigators discerned suggestion everywhere without ever having been able to say precisely what suggestion was. Babinski likewise showed that Bernheim and his followers did not take enough account of hysteria, which in many of their cases played a larger part than they imagined.

In these skirmishes, the defenders of the Salpêtrière achieved a few partial successes. One of the most interesting was secured in the discussion concerning criminal suggestions. Gilles de la Tourette, in his book *L'hypnotisme et les états analogues au point de vue médico-légal* (1887), was the first, I believe, to make a very remarkable observation (p. 203). A number of persons of importance, magistrates and professors, had assembled in the main hall of the Salpêtrière museum to witness a great séance of criminal suggestions. Witt., the principal subject, thrown into the somnambulist state, had under the influence of suggestion displayed the most sanguinary instincts. At a word or a sign, she had stabbed, shot, and poisoned ; the room was littered with corpses, and Liégeois would have been in high glee. The notables had withdrawn, greatly impressed, leaving only a few students with the subject, who was still in the somnambulist state. The students, having a fancy to bring the séance to a close by a less blood-curdling experiment, made a very simple suggestion to Witt. They told her that she was now quite alone in the hall. She was to strip and take a bath. Witt., who had murdered all the magistrates without turning a hair, was seized with shame at the thought of undressing. Rather than accede to the suggestion, she had a violent fit of hysterics. The incident reminds us of a remark that had been made some years earlier by Maudsley. It is interesting to note, he said, that the hypnotised subject " will not commonly do an indecent or a criminal act ; the command to do it is too great a shock to the sensibilities of his brain, and accordingly arouses its suspended functions." [1]

Enlarging on this significant incident, Gilles de la Tourette makes a few reflections upon the ease with which purely fictitious crimes can be suggested, whereas it is difficult to make the subject carry out a suggestion of a much less serious char-

[1] The Pathology of Mind, 1879, p; 52.

acter when the suggested actions are real. These and similar arguments had an effect. Motet, G. Garnier, Brouardelle, and Maudsley were influenced by them, and were henceforward inclined to attach comparatively little importance to the theory that criminal suggestion might be a danger to society. Even Delboeuf, though he had been one of the first and most ardent defenders of the Nancy School, came to recognise that upon this point the teachings of the Nancy investigators had been much exaggerated, if not utterly fallacious. [1] Bramwell wrote bluntly : " While Bernheim considers the Salpêtrière subjects so abnormally acute that they can catch the slightest indications of the thoughts of the operator, . . . he, on the other hand, supposes the Nancy subjects to be so abnormally devoid of intelligence as to be unable to understand when a palpable farce is played before them." [2] Here were some successes for the Salpêtrière counter-offensive.

But everywhere else on the battlefield the Salpêtrière School sustained a defeat. Pitres reported that in Bordeaux he had been unable to find a single subject exhibiting the symptoms of classical hypnosis.[3] Régnard acknowledged that in certain cases the subjects in the state of lethargy could hear what was being said by the onlookers.[4] In 1886 I myself published an article in which I showed that many other hypnotic states could be observed in a hysteric besides the three states described by Charcot. [5] I shall return to this topic presently. For the nonce it is enough to say that my essay conveyed the idea that subjects could be drilled to exhibit all kinds of combinations of the symptoms studied at the Salpêtrière, and that there was therefore good reason to suppose these symptoms to be artificial. Pitres also recognised the possibility of such intermediate states.[6] Many, even among the partisans of Charcot, were prepared to agree with Tamburini and Soury,[7] that the three states included phenomena

---

[1] Delboeuf, " Revue Philosophique," 1887, vol. i, p. 133 ; ibid., 1889, vol. i, p. 510.

[2] What is Hypnotism ? Proceedings of the Society for Psychical Research, 1896–1897, p. 236.

[3] Leçons cliniques sur l'hystérie, 1891, vol. ii, p. 130.

[4] Régnard, op. cit., p. 234.

[5] Pierre Janet, Les états intermédiaires de l'hypnotisme, " Revue Scientifique," 1886.

[6] Op. cit., vol. ii, p. 132.

[7] " Revue de l'Hypnotisme," November 1891 ; Société d'Hypnologie, 1892.

belonging to hysteria rather than to hypnotism. Most other observers unhesitatingly accepted Bernheim's view, declaring that the phenomena observed at the Salpêtrière had been wholly due to injudicious suggestion and to the involuntary drilling of the patients.[1] Even Charcot's pupils recognised this by implication, for they no longer tried to defend the old positions, and withdrew from the field; but they have never frankly acknowledged their defeat, and I think that the day for such an acknowledgment is overdue. It is possible that a few hypnotised hysterics may manifest natural modifications of sensibility, abnormal motor reactions giving rise to cataleptic states, and a remarkable inclination to develop contractures under the influence of trifling stimuli; but the regular arrangement of these modifications in successive phases, as demonstrated in the dozen Salpêtrière patients, was unquestionably due to an injudicious drilling. As Bernheim first ventured to declare in 1884, Charcot's hypnotism in three phases was never anything more than a cultivated hypnotism. In this dispute between Bernheim and Charcot the former won the battle.

As far as pure science is concerned, this conclusion suffices, and " major hypnotism " has lost all semblance of interest. But from the historical outlook there is still a question to be considered, seeing that the foregoing conclusion does not explain why those who directed the Salpêtrière clinic should have compromised themselves in so strange an adventure. Let us admit that the three states were the outcome of suggestion and drill. Does it follow that Charcot, one fine day, deliberately made up his mind to invent the three states, and set himself to realise his mental picture of them by drilling Witt., Bar., and Glaiz. ? The contention would be absurd! What then, actually happened ? A first factor in the explanation can be found in the peculiar method of work which, unfortunately, is still in vogue at many of the Parisian medical clinics. The visiting physician rarely sees the patient in private. As a rule there is a public sitting. The chief has a circle of auditors, and the patient is presented by a house physician or by senior students who have carefully studied the case and have prepared the ground. Such a method may perhaps be tolerated where we have to do with a broken leg, but they

[1] Cf. Stanley Hall, 1890; Crocq, 1893.

are preposterous when we are concerned with psychological troubles. It is a remarkable fact that Charcot, whom the public believes to have been an arch-hypnotist, never hypnotised any one. The subjects brought to him for examination had been hypnotised time and again by others, and had been drilled to undergo a change of state at a sign from the professor. Charcot merely gave this sign. The subject, when apparently obeying Charcot, was in reality still under the tutelage of another person, under the direction of the true and only hypnotist. The first hypnotised subjects presented to Charcot had already been studied, and, therefore, mentally modified, by various medical practitioners whose names have previously been mentioned. Charcot had never studied psychiatry, but had been an anatomist and neurologist, and was blind to all the dangers of such a method. He had no notion of the proper way of studying anyone's mental condition. In his simplicity, it seemed to him that the best way would be to begin by examining sensation and reflex action, while leaving to a later stage the examination of the mind. But it is really impossible to study the sensations of a neuropath, his dispositions, even his most elementary actions, unless we know his mind, his sentiments, his ideas, his education, his relationships with other persons. Charcot's primary error in method played a considerable part in generating and perpetuating all the subsequent confusions.

But we have merely thrust the problem back a stage, and if we leave it there we shall be attributing to Charcot and his fellow-workers an absurdity which we have no wish to impute. Can we suppose that Charcot's collaborators, who have since then done much excellent scientific work, deliberately invented the three states, and drilled the subjects to exhibit them—thus not only deceiving Charcot but compromising themselves ? The theory cannot be sustained for an instant ; and we still have to enquire, What was the origin of the three states ?

If the reader will permit a personal reminiscence, I shall be able, I fancy, to throw some light on the problem. At this date, from 1883 to 1889, I was teacher of philosophy in the State secondary school at Havre. I was studying all the phenomena of pathological psychology, and in especial those of hypnotism, sometimes at the hospital, where M. Powilewicz was good enough to give me the run of his clinic, and sometimes in connexion with the private practice of M. Gibert. Not having received any instruction from the exponents of either the Salpêtrière School or the Nancy School, I independently came to the conclusion that Charcot was wrong. Upon many of the patients I was able to examine, I found it possible to verify Bernheim's assertion. Major hypnotism was not a natural product. Those who wished to rediscover it must suggest it to patients, and must drill them in a peculiar way. I expounded this view as early as 1889, in my book *L'automatisme psychologique* (p. 47). But certain doubts were left in my mind by the observations I had made in one of my subjects, only one, a woman of forty-five who passes in my writings by the name of Léonie. She was one of Gibert's patients, and before she came under my observation she had been hypnotised by him by the methods of animal magnetism. In this patient I was able to note definite phases of hypnotic sleep ; phases in which various reactions could be induced, such as cataleptic postures, and contractures brought about sometimes by the percussion of muscles or tendons and sometimes by merely stroking the skin. No doubt, many of the details were not wholly accordant with those that had been noted at the Salpêtrière. Stimulation of the muscles during the cataleptic phase did not bring about paralyses ; there were no " etats dimidiés " ; the phases were more complex, and there were transitional forms in which the symptoms of the two states tended to become confused. It was when studying these transitions that I became aware of the existence of intermediate states, such as a state half way between lethargy and catalepsy, in which the patient would remain for a considerable time, while exhibiting symptoms both of lethargy and of catalepsy. This was the topic of my paper contributed to the " Revue Scientifique " in 1886. Still, Léonie certainly presented the essentials of Charcot's three states, and I could not deny the reality of these unless I could account for Léonie.

The most obvious explanation would be to suppose that I had myself, inadvertently, drilled the subject to produce them. I should have no false shame in admitting the fact, for I know how hard it is to avoid such mistakes ; but unfortunately the explanation lacks credibility. In a great many other subjects, studied in exactly the same way, nothing of the kind had happened. Moreover, I had already acquired the habit of taking full notes of what occurred at such séances, recording not only my own utterances but also the doings of the subject ; and I can find nothing in my notes indicating that Léonie was drilled in any way by me. I do find definite indications in my notes which lead me to suppose that I may have encouraged the subject to give a clearer demonstration of these transitional phases between the phenomena of lethargy and those of catalepsy. But I did actually record the existence of these transitions, of these peculiar neuromuscular symptoms, at the very outset of my study of Léonie. At the first sitting, when Gibert was demonstrating the case to me, before I had taken a hand in the game, I noted the spontaneous stages of lethargy and somnambulism. In subsequent sittings, directly I began to touch the subject, I was able to observe induced contractures and catalepsy. If I were not responsible, can we attribute the drilling to Gibert, who had repeatedly thrown the subject into the somnambulist state long before I first saw her. This hypothesis, likewise, lacks plausibility. Gibert was interested in very different problems. He disdained the study of the elementary phenomena presented by somnambulists, and had known nothing about Charcot's teaching when Léonie first came under his notice. He was very much surprised when Léonie passed into the cataleptic state because her eyes were opened. How could he have taught the somnambulist to play such tricks ? By these considerations I was led to think that the training, the drilling, of Léonie must have taken place, not only before she came into contact with me, but before she came into contact with Gibert. I realised that we ought to know the entire life history of an individual whom we wish to use as a subject in psychological researches.

Now Léonie, who had been born in the neighbourhood of Caen in the year 1838, had had a strange and eventful life If I had been able to collect all the necessary data, I should have written her biography, for it would throw much light upon a remarkable period in the history of magnetism in France. A sleepwalker since early childhood, she began at puberty to exhibit graver hysterical symptoms. Soon she attracted the attention of certain medical practitioners interested in animal magnetism—for, as I said above, there was a flourishing school of magnetism at Caen towards 1850. She had played the part of an ultra-lucid somnambulist, and had even been employed to guide some treasure-hunting excavations among the foundations of an ancient and ruined castle. In an extraordinary little book by de Baïssas, entitled *Les trésors du Château de Crèvecoeur*, 1867, the inquisitive may read how Léonie was half buried in the cellarage so that she might feel more acutely the proximity of the hidden gold. Later, she had been exhaustively examined by Perrier of Caen, who had found her one of his most instructive cases ; and she had even had the honour of being magnetised and exhibited by Dupotet.

To solve our problem, we should have to know exactly what happened at the sittings with Perrier, and what symptoms Léonie presented at that epoch. In conversation with me, she insisted that Perrier had written a book on her case, that it had been published somewhere about 1863, and that its title had been " Exercise somnambulique par le Docteur X." The frontispiece had been a portrait of " Léonie, the Somnambulist." Despite my best endeavours, I have been unable to find any trace of such a work, and I am inclined to think that it can never have existed outside of Léonie's imagination. But I am greatly indebted to Perrier's son for having placed at my disposal a number of records of the father's sittings, manuscript notes taken with scrupulous care by the magnetiser during the actual progress of the observations. I have also had the advantage of reading the articles contributed by Perrier to Dupotet's " Journal du Magnétisme." I have thus been able to learn that in 1860, and even earlier, Perrier was distinguishing phases in the hypnotic sleep of his subjects, and was already characterising them by modifications of sensibility, by cataleptic postures, and by reflex contractures initiated by various stimuli. The hypnotic phenomena exhibited to me by Léonie in 1884 were vestiges of the "somnambulic exercises" that had been made under Perrier's guidance in 1860.

A new and amazing outlook on the problem is thus disclosed. The phases of major hypnotism existed long before Charcot turned his attention to the matter, and on further enquiry we learn that the early animal magnetisers must have been familiar with them. Beyond question, traces of these phenomena can be discovered in very early books indeed. In 1787, Petetin was describing three phases of the magnetic state, one of them being an artificially induced catalepsy. Charles Despine, in 1840, divided the crisis displayed by his subject Estelle into three periods : dead or passive somnambulism ; catalepsy, with the maintenance of postures, the imitation of movements, and echo-speech (echolalia) ; and active somnambulism with spontaneity and an understanding of spoken words.[1] Teste, in his *Le magnétisme animal expliqué* (1845, pp. 304 and 329), likewise distinguishes three phases : dreams with immobility ; somniloquence ; and lucid somnambulism. Sensory and motor conditions differed in these three states.

The same classification was adopted by Baragnon (*Etude du magnétisme*, 1853). Hébert, of Gurnay, in his *Petit catéchisme magnétique* (1855, p. 29), describes five states, the last three of these being lethargic drowsiness, somnambulism, and ecstasy with the maintenance of postures.[2] Nay more, in Puel's treatise, *De la catalepsie* (1855) we find the description of a paralysis which can be brought about in the cataleptic state by rubbing the muscles and tendons, the symptoms being identical with those described by Paul Richer.[3] Dupotet, in his *Manuel de l'étudiant magnétiseur* (1846), describes analogous phases, and tells us that the rubbing of various parts of the head (especially the vertex) is a good way of inducing the change from one state to another. To sum up, though we do not find a verbatim anticipation of Charcot's teachings in these books on magnetism, we find a sufficient number of the elements of that teaching to enable us to affirm that the doctrine of the three states and of the physical modifications characteristic of them derives from the old theory and practice of animal magnetism. Is it not rather quaint to find that during the years 1878 to 1882 Charcot was presenting to the Academy of Sciences what he believed to be fresh physiological discoveries destined to discredit for ever the claims of the magnetisers, when in reality he was merely reproducing the

---

[1] Op. cit., pp. 45, 146, and 169.
[2] " Journal du Magnétisme," vol. xiv, p. 364.
[3] Cf. "Mémoires de l'Académie de Médecine," xx, 1856. Pitres, op. cit., vol. ii, p. 122, has been beforehand with me in drawing attention to this remarkable little treatise.

century-old teaching of these same magnetisers? It would be very difficult to ascertain how these doctrines came to form a part of magnetist teaching, and perhaps the research would be of little interest. Probably the magnetisers began by studying the degrees of drowsiness, and by examining the gradual advance of lucidity in the more and more intense phases of somnambulism to which Puységur and Deleuze were already referring. The theory was given definite shape by the noting of certain hysterical phenomena that are apt to accompany the phases of sleep or awakening. A certain fixity was then given to the doctrine through the handing on of the teaching, and probably also by the drilling of the subjects. What we are really concerned to know is how the teaching of the magnetisers had been able to make its way into the Salpêtrière. The fact is, that the intrusion had taken place long before Charcot's day. Husson, and subsequently Dupotet and many others, had made experiments in various clinics, although the visiting physicians were not always aware of what was going on. Enquiring and critical students attended lectures on magnetism, and particularly those of Dupotet at the Palais Royal. A noted magnetiser, the Marquis de Puyfontaine, had even been introduced into Charcot's own clinic, and had been in touch with several of Charcot's collaborators. It was with Puyfontaine's aid and under his guidance that were made the preliminary experiments to which I have already referred. The experimenters wanted to be in a position to show Charcot the most characteristic phenomena, to demonstrate the ones that would be most striking to a man accustomed to precise neurological observations. Certain changes of state, certain simple and interesting reactions, were induced again and again in the subjects by persons who were quite unaware that they were drilling their patients. Charcot, when the subjects were finally exhibited to him in public, discussed the phenomena openly in their presence, and this served to fix the symptoms yet more firmly. The results are on record.

The struggle between the Salpêtrière School and the Nancy School was but an episode in the great war that began in 1787 between the fluidists and the animists. The animists were the winners in this bout. When will the next bout come, and who are to be the winners in the long run?

5. RISE AND FALL OF HYPNOTIC SUGGESTION.

For the time being, the conquerors made the most of their victory. Everywhere, abroad as well as in France, there was from 1888 to 1896 what may be called a luxuriant blossoming of suggestive therapeutics. In France, there were now periodicals specially devoted to the question, such as Bérillon's " Revue de l'Hypnotisme," and the " Revue des Sciences Hypnotiques," which began publication on July 1, 1887. Furthermore, in the neurological, general medical, and philosophical press, in medical theses, and in numerous volumes, there were now reported a multitude of cures of all possible diseases by simple verbal suggestion, sometimes under hypnosis and sometimes in the waking state.

Many of the cures were still cases of neuropathic troubles. Joffroy cured hysterics suffering from convulsions or paralyses ; Blanche Edwards was successful in relieving hitherto intractable vomiting ; Babinski dealt with cases of abasia associated with agoraphobia, and wrote interestingly about the alternation of hysterical and hypnotic states.[1] Gilles de la Tourette showed how readily hypnotism could cure spontaneous sleepwalking. Pitres stressed the importance of suggestion in the treatment of hysterical anorexia. In " Brain " (1893, p. 207), he gave an interesting report on the treatment of an attack of lethargy ; from the outset of the attack he induced hypnosis, in which the patient remained subject to his guidance, and which he was able to interrupt at will. Fontan and Ségard, in a volume devoted to suggestive therapeutics,[2] noted that in neurotics physical troubles were more amenable to treatment than mental troubles. Ballet, Dumontpallier, Cullerre, Sollier, Briand, Laloy, and many others, reported cures of all kinds of seizures, delusions, and paralyses. Mesnet described the performance of surgical operations under hypnosis.[3]

Voisin, in especial, continued the application of suggestive therapeutics to the relief of mental disorders. At the Munich Congress, in 1892, he gave an account of the treatment of certain forms of mental alienation by hypnotic suggestion. Cullerre reported similar facts. Goroditche used the method

---

[1] Congrès de Psychologie, 1889 ; " Gazette Hebdomadaire," 1891, p. 15.
[2] Elements de médecine suggestive, etc., 1887.
[3] Académie de Médecine, July 30, 1889.

in claustrophobia and other forms of obsession, declaring that almost all neurasthenics could readily be hypnotised. Bérillon and Mavroukakis were equally successful in the treatment of agoraphobia in degenerates.

Although it was not contended that organic diseases of the nervous system could in every case be perfectly cured, still it was claimed that they could be much mitigated, and that the majority of their most painful symptoms could be entirely relieved. Fontan and Ségard cured attacks of hemiplegia consequent upon cerebral haemorrhage, and paralyses due to different forms of myelitis. At the Alienists, Congress in Bordeaux, on August 5, 1895, Bérillon read a paper on the treatment of locomotor ataxia by hypnotic suggestion.

Nor did the enthusiasts for suggestive therapy confine their attention to nervous disorders. All kinds of other visceral diseases were treated in like manner. Gibert of Havre, and after him a good many others, described the cure of warts by suggestion. Auguste Voisin, in especial, extolled the use of suggestion in uterine troubles ; surgical operations could be facilitated by suggestion, which induced anaesthesia and had a calmative influence ; childbirth ran an easy course under hypnotic suggestion ; and so on.

There was also a noteworthy movement in favour of applying hypnotic suggestion to children for educational purposes. Guyau was one of the first to point out the analogy between suggestion and instinct, and to speak of the possibility of utilising suggestion as a form of moral therapeutics for " the correction of abnormal instincts, or for the strengthening of normal instincts, that are too weak." Every suggestion, added Fouillée, was an instinct created by hypnotism, but in the nascent state.[1] Delboeuf, too, regarded hypnotism as a potent means of education and moralisation.[2] Bérillon took this notion to heart, and became a propagandist in favour of suggestive pedagogy ; he treated the bad habits of children by suggestion, dealing thus with nail-biting, incontinence of urine, idleness, untruthfulness, etc. P. F. Thomas confirmed the statement that suggestion had an important part to play

[1] Fouillée, Enseignement, p. 5.
[2] " Revue Philosophique," 1888, vol. ii, p. 171.

in education [1]; and as late as 1897 Pigeaud penned a thesis on the pedagogical use of suggestion. Bourdon of Méru wrote of the use of suggestive pedagogy in various difficulties of speech and aberrations of character.[2] These pedagogical applications reinforced the importance of suggestive therapy.

From France the movement spread rapidly to neighbouring lands. We have already noted Delboeuf's activities in Belgium, which led many other doctors to experiment with the new cure-all. In Switzerland, hypnotic suggestion was first turned to account by Auguste Forel; then by Ladame, who paid particular attention to the treatment of topers and dipsomaniacs by hypnotism.[3] Forel's important work, *Der Hypnotismus, etc.* (1889, third edition 1895), did much to spread Bernheim's teaching in Switzerland and subsequently in Germany, undermining faith in Charcot's doctrine, which had at first secured general acceptance.

In Germany there was now an extensive spread of interest in the topic. Albert Moll's important book supplemented that of Forel, and accelerated the impetus of suggestive therapeutics. In the " Neurologisches Zentralblatt " (1887), Richard Schultz drew attention to the curative efficiency of hypnotism, and recorded the cure of a patient who had suffered from hysterical paralysis for two years. In 1888, Max Dessoir published a bibliography of recent works on hypnotism; it was already extensive, enumerating 800 books, written by 500 authors.[4] Ewald Hecker of Wiesbaden, writing in 1892, advocated the complete distraction of the patient's mind from every thought of illness; this, he said, would cure all the sufferer's troubles. Schrenck-Notzing especially recommended the use of suggestion for the relief of neurasthenia; he sent out to medical practitioners a well-designed questionnaire asking each of his correspondents to report upon the method employed to induce hypnosis, the effect of this, cures, relapses, etc. In 1892, J. Grossmann founded the " Zeitschrift für Hypnotismus, Suggestionslehre, Suggestionstherapie und verwandte psychologische Forschungen," which played a considerable part in the German development of hypnotism. Among its

[1] " Revue Philosophique," 1895, vol. ii, p. 97.
[2] " Revue de l'Hypnotisme," 1897, p. 45.
[3] " Revue de l'Hypnotisme," 1888, pp. 129 and 165.
[4] Bibliographie des modernen Hypnotismus, Duncker, Berlin, 1888.—In 1890 there was a supplement, containing nearly 400 additional entries.

contributors were Forel, Freund, Hirt, Möbius, Moll, Schrenck-Notzing, and Sperling. In 1894, Grossmann, having circulated a questionnaire, published the answers in a work entitled *Die Bedeutung der hypnotischen Suggestion als Heilmittel.* Here we find declarations from twenty-eight specialists in diseases of the nervous system who extol the curative value and the moral worth of the new method of treatment. Works by a number of other authors might be added to the list, to give an adequate idea of the vogue of suggestive therapy in Germany at this epoch. Suffice it to mention the names of Hugo Harck (1896) ; Jolly (1894) ; Tatzel (1894) ; Tauscher (1898) ; Hoffmann (1899) ; Falk ; Schupp ; and Weygandt.

Turning to Holland, I must speak of Arie de Jong's *Het Hypnotismus,* and must above all refer to the work of Van Eeden and Van Renterghem in Amsterdam. A statistical account of the remarkable cures obtained by the two last-named was read at the Congress of Hypnology held in Paris in the year 1889. It need hardly be said that to these authorities hypnosis was a condition entirely free from morbidity ; there was nothing in suggestive therapy of which patients need be afraid. Cure was achieved simply by the ideoplastic force of ideas. " Mind is not subtilised matter ; psychic forces are new and unknown forces, the attributes of living matter." In 1894, Van Renterghem established a clinic whither numberless patients came in search of health. At first he worked in public, hypnotising his patients in batches. After a time, when the well-to-do began to seek his aid, he found it desirable to split up the room into cubicles, and to treat each patient separately. The results were equally good in either case. In 1907, at the last Amsterdam Congress, Van Renterghem, still faithful to his principles, continued to maintain that in medicine an important place must be assigned to suggestion, which made its appeal to a normal and universal faculty of the brain ; that of suggestibility. " We must put into the sufferer's mind the mental image of cure, for that will disperse his functional troubles ; this is nothing more than an application of ideodynamism, the capacity of the brain to receive and evoke and realise ideas." [1]

At a later stage, in connexion with the topic of artificially prolonged sleep [hypnosis], it will be necessary to allude to

---

[1] Comtes rendus du Congrès de Neurologie d'Amsterdam, 1907, p. 858.

the important work of Wetterstrand in Sweden. In Italy, Bianchi and Sciammana found hypnotism of little value in hysteria, but extremely useful in other diseases. Fianzi took the precisely opposite view, regarding hypnotic suggestion as indispensable for the cure of hysterical disorders.[1] As far as suggestive therapy in Greece is concerned, I may mention the names of Rinaldi and Caryophilis. Turning to Russia, in 1893 Theodor Shogentsy recorded the cure of cases of astasia-abasia by suggestion. At the same date, Tokarsky discussed the role of suggestion, and stated that in many cases the method was ineffective. The most important Russian contribution to the topic was one published by Bechterew in 1894, on hypnosis and its importance as a method of treatment. This author regarded hypnotism as essentially a means by which physiological changes in the respiration and circulation could be induced. Also he noted that hypnotic suggestion had a marked influence upon menstruation, upon all diseases of the nervous system, and even upon infectious disorders; he likewise employed it in a case of tubercular lesions of the lumbar region of the spinal cord. In 1895, Bechterew studied the difficulties that may arise in the induction of hypnosis,[2] and described the effects which he had found hypnotic suggestion to have upon all kinds of neuropathic symptoms. In 1899 he was still insisting that hypnotic suggestion was the only dependable way of treating obsessions and unhappy illusions. Before closing the list of Russian investigators I must add the names of Rybakoff, who wrote concerning hypnotism in the treatment of mental disorders; Orlitzy, of Moscow; and Zagailoff.

I think that treatment by hypnotic suggestion made its way tardily into English-speaking lands, and that this may be the reason why the wave subsided there rather more slowly than elsewhere. I will mention first a book published in 1893 by R. Harry Vincent, entitled *The Elements of Hypnotism, its Danger and Value*. Very important was the work of Charles Lloyd Tuckey. This author began with a study of the value of hypnotism in the treatment of chronic alcoholism.[3] Then came his book *Treatment by Hypnotism and Suggestion*. Con-

---

[1] Comptes rendus du Congrès de Rome, 1895.
[2] " Revue Neurologique," 1895, p. 47.
[3] Comptes rendus du Congrès de Munich, 1892.

siderably later, in Parker's symposium *Psychotherapy* (1909), we find him among the rare authors who are still defending hypnotic suggestion ; it can be used to annul fear, which, as Mrs. Eddy rightly contends, is a potent factor of disease; it can influence for the better the distribution of nervous energies. Milne Bramwell's admirable studies began with a contribution to " Brain " in 1896, and to the Proceedings of the Society for Psychical Research in the same year (p. 178) ; he contributed to the discussions at the Brussels Congress in 1897, and to Parker's *Psychotherapy* in 1909 ; and his *Hypnotism* (1903, etc.) is a standard work which has run through several editions. Bramwell stresses the historical outlook, which is so often neglected, and he has devoted considerable attention to the work of James Braid. He is, however, also interested in the practical use of hypnotism, concentrating attention upon morbid dreams in order to teach the patient how to disregard them, and in order to inculcate calm and concentration of mind.

In the United States, hypnotism properly so called has had much less vogue than Christian Science and psychotherapy by moralisation. Still, it has its place in the writings of Russell Sturgis,[1] S. Warren,[2] Sydney Flower,[3] and Osgood Mason.[4] These researches have been continued of late years by Boris Sidis and Morton Prince, whose works we shall have to study presently when we come to consider the practical application of such methods. In South America, in 1894, A. Moraga described the cure of a case of hysterical facial paralysis by suggestion. Quite recently, J. Antonio Agrelo, in the " Archivos de Psiquiatria " of Buenos Ayres, gives a definite place, though not a very large one, to hypnotic suggestion among psychotherapeutic methods.

In this cursory and fragmentary review I have made no attempt to mention the names of all of those who have published important works during the period under consideration. My only aim has been to give the reader an impression of the vast development undergone for a dozen years by the

[1] The Use of Hypnotism in the First Degree as a Means of Modifying or Eliminating a Fixed Idea, " Boston Medical and Surgical Journal," 1894.

[2] Autohypnotism, " Medical News," 1898.

[3] Hypnotism or Psychotherapy ?, " Pacific Medical Journal," San Francisco, 1898.

[4] Hypnotism and Suggestion in therapeutic Education and Reform, New York, 1901.

therapeutic method first formulated at Nancy. It spread all over the world ; and if we are to believe the authors who have reported on the subject, numberless cures must be placed to its credit.

The reader must not imagine that the numerous works on hypnotism poured forth from the press during the period we have been considering were written with a sole eye to treatment, or that all those who were studying hypnotism were blind adherents of one or other of the rival schools, were partisans of Charcot or of Bernheim. I have already pointed out that towards the year 1880 there appeared a new trend which might be called the school of Charles Richet were it not that the members of the school preserved their independence too fully to be labelled in this way. Like Richet, they wished to study suggestion and hypnotism for themselves, to understand it for themselves, and by their own exertions to discover its psychological laws. The history of this school belongs rather to the history of psychology than to that of psychotherapeutics ; but in due course it came into close touch with the science of medicine, for an intelligent application of hypnotism to the treatment of disease was only rendered possible by the work of psychologists. The most notable names among those who followed up this line of investigation, after Richet, are those of Myers, Gurney, Stanley Hall, Möbius, Ochorowicz, Forel, Beaunis, Binet, and Féré. I should like to associate with the work of this group my own studies published in the " Revue Philosophique " from 1886 onwards, and summarised in two of my books, L'automatisme psychologique, 1889, and L'état mental des hystériques, 1892. These studies were concerned with the relationships between the modifications of sensibility on the one hand, and those of attention, memory, and personality on the other ; with the various conditions in which transformations of the personality are to be observed ; with dreams, and all the varieties of somnambulism ; with the nature and factors of suggestion ; with subconscious actions, automatic writing, and so on—in a word, with all the varieties of psychological automatism.

The investigators just named, myself included, in their study of normal and pathological psychology, did not wholly approve what they regarded as the immoderate claims of the healers, what they regarded as premature attempts at the immediate application of half-developed notions to the cure of all diseases. But they thought that these applications of hypnotism were only in an initial stage, and that by degrees they would be modified so as to become more scientific. They fancied they were working at something which, though it had the imperfections of youth, had also the advantages of youth, and was destined to be long-lived. But something happened which neither the healers nor the psychologists had foreseen. Hypnotism had no time to undergo the expected modifications ; it speedily perished, or vanished from the stage.

After Charcot's death, which occurred in 1892, it seemed as if the rival doctrine of Bernheim ought to undergo enormous expansion. Nothing of the kind happened. After hypnotism had remained in a stationary position for a few years, it under- went a rapid decline. This decline began in France and the neighbouring lands of Belgium and Switzerland, the three countries where hypnotism had taken its rise. It was natural that those who were working at the Salpêtrière should have nothing more to do with studies that had turned out so badly, and after Charcot's death I was almost the only one to retain interest in the matter. But the astonishing fact is that the same thing happened in other medical circles. No one repudiated hypnotism, no one denied the power of suggestion ; people simply ceased to talk about hypnotism and suggestion. The number of publications devoted to these topics declined enormously, as may be learned from the indexes compiled and published annually by Ebbinghaus and by Baldwin. Whereas in previous years the books and articles concerning hypnotism, suggestion, and allied subjects had been numbered by thousands per annum, the number now fell to a few dozens. The German and Belgian periodicals which had proudly styled themselves " hypnological reviews," realising that the wind had changed, hastened to modify their titles. They became " neurological reviews," though a sense of shame led them to retain "hypnology" in a subtitle for a time. But, after a while, the subtitle was quietly dropped.

The vogue of hypnotism continued somewhat longer in foreign lands, which are apt to lag behind in their adoption of the Paris fashions. In Switzerland, Forel was still writing about suggestive therapeutics in the " Revue Médicale de la

Suisse Romande" as late as the year 1899. Even at the time when I am writing, Bonjour of Lausanne continues to treat his patients hypnotically, and fights vigorously against Dubois' rationalising psychotheraphy.[1] In Great Britain, Milne Bramwell stands almost alone to-day in defending hypnotic suggestion under its true name. In the United States, Boris Sidis, writing in the " Boston Medical and Surgical Journal" for August and September 1909, still speaks of the psycho-therapeutic value of hypnotism; but, as we shall see presently, he does not rate its worth very high. In Germany, Müller, Vogt (1909), Frank (1902), and Gumpers (1903), have not ceased to speak of the curative efficacy of hypnotic suggestion. In Russia, Bechterew and Narbut champion hypnotic sugges-tion, and so does Ingegnieros in Buenos Ayres; but these are brave and isolated devotees.

Still more characteristic of the decline of the method is the tone apt to be assumed by medical practitioners, and even by those who are specially interested in psychotherapeutics when they have occasion to speak of hypnotism. We used to be told that hypnotic treatment was simple, harmless, universally assessible. Now we learn that it is a dangerous method, though useful for the relief of certain neuropathic disorders. It would be a mistake to condemn it openly, but we must be slow to commend it. In 1902, Raymond was insisting on the dangers of hypnotism; next year, Cullerre drew up a more formidable indictment.[2] Especially quaint were the accusations of immorality which even medical prac-titioners brought against hypnotism. In 1890, those of us who wished to hypnotise our patients had sometimes to contend with the moral or religious prejudices of his relatives, and perhaps found it necessary to ask leave of priest or pastor. These latter, as a rule, were liberal enough, for they soon came to realise that the use of hypnotic suggestion was no more immoral than the use of chloroform or morphine. Yet, a few years later, our medical colleagues were proving less liberal-minded than the churchmen had been, and were accusing hypnotism of all kinds of immorality. Poor old hypnotism !

Most of these moralists charge hypnotism with lowering the moral dignity of the patient. Paul Dubois tells us that

---

[1] " Revue de l'Hypnotisme," 1906, p. 359.
[2] ' Annales Médico-Psychologiques," September 1903, p. 247.

suggestion appeals only to the automatic tendencies of the patient ; not to his reason, to his will, to the most exalted elements of his personality. Since, we gather, the automatic tendencies are much lower than reason and will, hypnotic treatment stands at a very low level from the moral point of view. Camus and Pagniez declare : " The cure of the patient who has been treated by suggestion will not be voluntary enough or meritorious enough ; the patient will not have learned to perform Actions in the full sense of the term, and we therefore run the risk of degrading him." Nay more, we are led to infer that such methods of treatment lower the moral dignity of the doctor too, since he makes use of a base and vulgar method. Dubois considers that suggesters are posing as miracle-mongers ; and we may remember that he is inclined to blush because he has himself had recourse to suggestion in the case of a child given to bed-wetting. Richard C. Cabot has an uneasy conscience. He asks whether the administering of bread pills and similar placebos is not a subtle form of lying. Even to save a man's life, Cabot would hesitate to assure him that a pill contained an active medicament when it really contained nothing of the sort.[1] Parker's *Psychotherapy* is full of similar attacks on hypnotism. One more pearl will suffice. J. R. Angell of Chicago sadly remarks that there is great danger attaching to such methods of treatment, for there is a serious risk that the patient may have recourse to a quack.[2] It would seem, then, that there is no such danger as far as other methods of treatment are concerned ?

Attacked in this way and abandoned by its own supporters, poor old hypnotism was unable to defend itself. It took to wearing a mask, or made itself very small, in the hope of being tolerated. Boris Sidis thinks that hypnosis, being difficult to induce and having a bad name among patients, may usefully be replaced by an equivalent state which he terms " hypnoidisation," and describes as being characterised by a restriction of the activity of the brain. The condition is remarkable for instability ; it is a light sleep whose intensity varies from moment to moment.[3] Paul Emile Lévy renounces hypnotism ; he is content to place one of his hands on the patient's forehead,

[1] Veracity and Psychotherapy, in Parker's Psychotherapy, I, iii, 23.
[2] Psychotherapy, I, i, 68.
[3] Sidis, The psychotherapeutic Value of the hypnoidal State, see Psychotherapeutics, a Symposium, p. 124.

while recommending the sufferer to lie still and to concentrate the mind. He goes too far for the strict moralisers. Dubois is dissatisfied, and says that these methods, modest though they may seem, betray the influence of Bernheim's teaching.[1] But even Bernheim has given up the game. No longer does he speak of "rotatory automatism" or of "negative hallucinations." The man who was always repeating that hypnotism was everything, now declares that hypnotism is nothing.[2] Indeed, he admits (with good reason) that there was a certain lack of precision about what he used to understand by the term suggestion, that a great many other kinds of moral influence played their part. He reminds us that he had himself written : " Mere words do not always suffice to impose an idea ; sometimes we must reason, demonstrate, convince ; some patients require forcible affirmation, whilst others are more powerfully influenced by gentle insinuation."[3] Is not this identical with the "persuasion" of to-day ? Bernheim, the arch-hypnotist, has become a simple moraliser, and is towing in the wake of his whilom pupil Dubois.

In these circumstances, why go on talking about hypnotism and suggestion ? Now and again a patient with an intractable malady, one suffering from delusion of persecution or some other form of obsession, one belonging to the very type of those who are not hypnotisable, will come to a doctor and ask to be cured by hypnotism. The doctor will receive such a patient with indulgent contempt, feeling that he would compromise himself to-day by a practice which twenty years ago was a cure-all. As a final catastrophe, Bérillon's "Revue de l'Hypnotisme" abandoned the name it had borne with so much courage for twenty years. With the July issue of 1910 it became a commonplace psychotherapeutic periodical. Hypnotism is quite dead—until the day of its resurrection.

Such a decadence, so rapid a disappearance after such high enthusiasms and such extensive developments, is certainly surprising. Those of a future day who are interested in the history of medicine will study this period with much curiosity, and will discover many cogent reasons to account for the sharp

---

[1] Parker's Psychotherapy, II, iv, 22 and 25.
[2] Bernheim, Congrès des Sociétés Savantes, Nancy, 1901.
[3] La suggestion, p. 227.

curve in medical theory and practice. For my own part, I have no such ambition, and am content to regard the decline of hypnotism as one of those transient eclipses to which the whole psychotherapeutic movement has been prone. But I can see two likely factors of this particular eclipse.

In the first place there can be no doubt that the struggle between the Salpêtrière School and the Nancy School was most unfortunate for hypnotism. Why it was disastrous will become plain if we consider the actual results of the struggle. Charcot had undertaken the study of hypnotism in a frame of mind which had been lacking to the magnetisers of a generation or two earlier ; he had a scientific bent, a fondness for accuracy and method, a sense of determinism. It seemed to him essential that we should know what we were talking about, and be able to understand one another when we were speaking of these obscure phenomena, and for that reason he insisted upon studying clear-cut symptoms with the aid of strict definitions. He wanted to be able to make scientific predictions ; and he aimed at formulating the laws in accordance with which one phenomenon appeared as the sequel of another.[1] These were good intentions. Other persons with a scientific spirit were charmed, and for a brief space forgot their dislike for induced somnambulism. Unfortunately, Charcot had made a very serious mistake in believing that hypnotic phenomena were simple physiological happenings akin to those he was used to studying in cases of insular sclerosis or locomotor ataxia, and in believing that an examination of the modifications of the reflexes that occurred in his hypnotised subjects would provide the data on which he could base the definitions and the laws of which he was in search. Bernheim, on the other hand, guided by the successors of the old-time animists, was well aware that hypnotism was a mental phenomenon and that its problems were psychological. Upon this fundamental point, right was on his side, and that gave him an easy victory.

The victory was unwelcome, to the scientific world at any rate ; it was recorded, but with regret. Charcot's doctrine, which had been overthrown, had been clear, simple, and easy to study. Charcot's subjects had had their symptoms

---

[1] In this connexion I may refer the reader to my essay on Charcot in the " Revue Philosophique," 1895, vol. i, p. 569.

controlled by registering apparatus of the familiar type. Charcot had seemed successful in including animal magnetism within the domain of physiology. To the science of the day, that had appeared a great advance ; but now the gains had to be discarded. What had the Nancy School to put in place of this fine fancy ? Hypnosis was a moral state in which suggestibility was enhanced ; it was the outcome of suggestion. As for suggestion, this was the manifestation of a general faculty of the human mind known as suggestibility or credivity. Suggestibility meant that ideas entered the mind and were accepted by it. All this formulation seemed simultaneously true and void. It seemed superficial, and not really scientific teaching.

To discuss these things, merely to study them, the observer had to leave the familiar ground of physiology ; he had to learn a new language ; he had to make acquaintance with a new sort of science, to learn psychology. But psychology was not favourably regarded by the leaders of the medical profession, who remembered that they had heard vague talk of the subject in the later days of school life, and who fancied that it was a mishmash of literature and ethics. Besides, what was there in the psychology of the time worthy of being carefully studied by medical practitioners ? I was always painfully aware of the futility of our psychological science when I tried to teach it to doctors. Empty discussions concerning the origin of ideas and the principles of intelligence, theoretical disquisitions anent the purely logical mechanism of thought—what bearing had they on real, practical life ? How could the physician find in them any explanation of his patient's behaviour ? Psychology ought to have been nothing else than the science of behaviour, but behaviour was the very thing that the psychologists ignored. Bernheim's supreme merit was that he disclosed the need for a pyschological science made for physicians and not for philosophers. But since this science did not yet exist, enquirers were repelled from a study for which such a science is indispensable. There was a revival of the old prejudices against induced somnambulism, which for a little while Charcot had dispelled.

The other main reason of the decadence is to be found, I think, in the difficulty practitioners had to face when they wanted to apply the teaching of the Nancy School. They had repeatedly been told that the faculty for being hypnotised was practically universal, that a good hypnotiser will hardly find more than twenty-seven insusceptible persons in a thousand. Bernheim had declared that a doctor who could not hypnotise 95 per cent. of his patients at the first attempt was a doctor who did not know his business. The would-be hypnotists therefore set to work bravely, endeavouring here and there and everywhere to hypnotise all who came to consult them, whatever the nature of the disease. The patient was often reluctant to be hypnotised. The new method seemed mysterious and alarming. Despite all the reassuring words of the doctor, the patient was on the look out for something strange or peculiar. Still, after talking matters over in the home circle, and perhaps after an interview with his spiritual adviser, he would make up his mind to be hypnotised, and the doctor would set to work with the usual formula. " Look at me fixedly, and think only about going to sleep. You will feel your eyelids grow heavy, and your eyes will become tired. Your eyelids are flickering." After a few sittings, the doctor would still be patiently repeating : " You feel your eyelids grow heavy ; your eyes are flickering." But the patient was obviously inclined to be annoyed, simply because he felt nothing at all. A patient, and especially a paying patient, does not like to feel nothing at all when he is being treated. I have seen patients extremely dissatisfied because a hypo- dermic injection had been painless ; they would rather suffer a little than feel nothing at all. Especially is this true when the patient has been expecting something extraordinary. The doctor would do his best to console his patient, saying : " You were wrong to expect anything extraordinary. Hypnotism is a simple affair, nothing more than what you have been experiencing. Don't say you have experienced nothing. You seem rather bored, and that is already some- thing ; we learn from the great teachers of hypnotism that a sense of boredom is the first degree. As yet, certainly, you have not been fully hypnotised. Don't expect too much at first. You have passed into a hypnoidal state, and that is an excellent beginning." In the end, the patient would become seriously annoyed, and would seek advice elsewhere. He would find a doctor who would at least give him a sharp purge. When patients grow weary of a method of treatment, doctors are always ready to admit that the treatment is open to many objections. Before long they found it necessary to account for their change of front by circulating the fiction that hypnotism was immoral.

The decline of hypnotism has no serious meaning. It has been due to accidental causes, to disillusionment and reaction following upon ill-considered enthusiasm. It is merely a temporary incident in the history of induced somnambulism.

CHAPTER FIVE

DEFINITION OF SUGGESTION

AT the close of this period of struggle and effort, and now that we have reached the period of calm which precedes rebirth, we shall do well to take stock, to ascertain precisely what we have gained, and to transfer the useful ideas to the reserve. Unfortunately this is a difficult matter, owing to the grave defects of medico-psychological observation, for in this field, more than elsewhere, there prevails a tendency to use vague and even inaccurate language. Nowhere else, perhaps, is a lack of precision more obvious than in works on psychotherapeutics and in the use of the words suggestion and hypnotism. I think it would be a good thing, therefore, to survey the writings of the recent decades in order to ascertain the meaning we ought to give to these two terms. Let us deal first of all with suggestion. An accurate notion of this phenomenon had always seemed to me a great desideratum, and I have more than once attempted a definition.[1] In these various definitions I have been guided throughout by the same general conception, but I think I may venture to say that I have been able to secure more psychological precision on each successive occasion. In the present work I should like to apply to the notion of suggestion the results of my latest studies on tendencies and their development.

1. INSTANCES OF SUGGESTION.

Every definition begins with the juxtaposition, the grouping, of a certain number of phenomena in accordance with their obvious analogies. Let us juxtapose here some instances as analogous as possible to those which the majority of the

[1] L'automatisme psychologique, 1889, p. 139; L'état mental des hystériques, 1892, p. 30; Rapport sur la définition de la suggestion au premier congrès de la Société Internationale de la Psychothérapie, 1910, published as Sonderabdruck of the " Journal für Psychologie und Neurologie," Leipzig, 1911.

before-mentioned authors have presented under the name of suggestions. In the choice of these there will obviously be a hypothetical factor, for this is an inevitable part of every classification. The worth of the supposition that there is an intimate kinship between the selected phenomena will only be proved if we succeed in discovering fairly simple general characters common to the phenomena of the group, and if these characters are manifest in all the leading instances of suggestion.

I consider that in our first description of the phenomena it will be important to exclude experimental suggestions, and above all to exclude therapeutic suggestions. These kinds of suggestion are the most complex of all, and in them errors of observation are most likely to occur. We must begin with the consideration of the far more simple phenomena of suggestion as it presents itself spontaneously and accidentally in the course of the neuroses.

In the descriptions furnished by suggesters, we find accounts of psychological phenomena, of actions, of perceptions, of sentiments of belief, appearing in the subject as a sequel of certain impressions, and in especial of certain words, and arousing surprise by their easy and rapid development. When we consider these phenomena we are inclined to think, either on the ground of our personal experience or on the ground of our previous knowledge of the subject, that we ourselves should not have reacted in like manner to these impressions or words, and that the subject was disinclined to react in this manner. Here we have nothing more than a general reflection on the foregoing observations, but it enables us to juxtapose phenomena of the same kind.

Rah. (f., 24) [1] suffered from somnambulist crises as a sequel of an attempted rape. In these crises, as usually happens in such cases, she related the incidents of the assault, or dramatised the scene, shrieking, and trying to run out of the room. One day, in her flight, she collided with an invalid chair and tumbled over the handles. This interrupted her delirium, and she said several times : " Hullo, it's an invalid chair ! " Then, with a complete change of manner, she took hold of the handles and began quietly to push the invalid chair round

---

[1] A conventional abbreviation for " female, 24 years of age." Similarly, " m " is used for " male."

the courtyard. She went on doing this for more than an hour, until the crisis was over.

Nof. (m., 19) would from time to time pass into a very peculiar state in which he was unable to resist the tendencies aroused in him by certain impressions. Thus (the incident was reported by himself and was also watched by his relatives), when in this condition, one day, he happened to pass a hatter's shop. Thereupon, he said to himself : " Hullo, there's a hatter's, a place where people buy hats," and he promptly went in to buy a hat of which he had no need. Another day, being in the same condition, he was passing the Gare de Lyon, and said to himself : " A railway station. This is the place one travels from." Thereupon he entered the station and, having read on a poster the name Marseilles, he took a ticket for that town, and set off by the Marseilles train. Not until he reached Mâcon did he come to himself, realise the absurdity of what he was doing, and quit the train.

A very interesting case, one which I have reported at considerable length,[1] was that of Irène (f., 21). Throughout a long illness brought about by the death of her mother, this patient refused to drink the water drawn from a particular tap, saying : " What flows from that tap is not water but red blood." This remarkable delusion began one day when the water was falling from the tap drop by drop, " like the blood from Mother's lips."

Mye. (f., 18) had a violent quarrel with her father on the matter of her betrothal. She talked very loud, and screamed for quite a long time, until she became hoarse. Still sobbing, she complained to her mother that the quarrel had made her seriously ill, and that she was certain she had broken one of her vocal cords. Thenceforward she suffered from aphonia, and was sometimes obstinately mute. The power of phonation only returned at night when she was dreaming, or for a moment or two during the daytime when she was in a rage. Directly she became consciously aware that she was speaking, she was once more unable to phonate, and could only whisper.

Lec. (f., 25), having just met a young girl suffering from chorea, observed : " That poor girl has become very ugly and ridiculous. How awful it would be if I were to have the same

---

[1] L'amnésie et la dissociation des souvenirs par l'émotion, " Journal de Psychologie Normale et Pathologique," 1904, p. 417 ; L'état mental des hystériques, second edition, 1911, p. 506.

illness. J. would no longer care for me." Shortly afterwards she began to writhe and twitch, and to suffer from a colourable imitation of chorea. The illness lasted a few days only, being speedily cured by suitable treatment.

Lqu. (f., 27) had been taken to the dead-house of a hospital that she might identify the father of one of her girl friends, the man having died of tetanus. She was much moved when she saw the corpse, and was terrified when she listened to an account of the symptoms of tetanus. She began to ask herself whether she had caught the disease, for she already felt a stiffness in the back of the neck. During the next few days she became affected with hallucinations, seeing imaginary hearses and corpses. Thenceforward, for three months (until the beginning of a course of treatment, which effected a speedy cure), she suffered from a spasmodic affection of the neck, so that her head was twitched backwards and forwards " as if I were saying how-do-you-do." Sometimes, instead of the nodding spasm, there would be periods of contracture during which the head would be drawn back for several hours.

Yz. (f., 17), attending the burial of her father who had died as a result of hemiplegia, could not help dwelling on the thought that the illness was hereditary, and that she was already affected by it in the germ. On returning home she kept one of her eyes closed, had twitches of the left shoulder, and dragged her left leg as if it had been partially paralysed. These troubles soon became complicated by obstinate hysterical anorexia, and the illness lasted for more than a year.

Such instances are extremely common, and the record of them might be extended indefinitely. The study of them underlay Bernheim's notion that the multiform symptoms of hysteria are due to autosuggestions of this character. In my book *L'état mental des hystériques* (1892), I classed these multiform paralyses and contractures among fixed ideas, while making, however, certain necessary reservations. At the time, my notion was not favourably received, but to-day it has been revived with a good deal of exaggeration. I shall not dwell on the matter now, for this would necessitate a detailed study of the complex pathogenesis of hysterical symptoms. Suffice it to have recalled here a few instances in which ideas and beliefs arising antecedently to the appearance of certain symptoms would seem to have played a part akin to that played by suggestions.

Now we come to cases in which actions are induced by the words of persons present, this being a somewhat more complicated matter. Elsewhere I have recorded the case of Justine (f., 40), who, in one phase of her illness, was unable to withstand the influence of words uttered in her presence, even when these words had no bearing on her own situation.[1] She conceived a hatred for a servant lad, being convinced that he designed to rob and murder her. At length she sent him away because, when going to market, she had heard some one say that it was dangerous to have servants living in the house. Among different fancies, she would refuse to have a fire lighted, would refuse to change her underclothing, would believe that her husband was unfaithful, and so on—while recognising, from time to time, that these notions were absurd, and that her fixed ideas had been the outcome of chance words she had heard.

Ne. (f., 26) [2] led a very irregular life, and passed a good deal of her time in certain cafés where she met with merry companions. These found it great fun to tease her because she had a trick of crying out loud, and especially of crying " Maman," when emotionally stirred. They noticed that under certain conditions, as when she had had a little more wine than was good for her, she would repeat in the most casual way any words uttered softly in her hearing. Of course the words these scapegraces chose to instil in place of the innocent exclamation " Maman " were shrewdly selected. At length, without saying anything about it to her persecutors, the poor girl applied for help to the Salpêtrière, asking how she could be freed from the trick of involuntarily punctuating her speech with some gross expletive whenever she was startled.

X. was a woman of thirty-three. Her husband noticed that she had a way of talking in her sleep. It occurred to him to turn this tendency to account. Without waking her, he would say to her in a low tone: "Tell me what you have been doing to-day." She would promptly comply. She soon came to realise in her waking hours that her husband knew all her doings, even things she would rather have kept to herself;

---

[1] Histoire d'une idée fixe, in Névroses et idées fixes, vol. i, 1898, pp. 156-172.   [2] Ibid., p. 370.

and she came to the hospital to ask me if I could safeguard her against these involuntary indiscretions.

We now come to experimental suggestions, and I shall choose a very clear instance. The day before, Marguerite had had a quarrel with her mother, and had made up her mind that nothing would induce her to tell me what it was all about. While she was still uttering loud protests to this effect, I put a pencil into her hand, and she wrote : " Mother did not want me to go to see my young man." Although she had written these words, she continued to behave as if she had kept her own counsel, and I have every reason to believe that she was really satisfied as to my ignorance.

As an example of simple therapeutic suggestion I may recall one published long ago in *L'automatisme psychologique*. A woman thirty years of age was suffering from complete paralysis of the lower limbs after being bedridden for years. While she was seated in a chair, and while Dr. Piasecki of Havre, who had taken me to see her, was standing in front of her talking to her on indifferent matters and apparently engaging her whole attention, I told her in a low tone to get up and walk. To her amazement, she did as she was told, and was cured from that time (p. 359). Very soon, in connexion with the therapeutic use of suggestion, we shall have to consider a number of like instances.

I might add numberless examples to the foregoing. The various works enumerated in the previous chapter are full of them. The psychological problem of suggestion is : How, from these descriptions, can we isolate the common and essential elements, which are found in all the instances, and which comprise suggestion properly so called ?

2. Unduly General and Inaccurate Interpretations.

Many authors have attempted to answer this question, and their replies must be classified in groups. A first category of answers is, I think, of great importance historically speaking, for it comprises the opinions which are the most widely held of all, and in my view the most unfortunate ones, for they have contributed greatly to confuse the issues. I refer to the definitions of suggestion which, in the phenomena we have been considering, stress only one trait, the psychological or moral trait, and make no attempt to clarify any of the others. This outlook was favoured by Bernheim, who, at any rate in his earlier writings, sought to give the word suggestion a boundless significance: " I will define suggestion as the action by which an idea is introduced into the brain and accepted by it " (p. 24). " Everything which enters the mind by any of the senses, everything which is aroused by the association of ideas, by reading, or by education, everything which is invented by the subject himself, all actions, all beliefs, whatever their origin—everything is suggestion." If we proceed to examine the way in which Bernheim uses the word suggestion, we shall find that he expands its significance yet more, including within the scope of the term all the sentiments, all the emotions : " Whatever the mode of penetration, every idea which activates the brain cells constitutes a suggestion." [1] To sum up, it is obvious that for Bernheim the word suggestion is a synonym of the hoary general terms " thought," " psychological phenomenon," " phenomenon of consciousness."

I do not contend that this conception is utterly mischievous. There was a certain justification for it at the time when Bernheim wrote, and in view of the end at which he was aiming. What he mainly wanted was to draw the attention of physicians to the importance of psychological phenomena, and to show that a great many morbid conditions ought to be considered from a mental or moral standpoint rather than from a purely physical standpoint. He achieved his end ; and, more than any other person, he was successful in leading the medical public to study psychology. Moreover, there used to be a school of persons, among whom Heidenhain and especially Prosper Despine [2] were the most conspicuous, who took no account of the psychological character of these phenomena, considering them to be perfectly explicable in terms of nervous mechanism. I discussed the notion at great length in L'automatisme psychologique. Bernheim gives the idea its quietus, for he certainly succeeds in showing one of the most essential characteristics of suggestion to be the fact that we have to with a psychological phenomenon.

[1] De la peur en thérapeutique, " Bulletin Général de Thérapeutique, Médicale et Chirurgicale," September 30, 1886.
[2] Despine, Psychologie naturelle, 1868 ; Etude scientifique sur le somnambulisme, 1880.

Is this sufficient ? In these medico-psychological studies, can we rest content with so vague a designation ? A good many writers used to think so, and a good many still seem to think so, for in quite a number of books the word suggestion is used without giving it a more precise significance. The results are most unfortunate. Bernheim himself brings the fact to light when he shows us that the most diversified and the most sharply distinguished psychological phenomena have long been confounded under the name suggestion. He writes : " Everything which enters the understanding through the ears, everything accepted by the mind whether with or without preliminary examination, everything that persuades, every-thing that is believed, constitutes a suggestion by the sense of hearing. Lawyers, preachers, professors, orators, men of business, quacksalvers, seducers, statesmen, are all suggesters." [1] This amounts to saying that everything is suggestion, and that every one is continually acting as a suggester. Such a formula-tion is extremely simple, but its acceptance would put an end to mental and moral science, and above all would put an end to psychotherapeutics. In reality, the very authors who seem to adopt such vague formulas are careful not to apply them. When, for the first time, they come across the phenomena of suggestion, they believe that they have made a discovery, and they are satisfied that they are going to exhibit something which is both peculiar and unfamiliar. Bernheim writes : " I regard it as my duty to make known the phenomena which have been shown to me at the Maréville asylum." If he had nothing more to disclose than undefined phenomena of consciousness, nothing more to describe than persuasion by a shrewd barrister (Cicero described this long ago), Bernheim need not make so much fuss about the matter. These authors have to encounter contradiction, and they strive to make people admit the reality of their discovery. Nay more, they hold séances to demonstrate the phenomena of suggestion, and make definite experiments for this purpose. Why should they take so much trouble if they were concerned with nothing more than undefined phenomena of conscious-ness ? Finally, when medical treatment is in question, they wish the patients to apply to particular physicians, who are able to recognise the phenomenon of suggestion, and to set

[1] Hypnotisme, etc., 1891, p. 26.

suggestion at work in a suitable manner. Do not all these things show that, despite the vague generality of their formulation, they are really convinced that suggestion has particular characteristics ?

I showed in earlier years that in certain instances the subjects themselves are well aware that suggestion has peculiar characteristics by which it is sharply distinguished from other psychological phenomena. A woman to whom I was trying to make suggestions interrupted me, saying : " That's not caught on this time." Yet she had understood me perfectly well, she had accepted the idea I had expressed, for she added : " You tell me to do this, and I will do it if you like, but I warn you that what you say has not caught on." She felt that the action would be done by her voluntarily after acceptation, but that it would not develop spontaneously as had done the actions following previous suggestions. Delboeuf records observations of the same kind. To such subjects, as to the suggesters themselves, suggestion is unquestionably a particular phenomenon.

I have been repeating these simple remarks for five-and-twenty years, and have as yet encountered only one objection. At the last meeting of the Société Internationale de Psychothérapie, Bernheim appeared to dissent from my view that suggestion is a particular psychological phenomenon.[1] He was unwilling that suggestion should be regarded as " an unusual action," as one out of keeping with the habitual mentality of the subject. In support of his own view, and against mine, he spoke of the jury carried away by the barrister's pleading, the buyer overpersuaded by the salesman's glibness. " Here," he said, " are customary phenomena, which are nowise unusual." Even if we admit that these examples are really instances of suggestion (which remains to be proved), they merely show that suggestion is not rare and exceptional, but is of frequent occurrence. This is not the question in dispute. I have never used the word " unusual " to describe suggestion ; I have used the word " particular." Sight is a particular phenomenon, distinct from smell, and we shall not annul this elementary difference by declaring that sight is not an unusual phenomenon.

[1] See my paper in the Sonderabdruck of the " Journal für Psychologie und Neurologie," Leipzig, 1911, p. 472.

Bernheim's answer misses the point. It is still necessary to ascertain precisely what we mean by suggestion, precisely what distinguishes suggestion from the thousand-and-one other phenomena of thought.

The majority of those who have studied the question have come to share the view I maintained in 1889 when I said that the phenomena of suggestion must be distinguished from other mental phenomena. Babinski wrote in 1891 : " According to Bernheim, suggestibility is the aptitude for being influenced by an idea. . . . But, if this were all, every reasonable person would be suggestible ; . . . it would be enough to say that every one is inclined to follow advice—a true statement, but not a new one. To define hypnotism and suggestion in so comprehensive, or rather so vague, a fashion, is tantamount to denying the existence of particular mental states." [1] Grasset, in his work *L'hypnotisme et la suggestion* (1903), also accepts my view. Camus and Pagniez, while disdaining suggestion, regard it as a particular mental phenomenon. At the Munich Congress of Psychotheraphy (1910), when I presented my report on the definition of suggestion (see footnote p. 208), most of those who took part in the discussion were prepared to accept this initial point in the report.[2] Besides, how could we have gone on to discuss the other points if we had begun by asserting that the word suggestion denoted an undifferentiated psychological phenomenon, not distinguishable from any other ?

If this be accepted as a matter of principle, we must draw the logical conclusions, and must exclude from the definition of suggestion such general characteristics as are common to all the phenomena of thought. This consideration enables us to reject certain definitions which, though ostensibly precise, are really invalidated by being based upon the vague conception we have just been discussing.

In common parlance, and sometimes even in medical terminology, suggestion is taken to mean incitement to thought, the awakening of thought. Haberman says : " A touch is eminently suggestive ; a clasp of the hand arouses

---

[1] " Gazette Hebdomadaire," July 1891, p. 21.
[2] This applies to Forel, Vogt, and Seif. Cf. " Journal für Psychologie und Neurologie," 1910, p. 334.

the idea of friendship; a caress arouses the idea of affection or love."[1] In Parker's *Psychotherapy*, Richard C. Cabot writes (II, iii, 21 et seq.) : " Rooms, places, colours, odours, and the quality of atmospheres—literal or metaphoric—all these, too, act most powerfully upon us through the back doors of our minds. One receives suggestion from the shape, arrangement, and colour of a room, the softness of the carpet on which one treads, the leap and sparkle of the fire on the hearth, the glitter of glass and metal. . . . Perhaps the most powerful impression I have ever received through suggestion was that of the lines, colours, and odours of the Cathedral of Seville. . . . Not a rational element in the whole—only instincts, feelings, deep-buried impulses were appealed to. . . ."

No doubt these are real factors, and they play a part in all the instances of suggestion we have considered in the foregoing pages. The sight of the invalid chair aroused the thought of pushing it ; the sight of the railway station aroused the thought of the journey ; the father's burial aroused the thought of his fatal illness ; chance words heard on the way to market aroused the thought of necessary precautions. But such phenomena are not peculiar to these suggestions, for we meet them in connexion with all other mental operations. From moment to moment, one or other tendency is being awakened in us by impressions received from without. The sight of a pencil arouses the tendency to write ; the sight of a staircase, the tendency to go upstairs ; the sight of a tumbler, the tendency to drink. The corresponding actions may or may not be performed ; they may be performed as suggestions, or in a very different way ; and if they are performed, this may be in various different fashions. If we understand suggestion thus, we are back in the realm of confusion. Moreau de Tours, at the opening of a lecture on impulses, related that on the previous day, when returning home after dinner, he could not look at any front door without having the thought of ringing the door bell. But, he added, " I did not ring any of them, and therefore I had no impulse." We see that Moreau's terminology was already far more precise.

[1] Hypnosis, its psychological Interpretation and its practical Use in the Diagnosis and Treatment of diseases, "Clinical Lectures in the Department of Neurology at the College of Physicians and Surgeons," New York, March 17, 1910.

Often, again, and especially in the writings of the Nancy School, suggestion has been confounded with the association of ideas in the widest sense of that term. By association we understand something akin to the mechanism which, in connexion with each of our tendencies, leads to the occurrence of a series of movements or actions succeeding one another in a definite order. The utterance of the opening words of a poem may be followed by the recitation of a hundred verses or more. This is what I used to call " a psychological system " ; what the Germans, following Freud, term " a complex " ; what to-day is generally spoken of as " a tendency." The law of association certainly plays its part in suggested ˏactions, but only on the same footing as in other actions, for the mechanism of association works in exactly the same way in actions of every possible kind. When any one writes a letter in fulfilment of a resolution arrived at after mature reflection, the mechanism of the act of writing is just the same as if the letter were being written under the influence of a suggestion. We do not draw a distinction between an epic poem and a comedy when we say that in the epic poem the words are composed of separate letters. Those who speak of the general automatism of thought as an essential part of the definition of suggestion, are, just like the writers previously considered, confounding suggestion with an undifferentiated psychological phenomenon.

The same criticism applies to the theories of those who hold that suggestion has an important part to play in social phenomena, and in the general influence exercised by one human being upon another. The idea is already to be found in the writings of Joseph Pierre Durand, for he distinguished between allonomy, or obedience to another, and autonomy, or self-determination. The same idea occurs in Forel's book (p. 15) : " The concept of suggestion is liable to be confounded with the concepts instinct, habit, reflex action, automatism. In fact, the distinction is difficult ; but it is made more obvious by the activity of the hypnotiser, and by the mutual influence of human beings on one another." The same idea is found in Moll's book, for that author is continually speaking of the way in which actions are modified owing to the influence of one human being upon another.

All this is true enough. In suggestions, or at least in

some suggestions, we can trace the effect of the influence of other persons. But such an influence is universal, for three-fourths of our actions are determined by social relationships. Orders, requests, prayers, instruction, and advice, betray the same influence. Are we, then, to say that these things are nothing but suggestion ? To do so would be to relapse into the confusions we have just been trying to escape.

Is it possible to eliminate in like manner other views of suggestion, less hazy perhaps, but defective in another way, since they approximate suggestion to very different phenomena, which ought to be considered from another outlook ? This fault is especially conspicuous in all the definitions which assimilate suggestion to emotion. Milne Bramwell draws the distinction between the two phenomena very clearly. He points out that emotion is a disturbance of the whole mentality, whereas suggestion is often a trifling matter, and one which causes practically no disturbance ; various distinct emotions cannot coexist, but several distinct kinds of suggestion can operate at one and the same time. " Emotional phenomena cannot be terminated at will," and cannot in an instant be changed in type, whereas a mere sign will change or check a suggestion.[1]

I think this important distinction between emotion and suggestion can be greatly clarified if, to begin with, we endeavour to form a more distinct idea of the nature of emotion.

In a report to the Société de Neurologie and to the Société de Psychiatrie de Paris, presented on December 9, 1909, I described emotion in the following terms : " There are circum-stances to which the individual is not adapted by his previous organisation, and to which, for one reason or another, he is incapable of adapting himself at the moment, although he is aware of these circumstances and is conscious of the necessity to react. In such instances we perceive, instead of a useful reaction, a multiplicity of disorders of function, and I propose to give the name of emotion to this multiplicity of disorders occurring under such conditions." Having studied these different disorders, modifications of feeling, diffuse or systema-tised mental agitations, disturbances of the visceral functions,

---

[1] Proceedings of the Society for Psychical Research, 1896, p. 220.

disturbances of the motor functions and of actions, and so on, I tried to subsume them under the dynamic theory of emotion, which renders conspicuous the systematic insufficiency of action and the disorders resulting therefrom. " We find such a suppression or degradation of action at the starting-point of every emotion. This insufficiency, which depends on various causes (the novelty of the situation, undue rapidity of the happenings, the weakness of the subject, etc.), is always a false step of the mind, an arrest of evolution, a decline of psychological tension. This initial phenomenon induces an effort of adaptation and a derivation. Energy, which is almost always expended in excess, and which is not properly utilised for a phenomenon of a higher order, is dispersed, and discharged upon phenomena of a lower order." [1] In a word, the essential characteristic of emotion is a quasi-negative phenomenon, the suppression of well-adapted actions, disorder, and an impotent effort to remedy it. In suggestion, on the other hand, what especially strike us are its positive characteristics, the performance of an action in a way which is indeed abnormal, but is none the less complete and fairly regular. Let us suppose that some one comes to reproach us. If he does so under the influence of a suggestion, he will speak clearly and forcibly ; but if he is under the influence of emotion (that of fear, for instance), he will tremble, choke, or weep, but he will not be able to speak. Obviously, we are concerned with very different phenomena in these two cases.

In my report to the Munich Congress of Psychotherapy in 1910, I pointed out these differences between suggestion and emotion. A number of those present, Trömner and Vogt, for instance, shared my views and defended them. But some of the contributions to the discussion were very remarkable. Several of those who took part in it protested against my making a psychological distinction between suggestion and emotion, pointing out that persons in a strongly emotional state became more suggestible, and that if we wish to act on people by way of suggestion it is often useful to stimulate their emotions. How fond people are of sowing confusion in our ideas ! We are not now concerned with elucidating the causes or factors of suggestion, which will have to be considered

[1] Rapport sur le problème psychologique de l'émotion, " Revue Neurologique," December 30, 1909, p. 1551.

presently. At the moment we are merely trying to ascertain the nature and characteristics of a phenomenon, and to decide the meaning of the terms we are using. Suggestion may be accompanied by emotions; it may develop as a sequel of emotions, and may even be caused by them; but we must not confuse suggestion with emotion. A sugar factory produces sugar, but is not itself sugar. Emotion may at times produce suggestions, but in essence it is quite different from suggestion.

We now come to a far more delicate question, one which has puzzled a good many writers, namely that of the relationships between suggestion and error. Quite a number of authors have fallen into a serious confusion through assimilating the two phenomena. An experiment made a long time ago by Emile Yung [1] of Geneva has been repeated again and again with very unfortunate results. About twenty young fellows had just been listening to a lecture on diatoms, and Yung told them that he would show them some diatoms under the microscope. He made them look through the microscope at a slide on which there was nothing but some dust and irregular fibres. Two-thirds of the young men, after having glanced at the preparation through the microscope, expressed themselves as greatly pleased at the sight of the diatoms, and when pressed, they gave vague descriptions of these imaginary diatoms. For my part, all I should have inferred from this little experiment would have been that the lecture had been badly delivered, or that the audience had been inattentive, or that these young fellows were inexperienced in the use of the microscope. But Yung was not content with such simple inferences. He decided that all the students were highly suggestible, and that he had made an admirable experiment in suggestion. Since then, the experiment has been often repeated, with variations, and has been described as " suggestion by error." Lipps tells us that suggestion depends upon the acceptation of ideas on inadequate evidence, and not as the outcome of a truly logical conviction. J. V. Haberman of New York adopts the same interpretation: " Suggestion is a phenomenon in which, under inadequate conditions, certain sensory perceptions are created, certain ideas are generated, and their motor consequences are hastened,

[1] Le sommeil normal et le sommeil pathologique, 1883, p. 58.

through the awakening of certain signs in the consciousness." [1] Quite recently, Babinski has distinguished persuasion from suggestion by saying that in the former the idea inspired is good, and leads to sound actions and true opinions, whereas in the latter the suggested idea leads to bad actions and false notions.

In my opinion, these conceptions are based upon linguistic fallacies, for they approximate words which are not comparable and which apply to totally distinct points of view. The word " error " like the word " truth " is a logical term describing a relationship between an idea or an action, on the one hand, and external reality, on the other ; it concerns the worth of the action or the thought. " Suggestion " is a psychological term which has to do with the characteristics and the mechaniŝm of a moral phenomenon regardless of its worth in relation to the outer world. To define suggestion by error and persuasion by truth is as unreasonable as it would be to define imagination as a sin and memory as a virtue. It is quite true that some suggestions are errors. When Nof. sets out for Marseilles though he has no business there, and when Irène runs away from a water-tap because she fancies that blood is flowing from it, the actions are based upon suggestion, and they are also mistaken actions. But when Marguerite tells me the truth about her behaviour, and when Marceline, who is dying of starvation, eats without noticing it, these actions, which are also due to suggestion, are anything but mistaken actions. Nay more, the same action may be an error or a truth as time and other conditions vary. Crocq of Brussels retorted to Babinski : " My banker advises me to buy certain shares. If they rise in value, you will tell me that I have acted on persuasion ; but if they fall, my banker has made me a suggestion ! " Some mistakes may be due to suggestion, but other mistakes are the outcome of voluntary action, or of passion, or of anything you please. I ask a passer-by the way, and, since I have no better advice, I take the road he points out. Let us suppose that he is " pulling my leg " and that he puts me upon the wrong road ; none the less, my action has been a voluntary one, and the outcome of deliberate reflection. All that Yung's experiment shows is that the young men made a mistake ; it tells us nothing as

[1] Op. cit.

to the nature of the action which led to the mistake. To
attend carefully to what we are taught, to repeat what the
teacher has said, to see as far as we can what he tells us to
see, and to believe that we have actually seen it, may all be
reflective actions. A special psychological analysis of the
behaviour of Yung's students would be essential to show that
their actions were not reflective, but were the outcome of
suggestion. In a word, the quality, the logical or moral
worth of an action, does not change its nature from the
psychological standpoint. If we define suggestion by error,
we are still within the orbit of the hazy definitions already
considered, and we are still confounding suggestion with all
other psychological phenomena. The only way out of this
difficulty is to analyse the actions which are regarded as
suggestions, and to understand their mechanism.

3. Automatism in Suggestion.

In my earlier writings on suggestion I emphasised two
points : First of all, I endeavoured to show that we must
consider these phenomena solely from the outlook of action ;
and, secondly, I contended that we must recognise the actions
in question to be incomplete, unfinished.

That we are concerned with action is obvious in most of
the examples previously quoted. We have to do with persons
who make purchases, set out on journeys, adopt special attitudes, utter certain words. We might hesitate to accept this
limitation when we think of the suggestion of sentiments and
hallucinations, but a moment's reflection will show that one
who has a certain sentiment is in reality one who adopts a
certain attitude and follows a certain line of behaviour. One
who is really grieved or angry, is affected throughout his body
by the motor, circulatory, and secretory modifications of
grief or anger. In hallucinations, too, there are dispositions,
present actions, and preparations for future actions. Irène
runs away from the tap ; when she sees a glass of water, she
makes gestures of terror and disgust ; at meals she insists
on having a bottle of water which has been brought from
elsewhere.

I need hardly say that like considerations apply to what
are termed negative suggestions, to suggestions of paralysis or

systematised anaesthesia. To refrain from action in particular circumstances when action might be expected, is still to act after a fashion, though not in the expected way. We have a particular way of moving, a particular carriage, a special way of breathing and of thinking, when we are alone, and when we are in company, respectively. Nay more, it is probable that we have a special attitude when we are in the company of this person or that, perhaps a special attitude in relation to each one of all the persons with whom we are acquainted ; and we may say that our acquaintanceship with each person consists in this peculiar attitude. If we think that X. has gone away, we abandon the attitude characteristic of the presence of X. in order to adopt that which corresponds to the person whom we believe to be present ; and if we believe that every one has gone away, we return to the attitude which is customary to us when we are alone. These are certainly actions. We even have a particular attitude in relation to the presence of a particular object, and we abandon the attitude when we believe that the object is not there. A woman does not comport herself in the same way in a room when she thinks that the walls are lined with mirrors as when she thinks that the mirrors have been taken away. I have often shown that negative suggestions cannot be understood without the supposition that a large number of positive perceptions and positive actions are involved. Similar considerations apply to the deferred suggestions which I have often studied in the same way. In a word, there is a component of action in all suggestions.

Furthermore, the same outlook must be taken in the case of all the phenomena of the mind. The scientific study of psychology is only practicable if we look upon all the phenomena of mind as actions, or grades of action. The mind appears to consist of an aggregate of tendencies. It is composed of dispositions to produce definite series of movements in response to stimuli applied to the periphery of the body. But these tendencies are activated to a different extent in different cases, and therein lies the diversity of psychological phenomena.

The second point we have to note is that in the case of suggestions this activation of tendencies is carried to a fairly advanced stage. We are not concerned with a mere disposition to action, or with a mere preparation for action. In most cases, the activation gets beyond the phase of desire. In some instances, indeed, when suggestions are made, the action does not get beyond a wish. " I want to pick up your hat and to put it on ; how stupid of me ! " Here we have to do with incomplete suggestions, whose development has been checked. But in the cases we have been considering in this chapter, the subject has really bought a hat, has really taken a journey, has really acquired an illness lasting several months.

Nevertheless, we must not make the mistake of thinking that such actions are wholly completed. In every normal action, a large part is mechanical, being the reproduction of similar actions previously performed, the manifestation of a tendency which has come into being within us long since. But there is a lesser part, dependent upon an original activity, and the outcome of an effort towards adaptation to the new features of the extant situation. The action has not merely to be adapted to the outer world ; it has also to be adapted to our own individuality. Every action is an addition to our personality, which not only preserves a memory of the action, but assimilates the action and considers it as a part of itself. This means that in the case of every action there must occur a series of psychological operations which, first of all, transform the action so as to harmonise it with the tendencies and interests of the doer ; and, secondly, transform the individuality of the doer in so far as the memory of the action becomes part of the individual's archives, and in so far as the personality of the doer is augmented and transformed by the addition of this new element.

Can we say that the actions described as instances of suggestion in the earlier part of the present chapter are thus complete ? Obviously they are nothing of the kind. They are maladroit actions, being almost always performed rapidly, negligently, and indifferently ; they are repetitions of actions formerly done, and repetitions which are not brought into relationship with extant circumstances. Nof. buys a hat or gets into a train just as he has done before, but he ignores the important fact that at the moment he does not need a hat or has no occasion to go to Marseilles ; his action lacks precision, lacks adaptation to the present. This element of misfit is all the more striking inasmuch as it is out of keeping with the subject's ordinary behaviour and with his education or past experience. We are amazed at the foolishness of these persons, and we say that their absence of mind goes too far. The patients say the same thing, as soon as they have emerged from the strange mental condition during which the action was performed.—" How could I have been such an idiot as to buy something I don't want ? I'm very careful of my money as a rule."—" Why on earth, when I was talking to Father did I come to think that I had broken one of my vocal cords ? There was no blood in my mouth, and I had no pain."—" Why should I have fancied that I was paralysed like my father ? I am so much younger than he, and I had not been ill before as he had. It's not my way to be so stupid." —It is because of this characteristic maladaptation that suggested actions are so often blunders.

But suggested actions are especially defective in the matter of their adaptation to the personality of the doer, and as concerns the reorganisation of the individuality after the performance of the action. Many of my earlier studies were devoted to the elucidation of this. First of all, the suggested actions do not harmonise with the subject's individual tendencies. We know perfectly well that the subject has no interest in the performance of the suggested action ; that he does not want to do it ; that, a moment before, he showed a wish to do the very opposite. The reader will recall how Marguerite was refusing to tell me her secret at the very time when, by suggestion, I made her write it. Strange, indeed, is the way in which, under the influence of suggestion, the individual will speedily perform actions or asseverate opinions opposed to all that we know of his character, his tastes, and his beliefs.

Let us consider the sentiments which the subject feels towards the actions which he performs in this way. We find that he is in a very peculiar state of mind. Many authors have studied the matter, especially in relation to the carrying out of posthypnotic suggestions. I may refer, in especial, to the works of Noizet,[1] Liébeault, Gurney (1887) ; to my own writings (1886–1889) ; to the books of Forel, Pitres, and Delboeuf. All these authors give similar descriptions. In many instances, the action is completed without the subject's appearing to be

[1] Op. cit., pp. 12, 119, and 320.

aware of what he is doing, for he will continue to talk of something else, to concentrate his attention and his consciousness on something quite different. The suggested movements of his limbs, and, above all, the suggested visceral modifications, seem to take place all unwittingly, " by a sort of instinctive intelligence," to quote Noizet's phrase. If we speak to the subject, if we compel him to attend to what he is doing, he is greatly astonished, and can hardly believe that he is actually at work upon something he had refused to do a moment before. To express his feelings, he will use such expressions as I have already recorded in connexion with my study of sentiments of incompleteness.[1]—" I feel as if some one were pushing me." —" It is not I who does this."—" My hands are acting, not myself."—" I can't think who is holding me back."—" Some one is stealing my thoughts."—" Some one else is writing down what I am thinking."—The subject will stop the performance of the action for a moment, to resume it as soon as his attention is elsewhere. But in exceptional instances, the subject will adopt the suggested action, and will tell us that he wished to do it for this reason or that, which is invented for the occasion.[2] We must note that when this happens, the adoption occurs at a late stage. It does not occur at the outset of the action in order to aid in the development of a tendency that is still feeble ; it occurs at the end of the action, when the suggested tendency has acquired a considerable impetus ; and it sways the individual's tendencies instead of being adopted by them.

Finally, when the suggested action is finished, we often note a phenomenon of which one of the first and best descriptions was given by Beaunis [3]; I refer to the forgetting of the suggestion, and of the fact that it has been carried out. Marguerite, for instance, never realised that she had disclosed her secret. Sometimes the subject is forced to recognise that he has performed the action. Then, as I have shown, he is astonished ; and in many cases he will try to annul the action, to suppress its consequences. Elsewhere I have described the case of a patient who could not see a bright object without stealing it, and who, when he found it in his pocket, would

[1] Les obsessions et la psychasthénie, 1903, vol. ii, p. 278.
[2] Cf. Charles Richet, " Revue Philosophique," 1886, vol. ii, p. 326.
[3] Le somnambulisme provoqué, 1887, p. 123.

restore it in a very contrite mood. Another kind of forgetfulness is that which we considered a moment ago in which the
subject adopts the action after it has been performed and
invents ridiculous reasons to account for it.[1] It is apropos
of this that writers have quoted Spinoza's saying : " Freedom
is nothing but ignorance of causes."

These characteristics of the performance of suggested
actions have often received specific names. Delboeuf proposed
to speak of the state in which they were performed as a
" paraphonic state." I myself have generally used the expression " automatic " actions or beliefs. In my more recent
writings, I have tried to show the place occupied by automatic
actions among the degrees of the activation of tendencies.
These tendencies, these dispositions to the performance of an
aggregate of coordinated movements, may remain in a " latent
condition," or may be " activated " more or less completely
by passing through the stages of " erection," " desire," and
" effort," in order to reach at length the stage of " completed
action," or the stage of " triumph." Between desire and
effort, and sometimes between effort and completed action,
I have placed a very interesting stage of activation. This is
characterised by the complete or almost complete performance
of the movements proper to the action, a performance complete
enough to generate the illusion of the action in the spectator
or the performer ; and nevertheless characterised also by a
certain insufficiency, so that the action cannot produce the
appropriate outward effects, since there is a more or less
complete suppression of those perfectionments of the action
which would render it psychologically real. This is the stage
of " quasi-action " (Baldwin), or of " ludic action." If the
insufficiency relates especially to the outward characteristics
of the action, to its objective consequences, we have to do with
" play " properly so called. If, on the other hand, the
insufficiency relates especially to the subjective modifications
of the individual, to the adaptations of his own personality
to the action, then we have to do with " automatic action."
When the alterations of individual sentiment are pushed to an
extreme, and when the automatic actions are performed by
one who does not remember what he has done and is unaware

[1] Cf. Beaunis, op. cit., Charles Richet, L'homme et l'intelligence, 1884,
p. 255 ; Binet and Féré, Le magnétisme animal, 1887, p. 217.

of what he is doing at the time, we term such actions " subconscious actions." The last-named form an important group of automatic actions. Suggestion, which belongs to the group of ludic activities, is especially akin to the group of automatic actions or to the group of subconscious actions.

Such reflections as these led me to attempt a definition of suggestion in all my writings on the subject, whether I was dealing with psychological automatism and hysteria or reporting to the International Society of Psychotherapeutics. The definition may be formulated as follows : *Suggestion is a peculiar reaction to certain perceptions ; the reaction consists in the activation, more or less complete, of the tendency aroused by the suggestion, in the absence of a completion of the activation by the collaboration of the remainder of the personality.*

This conception of suggestion, which brings it into line with the group of automatic actions and with subconscious actions, appears to me to have been adopted, at least implicitly, by many authors. Grasset, in especial, has made it his own, and has given it picturesque expression in his theory of the mental polygon and of the centre O. This symbolisation is merely another way of expressing what I set forth in my *Automatisme psychologique* (pp. 306 and 308) and in my book *L'état mental des hystériques*. In the diagrams printed in these works, the different points placed either on a straight line or at the angles of a polygon represent the different elements of the action as they have been organised by previous activity ; the centre O represents the personal consciousness which at one time will seize hold of, perfect, or control these elements, and at another time will ignore them, will allow them to develop in isolation just as they are. The activities of such tendencies left to themselves constitute what Grasset terms " inferior psychism," whereas the activities resulting from the intervention of O constitute what he names " superior psychism." Suggestion is thus regarded as an exclusively polygonal activity, and is consequently " inferior."

Certain authors have, since those days, expressed disdain for suggestion, considering that treatment by suggestion is degrading, and *morally* inferior ; such physicians have, unwittingly, adopted Grasset's theory without troubling to discuss it. Richard C. Cabot, like Paul Dubois, maintains that to suggest is " to introduce an idea by the back door of the mind." [1] All these interpretations recognise the part played by automatism in suggestion.

4. SUGGESTION AND IMPULSE.

Unfortunately a precise definition of so complex a matter is wellnigh impossible ; and my recent studies of phenomena which have been presented as being due to suggestion have made me feel that all the foregoing formulas are, if not incorrect, at least lacking in precision. I am tempted to make the same criticism regarding myself that I have so often made concerning Bernheim. I endeavoured to define suggestion in terms which, doubtless, are applicable to it, but which are likewise applicable to many other phenomena. Such definitions are, therefore, much too superficial.

Suggestions are certainly automatic phenomena, are actions which have been almost completed but to which the last stage of perfected activation is lacking ; but the trait is found in many other psychological phenomena. Reflex movements may be regularly performed without control or personal synthesis. Should we say that the withdrawal of the hand in response to a prick is due to suggestion ? Elementary tendencies, whether sensory, perceptual, social, or intellectual, often find expression in analogous actions. The simple fact of spelling correctly as we write, without being aware, or having a personal consciousness, that we are spelling the words correctly, must not, however, be attributed to suggestion, or we shall be admitting that all habitual actions are due to suggestion, and shall thus come back to the theory of the Nancy School. Actions that form part of games are closely similar to automatic actions. Suggested actions are in many ways closely akin to the actions that occur in games. The criminal suggestions brought forward by the Nancy School, and the localised suggested contractures of the Salpêtrière School, cannot be understood without having recourse to the theory of ludic action. And yet suggestion is very different from games, were it only in the matter of the constraint put upon the individual under suggestion, as contrasted with the liberty exercised by the individual at play. It is quite obvious that

[1] Cf. Parker's Psychotherapy, II, iii, 17.

our definition of suggestion as automatism does not clinch the matter satisfactorily.

I have always implicitly admitted that there was an element of suggestion in every possible action, that very elementary as well as highly complex actions can be suggested. But herein lies an error which renders all our definitions inaccurate and vague. Certainly the arm may be raised or the mouth opened under the influence of suggestion. But these actions are carried out after we have said to the subject: "Raise your arm"; "Open your mouth." The action is performed through the intermediation of speech, a fact which immediately annuls its "elementary" character. If we reflect for a moment, we shall realise that the majority of suggestions are made through speech, or by signs which correspond to speech; that such suggestions give rise to action which must be placed in a category apart; and that these suggestions occupy a field of activity far more circumscribed than we had imagined.

My study of the hierarchy of the tendencies has led me in recent years to the investigation of particular tendencies. I have named these tendencies "realist tendencies," endeavouring to introduce into the French tongue the very interesting significance attached by the English to the verb "realise." Here we are faced with the relationship between speech and action, a relationship which plays an important part in mental disorders, and which helps us to understand the essential content of the phenomenon of suggestion. For this reason I think it will be well to summarise the lectures I delivered at the College of France. The course dealt with "realist tendencies" and "rational tendencies," and was delivered during the sessions 1913–1914 and 1914–1915.[1]

In these lectures I portrayed as transformations of the act of speech, all the operations which go to make up the many varieties of consent and give rise to will and to belief. Such operations consist of special forms of behaviour whereby associations are established between speech and the complete actions of the limbs. Of course, speech itself is an action produced by specific movements; but the movements of the larynx and of the lips, etc., are very small compared with those

[1] This summary is made from the "Annuaire du Collège de France," 14th and 15th year of issue.

of our limbs; they do not necessitate so great an expenditure of energy, have not so great an effect on the material world, only produce a reaction in those who resemble us, and have little by little become distinct from other movements. Speech has become a highly specialised form of activity, and its relationships to the actions of the limbs have generated very important types of behaviour.

At the outset, speech was intimately bound up with the action of which it formed a part. The gestures which gave birth to language were nothing more than particular movements which were an integral part of the action, and which made their appearance especially at the beginning of the action. But already in the *command* (which was the starting-point in the creation of language), the gesture is separated from the remainder of the action. The chieftain learns to do no more than give the sign, and to stop there without continuing the action himself; the subordinate learns not to repeat the sign, but to complete the action of which the sign was the first stage. Already, now, speech and action have become partially separated, seeing that each phase is the work of a specific individual; their union is, however, still very intimate, and speech does not yet exist completely detached from action.

As time went on, the separation between the command, and the action fulfilling the command, became greater. A word was no longer attached to one precise and individual action; it became associated with many actions, each action differing slightly one from the other; words became generalised *symbols*. *Memory* built up a language which was independent of the events and actions amid which it had come to birth, a language capable of being reproduced in other circumstances and resulting in different actions. Men have, in the form of jokes and conversation, learned to play with language, to enjoy the excitement of language for its own sake quite apart from the action to which it was primarily linked. Doubtless the separation between the word and the deed has never been complete; otherwise the word would have lost all meaning. But the separation is sufficiently wide to make language often inconsistent, as can be heard in the babble of many a sick person. The patient will modify his words at the slightest provocation, without attaching importance to the most absurd contradictions, and without turning a hair at the discord existing between his actions and his words. This evolution has gradually led to the emergence of the *idea*, for the idea is essentially a form of inconsistent language. The word, or the phrase, which constitutes the main part of the idea, still retains a meaning, it evokes an action ; but this evocation is reduced to a minimum, and the tendency to perform the deed in actual fact has now become greatly enfeebled. Such methods of expression have degenerated into little more than parrot cries, and have lost the greater part of their efficacy.

A reaction against this growing independence of language, and an attempt to restore its stability, became essential. Men have striven to make their own words become once more commands unto themselves ; hence arise such things as *promises, pacts, affirmations*, and various kinds of *assent*, which are at the root of *belief*. Here we have attention working upon a portion of the foregoing action (understanding by "attention" the control exercised by a superior tendency over an inferior tendency).

Assent is a reaction to a special kind of stimulus, such as a *question*. It matters not whether the question is asked by the subject himself or is put to him by another. " Will you go for a walk with me ? "—" Is it raining ? " When the reaction of assent has been awakened in a mind capable of responding, the forms of response will vary according to the nature of the action associated with the words in the query. *Will* (taking the word in its general sense) is an assent which relates to an immediate action whose conditions of execution are actually realised, and which may be begun at the very moment when the speech is uttered. " Will you go for a walk with me."—" With pleasure." Forthwith I initiate the action of going out with the person who has invited me.

Belief is more difficult to understand, and has given rise to many misunderstandings owing to insufficient psychological analysis. Many writers, whose works on the subject are too numerous to mention here, have shown that belief is a compost of innumerable actions. The most important point seems to me to be this—that, in belief, the reflective action cannot be instantaneously performed, because the conditions needed for the performance of the action are not present. " I believe it is raining." Here we have to do with specific behaviour, the behaviour of the man who is threading the streets while a shower is falling, a man who steps warily, who holds up an open umbrella. When I say, " I believe it is raining," I make up my mind to take an umbrella, to behave in the street in much the same way as the man already described ; but I am not going to perform these actions immediately, for I am still in my room, where it is not raining. The decision is a conditional one : " If I go out, if I should have to walk about the streets, I shall behave in such and such a way." All belief is of the same kind ; it is an assent that bears upon the conditional performance of various actions.

These assents of will or of belief have remarkable results, for they furnish us with important notions of reality and being. Just as a " fact " is the record of a happening, so a " being " is what one wills and believes him to be. It is thus that the feeling of reality, and even hallucinations, are offshoots of will and belief.

Apart from these two varieties, which depend on the nature of the act, assent provides other essential results : the affirmation or the negation which may be applied to will or to belief. The former links up in a positive way the word and the corresponding deed : " I shall at once, or I shall when circumstances allow, perform the action of which I speak " ; this is affirmation. Specific expressions, and particularly the use of the personal pronoun (these duplicates of the Christian name), become formulas of affirmation. Or, on the other hand, we may detach the word from the deed as completely as possible by not performing the particular deed at the particular instant, but by performing a deed of a totally contrasted nature, in order to show more clearly the action of negation ; or we may take our oath that we shall not perform the deed later, even if circumstances should prove favourable. " No, I will not go out ; I'll sit in my armchair."—" No, I don't believe it is raining ; if I go out I shall not take an umbrella." In this case we have the formula of negation.

If this reasoning is correct, a further question arises : How is the choice between affirmation and negation effected ? How, as the sequel of a question, is the subject led to give a positive assent or a negative assent to the immediate or conditional actions proposed to him ; nay more, how does he come to give any assent at all ? It is obvious that in certain cases the assent, or the choice from among a variety of assents, takes place instantly and directly. The tendency which has been aroused by the verbal process fights against the tendencies which have been aroused at the same moment by other circumstances ; if the tendency aroused by the verbal process has sufficient strength and sufficient tension, it will triumph over the other tendencies ; otherwise the former will be overpowered by the latter. The action of assent or of negation comes along simply to register defeat or victory. " One wills and one believes what one desires " ; and all the influences which depend on exterior actions at the moment, on the prestige of persons who happen to be present, on the subject's previous experience, may, according to chance circumstances, play a part in guiding the assent into such and such paths.

There are probably many persons, especially among the weaker brethren, who are possessed of no other power of assent than the foregoing. Dr. Powilewicz (of Havre) and I had a girl of eighteen under observation a good many years ago. In *L'automatisme psychologique* I describe her case on p. 173. Blanche was a typical specimen of this mental state. She was epileptic and feeble-minded, but was not incapable of accomplishing all the functions of realisation ; she understood words, and was able to affirm or deny. But she obstinately denied that which displeased her, or affirmed with equal pigheadedness if we asserted anything in an authoritative voice. " Hullo, an elephant has got into the room ! "— " Yes, sir ; I'll put a piece of bread in his trunk." I found two similar types in Nageotte's clinic at the Salpêtrière, and I studied their sayings during the course of my lectures at the College of France. As the fancy moved them, they would affirm or deny anything and everything irrespective of difficulties or contradictions. We have here probably the inferior form of assent, a form especially characteristic of the feeble-minded, but which may on occasion even be met with among those who are not feeble-minded.

Among the latter, this ready assent is not a perfectly simple phenomenon, for the choice between affirmation and negation is made under a specific form which has been named " reflective assent." The essence of reflection is arrest, a slowing down of assent, which allows the subject to test the awakened tendency by a comparison with a number of other tendencies. In order to allow such a prolongation of the struggle between the tendencies aroused by speech, reflection, by introducing a temporary element of *doubt*, helps to clarify the subject's ideas. Not only does the phrase embodying the idea and implying an action contain little impulse towards the accomplishment of the action, but there exists at the very moment when the phrase is uttered a whole series of precautions and inhibitions ready to prevent us and others from over-stepping this minimal degree of activation of the tendency. The cleavage between the word and the deed is not in this case accidental. On the contrary, it is sought for, and is determined by a special action which consists in an endeavour to avoid assent, whether affirmative or negative : " It is no more than an idea, I'll say nothing more."

When we feel that the phrase is no more than an idea, we are usually not content with suppressing as far as possible the corresponding action, for we go so far as to reduce even the utterance of the phrase ; we speak so softly that the words do not reach the ears of those present, and can only react upon our own organism. This is a *thought*, which is simply conscious. Consciousness is, in fact, nothing else than a reaction of our organism to our own actions. Thought is a language which determines reactions within ourselves. Various degrees of assent are attached to the idea and to thought. Such are : *imaginings, fictions, sentiments*. These correspond to the beginning of vague activity incapable of applying itself to any definite and organised action, and they can only be explained through the medium of comparisons and metaphors.

It has been easy to study the utility of ideas thus under-stood, to study internal thought, the importance of *dissimula-tion* and of *falsehood*, the preparation for accomplishing action while nothing can be noticed from without, the first attempt at action under the guise of thought (which means under the most economic guise possible). The countless changes which internal thought undergoes during the course of mental disorders have been particularly instructive on all these points. Other important notions, such as the notion of *phenomenon* and the notion of *mind*, have issued from the idea and from thought. A mind is an entity capable of dissimulation and of falsehood, i.e. of thought.

But the main function of the idea is to permit of reflection. Here we have to do with a complicated process of behaviour which arrives at assent in two stages, which achieves realisation in two successive actions, just as many elementary mental operations are accomplished by two simultaneous actions. The first process consists, as we have seen, in giving to the verbal expression of the evoked tendency the form of an idea, and in keeping it for some time in this form. The second process consists in confronting this idea with other ideas which likewise represent, in a verbal form, a considerable number of other tendencies.

This work presupposes the approximation of other ideas to the initial idea, and that is what we name the *course of ideas*. The intrusion of these other ideas might be said to be due to the law of the association of ideas. But I feel that the importance of this law has been greatly exaggerated. More often we find that what determines these evocations are definite actions, similar questions to those we utter when asking for orders from an actual commander. This is often to be witnessed in the pathological exaggerations of reflection. Such queries lead to responsive actions, i.e. to fresh ideas ; and this is what constitutes the inward conversation which underlies all reflection.

Among the ideas thus evoked, a certain number will aptly respond to the craving for guidance, and will issue genuine commands. Moral duty (a subject of study hitherto neglected by psychologists) is a combination of the two attitudes aroused by the command ; the attitude which consists in receiving an order, and the attitude which consists in issuing the order oneself. This mixture of attitudes is the result of inward discussion, and constitutes the originality of the moral imperative. Aesthetics and logical rules are evoked in the same way. One of the fundamental rules of logic, the law of universal consent, as Garnier observed, constrains us to think the same way as our neighbours, and puts the veto on any belief which might be in opposition to the common thought. As an outcome, we have the principle of contradiction, for we always repeat in relation with ourselves the social behaviour we display towards others, and we shrink from contradicting ourselves precisely in the same way as we are inclined to avoid a clash with the thoughts of others. These fundamental rules of logic play in relation to beliefs a part similar to that played by moral ideas in relation to will.

Other ideas represent the particular influence of such and such a person according as, during the course of our inner colloquy, we are led to desire their blame or their approval. Nor must we forget that all the primitive tendencies relative to feeding, to the sexual function, to the instinct of self-preservation, to the instinct for construction, to conserving and developing the personality, to the intellectualisation of the individual, to the organisation of his own history, and so on, and so on, are likewise called forth by a question, and are transformed into ideas which become ideas of personal interest. Just like moral ideas, such ideas, too, will assume the force of an imperative. All these commands, setting themselves up in opposition one to the other, constitute the aggregate of motives.

The tendency primarily evoked, and then arrested in the stage of the idea, is subjected to the control of all these commands, and is compelled to adapt itself thereto. When this work is a preliminary to voluntary action it is termed *deliberation* ; and when it is a preliminary to the passage of ideas into belief it is termed *reasoning*. The presentation of alternatives and the estimate of their comparative worth must be regarded as imaginative trials of the action in the form of internal speech. Such a trial gives rise to social reactions within us. In these internal discussions, we recall moral rules, praise or blame the various witnesses and ourselves, or revive the memory of similar actions and their favourable or unfavourable consequences. As Rignano has well shown, reasoning is closely akin to this deliberation, for it, likewise, consists of a series of mental experiences in which ideas which come into collision with contradictions are eliminated. These experiences are much less expensive in the world of thought than in the world of reality, and as an outcome of them there ensues either an increase or a reduction in the tension of the tendency that forms the subject of deliberation.

After a very remarkable intermediate stage, which takes the form of a shorter or longer arrest of mental work (it may be very long in certain patients), comes a *decision* or a *conclusion*. Positive or negative assent results ; either the idea is definitely rejected, or else it is transformed into reflective will or reflective belief. But we must not fancy that the idea is still what it was to begin with. The decisions that are the outcome of such work are by no means identical with voluntary actions and beliefs that are the outcome of immediate assent. They are essentially different, for the original tendency has been transformed ; it has undergone evolution through adapting itself to all the commands it has encountered in the course of the reflective process. Furthermore, they represent a far more stable union between word and deed, for the union has been subjected to legal verifications ; primary assent is a simple certificate, whereas secondary assent is a certificate that has been legally stamped. We are no longer concerned with simple voluntary actions, but with *resolutions* : no longer with simple belief but with *knowledge* ; seeing that knowledge is nothing but belief that follows upon accurate reflection, nothing but legalised belief. Finally, the decisions in which there has been an adaptation of the act to individual tendencies, and an adaptation of the entire personality to the action, give birth to the *sentiment of action* (which is of immense importance), to personal memories, and to the adoption of the action by the personality which has played a part in the decision and had been transformed thereby. Action has become *personal*, just as belief has become *real* ; the things in which we believe after full reflection have become for us, not merely entities, but realities.

Manifestly this labour of reflective assent is long and difficult ; it is an operation of a superior category, needing the maintenance of a high tension of the psychological forces throughout a definite period of time. Naturally, therefore, the process does not always run its course without disturbance. One of the commonest among the disorders that arise is an incapacity to bring the reflection to its term, to culminate in a decision, in a conclusion that differs from the premises. Certain patients, abulics, and doubters, perform the action of ideation, and begin interrogation and discussion, but can get no further. They never reach the stage of reflective affirmation or negation ; they never get beyond ideas and imaginations, never achieve resolution or knowledge. That is why, in such persons, will lacks a personal character, and belief lacks reality. " It is not I who wills, and I am no longer in a real world."

But there is another form of disorder of reflective assent, and one of great interest to us in this connexion. I refer to *impulse*. In this phenomenon, there is at first a reflective attitude, wherein the tendency that has been evoked is arrested at the stage of the idea; memories are called up; there is interrogation, and there are the beginnings of discussion. But none of these things reach their climax, for the operation is suddenly checked. We can understand the nature of this arrest better if we compare it with another very remarkable phenomenon, namely the way in which certain patients suffering from depression carry on a discussion with the persons of their immediate circle. They vigorously express an opinion of their own, and when this opinion encounters contradiction they want to defend it and to contest the opposite view. We shall notice at once that they argue badly, that they do not listen to the statement of the other side of the case, that they themselves adduce no new arguments worth mentioning, and that they are content to reiterate their own opinion (sometimes with growing anger). The typical point is, that they never reach the end of the discussion. The end would be a modification of the two opinions, to attain a result which might be more akin to one or to the other of the original statements, but which would represent such a modification of both as to enable the two interlocutors to unite upon a common thought. Long before this final stage is reached, our subject suddenly stops the operation. In some cases he may angrily quit the scene, while reasserting his own opinion unchanged, and quite unconcerned as to what his adversary's view may be. In other cases he appears to accept the adverse opinion fully, without discussion, saying: " At bottom, I really agreed with you; I thought exactly as you think." Now, in internal discussion, the same sort of thing may happen. The subject will suddenly give up deliberating or reasoning, and will assent more or less fully to one or other of the conflicting ideas, according as either may chance at the moment to preponderate in his mind. Here we have a sudden return to immediate assent, after a stage of reflection which remains unfinished.

In this phenomenon we discern once more the characteristics of automatic action, that is to say, of unfinished action, which lacks the perfect adaptation which might have been achieved had it been finished. But we are concerned with a peculiar form of automatism, with an automatism of will and belief understood as functions of realisation, as functions which establish a tie between word and deed.

The important thing to note, in this connexion, is that suggestion is only a variety of impulse. First of all we have to realise the important fact that suggestion always has speech and the idea as starting-point. Sometimes, as in many of the cases previously recorded, the subjects have themselves given expression to the idea at the outset.—" It's an invalid chair."—" There's a hatter's."—" A railway station. This is the place one travels from."—" The water is flowing from the tap drop by drop like the blood from Mother's lips."— Sometimes, in the subject's presence, other persons have spoken of the danger of having servants in the house, of the symptoms of tetanus, and so on, thus arousing the idea which acts as a suggestion. We have no right to speak of suggestion unless we can find evidence that this preliminary phase of ideation has occurred in the subject's mind. That is why we must not overstress the explanation of hysterical symptoms by suggestion, for a great many hysterical symptoms arise before the subject has entertained any ideas about them, or they are quite independent of the subject's ideas.

We must not forget that the persons who have such ideas are fully capable of reflecting about them. In most of the circumstances of life, they reflect with a fair degree of ability. We expect them to reflect with the same ability now, and the subjects expect it of themselves. But what is typical of suggestion is that they fail to do what we and they have expected. Concerning the suggestive idea, they have the beginnings of reflection, so that we often note a period of deliberation and an attempt at reasoning. Justine told us about the character of her servant. Lqu. asked whether tetanus was so contagious that it might attack some one who had merely gone near the body of a person who had died of this disease. But such deliberation is brief, and does not culminate in a decision. The subject continues to keep the same idea in mind, without modifying it and without adopting it. Even in the cases which I have termed " suggestion by distraction," we often find that the subject has rejected the idea without any kind of deliberation. In either case, reflection is soon over; the subject no longer questions or discusses the idea. But the idea, now left to its own devices, has not been annulled ; the tendency appears to be equipped with an adequate charge of energy, and it develops independently. Complete realisation in the form of voluntary action and belief occurs, but there is always a lack of the last touches which reflection could have added. That is why the action continues to seem strange to us, and that is why the subject himself is fully able to distinguish an action he performs under the influence of suggestion from an action he performs as the outcome of voluntary assent.

We have, however, to note other qualities in the impulsive action, over and above the defects just described. In certain patients suffering from depression it is easy to detect remarkable differences between inferior automatic actions and actions belonging to a more exalted type. For example, Adèle, thirty years of age, has gradually arrived at the ultimate stage of reduced psychological tension commonly designated dementia praecox, which I myself am inclined to regard as psychasthenic dementia. She has become practically incapable of action, but is continually chattering to herself. Her violent recriminations against all the other members of her family are uttered very rapidly, out loud. Sometimes the observer can attract her attention for a moment, can check the flow of words, and can secure a brief answer to a definite question. But when this happens, the answer is uttered slowly and with difficulty, and in a very low tone. There is a remarkable contrast between the comparative inaudibility of these reasonable answers to questions, and the loud automatic recriminations which are resumed a moment later.

A good many years ago, I made the same observation in connexion with suggestions made to an abulic suffering from depression.[1] " If I ask Marcelle gently and politely to perform an action, she says : ' All right,' and tries to do what I ask ; but she does not do it. If, on the other hand, standing in front of her, I bluntly order her to perform the action, she is surprised and refuses ; and nevertheless she does what I tell her, unhesitatingly." Posthypnotic suggestion enables us to demonstrate the contrast between the movements that are lost and the movements that are preserved. While the subject was in the hypnotic sleep, I made the following

[1] Névroses et idées fixes, 1898, vol. i, p. 10.

suggestion : " When I tap the table, you will pick up this hat, and you will hang it up on a hat-peg." Then I awakened her. A little later, I spoke to her in the tone used when asking any one to perform some little service : " Would you be good enough to relieve me of this hat, which is in my way when I am writing ? Please hang it up on the hat-peg."—" Certainly," she answered. She tried to rise, shook herself, stretched out her arms, made incoordinated movements, sat down again, got up once more, and so on. This continued for twenty minutes, during which she was unable to do the simple thing I had asked. Then I tapped the table. Instantly she rose, picked up the hat, hung it on a peg, and returned to her seat. Under the influence of suggestion, what she had been trying to do by reflective volition for twenty minutes in vain, was done in a second or two.

The contrast between the speed and energy of the inferior type of action, and the sluggishness and weakness of the superior type of action, would appear to depend on the working of a law with which we shall become more fully acquainted thanks to numerous instances that will be given in the course of the present work. The law is that actions which are the outcome of a higher tension need much more energy for their performance than actions which are the outcome of a lower tension. The subject may have quite enough energy for the lower-grade action, although a sufficiency of energy for the higher-grade action may be wanting ; it would even seem that there is a sudden release of tension when the subject passes from the attempt to perform the higher-grade action to the performance of the lower-grade action. This feature is important. Here I merely note it in passing, but we shall have to reconsider it when we come to discuss the practical use of suggestion.

Finally, this approximation of suggestion to impulse facilitates the distinction between suggestion and other phenomena with which it is apt to be confounded. There is certainly some analogy between a suggestion and a command, for both phenomena are based upon the fundamental association between the verbal sign and the corresponding action. The words " command " and " obedience " may have different significations when we are dealing with minds at different stages of development. For the lowest grades of mind, when language is in its initial stages, a word is nothing more than a fragment of the action, a fragment which, in accordance with the laws of imitation and hierarchy, entails, the instant it is perceived, the performance of the complementary part of the action. We may say that at this stage an order is almost identical with a suggestion, seeing that as yet the phenomena that will ultimately undergo differentiation are still confounded. But we are not concerned here with the practical form of suggestion that we can study in individuals who have attained a much higher mental level. When an idea comes to act as intermediary between command and performance, we are confronted with realist tendencies. The command may be carried out after deliberation, acceptation, and decision, whether these operations are repeated in the case of each specific command, or whether they have been made once for all as regards certain categories of commands so that nothing more is requisite than the feeling that the specific command belongs to a group of commands which have already been accepted in advance. I may give an example which has interest in connexion with the history of the topic we are studying. The patients in hospital are quick to realise that it will be of advantage to them to comply with the doctor's whims. They understand that they will do well to perform rapidly, for the delectation of admiring spectators, any little tricks the doctor may order, thus displaying a voluntary obedience which has often been mistaken for the outcome of suggestion. But in other instances the tendency to obedience represented by the idea of the command is not subjected to reflective acceptation ; it is automatically realised. Thus a command may take effect through suggestion, just as any other sort of idea may be transformed into an impulse.

Demonstration and persuasion are often, and with good× reason, contrasted with suggestion. Their aim is to guide reflective assent towards a particular end. Whereas, in the case of suggestion, there is an attempt to suppress the intervention and discussion of motives, the object of demonstration and persuasion is to supply motives and to guide their action. In fact, they are deliberative processes. No doubt, after a long course of persuasion, the subject may cease to reflect, may renounce the attempt to come to a decision, and may surrender to the impulse engendered by the persuasion.

Here, obviously, persuasion and suggestion are mingled, and persuasion is transformed into suggestion. But it is none the less true that, in most instances, persuasion, which aims at inducing the subject to come to an individual decision, must be contrasted with suggestion, which aims at generating an impulse.

Thus we rediscover in suggestion all the characteristics of impulse, if we regard impulse as an automatism of reflective realisation. Suggestion can then be looked upon as *the induction of an impulse in place of reflective realisation.* This view of the matter brings us in touch with certain writers who have expressed the same idea more or less clearly. Bernheim, who had so many flashes of insight, was in his first book already writing of " natural credivity." A good many years later he laid stress upon the notion of " a psychical image which tends to realise itself." [1]   Others, like Lloyd Tuckey and Münsterberg, have spoken of an idea which is accepted too quickly, and is uncritically transformed into an action. I think there is good reason for stressing the automatic character of this realisation, and for approximating suggestion to the category of impulses.

[1] Bernheim, " Journal für Psychologie und Neurologie," 1911, p. 473.

CHAPTER SIX

CONDITIONS UNDER WHICH SUGGESTION OCCURS

IF suggestion be thus a phenomenon with definite charac- teristics, we may opine that it will occur under special circumstances, and that in the absence of these circumstances suggestion will not ensue. Manifestly a knowledge of the suitable environing conditions is indispensable to those who wish to apply the therapeutic method in practice, and it is surprising that so little attention should hitherto have been paid to the conditions in question.

The neglect is explicable as the outcome of an unfortunate conception associated with one of the notions we have been studying. A whole school of investigators has confounded suggestion with thought in general, with psychological pheno- mena of any and every kind. The necessary inference was that suggestion was a commonplace matter, occurring in every one, and at all times, so that a study of the precise conditions under which it occurs would be superfluous. For these authors, belief depends on credivity, and suggestion on sug- gestibility. They are general qualities of the human mind, and there is no more to be said. Strange as the assertion may appear, it has been supported by remarkable statistics, according to which suggestion can be assertained to occur in 97 per cent. of human beings, or (some say) in 92 per cent. I have collected a great number of these statistics, designing to publish them as items of interest ; but really they are futile, and their publication at the present day would be ridiculous. The error underlying such imaginary estimates is obvious. The compilers of these statistics never took the trouble to formulate a definite idea of the phenomenon under investi- gation, and all was grist which came to their mill. Some of them confounded suggestion with emotion or error ; others, with docility or complaisance ; most, with the evocation of tendencies and with the association of ideas. Statistics compiled upon so hazy a basis are valueless. It is far from easy to ascertain the frequency of suggestion, and the first step must be to study the conditions under which suggestion occurs.

1. HYPERTROPHY OF A TENDENCY.

I do not stand alone in realising the importance of the conditions in question. Several theories, all of them interesting, have been formulated concerning the matter. One theory will lay stress upon one special phenomenon which seems to be a determinant of suggestion ; another theory will try to explain everything by a different phenomenon. We draw the inference that suggestion is a complex matter, dependent upon the conjuncture of quite a number of circumstances.

Unfortunately it is impossible, as yet, to decide what are the precise physiological conditions under which suggestion occurs. Several attempts of the kind have been made. J. P. Durand used to speak of " nervous congestions " ; Jendrassik referred to "modifications of the cerebral circulation " ; [1] Milne Bramwell quoted John Hughes Bennett's theory that the phenomena of hypnosis were due to a physiological suspension of the functional activity of the " association fibres " in the brain.[2] These theories are neither true nor false—we know nothing about the matter. In my opinion, physiological theories of suggestion will only become possible after precise psychological theories have been elaborated.

One of the simplest among the psychological theories has arisen in connexion with the view that suggestion is a normal phenomenon, common to all mankind. Since suggestion is the rapid and almost complete activation of a tendency, does it not seem reasonable to associate it with an undue development of this particular tendency, which may be regarded as too powerful, too ready to respond to a trifling stimulus. This is undoubtedly the state of affairs as regards certain impulses which we have assimilated to suggestion. A toper will immediately have an impulse to drink if he is offered a glass of liquor ; an amorous or a jealous person will yield

---

[1] " Archives de Neurologie," May and July 1886.   [2] See next note.

to impulse should we speak to him of love or of vengeance. The potency of the hypertrophied tendency leads promptly to the annulling of superior tendency (the tendency to reflection). This is what happens in the familiar surrender to a passionate impulse.

But some careful observations made by Milne Bramwell [1] a good many years ago have shown that this explanation, in its simplest form, is not generally applicable. He proved that we may suggest to a subject actions that differ greatly one from another. In experimental work, we may by suggestion make the subject walk, or eat, or talk, or sleep. In the natural instances of suggestion previously described, Nof., when he passes a hatter's, has an impulse to buy a hat, and when he catches sight of the Gare de Lyon he has an impulse to set out for Marseilles ; Justine was equally ready to obey the words which impelled her to discharge her servant, and those which prevented her changing her underlinen or speaking to her husband. If we were to accept the explanation now being considered, we should have to suppose that in these subjects there is a medley of hypertrophied tendencies and contradictory passions, and this would be absurd. Genuine passionate impulses cannot be thus transformed. If we have to do with a toper, a lover, or a jealous person, we cannot arouse in any one of them some impulse different from the ruling passion by talking about buying a new suit or taking a railway ticket.

For this reason, the advocates of the theory we are discussing supplement their explanation by associating all the suggested actions with a single tendency. They contend that these actions have one common characteristic, in that they are all acts of obedience, of complaisance to some particular person. When the subject walks or lies down, eats or writes, at the least sign from the doctor, he is not activating as many different tendencies. We have seen that there is an element of incompleteness in these suggested actions, that the activation of the tendency has in it, in every case, an element of make-believe. The important part of the action, in the cases we are now considering, is the prompt obedience to the signal of the suggester. Thus it becomes needless to postulate the existence of a multiplicity of hypertrophied tendencies, a

[1] Proceedings of the Society for Psychical Research, 1896, pp. 216–226.

multiplicity of passions. Enough to assume the hypertrophy of one tendency only, the tendency to submission.

Interesting though they are, these social theories of suggestion have seldom been formulated clearly. Liébeault has remarked that "manual workers, agricultural labourers, children, and soldiers, trained to obey, are extremely suggestible." In 1884, Bernheim confirmed this observation, writing : "The common people, men who have been subjected to military training, manual workers, all whose mode of life has accustomed them to passive obedience, seem to me, as they seemed to Liébeault, more readily suggestible than persons of a more refined and reflective temperament, in whom there is apt to manifest itself a certain amount of moral resistance (often unconscious) to suggestion." This thesis has seldom been expounded so clearly. I am given to understand that I was wrong in ascribing it to Forel and to Vogt. On the other hand, both Hattingberg and Seif are inclined to accept it, and to regard an exaggerated obedience as the essential factor of suggestion.[1]

Similar ideas underlie the theories of suggestion which have been put forward by certain members of the Freudian School. We shall return to the important ideas of the Freudians in a subsequent chapter, and for the moment we need concern ourselves only with what they have to say anent the topic of suggestion. I think especially of the thesis expounded by Ferenczi in his essay *Die Introjektion in der Neurose und die Rolle der Uebertragung bei der Hypnose und Suggestion*.[2] The physician's care for his patient, and the simultaneously authoritarian and benevolent nature of his attitude towards the patient, arouse in the latter's mind the powerful tendencies which used in childhood to determine the behaviour towards the parents. Now these tendencies are (according to the Freudians) fundamentally amorous. Therefore, the tendencies evoked in the patient by the physician are tendencies to amorous submission. "Credulity and hypnotic docility are rooted in the masochistic element of the sexual tendency." Ernest Jones, in an article entitled *The Action of Suggestion in Psychotherapy*,[3] unhesitatingly propounds this

---

[1] Congrès de Psychothérapie, 1910, p. 341.
[2] " Journal für psychoanalytische Forschungen," 1910, vol. i, p. 1.
[3] " Journal of Abnormal Psychology," 1910, vol. v, pp. 215–254 ; Papers on Psychoanalysis, third edition, pp. 340–381.

interpretation, contending that unconscious sexual attraction lies at the foundation of suggestion and hypnotism. He writes : " Warm affection, dread, jealousy, veneration, exactingness, are all derivatives of the psychosexual group of activities. . . . Janet himself does not fully agree with the sexual interpretation, evidently because he adopts an extremely limited conception of the sphere of sexuality in all his works." [1] Seif, at the Congress of Psychotherapy in the year 1910, maintained the same view, regarding suggestion as the transference of an infantile tendency towards amorous obedience.[2] " In fine, the subjects obey the suggester because they are more or less in love with him." If I understand this theory aright, suggestions are carried into effect in order to please a beloved person, to win his favour and to inspire in him a reciprocal affection. Thus the two theories we have been considering are akin. They may be summarised by saying that the first explains suggestion as due to an exaggeration of obedience, and that the second explains it as due to an exaggeration of complaisance.

To appreciate the worth of these interpretations, we must know exactly what the authors understand by the terms obedience and complaisance respectively, and of what psychological nature these qualities are supposed to be. This, unfortunately, is by no means easy to learn. Are they thinking of reflective and voluntary obedience and complaisance, in which the subject is aware that he is obeying, and is of opinion that obedience will promote his interest or advantage him in his love ? It is not difficult to find cases of this kind. I have attended a hospital clinic where the physician (who was an excellent man but a poor psychologist, and a firm adherent of the Nancy School) boasted his ability to influence all his patients by suggestion. He would make a triumphal progress through the ward, and at each bed he would order the patient to perform some ludicrous action. The order was instantly carried out, but behind the worthy doctor's back the patients would make fun of him, explaining that they had played off these tricks so as to be rewarded with a glass

[1] " Journal of Abnormal Psychology," vol. v, p. 243 ; Papers on Psychoanalysis, third edition, p. 366.
[2] Seif, Congrès de Psychothérapie, 1910, p. 341.

of wine. Again, psychasthenics suffering from abulia often appear extremely docile. They do whatever they are told to do, even when the actions are distasteful ; they seem to agree with everything said to them in conversation, even when the interlocutor is obviously less intelligent than themselves, and when they know him to be mistaken. The reason is that they want peace at all costs, and that they dread effort and struggle. Furthermore, they want people to have a kindly feeling towards them, and there is nothing of which they arc so much afraid as arousing animosity which would be likely to involve them in subsequent strife. If the authors I have been quoting were thinking only of obedience and complaisance of this calibre, there is a ready answer to their arguments. Such phenomena are not instances of suggestion at all. I need not stress the point, since I have already expounded the characteristics of genuine suggestion.

When we are criticising a theory, we shall do well to put it in the best possible light, even though the author has not succeeded in doing this for himself. We may take a different view of the obedience and complaisance of which they speak. Let us suppose that, for special reasons, and in certain cases, the obedience or complaisance is no longer wholly voluntary and reflective, but has become impulsive owing to an overdevelopment of the corresponding tendency, as happens in the case of the various passions. Let us think of one in whom the circumstances of education, and the prolonged practice of an occupation in which he is subjected to a rigid discipline, have developed an overwhelming habit of obedience. In him, the tendency to passive obedience may have been so greatly hypertrophied that the instant it comes into play it is realised impulsively, and quite independently of the will. Richard C. Cabot, in his essay *Suggestion, Authority, and Command,*[1] quotes instances of this kind. Such a person, directly he receives an order, or fancies he has received one, will obey on impulse, and will even attempt to obey conflicting orders simultaneously. Is not this precisely the attitude of one under the influence of suggestion ? In like manner we may suppose an individual to have retained infantile characteristics, and to suffer from extreme hypertrophy of the need for paternal guidance ; or we may suppose an individual

[1] Parker's Psychotherapy, II, iii, 19.

affected with hypertrophy of the amorous tendencies.   In such persons, obedience and complaisance will take an impulsive form.   In these cases, likewise, the phenomena resemble those of suggestion, and we may presume that this is how the facts are understood by the authors whose views we are considering.

Familiar facts may be quoted which seem to favour such an interpretation.   We know how great a development of suggestibility is apt to ensue in those who are treated by suggestion for a long time and by the same person.   Here it is obvious that exercise has promoted the growth of the tendency to unreflecting obedience.   Nor is it difficult to note that certain subjects manifest a growing need for the presence and the guidance of their doctor, and to realise that this need has a definite resemblance to love.   It is a need which we shall often have occasion to study in the course of this book. Various and complex conditions combine to arouse it, but we can certainly agree that its effect is to create a tendency to obey orders with a minimum of reflection.   I cannot say that, like Bernheim, I have noted any preponderant inclination to accept suggestions among the common people, among servants and soldiers and manual workers.   It seems to me that excessive suggestibility is not peculiar to persons of any particular class or occupation.   Still, I am quite willing to admit that young people are as a rule more suggestible than adults, women than men ; and this is in keeping with the interpretation we are discussing.

Are we entitled to generalise on the topic, and to declare that no suggestion is anything more than a passionate impulse, dependent solely upon a hypertrophy of the tendency to obedience or to complaisance ?   I do not think so, for a great many objections instantly present themselves to my mind. In numerous patients, suggestions can be made effectively at the very first interview, before they have had time or opportunity for appreciating and loving the doctor.   Are we to suppose that in such patients, before we came in contact with them, there already existed a well-marked tendency towards obedience in general, and towards veneration for the doctor in particular ?   If we make enquiries of their relatives, and if we study the characteristics of these patients, we shall not, as a rule, discover anything of the kind.   On the contrary, we shall learn that they have not been famous either for docility or for complaisance. I have emphasised the fact in the records of a good many cases, and my contentions have not been challenged. Exceptionally suggestible individuals are not necessarily persons who have been broken in to obedience, are not necessarily soldiers, or servants, or common sailors. In actual fact, they are neither exceptionally docile nor exceptionally confiding, provided that the circumstances are such as to enable them to form their own judgments, and provided that they are not carried away by the automatism of a successful suggestion. Indeed, they are apt to be undocile, undisciplined, incapable of reasoned obedience and reasoned trust. I have frequently had occasion to note that they are temperamentally cold, and that they themselves complain of their inability to feel deep affection. Ferenczi and Ernest Jones seem to fancy that it is easy to be too affectionate ; to believe that all suggestible persons are capable of unbridled love and infinite complaisance. For my part, I am much more sceptical, and I think that these weak and suggestible individuals are as incapable of loving as of obeying. Their daily associates are usually astonished when the patient is promptly influenced by suggestion. " As a rule, X will not listen to any one, and he has been to doctor after doctor without putting faith in a single one of them."

Another thing which shows that suggestibility cannot always be dependent upon a profound disposition of the character, is that it is sometimes transient. We see people who, during some particular phase of life—after giving birth to a child, for instance, in the course of a serious illness, during an attack of typhoid, during convalescence, or as a sequel of some grave emotional shock—become amazingly suggestible. They will take suggestions from any one. No matter who is talking to them, man or woman, inferior or superior, the interlocutor can make them believe all sorts of absurdities. Their habitual associates will discover that it is possible to play tricks with such persons, owing to their extraordinary credulity. Pk. (m., 28), hitherto an energetic man, had undergone a change of character when he returned from the colonies after a severe attack of malaria. It was for this change of character that he sought advice. " Any chance comer can do what he likes with me. I have an irresistible tendency to do the most ridiculous things when any one speaks of them in my presence ; and often I have no remembrance of what I have been doing in this way." In such cases, after a brief course of treatment, and even, in certain instances, after nothing more than a few days' rest, the undue suggestibility will vanish. Pk. had recovered from his suggestibility after spending two months in hospital. A great many women are suggestible during menstruation, and especially during the days immediately after the cessation of the flow, but exhibit no tendency to this type of reaction during the remainder of the menstrual cycle. In the present work we shall frequently have occasion to consider an important phenomenon, namely the disappearance of all disposition to hypnotism and suggestion after the cure of certain nervous depressions, whereas these phenomena were characteristically present during the persistence of the malady. For the nonce it will suffice to point out that the appearance and disappearance of suggestibility in this fashion are hardly in keeping with the idea that the phenomenon depends upon the existence of a profound and permanent disposition. Can we understand how a disposition to loving obedience, to excessive complaisance towards the kindly doctor who reminds the patient of his parents, could disappear in this way after a few days' rest ?

In cases of this kind it would seem that during the periods of suggestibility there has been a transformation, that the tendencies to obedience and complaisance must have been modified by a superadded influence. Presumably these tendencies have existed for a long time ; they continue to exist after the cure ; and we may suppose that ordinarily, just like any other tendency, they are subject to the control of reflection. But during the period of illness, they seem to get out of hand and to become impulsive ; in a word, they behave like suggestions. Far from explaining suggestion, these impulses to obedience and complaisance seem to me to be themselves remarkable instances of suggestion ; and their abnormal development brings us face to face once more with the original problem, instead of helping us towards a solution.

Finally, we must not forget that suggestions may originate from things as well as from persons. At the beginning of this chapter we saw how suggestions could be induced by inanimate objects or accidental circumstances. Surely we are not entitled to say that the sight of an invalid chair, a hatter's shop, or a railway station, must have aroused a vigorous tendency towards obedience or towards amorous complaisance. I am well aware that at the sight of these objects the subject talks to himself, and that we are still entitled to say that language is exerting its influence. But in this case, the words are the subject's own. If he had an overmastering tendency to obey another, he would be affected with self-doubt, and would not obey his own words. Suggestions of this very interesting kind are certainly not explicable as being the outcome of the hypertrophy of some social tendency.

In conclusion, however, we may agree that in the case of most suggestions the tendencies to obedience and complaisance must be important factors. We know that these tendencies become more and more strongly operative in the course of prolonged treatment, and that when developed by exercise they may play a great part. We know likewise that, in certain persons at any rate, they may from the first facilitate suggestions by undergoing transformation into impulses. But I do not believe them to be sole and sufficient explanations of the phenomena of suggestion, which may occur in their absence, and which can never occur without the cooperation of certain superadded influences.

2. SUBLIMINAL TENDENCIES.

There is yet another theory of suggestion based upon the notion of impulses rooted in the hypertrophy of tendencies. I refer to that of F. W. H. Myers, of which a detailed account is given by Milne Bramwell in his *Hypnotism*. We may speak of it as the theory of *subliminal tendencies*—tendencies below the threshold of the individual consciousness.

Substantially these authors accept the view of suggestion put forward by myself in the years 1886 to 1889, and agree with me in regarding this phenomenon as the development of an inferior tendency emancipated from the control of reflective and personal tendencies, its development in the form of an impulse. Having gone so far, they separate themselves from me by associating this development and emancipation, not with weakness of the superior individual tendencies, but with a peculiar energy of the inferior subliminal tendencies. J. P. Durand used to say that we have within us a number of lower-grade minds in the brain and spinal cord at various levels below that of consciousness. In like manner, Myers' hypothesis is that there exist numerous tendencies equipped with wonderful energy and perfection below the individual consciousness. He reaches out towards the conception of a sort of submerged ocean of subconscious mental activities, the crests of whose waves are sometimes visible and sometimes hidden, so that we have no reason to be surprised if, from time to time, certain influences act more powerfully upon this hidden mind than upon the waking intelligence. He writes: " My view is that a stream of consciousness flows on within us, at a level beneath the threshold of ordinary waking life, and that this consciousness embraces unknown powers of which these hypnotic phenomena give us the first sample, the scattered indications." [1] This subliminal thought, says Myers, has wonderful powers. In the physiological domain, it can act upon the viscera and upon the circulation; it can modify the various layers of the skin in all sorts of ways; we can unhesitatingly ascribe to it all the cures of visceral diseases, all the blisterings, and all the cutaneous stigmatisations, which the magnetisers and suggesters have described. In the moral or psychological sphere, these subliminal powers can give rise to all kinds of energetic and ingenious activities. Myers and Bramwell add that such activities are, in addition, thoroughly moral in the ethical sense of that term, for, whereas they agree that cutaneous stigmatisation can be brought about by suggestion, they will not for a moment admit the possibility of effective criminal suggestion. In this respect, they strenuously oppose the teachings of the Nancy School, and pour ridicule upon the laboratory crimes of Liégeois. The subliminal tendencies are also able to intensify images to the degree of hallucination, but this, we gather, is a merit. They can keep us informed as to the time without the use of timepieces or of calculations; they enable us to perceive the thoughts of others without the intermediations of our sense organs; they can help us to see objects outside the range of physical vision, to predict the future, and so on. [2]

[1] The Subliminal Consciousness, Proceedings of the Society for Psychical Research, 1891–1892, p. 350; see also Bramwell, Hypnotism, 1913. pp. 358–398.
[2] Myers, Proceedings of the S.P.R., 1895, p. 334 et passim.

Whence come these wonderful powers? It would seem that they were qualities possessed as a common heritage by all our ancestors, by primitive men, by the animals of the early ages. But we epigones, preferring an individual and intellectual development, have sacrificed the precious faculties. Our thought is so exclusively guided by an intelligent and scientific interpretation of the external world, that the simple and primitive faculties have lapsed. Still, they have not been completely destroyed. By good fortune they continue to exist hidden in the depths of our being, and in special circumstances they may reappear. Many of the disorders and many of the remarkable modifications of human thought are due to the activities going on in this subliminal stratum which, for a time, bursts through the alluvial strata of the intelligence to make its appearance as an outcrop. Automatism, says Myers, is not simply a regression, for it may be a manifestation of true progress. Hysteria is akin to genius. Hysteria is merely an irrational autosuggestion making its way into regions at depths below those to which the power of the will extends ; it is " a morbid or uncontrolled functioning of powers over the organism which effect profounder modifications than the empirical self can parallel." [1]

According to this theory, suggestion is an appeal which makes its way into the subliminal consciousness. The simultaneous results of this appeal are, first, the suppression of the comparatively unimportant superior consciousness, and, secondly, the intensification of the potent inferior tendencies. Instead of being a simple arrest of the functioning of certain normal centres, it is the cultivation of powers over which, as a rule, we can exercise little control. The subliminal consciousness and the unconscious memory have more power, both physiological and psychological, than the supraliminal consciousness, for the latter has its activities restricted by the demands of the struggle for existence.

These theories are very remarkable, and it is surprising that contemporary philosophers have paid so little attention to them. They have a strange kinship with those philosophies of the day which despise the intelligence and would have us put out our eyes in order to see better—inasmuch as by suppressing the intelligence we shall give free rein to wonderful

[1] Proceedings of the S.P.R., 1891–1892, p. 309.

instinctive intuitions. It seems to me, however, that the theories in question have little bearing upon the main problem, that of the conditions under which suggestion occurs. We are told that, during suggestion, there is a revelation of the wondrous powers of subliminal tendencies. For my own part, I am not wholly convinced of the reality of all these wonders, and the nature of some of them will have to be discussed presently. For the moment, that is beside the question. Our business at this juncture is, not to express our admiration for the results, but to learn how to produce them. How, under what conditions, can we set the subliminal tendencies to work? They exist, we are told, in all of us and at all times, seeing that we are the offspring of the marvellous primitive beings above described. Why, then, are the powers manifested only in certain persons and only at certain times? We must never forget that the essential problem of suggestion is to ascertain the conditions under which a particular phenomenon occurs in certain people at certain times. We do not explain it by talking about the general qualities of the human mind. The word " subliminal " is not an explanation ; it is merely a description of the fact that the individual consciousness plays little part in producing the suggested action. What we want to know is, why subconscious phenomena occur— under what conditions they appear. The only explanation given, in a very vague formulation, by the authors we have just been quoting, is that, in certain individuals, such as hysterics, the subliminal tendencies have undergone hypertrophy, and are prone to be set to work in response to comparatively feeble stimuli. We are back again at the query which had to be propounded in relation to earlier theories. What proof is there that the subliminal tendencies are hypertrophied in certain individuals? How can we recognise the existence of such hypertrophy except by the manifestations of suggestion which the hypertrophy is postulated to explain? Why do not these beneficent hypertrophied tendencies preserve us from all diseases, or why is it that they do not get to work in order to bring about a cure unless they are artificially stimulated in some particular way? Why do such potent hypertrophied tendencies disappear from time to time, so that the subject is no longer suggestible? Not one of these questions has been seriously studied. They cannot be seriously studied under the aegis of a conception which is far more philosophical than it is psychological and medical.

3. CONCENTRATION OF ATTENTION.

Some observers have had a clearer notion concerning the problem of suggestion, and have realised that we must try to discover the direct antecedent of the phenomenon.

One of the theories most frequently enunciated is that suggestion arises out of an effort of attention, is due to a sort of exaggeration of attention. This notion secures expression in the writings of Braid, Hack Tuke, and Liébeault ; more recently it has been formulated by Bleuler ; [1] but I think the first adequate exposition of the theory is to be found in Münsterberg's *Psychotherapy* (1909). The development of all the elements comprised within the awakened tendency, and the suppression of all the conflicting tendencies, are compared to the analogous phenomena which can be noted in mental work, during the concentration of attention upon a particular point. Suggestibility, says Münsterberg in the chapter entitled " Suggestion and Hypnotism," does not result from partial sleep. The diminution of function is due to excess of attention directed towards some particular point and towards its motor results. Normal attention serves merely to promote the clarity of perceptions, but this excess of attention induces a new motor attitude which opens the way for the realisation of one idea, and blocks the paths towards all other realisations (pp. 98–99, summarised).

No doubt there is some truth in this. Every tendency which undergoes activation gives rise to certain movements and suppresses certain others. We see these characteristics both in the impulse of the epileptic and in the work of the student. If Münsterberg wanted to draw attention to this commonplace characteristic of the coordination of movements, he could have contented himself with saying that the suggested action has the familiar features of attention. But, I repeat, the formulation is commonplace, and tells us nothing as to the causation of this particular aspect which is characteristic of the suggested action.

If such theories are to be of interest to us, we must give

[1] Affektivität, Suggestivität und Paranoia, 1906.

up playing with words, and must use the term " attention " in a definite sense. I cannot here attempt an exhaustive study of this thorny problem. To begin with, I will say, following Rignano, that attention consists of an arrest of a tendency in the first stage of activation, the stage of erection ; an arrest determined by the simultaneous activation of a second tendency which controls the first. When an animal is watching its prey, the tendency to pounce upon the prey is already awakened, and is ready to become fully active at the first sign ; but it is arrested at the stage of erection by some other tendency, that of fear or caution, for instance. During expectation, which is one of the elementary forms of attention, the tendency towards the actions bearing upon the expected event is likewise in a state of erection, but it is held in check by other tendencies which are related to the absence of this event. I may add that (especially when we have to do with the higher forms of attention) this arrest, this control, is effected by a tendency which, in the hierarchical table of the tendencies, occupies a higher place than that of the tendency which is checked. The social tendencies control the perceptive tendencies ; the tendency to reflection checks and controls the tendency to immediate assent. If we accept these definitions, what the authors recently quoted mean is that the work of checking and controlling, by its persistence and its exaggeration, itself brings about the impulsive development of the controlled tendency.

This seems a strange notion, and yet there are certain phenomena which appear to justify such an interpretation. The animal which goes on watching its prey indefinitely, will end by leaping at a shadow ; if we wait too long, we shall react at last although the phenomenon is not really present. The subjects who have exhibited the phenomena of suggestion have had their attention drawn to the idea of a purchase, the idea of travelling, the idea of danger from servants, the idea of the contagion of tetanus. We sometimes find that they have talked about this idea for a considerable time ; that their minds have been much concerned with it ; in a word, that they have paid attention to it. Besides, in experiments upon suggestion, we often directly aim at arousing the subject's attention : " Look carefully at my hand, it has the properties of a magnet, and will attract your hand ; attend closely to your feelings, and you will already feel a slight movement of your hand." It would seem that our authors are right in saying that some measure of concentration of the attention is the antecedent of suggestion.

In part, at least, we can readily understand this role of attention. A tendency which has just been awakened from the latent condition, has a very low tension. It has little energy, and unless it be promptly activated it will work feebly, and will be prone to be inhibited, that is to say counter-acted by any other tendency subject to a more intense activation. But if it be awakened for a certain time without undergoing discharge in the form of a completed action, if it be maintained in the special phase of erection, it becomes more energetic and is more readily capable of being activated. Every one knows that restrained longings are apt to grow stronger. Coquetry in women has as its main object a pro-motion of the energy of the sexual tendency of the male. During expectation we can note the increase in the strength of the arrested tendency, causing enhanced impatience, and agitation. Thus attention, by checking the tendency and by maintaining it at this first stage of erection, favours its increase ; and we can easily understand that it is paving the way for the transformation of the tendency into an impulse.

But we must not go too far ; we must not regard this concentration of attention as the sole determinant of sug-gestion. The comparison of suggestion to an exaggeration, a cramp, as it were, of voluntary attention, has been discussed by various writers : especially by Gurney in 1884 ; [1] by myself in 1889 ; [2] and by Milne Bramwell in 1896.[3] It is rather surprising to find Münsterberg reviving this old theory without saying a word about the objections which have already been raised. Apparently I must repeat them. Gurney was the first to draw attention to a remarkable characteristic of sug-gestion, its mobility. In very suggestible subjects, we can give numerous suggestions in rapid succession. They may all be carried out ; or the action may be begun, to be checked as soon as the operator passes from one suggestion to another. Milne Bramwell, who has paid much attention to experiments

---

[1] Proceedings of the S.P.R., 1884, pp. 274 and 276.
[2] L'automatisme psychologique, p. 180.
[3] Proceedings of the S.P.R., 1896, pp. 216 to 226.

of the kind, quotes with approval Gurney's formulation (op. cit., pp. 271–272) of the anomaly of this conception of a " cramp " when the attention is incessantly flitting from one object to another.

Long ago, Bertrand pointed out that the subjects' attitude during suggestion, their behaviour, their feelings, and their remarks, differed greatly from what is characteristic of an attentive person. " We note in them the most complete moral inertia, a lack of attention and reflection. . . . They are not surprised by the strangeness of their sensations, any more than we are surprised in our dreams ; the association of ideas seems to go on in them quite independently of the will." [1] Gurney makes the same observation (op. cit., p. 276) : " Even in the ' alert stage,' when the ' subject ' can be made by an occasional word to enact scene after scene with astonishing truth and vigour, the indications, if he be left alone, are of blankness, not of concentration." I have myself stressed this point, showing that the subjects are unaware of the preparatory work which is going on in their minds, that they have no sense of effort, that they do not retain a consecutive memory of the action and do not link it on to their personality ; that in many instances they are utterly unaware of it. This is the very reverse of what happens when attention is at work, for attention determines conscious efforts, the feeling of personal activity, definite memories.

Taking another standpoint, we must study the way in which these suggestible individuals behave in everyday life, apart from the phenomena of suggestion. Again and again I have pointed out that such persons, far from being endowed with the amazingly high powers of attention sometimes ascribed to them, are extremely absent-minded, and are incapable of will and of attention. Nay more, when we watch them closely we see that their suggestibility diminishes and disappears as soon as their attention comes into play. When they attend to real objects, they resist suggestions which would otherwise have influenced them readily. " No, that is not a bird upon the table. It is an inkstand. Now that I fix my attention upon the inkstand, I no longer see your bird." Conversely we may note that suggestion develops in periods when attention lapses. Here is a typical instance. Myb. (f., 64) has heard

---

[1] Bertrand, De l'exstase, 1820, p. 85.

during the day some talk about a band of hooligans who are alarming the people of her village. She is anxious, but keeps on saying : " Still, I don't believe it ; it's all nonsense." In the evening she goes to sleep, and then passes into a condition of delirious somnambulism in which she utters cries for help and hits out at any one who comes near her. On being awakened she exclaims : " I have had such a dreadful nightmare ; those wretched hooligans were really there."— Pkw., an epileptic girl of sixteen, complains that one of the other patients is being rude, and is continually exclaiming " cow " and " pig." She adds : " That woman is awfully vulgar ; I should never use such expressions myself." Shortly afterwards, Pkw. has an attack of epileptic vertigo, followed by a stage of mental confusion, during which she cries out " cow," " pig." In these remarkable cases we see that the tendency aroused by the conversations was checked by reflection and attention as long as the subject was awake, and that it only developed into an impulse during sleep. or mental confusion, when attention had lapsed.

That is why, for some time past, the general tendency has been to avoid arousing attention when making suggestions. Many authorities have noticed that in certain patients suggestions made by insinuation, made gently without attracting attention, succeed better than imperative suggestions. I have myself written at considerable length about suggestions of this kind, terming them " suggestions by distraction."[1] A great many subjects who are not ordinarily cataleptic will keep the arm raised if we raise it gently without their noticing it. In some subjects we can bring about the performance of complicated actions by standing behind them and suggesting the actions in low tones while they are talking to some one else. Let me recall the case of Ne., to whom the utterance of bad language was effectively suggested in this way. Suggestion by distraction is commoner than most people suppose ; and in many instances, instead of associating suggestion with excess of attention, we should be inclined rather to associate it with distraction or absence of mind.

How then are we to understand the phenomena quoted

---

[1] L'automatisme psychologique, 1889, pp. 185, 224, and 237 ; Les accidents mentaux des hystériques, 1894, p. 31 [this is part of the work now entitled L'état mental des hystériques].

at the outset of this section, which seemed to show that attention was the essential determinant of suggestion ? I think there is a misunderstanding. As long as attention is still very active, there is neither impulse nor suggestion ; there is an arrest of assent, and an effort towards reflection. It is at the moment when attention lapses that the tendency, which has hitherto existed only in the form of an idea, and has perhaps been concentrated during the period of arrest, undergoes discharge in the form of an impulse. A patient of mine once said to me : " I was attending carefully, and did not yield ; but I got tired, and had a moment's weakness and absence of mind ; it was then the thing happened." It follows that the intense and prolonged effort of attention does not exercise its influence directly, but paves the way for suggestion by keeping the tendency in the state of erection, by giving it time to undergo reinforcements, by concentrating it. But thereby it becomes a determinant of the forms of enfeeblement of thought which we have next to consider.

4. MONOIDEISM.

We find it necessary to return to a group of theories of suggestion which have been based upon an entirely different principle. Instead of associating the suggestive impulse with an unusually high development of certain tendencies, these theories associate it with a general weakness of the mind, and in particular with a weakness of the higher tendencies which constitute the personality. While maintaining the same essential character, the theories in question have assumed a number of different forms.

The first form, I think, is what is known as monoideism, the theory according to which an idea detached from other ideas will exercise an unusually powerful force in the mind. This notion was formulated long ago both by Descartes and by Condillac. The magnetisers were well aware that suggestion was more powerful when the subjects were " isolated," that is to say when they were apparently unable to perceive any phenomena except the personality of the magnetiser and his utterances. Braid gave a similar explanation of suggestion when he spoke of mental concentration in this connexion, but his views of the matter were vague, and his theory resembled that of those who regard suggestion as a manifestation of an excess of attention.[1] Subsequently, Liébeault formulated the same idea, but with rather more precision.

It is to Charles Richet, I think, that we are indebted for the best monoideistic interpretation of suggestion. He wrote in 1879 : " A trifling auditory or visual stimulus passes unnoticed by one in the auditorium of a theatre, whereas the same stimulus would have a great effect upon one who is alone in a silent place. A person in the ordinary waking state may be compared to a member of the audience at a theatre, whereas the somnambulist to whom a suggestion is made is like a man in a lonely and quiet place."[2] If a thought is to be checked, says Richet, another thought must put an obstacle in its way ; if a sentiment is to be hindered, a stronger sentiment must be at work. " We may suppose that, in suggestion, the phenomena we perceive are due to the absence of this simultaneous memory of two sentiments or two thoughts."[3] Charcot accepts this interpretation, writing : " In certain subjects we can give birth by way of suggestion, of intimation, to a coherent group of associated ideas, which become installed in the mind like a parasite, the group being isolated from all other groups, and disclosing its existence to the outer world through appropriate motor phenomena."[4] Again : " The suggested idea, or the group of suggested ideas, thus isolated, will be shielded from the influence of the great collection of individual ideas which has for so long been undergoing accumulation and organisation, and which constitutes the consciousness properly so called, the ego. That is why the movements which disclose to the outer world these acts of unconscious cerebration are distinguished by their automatic character, by what may be spoken of as their purely mechanical character. Thus we have in all its simplicity the man-machine dreamed of by Lamettrie."[5]

Thenceforward, this idea of monoideism secured almost universal expression. Ochorowicz, Schneider, Gurney, and Delboeuf, clarified and defended it. " In suggestion," said Delboeuf, " all other objects disappear ; a suggestion is as

---

[1] Cf. Bramwell, Proceedings of the S.P.R., 1896, pp. 214–215.
[2] " Revue Philosophique," 1879, vol. ii, p. 612.
[3] Richet, L'homme et l'intelligence, p. 529 ; cf. also " Revue Philosophique," 1888, vol. i, p. 506.
[4] Oeuvres, vol. iii, p. 336.   [5] Ibid., p. 337.

detached from surroundings as are the images of an ordinary dream. Like these images, the suggestion shows up against a black background, and is thus made conspicuous by contrast. What has been spoken of as the absence of shame in the dream and in suggestion, is often due to this alone." [1] Wundt may seem to have criticised these views of suggestion, but he hastened to reformulate the very same theory, while translating it into anatomical terminology. [2]

A great many cases could be quoted to illustrate the monoideism that characterises suggestion. Long ago, I myself described at considerable length the individuals who are taken prisoner by a suggested idea, so that they can see and think of nothing else. For the time they ignore their objective situation, and forget even their name ; and when they return to the world of reality they have no memory of what they have been doing. [3] On the other hand, we hinder the development of suggestions when we remain in rapport with the subject, and when we insinuate into his mind other ideas which oppose the first idea. When the subject resists a suggestion, we can note that the idea has, by association, awakened antagonising tendencies. We suggest to a youth that he should strip. He begins to do so, but then, remembering that his shirt is dirty, he stops undressing ; and if we persist, he has a nervous crisis. Suggestion ceases to act when monoideism disappears. Bramwell, criticising this theory, refers to his own experiments with multiple suggestions, made successively or even simultaneously. [4] We may answer that in these cases each system develops in isolation, and that there is no common consciousness ; we may also rejoin that in many such instances there is, at bottom, only one suggestion at work —the suggestion that the subject shall promptly obey the suggester's orders, whatever these may be. In that case, the suggested idea is substantially unique. Monoideism would seem, therefore, to be one of the important determinants of suggestion.

Unfortunately, however, illusory elements enter into this terminology and into these explanations. Concentration of

[1] Delboeuf, " Revue Philosophique," 1887, vol. i, p. 132.
[2] Wundt, " Revue Philosophique," 1892, vol. ii, p. 557 ; Hypnotisme et suggestion, 1893, p. 85.
[3] Janet, L'automatisme psychologique, 1889, p. 186.
[4] Proceedings of the S.P.R., 1896, p. 243.

thought and action are extremely common when a tendency is realising itself in action. We see this to a preeminent degree in the resolution that follows reflection, for this resolution is definitely characterised by a return to unity after the dispersal that has been going on during the discussion of conflicting motives. It is natural, therefore, that monoideism should be found in suggestion. If that is all the theory has to tell us, it is one which differs little from the theory of the concentration of attention. Unless we are told of some special characteristics of this monoideism, we shall assume it to be identical with the monoideism of reflection and with other manifestations of monoideism.

5. Suggestion and Psychological Depression.

If the theory of monoideism is to have a precise significance, we must go a step further. We must show that, as far as the monoideism of suggestion is concerned, we have to do with a special form of weakness owing to which an elementary idea is left in isolation, and is not combined with others to form a higher unity. Thus in 1889 I endeavoured to render the notion of this form of monoideism more precise by studies concerning " the restriction of the field of consciousness, the enfeeblement of psychological synthesis, and mental dis-aggregation." I tried to show by numerous observations and analyses which I need not recapitulate here the truth of the assertion that " it is a condition of natural and perpetual distraction, which prevents these persons from appreciating any other idea than the one which actually occupies their mind." [1] This condition is not disclosed only by suggestibility, for it gives rise to a special type of behaviour in the persons who forget the presence of others as soon as these latter cease to speak ; who exaggerate all their own thoughts, which very readily become transformed into hallucinations and impulses ; who are always absent-minded and heedless ; who are excessively emotional, and whose emotions are so readily modified by trifling influences.[2] " The restriction of the field of consciousness is shown by the lack of the number-less collateral thoughts which events ordinarily call up, and

[1] L'automatisme psychologique, 1889, p. 189.
[2] Ibid., pp. 189, 201, and 213.

which give to normal behaviour its balance and continuity."
Somewhat later, I resumed and completed this line of study
in my work on *Les accidents mentaux des hystériques*.[1] My
observations regarding this matter have never been seriously
discussed. I still regard them as of importance, for they
throw light on the conditions under which we can best
endeavour to induce suggestions.

To-day, however, it is possible to advance further along
the same road, and to understand this reduction in the power
of psychological synthesis by associating it with the general
lowering of psychological tension of which it is no more than
a particular form. We know that in a very large number of
phenomena regarded as lying in the No-Man's Land between
the normal and the pathological (phenomena of which fatigue
and emotion are typical instances), the level of mental activity
lowers. When this happens, difficult adaptations to new
situations can no longer be effected ; the higher tendencies,
those which are most complex and which have been most
recently acquired, can no longer undergo complete activation,
and remain in one of the initial stages of activation, or enter
the field of activity slowly and late. The more profound
the depression, the more numerous are the tendencies which
become affected in this way, and the more markedly does the
disorder extend to the elementary tendencies.

It is easy to ascertain that suggestion is related to these
phenomena of depression. We see suggestibility in connexion
with fatigue. The absence of mind of the man who is working,
and who is making or has just made a notable effort of attention,
is largely the outcome of fatigue ; and it is during such periods
of distraction that we can most often study the workings of
suggestion, elementary suggestion at any rate, in normal
persons. Lagrange and Tissié have recorded remarkable
instances of the suggestibility that is manifested after excessive
fatigue, as in those who have just been engaged in a long-
distance bicycle race, for example.

Still more obvious, in this connexion, is the part played
by emotion—and emotion, as I have tried to show elsewhere,
is in reality nothing more than a kind of fatigue.[2] A great

---

[1] 1893, pp. 45 and 52. See Bibliography
[2] Les problèmes psychologiques de l'émotion, " Revue Neurologique,"
1909, p. 1556.

many of the earlier writers on suggestion have insisted on this point. I may refer to Mesnet,[1] Liébeault,[2] Myers,[3] and Beaunis,[4] who lay stress upon the changes in the subject's facial expression at the moment when a suggestion is made, and upon the way in which emotion disorders his ideas. I myself have summarised the role of emotion and fatigue in every suggestion as follows : " When, to one of these hysterical women, we enunciate an idea which is strange and which conflicts with reality, she shows signs of surprise, seems to experience an emotional shock, and resists for a time ; that is to say, for a time she retains consciousness of the notion of her personality, and is still aware of external objects, so that these sound ideas oppose the contradictory thought. Then, since in these patients attention is speedily fatigued, she becomes unable to retain so many things in her mind at once. . . . Her narrow consciousness has no longer room for the antagonising memories and sensations, . . . and all the elements of the suggested idea are free to develop. . . . At the moment of suggestion there occurs a shock, there is felt an emotion which destroys the subject's enfeebled personal synthesis, so that the suggested idea remains isolated."[5] As little later, Bourdin gave an excellent summary of the same ideas : " A weakly and impressionable mind is predisposed by intense emotion, mingled simultaneously with genuine fear and secret pleasure, to submit to the will of the experimenter, to surrender to him for the time being—there is a true vertigo."[6] More recently Bleuler, Lipps, Münsterberg,[7] and Ernest Jones,[8] have returned to this question of the part played by emotion in suggestion. Finally, we can study the working of suggestion in certain mental disorders, which are merely permanent depressions of psychological activity. Suggestion has often been described in the course of various intoxications, and in dream delirium.

After the lapse of twenty-five years, I find it necessary

[1] Somnambulisme pathologique, 1874, p. 147.
[2] Du sommeil, etc., 1866, p. 144.
[3] Proceedings of the S.P.R., 1886–1887, p. 164.
[4] Le somnambulisme provoqué, 1886, p. 80.
[5] L'état mental des hystériques, 1893, vol. i, p. 53.
[6] De l'impulsion et spécialment de son rapport avec le crime, 1894.
[7] Psychotherapy, 1909, p. 123.
[8] The Action of Suggestion in Psychotherapy, " Journal of Abnormal Psychology," vol. v, p. 243 ; Papers on Psychoanalysis, third edition, pp. 340–381.

to reiterate an affirmation which has often been contradicted, but which I see no reason to withdraw. I refer to the statement that suggestion is an eminently hysterical phenomenon, being witnessed most often and most easily in this particular neurosis. Many of the earlier observers were convinced of this truth. Charcot, Beaunis, Delboeuf, and Gilles de la Tourette, defended the view ; but to-day it is sometimes discredited. At the Geneva Congress, Schnyder declared that suggestion can only be detected at work in a minority of hysterics, in 43 per cent., whereas it can be detected in 70 per cent. of neurasthenics. It seems to me amazing that any medical practitioner could have made such a statement. Happily Terrien, of Nantes, reversed the terms of the proposition, maintaining, as I have always maintained, that suggestion plays little or no part in neurasthenia, but plays a large part in hysteria.[1]

We thus come to a first conclusion. Suggestion is due to a mental depression, which may be transient and related to fatigue or to emotion, or may be long lasting as the outcome of one of those neuroses which are preeminently characterised by depression.

The great difficulty, and the most persistent, is that not all varieties of depression are competent to give rise to suggestion, so that we have to specify the degree and the kind of depression that can originate suggestion. The early writers on the subject had already pointed out that suggestion properly so-called does not occur in idiots and dements. In these patients, the various tendencies are dissociated, so that it is hardly possible for them to take the form of ideas and assents.

In melancholia, too, in mania, and in psychasthenic delirium, we find it difficult to detect any phenomena akin to suggestion. I think that these intense forms of depression affect and disorder the functions of immediate assent. Such patients have lost the power of willing and believing, even in a direct fashion. Their raptus (seizures, or paroxysms) are inferior forms of activation, resembling those reflexes in which tendencies are not checked at the stage of the idea or even of the wish ; they must not be confounded with impulses or

[1] Terrien, " Archives de Neurologie," 1907, p. 147.

suggestions. " Certain minds, then, are below the level at which suggestion is possible, just as certain patients in whom a microbic infection has occurred are incapable of a febrile reaction." [1]

I must add that there are lesser grades of depression in which suggestion is equally unknown. In my lectures at the College of France, when I was trying to describe and classify the various degrees of depression, I placed accesses of gloom and lethargy of mind at the beginning of the scale of depression, just below the mean level of normal tension. The depression of gloom or sadness affects only the lasts grades of activation, those which relate to the triumph, those which terminate and crown the act. Lethargy of mind, which touches a lower level, affects the regions of effort and all the tendencies which (like work) are derived from effort, all the operations in virtue of which action passes from decision to performance. But suggestion, as we have seen, has no need of operations of this sort, for it maintains itself at the level of the realist tendencies, of the tendencies that bring about assent, and these are not affected in the first grades of depression. Thus we do not observe suggestion in sad persons or in idle persons. They are, if we like to phrase it thus, above suggestion.

Suggestion belongs to a very special group of depressions, those which bear almost entirely upon the realist tendencies, especially in their complete form of tendencies to reflective assent. This is the grade of depression characteristic of the psychasthenic state, wherein, independently of suggestion properly so called, we can observe all the most interesting disorders of will, belief, and the sense of reality.

This special kind of depression is met with under two forms : that of psychasthenia in the strict sense of the term ; and that of hysteria, which I am more and more inclined to regard as merely a variety of the former. In psychasthenia we can generally detect the presence of obsession, which, more often than is commonly supposed, has interesting relationships with suggestion ; but obsession in psychasthenics does not usually manifest itself in the form of impulse. There are, I think, several reasons for this failure of obsession to take effect as impulse. First of all, the tendencies underlying the obsessive idea are endowed with little energy. We shall see

[1] L'état mental des hystériques, vol. ii, p. 48.

later, when studying the tendencies that take the form of a search for excitation, that certain psychasthenic obsessions may assume a definitely impulsive form as suggestions when they depend upon a vigorous tendency such as the need for excitation. In the second place, the obsessive idea has to encounter resistances, such as habits of doubt, hesitation, and disquietude. Finally, in psychasthenics, while it is certain that the powers of reflection are disordered, so that the mind can no longer reach a conclusion, still, reflection is never completely arrested, and therefore the obsessive ideas are never allowed a perfectly free rein.

In hysteria, on the other hand, we can discern, underlying the idea, certain tendencies which have retained more energy ; we can discern a considerable inclination to obedience and complaisance, instead of disquietude and doubt. But reflection, which is disordered in hysteria as well as in psychasthenia, though in another way, does not now persist indefinitely. It is suddenly checked. The hysteric relinquishes internal discussion, just as the patient I was describing a few pages back relinquished the discussion with his adversaries—but the hysteric abandons discussion without making any inward reservations. The hysteric ceases to question himself, ceases to call up new pros and cons, ceases to surround the evoked idea by other ideas. If the circumstances or the words of an individual who is on the watch continue to evoke and strengthen this idea, it remains alone, isolated, and powerful. It is then transformed by automatic assent, of which the subject is still capable, so that it becomes a suggestion. The curtailment of the mental field, monoideism, is not now the outcome of a synthesis which has transformed the primitive idea by adapting it to others. It results from the disappearance of all other ideas (which are no longer called up by the enfeebled powers of reflection), and from the survival of the primary idea just as it existed before reflection began—the idea which has now become impulsive. Further back I was describing the passionate impulses in which the transformation of an idea into an impulse was due to the inherent energy of the underlying tendency. In the present case we are concerned with genuinely suggestive impulses wherein the transformation of the idea into an impulse is due to the insufficiency and suspension of reflection.

To conclude the account of the conditions under which suggestion occurs, I must say a few words anent a matter which used to be considered very important, and concerning which a vast amount has been written. Are the conditions under which suggestion occurs part of the normal equipment of the mind, or is suggestion a pathological phenomenon ? At the Congress of Psychotherapy in the year 1910, although nearly all my inferences (those I have just been expounding) as to the nature of suggestion and the conditions under which it occurs had proved acceptable, there were indignant protests when I drew the final conclusion that suggestion is a pathological manifestation. Sentiment plays its part here. Doctors who want suggestive treatment to be accepted by the public, by the whole public, are naturally unwilling to have it described as an abnormal phenomenon, as one peculiar to certain types of patient. There are, moreover, many misunderstandings attaching to the use of the terms " suggestion," " health," and " disease."

Even though the term " suggestion " be used with a precise significance, we have to recognise that suggestive phenomena can be witnessed in persons whose condition is normal. Pathological phenomena are only exaggerations of normal phenomena ; and distraction, fatigue, and emotion are, to a certain extent, compatible with what is termed normality. It is, therefore, always easy to quote instances of suggestion in the normal state. These instances are always the same : keeping step ; contagious yawning ; the way in which we incline to raise our eyes when we see others staring at something above the ordinary line of vision ; the way in which people will scratch themselves when they hear any mention of fleas ; and so on.[1] I quite agree that these actions are sometimes truly suggestive in nature, although they occur in persons who are perfectly normal. But such suggestions take effect in the production of insignificant actions only, and are promptly suppressed if the action becomes important. If we feel that we are being watched, we check the impulse to yawn or to scratch.

The fact is that, in the normal human being of our days, the inclination to reflect is always ready to be awakened.

---

[1] Cf. Haberman, op. cit., p. 7.

Reflection supervises our actions so that these may conform to certain elementary rules, and, in especial, may conform to our own personal interest. Thus, reflection comes into play whenever actions of any importance have to be performed. No doubt it is easy to make amusing experiments which show that reflection of this kind is sometimes in abeyance. Binet, in his *La suggestibilité,* and Münsterberg, in his *Psychotherapy,* mention some experiments of the kind. Here is a remarkable one. Show any one a drawing of two circles of precisely the same size. In one of these circles are written the figures 14 ; and in the other, the figures 19. On being asked which of the two circles is the larger, the majority of persons will point to the circle 19. But in this we have to do with exceptional conditions, and with matters of trifling importance. Every instinct is liable to be deceived.

The suggestion with which we have to do in medical science is of a very different kind. It cannot be serviceable unless it induces actions which are fairly important, which persist for a considerable time, and which do not cease because of some minor incident. But these conditions can only be fulfilled if there is a rather serious suspension of control and reflection, a suspension incompatible with a normal state of mind. What we have to ask ourselves is, whether this peculiar condition, which affects the level of reflective assent and does not extend into lower levels of the mind, can exist apart from hysteria. A precise answer can hardly be given, seeing that hysteria, like most other disorders of the mind, can only be defined by its psychological symptoms. " Hysteria " means this particular form of depression. We may agree that such depression may arise accidentally in certain persons, and may not affect them for so long a time as to constitute a neurosis properly so called. That is the explanation of the periods of transient suggestibility in the course of various diseases, or as a sequel of fatigues or emotion. In the next chapter we shall have to enquire, apropos of hypnotism, whether it is in our power to produce these abnormal phases artificially.

For the nonce it will suffice to summarise some elementary notions concerning the mechanism of suggestion and the conditions under which it occurs. In my view, suggestion, far from being a simple and commonplace phenomenon, is a very definite phenomenon indeed, and one which is induced by the cooperation of several factors.

1. Suggestion is only possible in the minds of those who, it may be for a very brief period or it may be for a considerable time, suffer from a depression of an average degree of intensity, affecting the level at which the realist tendencies work, and rendering reflection slow, difficult, and brief.

2. It can only supervene when some circumstance or other has given birth to an idea at a moment when reflection cannot awaken ; or when some circumstance or other has made an idea penetrate so rapidly that the sluggish process of reflection has no time to become active.

3. It may also arise when an idea has remained in the mind so long that the tendency to reflection has been exhausted before a conclusion has been reached.

These conditions do not often occur in natural circumstances, although at the beginning of the present chapter I have recorded a few instances of the kind. Generally speaking, the operator who wishes to make use of suggestion must artificially assemble the requisite factors.

CHAPTER SEVEN

PROBLEMS OF HYPNOTISM

THE same questions have to be asked as regards hypnotism. We have to do here with a psychological modification which we are trying to bring about in the subject's mental state. What is its nature ? What are the conditions under which it occurs ?

The most obvious and indisputable characteristic is that we have to do with an *artificial modification of the mind*, which the operator can produce at the moment of election, and which he can terminate at will by bringing the subject back into the preexistent state. This characteristic is plainly manifest in all the practices employed to hypnotise or put to sleep, and in all those employed to dehypnotise or to awaken the patient. But as to the nature of the modification which is induced by these processes, there is far less general agreement.

I. HYPNOTISM AS A STATE OF SUGGESTIBILITY.

The study of hypnotism has always been closely linked with the study of suggestion. I believe the reason for this association to be as follows. The experimenters, while continuing to repeat that suggestion was universal, could not help noting that in actual fact their patients paid very little attention to therapeutic suggestions, and they tried to modify the subjects' mental condition in order to render this more malleable. On the other hand, little gain would accrue from inducing a permanent and perpetual suggestibility, for one who is persistently suggestible will be persistently exposed to all kinds of influence. He will always pay heed to the latest voice ; a beneficent suggestion he has just heard will be annulled a moment later by a counter-suggestion. Persistent suggestibility cannot provide the ideal conditions of treatment. Greatly preferable will be a suggestibility that shall be well marked but of very brief duration ; a definite state of mind which can be easily produced and just as easily annulled by the will of the experimenter, with the proviso that, when the state has passed away, the patient shall still be favourably influenced by the beneficial suggestions he has received, but will have become inapt to receive new suggestions. Unfortunately it is far from easy to bring about transformations of the human mind at will, and upon this matter we are ignorant and ill-equipped. For this reason it was natural to study a transformation of mind whose characteristics were already familiar, and one that could be induced with comparative ease ; and to study this condition in order to learn whether it might not provide the desiderated form of suggestibility. A century ago, the magnetisers used, by artificial means, to induce in their subjects a transient modification in the mental state ; then, by other means, they annulled this state, and restored the subject to his original condition. The hypnotists produced the same changes in the mind, though perhaps by different methods. Thus the means were known whereby it was possible to induce an abnormal mental condition of brief duration. Was it not desirable to make use of the condition ? On this line of reasoning, the attempt was made to employ suggestion when the subject was hypnotised, in the belief that hypnosis was peculiarly favourable to such suggestions.

It has to be remembered that hypnosis, or what the magnetisers termed induced somnambulism, had never been clearly defined, so that it was easy to ascribe to it any qualities the experimenter might wish. Charpignon said it was " a dynamic modification of the organism and a change in the distribution of its electricities." [1] J. P. Durand spoke of it as a form of nervous plethora. Braid, Bubnof, and Heidenhain called it nervous exhaustion. Some authorities termed it a condition of irregular and unequal distribution of the nervous fluid. Most hypnotisers said simply, with Paul Richer, that hypnotism was " a totality of peculiar states of the nervous system determined by artificial manipulations " [2]—a non-committal statement. In these circumstances, hypnosis

---

[1] Charpignon, Physiologie, médecine et metaphysique du magnétisme, 1848, p. 292.
[2] Richer, Etudes cliniques sur l'hystéro-epilepsie, ou grande hystérie, 1885, p. 512.

was, so to speak, void, and suggestion installed itself in the vacant space.

A great many writers have been inclined to identify suggestion and hypnotism. For them, hypnosis was a very simple notion, being the name given to a transient psychological condition induced by artificial means, and characterised solely by the possibility of making, in the hypnotised subject, any suggestions the experimenter might please. The way had already been paved for this notion. One of the magnetisers, Dupau, had said that the condition of his somnambulists was characterised by an impairment of will, by excess of imagination, and by imitativeness.[1] J. P. Durand was inclined to regard hypnosis as a "hypotaxic" condition preparatory to the "ideoplasty" of suggestions. Joly, in his little book *L'imagination* (1877), summarised the opinion of his day when he said : "Somnambulism is characterised by the moral inertia of the subjects, who accept every idea with which they are supplied."

Bernheim did more than previous writers to render this conception precise. For him, hypnosis was "a peculiar psychological condition capable of being artificially induced, and activating or intensifying suggestibility, by which is to be understood the aptitude for being influenced by an idea accepted by the brain, and the aptitude for realising it."[2] In an article in the "Temps," January 29, 1891, in which Bernheim gives an excellent summary of his own teachings, he writes : "Hypnosis is, then, not an induced sleep, but is suggestibility activated and intensified. . . . Hypnosis is not an unnatural condition ; it does not create new functions ; . . . thanks to a peculiar form of psychical concentration [?], it exaggerates the normal suggestibility with which we are all to some extent endowed ; it develops a new state of consciousness characterised by a predominance of the imaginative faculties and by a reduction of intellectual initiative—a state thanks to which we more brilliantly and clearly realise the ideas, the impressions, and the images that are induced." Beaunis formulates a similar definition.[3] Barth tells us that hypnosis is characterised by the suppression of the voluntary

[1] Dupau, Lettres sur le magnétisme, 1826, p. 88.
[2] Bernheim, De la suggestion, 1886, p. 166.
[3] Beaunis, Le somnambulisme, 1886, p. 230.

cerebral influx and the exaggeration of the automatic cerebral influx, and by paralysis of the conscious will with an exuberance of memory and imagination.[1] We find the same view in Schneider's book, in Babinski's article, in Lloyd Tuckey's book, and in the same author's contribution to Parker's *Psychotherapy*.[2] Tuckey tells us that the effect of suggestion is greater in proportion to the depth of the hypnosis. Vires' more elaborate definition has the same significance : " Hypnotism is a condition of the nervous system characterised by the slumber of all general or kinaesthetic sensibility, by the suspension of all intellectual activity, and by the uniting of all the sensory or intellectual elements under the command of an operator. It is differentiated from normal sleep by the fact that the sleeper neither knows nor hears what is going on around him."[3] Myers' views, which are reiterated by Bramwell, involve much the same definition of hypnosis, the only difference being that suggestion is regarded as more potent. According to Bramwell, the supraliminal consciousness of voluntary psychic phenomena, having been elevated in the course of evolution, has relinquished the power of guiding and controlling the phenomena of the organic life, and has entrusted these matters to the management of the subliminal consciousness. During hypnosis, the will resumes its influence over subconscious vegetative phenomena.[4]

Can we take these definitions in a precise and literal sense ? Can we write simply and intelligibly : Hypnosis is a condition in which suggestion exists alone, or preponderates enormously and determines all the other phenomena ; whereas the waking state is one in which suggestion plays no part. Obviously this will not do, seeing that so many observers, and especially Richet and Bernheim, have offered many proofs that suggestion occurs in the waking state. We have seen, moreover, that certain individuals are persistently suggestible, for periods lasting a number of years, although their condition is to all appearance normal. This permanent susceptibility to suggestion conflicts with our general notion of hypnosis as a state which is both transient and artificially induced. It is

---

[1] Barth, Du sommeil non naturel, 1886, p. 125.
[2] How Suggestion Works, Parker, II, ii, 5.
[3] Vires, L'hypnotisme et la suggestion hypnotique, 1901.
[4] Bramwell, The Evolution of Hypnotic Theory, " Brain," 1896.

impossible, therefore, to accept the foregoing definitions literally. If we adopt them at all, it must be in an attenuated sense, for we can say no more than that hypnosis is a condition in which an individual's suggestibility is considerably greater than in what is known as the waking state.

The definition thus becomes extremely vague, and hard to establish. Besides, even in this restricted sense, it entails numerous difficulties. First of all, it involves what I must regard as a very questionable affirmation, namely that during the state of hypnosis all the other important and characteristic phenomena are dependent on suggestion. I am well aware that this contention will be agreeable to certain contemporary writers who believe that all the psychological phenomena of the neuroses depend upon suggestion. I think that the assertion lacks confirmation. I cannot myself believe that posthypnotic amnesia, for instance, has always been suggested to the subject by a clumsy experimenter. The theory that everything depends upon suggestion (which is itself left entirely unexplained) is quite inadequate.

Moreover, there are other difficulties. The definition is so general and so vague that it becomes applicable to quite a number of things which are not hypnosis at all. There are a good many conditions in which suggestibility is greatly increased ; for instance, in intoxications such as that due to alcohol, in certain infectious diseases such as typhoid, in states of fatigue or emotion, etc. Are we to call all these " hypnosis " ? Are we to ignore the most essential characteristic of hypnosis, and the one which gives it its practical importance ; I mean that it is artificially induced, that it depends upon the experimenter for its beginning and its end ?

We still have the main difficulty to consider. As Lafontaine (p. 112) and Charles Despine, the magnetisers, pointed out long ago, the degree of suggestibility witnessed in what we now term the hypnotic state is very variable. All those who have practised hypnotism have described cases in which a resistance to suggestion has been manifest.[1] For many years I have been stressing accounts of hypnotic states in which there is no suggestibility ; of conditions in which the subject manifests powers of personal volition perfectly identical with those of the normal individuals with whom we rub shoulders

---

[1] Cf. Binet and Féré, Le magnétisme animal, 1887, p. 107,

in everyday life and whom we do not regard as hypnotised. The fact is all the more remarkable seeing that the subjects in question were patients, and that in the waking state they were characterised by well-marked distraction, mental confusion, and suggestibility. Have we to reverse our phraseology, and to say that in these subjects hypnosis is their ordinary and persistent condition, whereas the waking state is transient and artificially induced ? I have done this myself at times, quite aware that I was straining the sense of the terms, and was using them as metaphors to illustrate my thoughts regarding these remarkable conditions. Were we to adopt such language as a matter of routine, " hypnosis " would forfeit the characteristics of being artificially induced and of being a transient condition. A good many other writers have recorded observations adverse to the notion that heightened suggestibility is an essential feature of hypnosis.[1] Claparède, after having made some experiments to compare the mental condition of subjects during hypnosis and in the waking state respectively, came to the following conclusion : " It is very doubtful whether hypnosis can be regarded as increased suggestibility. Certain subjects are more suggestible in the waking state than during hypnotic sleep." [2] We thus come back to the conclusions which I formulated many years ago : " The phenomena of suggestion are independent of the hypnotic state ; well-marked suggestibility may exist quite apart from artificial somnambulism, and suggestibility may be entirely lacking in one who is in a state of complete somnambulism ; in a word, suggestibility does not vary simultaneously with somnambulism, and does not vary in the same direction." [3]

2. HYPNOTISM AS A STATE OF SLEEP.

We can now pass to a second group of definitions which are somewhat better than those we have been considering, seeing that they pay more heed to the transient and artificial characteristics of hypnosis. In these definitions, hypnosis is compared with normal sleep, and is regarded as a sleep

---

[1] Cf. Bramwell, Proceedings of the S.P.R., 1896, p. 218.
[2] Edouard Claparède and W. Beede, Recherches expérimentales sur quelques phénomènes simples dans un cas d'hypnose, " Archives de Psychologie," July 1909.
[3] L'automatisme psychologique, 1889, p. 171.

artificially induced in the midst of the waking state and in opposition thereto.

Such was the thesis expounded long ago by the philosopher Jouffroy, who wrote : " Perhaps the somnambulic or magnetic sleep does not differ so much from ordinary sleep as most people suppose. The majority of the phenomena presented by the former are no more than salient instances of the phenomena observed in ordinary sleep." [1] Maury advocated a similar notion. He compared dreaming with hallucination, and insisted that suggestion must occur during natural sleep, since it was possible to influence dreams. " In hypnosis," he wrote, " just as in sleep with dreams, there is a certain torpor accompanied by moderate excitement." Many magnetisers and hypnotists have compared the condition of their subjects to that of ordinary sleep ; among these I may mention Teste,[2] Noizet,[3] Liébeault,[4] Max Simon,[5] Carpenter, and Gurney.[6] Bernheim vacillates between this theory and the one expounded in the previous section. In that section we quoted the article that appeared in the " Temps " on January 29, 1891. Here Bernheim writes : " Hypnosis is not a sleep. . . . Some hypnotised persons have no sense of being asleep." But at other times, he writes the precise opposite : " Hypnosis is identical with sleep ; . . . the spontaneous sleeper is only a self-hypnotised person who receives suggestions from his own organism." [7] In later years, Bernheim seems to have adopted the view just expounded. In his report to the International Society of Psychotherapeutics, presented to the Munich Congress in September 1911, he wrote : " Hypnotic sleep has no special qualities ; when it is genuine, it does not differ in any way from natural sleep. . . . Hypnosis is nothing more than the sleep which has been induced by a suggestive process. . . . The words ' hypnotism ' and ' hypnosis ' might be suppressed, for it would suffice to speak of sleep induced by suggestion." [8] Let us disregard, for the moment, this

[1] Mélanges philosophiques, fifth edition, 1875, p. 236.
[2] Le magnétisme animal expliqué, 1845, p. 278.
[3] Mémoire sur le somnambulisme, etc., 1854, p. 93.
[4] Du sommeil et des états analogues, 1866, p. 144.
[5] Le monde des rêves, 1882, p. 201.
[6] Proceedings of the S.P.R., 1883–1884, p. 266.
[7] " Revue de l'Hypnotisme," 1887, p. 136.
[8] Bernheim, " Journal für Psychologie und Neurologie," 1911, Sonderab druck.

question of induction by suggestion, for it relates to the problem of the determinants of hypnosis. The residual point is that, for Bernheim, hypnosis is the same thing as sleep.

This opinion has been voiced by many contemporary authorities. We shall find it in various formulations in the writings of Forel, Vogt, Wetterstrand, Moll, Jong, Lehmann, Wundt, Voisin, Bérillon, Döllken, etc. This comparison of hypnosis and sleep was made for various reasons, which are interesting. Hypnosis was regarded as a peculiar mental condition occupying a definite part of the lifetime, and differentiated from the ordinary consciousness of the subject. Now, sleep seemed to be the only phenomenon endowed with such characteristics. It had been noticed that the hypnotic state, at the outset, frequently resembled a sort of swoon or doze. Certain subjects, in the opening phase of the abnormal period, exhibited some degree of torpor, found a difficulty in moving and sleeping, and complained of feeling heavy and sleepy. The end of the hypnotic state is very like an ordinary act of awaking, accompanied by a sense of the throwing off of torpor, and characterised by a gradual return to the normal condition, and above all by a forgetfulness of what has happened during the abnormal condition—this being closely analogous to what we see in one who awakens from ordinary sleep and forgets his dreams. In the case of all these manifestations and feelings we have, doubtless, to allow for the ancient traditions of the magnetisers and for the part played by the training of the subjects. Still, a considerable proportion of the phenomena is natural and spontaneous, for we see such phenomena also in subjects who have not been experimented upon or trained in any way, in accidental cases of illness, which can likewise induce dissociations, and can bring about conditions distinct from the waking state. Finally, we have to note that a good many of the more important phenomena of hypnotism are paralleled by the phenomena of sleep. Jouffroy had already observed this : " When the magnetiser's voice makes itself heard, the mind of the somnambulist, recognising the sounds which the somnambulist has determined to observe, will concentrate attention on these sounds, will understand them, and will respond to them. If this voice authoritatively orders the subject to attend to the feelings in particular parts of the body, the subject will obey, and will distinguish the most trifling sensations in these parts, while ignoring much stronger sensations in other parts. Well now, if, when you fall asleep, you have a fancy that there are bugs in your bed, the most trifling irritations will disturb your sleep. They will disturb you because they will attract the attention of your mind, and your mind will attend to them because it is forewarned. Were it not forewarned, it would disregard much stronger sensations. We can thus understand how it is that, since the mind has the power of awaking the senses or of not awaking them as it may please, the subject remains asleep as long as the magnetiser wishes, and awakens directly the magnetiser orders him to awaken or touches him in a prearranged manner." [1] We may add that dreams may be evoked by various impressions; and that they have frequently been compared, and then confounded, with hallucinations and with suggestions. These remarks and these facile comparisons have given rise to the prevailing opinion that the hypnotic state is a form of sleep, perhaps perfectly identical with normal sleep, or perhaps differing slightly from normal sleep in its production or in its course.

The theory is a fascinating one, but it has been subjected to criticism, not only by myself in 1889, but subsequently by many other writers, such as Ochorowicz,[2] Krafft-Ebing, Mendel, Babinski,[3] and Döllken. These criticisms may be summarised and amplified as follows. It is true that sleep is a phase of life differing from our normal state, but it has its own peculiar characteristics none the less. During sleep there occurs a marked slowing down of all the bodily and mental functions. The activity of the circulation, the respiration, and even the secretions, is greatly reduced; psychological tension is much lowered; movement and action are almost completely suppressed. External stimuli, which arouse action in the waking state, will, during sleep, either pass entirely unperceived, or else, if they evoke tendencies, will do so only to a minimal degree. The tendencies thus called into activity, but undergoing only a partial development, remain in the state of dreams, which perhaps represent a grade of activation inferior to that of the idea. If the stimulus be repeated, or if it be powerful enough to compel the evoked tendency to

---

[1] Op. cit., p. 236.   [2] Congrès de Psychologie, 1889.
[3] " Gazette Hebdomadaire," July 1893.

develop more strongly, the result is very remarkable. Now the sleeper stirs and awakens, for the state of sleep is incompatible with a very moderate rise in psychological tension. To employ an image I have often used, sleep may be compared to a condition of minimal expenditure, in which economies are made to facilitate great expenditure in the waking state ; just as people with a small income will sometimes live for six months of the year cheaply in a quiet country place that they may be able to spend freely in town during the other half of the year.

But if this description of sleep be accurate, sleep differs markedly from hypnosis, for in that condition the tension of bodily and mental activity is considerably higher. In hypnosis, unless special suggestions have been at work, we do not observe the reduction of functions which is characteristic of normal sleep ; there is no extensive slackening of the respiration, for instance, such as always occurs in sleep. Mental activity, above all, may display quite a high tension in the hypnotic state. In most instances, the subject remains capable of moving and acting spontaneously ; and in all cases he is able to understand what is said to him, and he himself speaks. When we come to the more inert forms of hypnosis, we witness the fundamental phenomenon of suggestion, namely, incitement to action, which does not occur during normal sleep. By the words we address to the hypnotised subject, we can make him perform complete actions without experiencing any change of state ; but in the sleeper we cannot induce any movement by speech, and, if we press the point, we shall simply awaken him. Here is an observation I have made several times. I wanted to hypnotise a woman in whom artificial somnambulism had often been induced, at a time when she was tired out after several nights of watching and hard work. She was sitting in an armchair, and fell into an ordinary sleep. When I tried to make her speak to me, as she usually did in the somnambulist state, she awoke with a start and rubbed her eyes, saying : " I was so tired that I fell into an ordinary dose."

A little difficulty arises in connexion with dreams, for we believe that in certain cases they may be determined in the dreamer by external stimuli. I think the occurrence is less common and less complete than most people suppose ; still, for the purposes of the present argument, we will agree that it really happens. Now, it is a grave mistake to confound the dream with suggestion and hallucination. A hallucination, as I have tried to show a good many times, is in reality an action, an impulsive action. The main characteristic of the visual or the auditory hallucination is not that the subject sees or hears something which has no objective existence. This is a minor consideration, for the subject's inner consciousness does not concern us, and does not concern science. What interests the man of science, and what interests the police, is the behaviour; is the fact that the hallucinated person behaves like one to whom signals are made, or like one who hears abusive language; that he strikes out at others, that he accuses others, or that he complains of having been insulted. If these objectively directed actions do not occur, if there be nothing more than an incommunicable phenomenon of consciousness concerning which no one has or will have anything to say, there may be an entity metaphysically considered, but from the point of view of psychological science there is nothing at all, and there is no occasion to speak of hallucination. Now the dream, in so far as it is really a dream, does not manifest any of these actions, these gestures, these words; the dream is accompanied by inward phenomena, and not by phenomena that are outwardly directed. In other words, a hallucination is a tendency activated by a high degree of tension; but a dream is a tendency which is not activated at all, which is only faintly called up, because it possesses such a minimal degree of tension. To confound a dream with a hallucination, is to confound evocation with action.

We conclude, then, that normal sleep and the hypnotic state are different both physiologically and psychologically. No doubt they are both distinct from the waking state, but that does not suffice to make them identical one with another. Unquestionably, they can influence one another, for sleep can be used to induce hypnosis, and hypnosis can be used to induce sleep. But they remain distinct, and it is unscientific to blur the distinction.

3. HYPNOTISM AS ARTIFICIAL SOMNAMBULISM.

If the attempt be made to relate hypnotism to a state which, though not normal, is at least spontaneous, it seems to me that it will be difficult to avoid the assimilation of the hypnotic state to somnambulism—an assimilation which had been made by the whilom magnetisers. Such an assimilation was made by Bertrand and by Deleuze ; it was once again made by Braid, Noizet,[1] and Liébeault ;[2] and was later taken up by Charcot's school. I, too, have laid stress on the resemblance,[3] and I will merely summarise the arguments

It has long been observed that subjects who suffer, or have suffered, from spontaneous somnambulist crises, whether by night, or during the daytime as a sequel of a fit of hysterics, are persons in whom the states which were first spoken of as magnetism and which subsequently came to pass by the name of hypnotism, are most easily induced. When a subject is in a natural somnambulist crisis, or has a fit of hysterics accompanied by delirium and babbling which resembles somnambulism, his condition may easily be transformed, and he may be made to pass into the hypnotic state. Mesnet [4] observed this phenomenon, and Beaunis in his *Le somnambulisme provoqué* (p. 33) emphasises the point : " Natural sleepwalkers pass very easily into the hypnotic sleep." Memory, which is a delicate reagent for the detection of the relationship between one psychological state and another, readily bridges the gap between spontaneous somnambulism and the hypnotic state. Azam long ago drew attention to this fact.[5] Here is another observation of frequent occurrence upon which I was wont to lay special stress : a somnambulist who, on recovering from the crisis, has forgotten the actions performed during the somnambulist state, will often recapture the memory of those actions if subsequently put into the hypnotic trance.[6] Or, again, a subject who, on awakening from the hypnotic sleep, appears to have forgotten all that happened during that state, may spontaneausly recall the incidents during a subsequent crisis of somnambulism attended by delirium. The same remarks apply to the phenomenon of automatic writing often exhibited by such patients. Most observers

---

[1] Op. cit., 1854, p. 103.   [2] Du sommeil, 1866, pp. 90–95.
[3] L'automatisme psychologique, 1889, p. 90 ; L'état mental des hystériques, 1894, vol. ii, p. 191.
[4] De l'automatisme, etc., 1874, pp. 53 and 76.
[5] Azam, " Revue Scientifique," 1883.
[6] Cf., among a number of other observations, the fugues of Rou., Névroses et idées fixes, 1898, vol. ii, p. 256. Concerning the term " fugue," see footnote to p. 56.

have confirmed these facts, which seem to reveal an intimate bond between the two states.

Some authors, however, have noted differences between the characteristics displayed by natural somnambulists and by persons in the hypnotic state. These differences may occur in their gestures, or in their spontaneous activity, or in their proneness to accept suggestions. As I have said before, such peculiarities are due to the individual character of the hypnotised subjects; they are due to the special disease from which such persons are suffering; and depends upon the amount of drilling the patients have undergone. They are of little importance. Certain so-called natural somnambulists are more suggestible in the somnambulist state than are many persons under hypnosis. Let me recall the case of Rah. During the somnambulist crisis, the objects she encountered became factors of suggestion. On the other hand, we find certain subjects who are particularly independent during the hypnotic state, and who exhibit more will of their own at such times than they do in the waking state. Bernheim [1] has another objection to make. He declares that most of the phenomena characteristic of hypnotism, and in special those which are characteristic of posthypnotic amnesia, may be brought about during the waking state by means of suggestion. I do not fancy that it would be easy to do this nor do I believe it possible to produce such results with every patient. No matter. If, during the waking state, you have produced through suggestion all the phenomena characteristic of hypnotism, including posthypnotic amnesia, you have simply brought about a hypnotic state by suggestion. We have to do here with a theory dealing with the production of hypnotic sleep through suggestion; but it is not a theory of the characteristics of hypnotism, nor is it a definition of hypnotism. Why should Bernheim wish to maintain that sleep brought about by suggestion is hypnosis, and at the same time refuse to admit that somnambulism brought about by suggestion is hypnosis? I am led to my erstwhile belief that hypnosis, no matter how it has been brought about, belongs to the group of somnambulist states, just as suggestion belongs to the group of impulses.

[1] Définition et valeur de l'hypnotisme, " Journal für Psychologie und Neurologie," Leipzig, 1911, p. 471.

Can we go further, and obtain a general idea of what somnambulism really is ? Somnambulism is a modification in the mental state of an unstable individual ; this modification consists of very varied alterations which are not the same in all individuals. I have, in the course of my practice, noted certain modifications in the predominant sensations, in the nature and the number of the tendencies which can be evoked, in the dimensions of the field of consciousness. Now I want to add to these modifications some important changes in psychological tension. These changes are often less considerable during hypnosis, when attention and will are feebler, than during the waking state, when suggestibility is increased ; or they may be more considerable, and one may obtain artificial states during which the individual will is strengthened and suggestibility has disappeared. Many other modifications, our knowledge of which is still imperfect, may be found in these states.

Such changes are constantly met with in the ordinary course of life, and do not induce somnambulism. The fact is that usually the modifications are slight, or are gradually brought about, or are compensated by other phenomena ; and they do not interrupt the continuity of personal memory. Though I may be weary and depressed at this moment, I can still remember what I was doing a while back when I was not weary or depressed. In certain cases, and for divers reasons (among which suggestion may play a part), these modifications in the mental state are accompanied by a modification in the continuity of personal memory, and by the interpolation of alternative memories. Such a phenomenon is very important, and it entails a mass of important consequences. As Gurney says " the combined features of breach of memory and special rapport with the hypnotiser are such common and such important characteristics of hypnotic trance, that cases which present them and cases which do not had better not be confounded under a single general name." [1]

Doubtless, the amnesia following somnambulism has specific characteristics : it is variable ; it may, up to a certain point, and at least momentarily, be influenced by suggestion ; it does not go very deep, and affects only personal

[1] Proceedings of the S.P.R., 1887, p. 281.

reminiscence and not automatic reminiscence; it may be brief, and may disappear in the course of time; or, in consequence of modifications in the disease, or as the result of a change in psychological tension. The memory of the hypnotic state re-emerges it is true, during the waking state after a certain lapse of time, just as memory ultimately reasserts itself in the case of somnambulism and of double consciousness; but this does not mean that the amnesia does not exist, or that it is not extremely characteristic. Thus somnambulism appears to be a temporary transformation of the mental state of an individual, capable of bringing about in this individual certain dissociations of personal memory.

A definition of hypnotism would seem to arise quite naturally from this conclusion. Puységur was probably the first to note that, by procedures whose action we do not fully understand, we are sometimes able to bring about similar transformations in certain individuals, to place such individuals in the somnambulist state. Hypnotism, which gradually arose out of animal magnetism, is nothing more than the artificial production of somnambulism. *Hypnotism may be defined as the momentary transformation of the mental state of an individual, artificially induced by a second person, and sufficing to bring about dissociations of personal memory.*

This definition will, I feel sure, help to clarify discussion. It is obvious, however, that such a definition is not perfect, and it might give rise to certain difficulties. It would constrain many authors to curtail their use of the words hypnotism and hypnosis, which they are apt to employ very loosely. My personal feeling is that it would be well never to use the word hypnosis to denote minor states of melancholy, of fatigue, or of torpor, which hitherto have been so lavishly beplastered with that name. All that would result from such curtailment would be that hypnosis would become a rarer phenomenon. The difficulty would be greater when describing states in which a mental modification evoked artificially is, nevertheless, real. In particular this difficulty would arise in those cases of accentuated suggestibility which are not followed by amnesia even when the operator tries to produce this condition. Such states may be related to hypnosis, and in certain cases they can be shown to be a prelude to the hypnotic state, for in a very little while after they are evoked we can produce complete hypnosis. I think we shall do well to study these states more closely, and to determine their characteristics. In so doing we might make use of such expressions as " state of suggestion " or " state of hypotaxy," following J. P. Durand ; or " state of charm," following Brémaud ; or " state of hypnoidisation," following Boris Sidis. In any case we should not allow ourselves to confound these states with true hypnosis. As Delboeuf remarked in 1886 : " Precision of languages is an indispensable prerequisite to psychotherapeutic investigations." [1]

4. Conditions under which Hypnosis occurs.

It is even more difficult to ascertain the conditions under which hypnosis, as thus defined, occurs ; but the foregoing studies concerning suggestion simplify our new task. It is needless, at the present date, to emphasise the futility of the dreams which prevailed thirty years ago as to the possibility of the universalisation of hypnotism. There was a time when doctors did not hesitate to claim that they were able to hypnotise 98 per cent. of their patients, and even the most modest among them would not admit failure in more than 20 per cent. of their cases. Lombroso made fun of these absurd statistics, and asked whether those who published them had run up against an epidemic. These witticisms were responsible for the subsequent neglect of the study of hypnotism, and the world has had to pay for them.

Nor need I dwell upon the hypotheses anent the physiological basis of the hypnotic state. Enough has been said about congestion or anaemia of the brain, about paralysis or stimulation of special regions of the cerebrum, about dissociations affecting certain nerve centres. Such theories, unfortunately, are of as little moment as were the fancies of the magnetisers relating to the " nervous fluid " which made its way through space to act upon those whom the magnetiser wished to influence.

The social theories of hypnotism may seem to be rather more interesting, but we have already examined them during our study of suggestion. Ferenczi believes that hypnosis is merely an old love passion of the subject transferred upon

[1] ' Revue Philosophique," 1886, vol. ii, p. 158

the physician. It is easy to answer that the patient may be passionately in love with the doctor, and may transfer upon him all antecedent sexual and affective tendencies, without being hypnotised. If the explanation is to have any validity at all, we must add that the patient enters into the hypnotic state through complaisance, in order to please the doctor—and we are back once more at the explanation of hypnotism by suggestion.

In actual fact, investigators have gradually come to recognise that clinical conditions are the most important determinants of hypnosis. They now know that hypnosis depends, above all, upon a special condition of the nervous system and of the thoughts of the individual whom they are trying to hypnotise. It depends, as Forel said more than thirty years ago, "upon the temporary disposition of the subject." [1] At one time, people were a good deal exercised by the debate as to whether hypnotism was morbid or normal. Bernheim insisted that in the hands of Charcot the hypnotic state was a neurosis, but that in his own hands it was perfectly normal. Beaunis, Forel, Van Eeden, and Wetterstrand, also declared that hypnotism, as they practised it, was a manifestation of perfect mental and moral health, and that individuals who were quite well could be modified in the same way. Myers and Bramwell outdid this contention by saying that the hypnotic state was actually superior to the normal state. Some investigators have adopted an intermediate position. Ochorowicz, Charles Richet,[2] Löwenfeld,[3] and perhaps also Crocq, of Brussels,[4] incline to regard the susceptibility to hypnosis as an abnormal mental disposition, or rather as an exceptional trend like a gift for music ; but they do not consider it pathological : these ideas seem to have been almost forgotten to-day. Hypnosis as an actual phenomenon, hypnosis as defined above, implies that, under comparatively slight stimulation, an individual has experienced a dissociation of consciousness and of personal memory ; that he has become capable of doing important actions for a considerable time, without retaining any memory of what he is doing, and with-

---

[1] Comptes rendus du Congrès de Psychologie, 1889, p. 61.
[2] Op. cit., p. 95.
[3] " Zeitschrift für Hypnotismus," 1899, vol. vi, p. 2.
[4] Comptes rendus du Congrès de Psychologie, August, 1900.

out being able to control these actions by his own thoughts. Manifestly, such a disposition runs counter to the normal organisations of thought; it may be dangerous; and unless we are playing with words, we cannot regard it as an indication of mental balance and moral health.

One of the favourite arguments of the before-mentioned authors is that hypnotism would seem to be sharply contrasted with certain mental disorders, seeing that it is often impossible to hypnotise persons suffering from such disorders. I quite agree that it is impossible to induce hypnosis in a great many cases of mental and nervous disease. We are absolutely unable to hypnotise idiots, and persons suffering from dementia due to organic disease of the nervous system. Although Auguste Voisin used to claim that he could hypnotise lunatics, sufferers from melancholia accompanied by delusions, and persons affected with mania or with systematised delusions of persecution, I think he has now abandoned his efforts in this direction. If it were easy, or even possible, to hypnotise such patients, the investigations would have been continued, for the results would have been of great value. Gilles de la Tourette had already pointed out that artificial somnambulism can rarely be produced in epileptics.[1] At one time I was myself interested in this problem, and I tried to hypnotise about a score of epileptics. Although the conditions were as favourable as could be hoped for, the results were minimal. Only one of these patients passed into a definite hypnotic state, but this was a woman in whom the diagnosis was doubtful, for, though she had epileptic fits, she also suffered from unmistakable hysterical crises. Bernheim used to say : " Neurasthenics are difficult to hypnotise." [2] I quite agree ; and I have made lengthy investigations on my own account, tending to show that psychasthenics cannot be hypnotised. Their mental condition is dominated by doubt, criticism, indecision, and agitation ; and all these conflict very strongly with suggestion and hypnosis. I therefore have no hesitation in admitting that there are many diseases whose symtoms do not include the manifestation of hypnosis ; but there is nothing remarkable about this, and it does not signify that the occurrence of hypnosis is an indication of health. But even

[1] Traité de l'hystérie, vol. i, 1891, p. 175.
[2] De la suggestion, etc., second edition, 1886, p. 220.

in the illness in which the occurrence of hypnosis is commonest, even in the hysterical neurosis, there are, it will be said, cases in which this neurosis seems to run counter to hypnotism. Bernheim, Forel, Moll, and, following these authorities, Bramwell,[1] insist upon the point that a good many hysterics are difficult to hypnotise. Once more, I am in full agreement. The hysterical neurosis is far from being as unstable as people are apt to suppose ; some of its symptoms will persist unchanged for years ; and we are not always able, in hysterical patients, to bring about the disturbance which leads to the onset of hypnosis. But though there be certain hysterics who cannot be hypnotised, the fact remains that there are plenty of hysterics who are susceptible to hypnotism ; and it is also true (this is the most important point) that persons who can be effectively hypnotised are almost always hysterics.

The weighty medical theory according to which the phenomena of the hypnotic state must be numbered among the symptoms of the hysterical neurosis, began to be formulated in the early days of the study of animal magnetism. Bertrand said that magnetism was the best remedy for hysteria.[2] Again, he said that it was in hysterical women that magnetism succeeded most quickly and could best assert its influence.[3] He reiterated the opinion in " Hermès." [4] Abbé Faria speaks even more definitely. " In hysterics, we do not produce a lucid sleep which did not exist before ; we merely develop it, for it already existed in them thanks to acquired predispositions." [5] Noizet was aware that the majority of those in whom he studied induced somnambulism were patients suffering from hysteria and other nervous disorders.[6] In Briquet I read : " We have to thank Monsieur Gendrin for having again attracted the attention of medical practitioners to a fact which has long been known, namely, that most of the persons who are called magnetic somnambulists are hysterical women." [7] Charles Despine said in plain terms that the effects of induced somnambulism are nil in persons whose health is normal. He wrote : " This condition is

[1] " British Medical Journal," September 10, 1898.
[2] De l'exstase, 1822, p. 428.   [3] Ibid., pp. 218 and 221.
[4] Issue for August 5, 1826, p. 224.
[5] De la cause du sommeil lucide, p. 41 ; cf. also Gilles de la Tourette, op. cit., p. 53.   [6] Op. cit., p. 157,
[7] Traité clinique et thérapeutique de l'hystérie, 1859, p. 413.

abnormal, essentially morbid ; it is obviously connected with hysteria." [1] At Strasburg in 1868, Baillif penned a thesis concerning magnetic sleep in hysteria. We see, then, that the theory of the hysterical nature of these phenomena was not invented by Charcot and his school. All that these observers did was to verify and confirm it in manifold ways.[2] I maintained the same theory in 1889, before I adhered to Charcot's school, and all my studies since then have strengthened my conviction of its soundness. Since then, a great many writers who have no connexion with the school of Charcot have come to the same conclusion. Yung declared that those who were generally affected with induced somnambulism, had, hitherto, been hysterical patients ; Donkin, Orlitzy, of Moscow,[3] and Crocq, of Brussels,[4] put forward similar views. The passion that used to rage whenever this topic was discussed has at length subsided, and it is now possible to examine calmly the arguments favourable to the hysterical theory of induced somnambulism.

I have already explained several times, and at considerable length, that the psychological characteristics of the hypnotic state are identical with those which can be observed in the somnambulism which occurs spontaneously in the course of hysteria, and with those witnessed in hysterical crises and the like. If we make a careful study of the mental state of any one in whom unmistakable hypnosis can be induced, or even if we merely study the clinical history of such a person, we shall find it easy to discover a good many symptoms of the hysterical neurosis. Such, at any rate, has been my own experience in all the cases of well-marked neurosis which have come under my observation. They are not very numerous, for I have no wish to compete with the writers who boast of hypnotising 4,000 persons every year. In my notes, I find the record of only 120 instances of unmistakable hypnosis, and in every one of these cases the patient was

[1] De l'emploi du magnétisme animal, etc., 1840, pp. 131 and 149.
[2] Cf. Gilles de la Tourette, op. cit., p. 61 ; Féré, Société Médico-Psychologique, May 1883 ; Pitres, Leçons cliniques sur l'hystérie, etc., vol. ii, p. 347 ; Barth, Du sommeil non naturel, p. 141 ; Régis, " Revue de l'Hypnotisme," 1896 ; Babinski, " Gazette Hebdomadaire de Médecine et de Chirurgie," 1891.
[3] Société d' Hypnologie et de Psychologie, April 26, 1904.
[4] " Revue de l'Hypnotisme, 1893, p. 339 ; Deuxième Congrès de l'Hypnotisme, August 16, 1900.

suffering from severe hysteria at the time, or else had previously manifested hysterical symptoms. Finally, we have to consider a remarkable and telling fact to which I have already referred in connexion with the topic of suggestion : " When hysteria is cured in actual fact, and not only in appearance, somnambulism and suggestion disappear." [1] The same fact had been noted long before by Charles Despine, in his account of the case of Estelle : " The best indication of the return of perfect health is that the aptitude for somnambulism vanishes." In 1887, Fontan and Ségard said that the subject became less hypnotisable as health returned. [2] During these periods when progress towards a cure is being made, we can note some very remarkable phenomena. The patients recover the lost memories of the periods of hypnosis, and find it difficult to understand how they could have allowed themselves to be put to sleep and why they should have forgotten the sittings. They are inclined, at this stage, to accuse themselves of having practised simulation when they were hypnotised—or magnetised, for the phenomena we are now considering used to play an interesting part in the quarrels that raged round the topic of animal magnetism.

Of course it is possible to raise an objection to this theory by introducing the question of incomplete and ill-defined hypnotic states, and by saying that hysteria is only present in those who are susceptible to profound hypnotism. [3] My own preference, as I have shown, is to restrict the use of the term hypnosis to denote the typical phenomena of somnambulism, and to separate from these, as more akin to simple suggestion, the conditions of " charm " which are sometimes termed incomplete hypnotism. In these circumstances, I think I am in agreement with most observers when I regard the hysterical neurosis as the leading factor of hypnosis properly so called. If a more precise statement is requisite, we may say that hypnosis is more readily induced in patients who have already exhibited the phenomena of psychological dissociation, spontaneous somnambulism, crises with apparent loss of consciousness, delirium with subsequent amnesia, subconscious actions, etc. This amounts to saying that

[1] L'automatisme psychologique, 1889, p. 446.
[2] Eléments de médecine suggestive, etc., p. 37.
[3] Cf. Haberman, Hypnosis, etc., 1910, p. 19.

hypnosis is more readily induced in proportion as the hysteria from which the patient suffers is well marked, and in proportion to the degree to which it has assumed its characteristic mental form.

While hysteria is thus the basic factor, other factors play an important part in deciding at what moment the hypnotic state will arise in one who is predisposed through the existence of a hysterical mental condition. These supplementary factors are identical with those which have already been considered under the head of suggestion. Fatigue is often the starting-point of unmistakable somnambulism, and Tissié has recorded a remarkable instance of this in a bicycle racer. Here exhaustion has brought about a lowering of psychological tension which mainly affects the comparatively exalted tendencies of the personality, so that the lower-grade tendencies can develop in isolation. But somnambulism induced by such a mechanism is especially the outcome of mental fatigue, of fatigue due to persistent attention. I have frequently had occasion to note this when trying to make hysterical patients cultivate the faculty of attention. In many instances, they appeared to become so greatly absorbed in their studies as to lose all sense of their surroundings and to forfeit the awareness of personality. They would pass into a dreamy state, or begin to talk in a rambling fashion. When I tried to shake them out of this condition and to bring them back into touch with reality, they seemed to awaken with a start, and were then found to have no memory of the brief period during which the mind had been clouded. In my patient Marcelle, a somnambulist state of this character was induced by nothing more than an explanation I made to her concerning the visual field. Such phenomena are commoner than most observers realise. A good many crises of somnambulism with delirium are initiated by fatigue due to the patient's attempt to perform a mental operation.

Without fully understanding the facts with which they had to deal, many experimenters have used fatigue of the attention as a means of inducing hypnosis. The passes of the magnetisers demanded a prolonged effort of attention on the part of the subject; so did Braid's plan of making the patient fix the eyes upon a bright object close at hand and in the upper part of the visual field; so did the method of self-hypnotisation employed by the Indian fakir, who persistently contemplated his own navel. Quite a number of observers have insisted upon the importance of concentration of attention in the initial stages of hypnosis, and have been well aware that hypnosis did not occur if the subject would not or could not fix his attention in this way. Heidenhain, J. P. Durand, Braid, Stanley Hall, Schneider,[1] L. Fischer,[2] and more recently Münsterberg, have laid much stress on the importance of " over-attention " in the induction of hypnotism. It is important that we should understand how this effort of attention acts. J. P. Durand gave a remarkable explanation of Braid's experiment. He said that the concentration of vision upon an unimportant object led to a notable secretion of nervous energy without any expenditure; consequently, there was a superabundant accumulation of energy, and it was upon this reserve of power that suggestion took effect. Most of the authors just mentioned, in agreement with Münsterberg, appear to believe that the hypnotic sleep, like suggestion, is directly determined by the effort of attention. We have seen, however, that this is very improbable, for in such patients the powers of attention are feeble, despite the best efforts at concentration.

I think that we must look for an explanation in the direction indicated a good while ago by Hack Tuke: " I regard it as impossible to exclude the act of attention from any of the physical processes that are employed to develop suggestibility. After a time, the will is exhausted, and becomes paralysed; then the involuntary action occurs, whether consciously or unconsciously." [3] Perronnet, a magnetiser, put the matter very well when he said: " When the conscious attention has been fixed for a long time upon one and the same groups of psychical phenomena, the nerve cells which function as the anatomical substratum of this act of attention gradually undergo an impulse towards the unconscious condition." The same view was advocated by Charles Richet; [4] by Fontan and Ségard, and, above all, by Féré. The last named wrote: " All the sensorial stimuli employed

[1] Die psychologische Ursache der hypnotischen Erscheinungen, 1880.
[2] Le magnétisme animal, 1883.
[3] Cf. J. P. Durand, Essais de physiologie philosophique, p. 77.
[4] L'homme et l'intelligence, p. 217.

to induce hypnotic sleep, though their first effect is stimulant, speedily led to the onset of exhaustion ; . . . all the methods really act by inducing fatigue." [1] The same ideas have been well expressed by Espinas : " If these weak and uniform sensations induce [hypnotic] sleep, it is because they bring about exhaustion of the corresponding sensory centres." [2] In this connexion, he lays especial stress upon " voluminous, massive, extensively irradiated sensations, which are especially exhausting." Similar notions are to be found in Madame Manacéine's book, *Le sommeil, tiers de notre vie* (p. 135). All these contentions are perfectly sound, but we must not forget that the individuals with whom we are dealing are not normal persons capable of resisting fatigue for a long time, and, above all, capable of withdrawing their attention from anything which causes distressing fatigue. The subjects with whom we are concerned suffer from a lowering of tension at the very outset of the fatigue, and are consequently incapable of making the little effort which is requisite for the withdrawal of attention from that which is tiring them.

Another very important factor is to be found in emotion, a phenomenon closely akin to fatigue. We know that emotion plays its part in causing spontaneous somnambulism, which is nearly always the outcome of a severe shock. This shock, as I have repeatedly tried to show, disorganises the mental syntheses, modifies the psychological tension, and induces mental conditions in which dissociation and the isolated development of the lower-grade tendencies are very apt to ensue. Many hypnotisers have tried to induce hypnosis by arousing emotion in their subjects, rather than by causing fatigue. Most of those who used to give public exhibitions of hypnotism made a practice of bringing young people on to the platform, would expose them quite suddenly to the glare of the footlights and to the gaze of the audience, and would add to their bewilderment by suddenly thrusting their heads back, or by giving them a smart blow on the nape of the neck (this was Hiram Jackson's method), or by twisting their heads rapidly from side to side. Charcot's abrupt procedures, such as flashing a light on the subject or sounding a gong, played a similar part in the early days

---

[1] Sensation et mouvement, 1887, p. 140.
[2] Du sommeil provoqué chez les hystériques, 1884, p. 9.

of his investigations. In all these cases, the emotions of surprise and alarm were predominant, and induced exhaustion more quickly than fatigue would have done. I am confident that even if we use much gentler methods we shall always arouse intense emotion when we try to hypnotise. Nor would it be good to attempt to reduce this emotion too much, for we should then forfeit a great part of our influence.

The effect of various intoxicants is of interest in certain cases. We know that alcoholic intoxication sometimes gives rise to increased suggestibility, and may cause manifestations of amnesia and alternating memory. Under ether and chloroform, similar phenomena may be noticed, and it is possible that in cases of the hysterical neurosis we may have to do with like phenomena of intoxication. It is not improbable that we could turn artificial intoxications to account, thus giving rise to conditions resembling the hypnotic state by methods analogous to the administration of chloroform and ether. Several observers have worked along that line. Bernheim, in this connexion, once referred to the effect of morphine, but I do not think he has laid much stress upon the matter. Fazio and Geoffredi, of Naples, have made a successful use of ether; and others have used chloroform. I tried chloroform in one case, and ether in three others. The results were interesting, but I do not think that they proved much, for the patients were hysterics whom I could have hypnotised in other ways, and in whom I simply revived the hypnotic state by the use of the anaesthetic. I have had no opportunity (perhaps I have been too timid) to repeat the experiment under more interesting conditions, namely upon subjects who could not be hypnotised in any other way. That is why I have been greatly interested in the experiments of Paul Farez, who made use of the hyponarcosis induced by the inhalation of a moderate amount of somnoform. His results seem to have been encouraging, especially as regards his attempts to transform the hysterical sleep of the " sleeping woman of Alençon " into a hypnotic sleep.[1] Experiments of this kind ought to be carefully repeated, for I think they might serve as the starting-point of a new form of hypnotism independent

[1] Farez, La dormeuse d'Alençon, " Revue de Psychothérapie," August and September 1910 ; Eden Paul, Pathological and prolonged Sleep, " Journal of Mental Science," July 1911.

of hysteria, whereas, to-day, hypnotism is entirely dependent upon this neurosis—or, if you like, upon this spontaneous form of intoxication.

Doubtless these states are important, but, if they acted alone, somnambulism would only occur from time to time, and very rarely. Such states of exhaustion only leave the field free for the invasion of all kinds of inferior tendencies, and these inferior tendencies, developing without guidance, would give rise to simple fits of hysteria or to other states in which no way resemble somnambulism. This is precisely what takes place occasionally when one is trying to hypnotise a subject. But such an accident may be avoided by the intervention of other psychological conditions which obviously play an important role.

Somnambulism is not only an arrest of the normal individual consciousness ; it likewise consists in the development of other tendencies. In order that hypnosis may occur, it is necessary that, at the moment of the depression, there should awaken and develop tendencies accordant with the hypnotic state ; that is to say, tendencies that shall not be in opposition to hypnosis, that shall enable the patient to sit quietly in the armchair, to listen to the hypnotist, to converse with him ; in a word to behave like a hypnotised person.

When we are dealing with persons who have previously been hypnotised, such a phenomenon is easily realised, for the previous sittings have prepared the ground for the adoption of a suitable attitude. The tendency to behave in the same way as on a previous occasion is all the more potent if there have been a considerable number of sittings. The tendency remains latent during the waking state ; it is inhibited by the development of the personality ; but at the mere sight of the hypnotist, or at the sound of his voice, the tendency reemerges, and realises itself as soon as there occurs a slight depression occasioned by fatigue or by emotion. For this reason, persons who have already been hypnotised are easily brought under the hypnotic influence, especially if the same procedures are resorted to as on previous occasions, thus calling up as associations which will tend to develop the subjacent tendency.

On the other hand, persons who have never been hypnotised but who are spontaneous somnambulists, or who suffer from fits of hysterics with such characteristic symptoms as delirium or babbling, are more difficult to deal with. At the moment of depression these symptoms arise, and the subject is inclined to fall into a fit of hysterics at the very time when the hypnotic state should develop. One of my patients suffered from crises of somnambulist delirium during which she rehearsed the scene of the death of one of her nieces, and wished to throw herself from the window as the niece had done. As soon as she was ever so slightly fatigued or emotioned by the hypnotist, the whole of the scene was recapitulated. In her crises, Irène would imagine herself present at her mother's deathbed, and would " help her to spit out her lungs which were suffocating her " ; then she would endeavour to throw herself under the wheels of an imaginary locomotive. I had merely to make her fix her eyes on a luminous point, and she would instantly become delirious, crying : " Oh mother, do you want me to go along with you ? "—Madame D., if taken by surprise, would immediately hear once more the words of a practical joker who had once told her that her husband was dead.—Numerous similar examples might be quoted.—Here we have to do with the moral components of hypnotism, that is to say, the development of complex states outside the personality ; but this factor of the hypnotic state cannot be turned to practical account ; the operator has to intervene in order to perfect the state. He seeks out the stimuli which will be capable of influencing the subject, which can arouse psychological phenomena in spite of the resistance imposed by the developing tendencies. Success is often achieved by the use of very simple stimuli, such as touching the forehead, clasping the hand, speaking softly, or commanding in a firm voice. Sometimes a circuitous route will have to be taken ; the operator will have to enter into the subject's fantasy, and call forth impressions which can easily be incorporated into the dominant tendency. Elsewhere I have related how Gu., when in a delirious crisis, would rave about the bunch of red everlastings that some schoolmates had laid on her father's coffin ; she would be quite unresponsive to cutaneous stimulation and to the uttered word. Yet one needed but to murmur : " I have brought a nosegay of violets," and she would immediately hear, and would express her thanks. Having gone so far, it was no longer difficult to modify the crisis, little by little to transform the dominant tendencies, in fact to turn the hysterical crisis into a phase of hypnosis. Here we have an education of the subject which has been scoffed at, but which is, nevertheless, inevitable. Doubtless it is foolish to train your subjects to talk familiarly with you while they are in the hypnotic state, to gaze about with terrified eyes, or to hold your hands and constantly rub your thumb-nail ; these are merely exaggerated forms of an excellent practice. Hypnosis is not only a subconscious state ; it is an artificial condition determined by the hypnotist, and, up to a certain point, determined by the temperament of the hypnotist. The hypnotist must, while the subject is in this state, provide the tendencies and the frame of mind he needs ; the state would not be worth producing if the subject were still to be as uneasy as in the waking state.

When we have to do with subjects who have never been hypnotised, and who have not hitherto suffered either from spontaneous somnambulism or from any sort of delirious crisis, the induction of the hypnotic state is certainly more difficult. If the subject had had no previous knowledge of this state, if he had had no tendency to adopt the attitude of a hypnotised person towards the hypnotist, it is probable that the before-mentioned procedures, should they succeed in lowering the tension and in temporarily suppressing the subject's powers of self-control, would only give rise to a convulsive crisis or to some indefinite form of somnambulism with delirium ; thus we should be back where we were in the case of subjects just described, and should have to give to this somnambulism its special form. But in many cases the subject already knows what a hypnotised person is like. Now, to know anything is to have within oneself a verbal form appropriate to the tendency to realise that thing. Under normal conditions, the tendency remains latent, or does not develop beyond the first degree, wherein it exists only as an idea. But in suitable circumstances, such as those produced by a depression of the personality, the tendency, being awakened and stimulated by the presence and the words of the hypnotist, undergoes realisation, and the subject then behaves like a hypnotised person. It is because particular ideas upon the topic are current at a particular time, that the somnambulists of any epoch present similar characteristics ; it is because the hypnotist is present at the outset of the hypnosis, that almost all states of this kind exhibit the phenomena of what used to be called "magnetic rapport."

At this stage we are faced once more with the problem of hypnotism by suggestion, which has too often been regarded as the typical form of the phenomenon. Obviously, there is a close relationship between suggestion and hypnotism. A suggestion which undergoes realisation is already an abnormal state, different from the waking state, and, as Beaunis said, it is apt to be followed by amnesia. It has been shown again and again that when posthypnotic suggestions are being carried out the subject has relapsed for the nonce into the hypnotic state. It follows that when we influence a person by suggestion we have already induced in him a condition of transient hypnosis. If the suggestions are numerous and complicated, and if they follow one another so rapidly that the subject has no time in the interim to resume the condition of normal consciousness, we induce hypnosis. A fortiori this happens when we suggest enduring attitudes of mind, general and long-lasting modifications of behaviour. Especially does this happen when we make the famous suggestion "Sleep!" devised by Abbé Faria in 1818. This particular suggestion is so successful in inducing hypnosis, that it has been extensively utilised, and it is often regarded as the only factor in hypnotism. It was the method employed by Noizet,[1] and J. P. Durand also made use of it.[2] Subsequently, following Bernheim's example, all the practitioners of the Nancy School induced hypnosis in this way.

If we are to appraise the method accurately, we must understand first of all that, although we tell the subject to sleep, to close his eyes, and so on, the result is not sleep at all, in the ordinary sense of that term. If the subject really went to sleep, he would not be hypnotised. As we have seen, he would wake with a start when the hypnotist touched him or spoke to him. In Faria's experiments, and in the experiments made by those who use Faria's method, the word "sleep" is understood by the subject as signifying a general change of attitude, a general relaxation. In certain cases, the subject understands that he is directed to "pass into the state of somnambulism." In this connexion I may point

[1] Op. cit., p. 88.   [2] Cours de braidisme, p. 152.

out that psychological depression, though mainly the outcome of exhaustion, emotion, or intoxication, can also to some extent be induced by various forms of voluntary activity. We can, to a degree at least, spontaneously relax ourselves; just as in other cases we can deliberately render ourselves tense, we can " buck up." " Going to sleep " and " waking up " have similar connexions. In Part Four of the present work, when we come to consider stimulant methods of treatment, it will be necessary to form more precise notions concerning these matters. Enough here to point out the obvious psychological fact that the suggestion of going to sleep, the suggestion of being hypnotised, understood in a specific sense, can arouse tendencies which undergo realisation in consequence of the mental dissociation induced by emotion.

Milne Bramwell is very critical of the Nancy theories concerning hypnotism by suggestion. He summarises Bernheim's views as follows : " In other words [according to Bernheim], every one is suggestible, and if you take some one and suggest to him to be more suggestible, that is hypnotism." He goes on to criticise at considerable length the assumptions underlying Bernheim's outlook.[1] The criticism is sound as directed against those who contend that suggestion explains everything. But here suggestion plays only a minor part, for it merely replaces the education of the somnambulist which we have shown to be requisite ; the somnambulist state ensues for very different reasons, and suggestion gives the somnambulism its specific form. The essential factor of hypnosis is depression, the arrest of the normal individual consciousness, the suspension of the special mental condition which we regard as the waking state—a state which is unstable in patients whose mental tension is very readily lowered so that it is annulled under the influence of fatigue and emotion. The suggestion of sleep, or the artless suggestion to be more suggestible, serves merely to guide the inferior tendencies which now replace the superior tendencies. To assemble all the requisite conditions is by no means easy, and that is why, in the practice of hypnotism, so much depends upon the operator's skill and experience.

Suggestion and the induction of hypnosis are two methods

[1] Proceedings of the S.P.R., 1896, pp. 217 et seq.

in which the doctor is able to turn pathological symptoms to account. The depressed patient has lost the power of reflective voluntary action, and is unable to give balance and continuity of his conscious life. But he can still act with a certain amount of energy when a lower-grade tendency has to be activated ; for considerable periods he can maintain certain forms of activity which are conspicuous though transient. This accounts for his impulsive actions and for his somnambulist crises. In ordinary circumstances, such actions and crises are useless or noxious. But in medical practice we often have to turn pathological symptoms to account ; this is what we do when we adminster an emetic or a purgative or a revulsant, and this is what we do when we use a vaccine. Suggestion and hypnotism are nothing more than the artificial employment of impulse and somnambulism. When we suggest, we induce an impulse in the place of a reflective voluntary action ; when we hypnotise, we induce somnambulism in the place of the waking state. What we now have to enquire is how the induction of these morbid phenomena can play a useful part in treatment.

CHAPTER EIGHT

APPEAL TO THE PATIENT'S AUTOMATISM

Now that we are somewhat better informed regarding the nature of suggestion and hypnosis and regarding the conditions under which they occur, we shall find it easier to estimate their practical worth. What is their real efficacy, and what service can they render? Are we entitled to make use of their influence, and is it practically possible to do so? Have we already achieved definite results which justify us in making such an appeal to psychological automatism?

1. SUPERHUMAN POWERS.

In answer to the first question, whether suggestion and hypnotism have real efficacy, enthusiasts are often inclined to reply in most exaggerated terms. They tell us that suggestion and hypnotism embody a titanic, a superhuman power, which greatly transcends that of the normal human will; that by suggestion and hypnotism it is possible to bring about physiological and psychological changes which the will could never effect under normal conditions. We have no right, a priori, to say that this contention is absurd. Suggestion gives rise to actions under conditions differing from those in which the will produces actions, and we are not entitled to say beforehand that the actions will necessarily be of the same kind in both cases. But before we can admit that suggestion is endowed with a wonderful power superior to that of the will, we shall ask for experimental proof, and it is here that difficulties arise.

The most important phenomena that have been adduced to substantiate the alleged power of hypnotic suggestion are the physiological modifications which suggestion is said to have caused. Normally the power we can exercise over our visceral organs and our physiological functions is greatly restricted, and is usually indirect. Hypnotic suggestion, we are told, can influence these organs and functions markedly and directly. The most extensive discussion has turned upon the question of vasomotor phenomena. The earlier magnetisers declared they could check or increase the flow of blood from accidental wounds or from those made for the purpose of blood-letting; [1] and since then many accounts have been published of flushings, swellings, local elevations of temperature, blisterings, stigmatisation, the cure of warts, etc., due solely to hypnotic suggestion. A precise verification of these phenomena, and the discovery of the exact mechanism of their causation, would do a great deal to demonstrate the power of suggestion. Unfortunately, however, science has not yet pronounced a definite verdict upon any of these matters. Very remarkable, very striking observations are still recorded from time to time. Among the most recent are those describing the production of burns by suggestion. The experiments were made by Konstamm, of Montel, and Vogt alluded to them at the Psychotherapeutic Congress of 1910. But no one has been able to reproduce the results under test conditions. Konstamm was unable to continue his investigations, and there remains nothing more than the memory of a remarkable phenomenon which does not form part of the accepted data of science. I have had similar experiences. In former days I was able to detect, or I thought I was able to detect, definite flushing and swelling of the skin as a result of a suggested mustard plaster or a suggested burn, but the symptoms did not appear until at least twenty-four hours after the suggestion had been made, and I am not confident that the subject was kept under sufficiently strict observation during the intervening period. Test conditions are by no means easy to enforce. When, subsequently, I tried to verify my earlier results, I did not succeed in obtaining satisfactory verification, and my failure naturally led me to ask myself whether, in my first experiments, I might not have been the victim of an illusion.

Since that time, I have had opportunities for the study of a very interesting case, that of a woman who suffered from a mystical delirium, and in whom from time to time there could be seen on the hands and the feet little wounds

[1] Cf. Charpignon, Physiologie, médecine et métaphysique du magnétisme, 1848, p. 361.

resembling the stigmata of Christ. This phenomenon reminded me of the burns due to suggestion, and I tried to subject the appearance of the stigmata to strict verification. As I have shown in my published report of the case, verification was a difficult matter, and I was unable to come to a satisfactory conclusion.[1] In these circumstances, we are hardly entitled to place much reliance upon such phenomena as evidencing the remarkable efficacy of suggestion. Even if they are genuine, they are probably the outcome of a peculiar condition of the circulation and the skin akin to that which accounts for the familiar phenomenon of dermographism. Suggestion, properly so called, would then play no more than an accessory part in their production.

Certain authorities such as Yung, Beaunis, and Bernheim, tell us that by suggestion they have been able to modify, and even to stop, the beating of the heart. I have tried to verify this, taking simultaneous graphs of the respiratory movements and of the heart-beat. In these observations, the modifications of the heart-beat were usually trifling. In the exceptional instances in which fairly extensive modifications occurred, it seemed to me that they were dependent upon respiratory changes, thus occurring in accordance with familiar physiological laws. The influence of suggestion upon the breathing is unmistakable, but it does not exceed the power of the will to affect the respiratory movements. It is possible that changes in the cardiac rhythm independent of changes in the breathing may, in certain cases, be directly induced by suggestion, but the phenomenon is quite exceptional, and presumably depends upon idiosyncrasy.

I think that changes in the rhythm of menstruation are the most satisfactorily attested among the circulatory modifications due to the influence of suggestion. A great many cases of this kind have been summarised in Schwob's thesis (1890), in Raciborski's studies (1865), and in an article by Auguste Forel published in the " Revue de l'Hypnotisme " for April 1889 (p. 298). I have myself recorded a number of phenomena of the same kind, but it is difficult to decide their evidential value. Apart from the possibility that mere coincidence may account for some of these happenings,

---

[1] Une extatique, conférence faite a l'Institut Psychologique, May 25, 1901, reported in the " Bulletin de l'Institut Psychologique," 1901, p. 219.

emotion, and many other psychological phenomena, are capable of influencing the menstrual flow.

Similar considerations apply to modifications of the gastro-intestinal functions. A great many writers speak of vomiting suggested by the idea of sea-sickness, and of purgation following the administration of a bread pill. A. Mathieu and J. C. Roux insisted once again, a few years ago, upon the influence of ideas upon the digestive functions in hysterical patients.[1] Summarising the opinion to which I have been led by my own experience, I am inclined to say that the phenomena are real enough, but that they occur less frequently than people are apt to suppose. We must not forget that the functions in question are readily disturbed by sentiments and emotions, and that suggestion is apt to work through the intermediation of these. The better acquainted we are with the mechanism of such nervous phenomena, the less will it seem to us that there is anything wondrous about the effects of suggestion.

The so-called criminal suggestions offer a similar problem in the domain of moral behaviour, and this accounts for the great interest with which they have been studied. Some have contended that such suggestions would speedily induce dreadful changes in the mind of the subject, and could force him to perform actions which he would never have performed but for this. Apart from their social importance, experiments of this kind are supposed to have furnished a signal demonstration of the marvellous power of suggestion. It is a good many years since J. P. Durand insisted upon the reality of criminal suggestion, and he was well aware of the importance of this matter from the theoretical point of view. " If it be proved," he wrote, " that the crimes committed under the influence of hypnotic suggestion are pure comedy, the whole foundation of hypnotism is undermined, and the entire edifice will crumble." Milne Bramwell adopts the same view, for, when he is trying to show the absurdity of criminal suggestions, he declares that the problem is one of primary importance to those who are coming to a conclusion as to the value of hypnotism. I think these writers overstate their case. Hypnotism would still be important even if there were no such things as genuine criminal suggestions ; but we should no longer be able to ascribe such marvellous powers to the hypnotist.

In any case, the members of the Nancy School, relying on the striking experiences already recorded, declared that the utterance of a mere word before a chance comer might bring about a complete realisation of ultra-criminal tendencies. The critics hastened to insist that experiments concerning imaginary crimes had no significance whatever, for the subjects were well aware that the whole thing was play-acting, and would not have done what they did had serious issues been at stake. The inference of the critics was that criminal suggestion had no real existence. I think that the whole of the argumentation on both sides is faulty, for lack of an adequate psychological analysis. I agree that the magnetisers experiments, which were uncritically repeated at Nancy, had little significance. The carrying out of an idea as a mere piece of play-acting is no more than the first stage of realisation ; and the tendency which is activated in this way has acquired nothing more than a minor degree of tension. That is why neurotics, whose mental tension is low, are so fond of play-acting, simulation, humbug. Still, the critics were mistaken in their inference that, under other conditions, and in certain subjects, it would be impossible to induce criminal and dangerous actions through the mechanism of suggestion.

If we study the real activities of our patients, we shall find that there are times in their lives when casual suggestions, or even deliberate or malevolent suggestions, will induce actions with grave consequences, will lead to the commission of crimes. Among my notes I find the records of five cases in which rape took place in hypnotic sleep and under the influence of suggestion. In another of my cases there occurred what I cannot but regard as a theft on the large scale which was effected solely by the instrumentality of suggestion. A person who gave himself out as a doctor and hypnotised an ailing woman was able to suggest her handing over to him a fairly large sum of money on which he was able to keep his clutches. In another instance, a pregnant woman had abortion procured under the influence of the suggestion of her lover. Finally, for a long time I had under observation a woman who was practically enslaved by the power of suggestion. She had been hypnotised by another woman, a hotelkeeper, and had been persistently subjected to the influence of suggestion, this leading her to take to drink, and to practice a most degraded form of prostitution. When she had been enabled to free herself from the other woman's domination, she showed that her true character was very different from that which had been imposed upon her by suggestion. For years, thenceforward, she lived an orderly life, and was amazed at herself whenever she recalled the things she had been wont to do. But we should make a great mistake were we to record these observations without promptly adding that the persons to whom they relate were seriously ill, that they displayed all kinds of neuropathic symptoms, that they had no will of their own, were incapable of guiding themselves and of resisting the will of others. The interesting point from the medico-legal outlook is that we should ascertain whether, in such patients, suggestion was a more potent and more dangerous force than the persuasions and the threats that are ordinarily employed. Psychological considerations make us realise that suggestion could not have been the sole factor. Disorder of the will must certainly have been a contributory cause of the crime. Interesting though these cases are, they do not prove that suggestion has any wonderful powers.

Similar considerations apply to the induction of paralysis, contracture, and even anaesthesia, by suggestion. A good many writers, after pointing out that these phenomena are not attended with extensive modifications in the reflexes and in the condition of the organs, go on to declare that they are inclined to regard such functional troubles of movement and sensibility as nothing more than phenomena of a simple kind which can easily be reproduced by the normal will. I am far from agreeing with this contention. Hysterical paralysis is something more than voluntary immobility ; and hysterical contracture is something very different from the voluntary assumption of a particular posture. There can be no doubt that in the future we shall be able to detect in these syndromes the existence of interesting physiological modifications which the normal will cannot cause. In any case, in the durability of such phenomena, in the way in which they persist notwith-

standing the demands of life and notwithstanding the action
of various stimuli which ought to have brought about other
movements, we can discern fundamental characteristics. With
considerable effort, and with manifest disturbance, the will
can roughly imitate these characteristics ; but it cannot
reproduce them accurately. It would seem, then, that suggestion, since it can cause such phenomena, must in this case
manifest a power greater than that of the normal human will.

Now, first of all, we must point out, that the production
of such phenomena by suggestion is not so common an occurrence as people are apt to suppose. When, at a public
demonstration, a doctor suggests that a subject shall have a
paralysis or a contracture of the right arm, the subject knows
perfectly well that the doctor has no wish to make him an
invalid ; he knows that the inertia of the arm is only a game,
that it will not interfere with any of the important acts of
life, and that the trouble will have passed away long before
the next meal when he will want to use the arm for practical
purposes. In such suggested paralyses there is an element of
comedy, just as there was in the laboratory crimes. The
danger of suggestions of the kind has been greatly exaggerated
by those who are continually telling us that suggested paralyses
will become permanent and incurable unless we hasten to
terminate them by suitable suggestions. It has often happened in my own experience that, after having induced a
contracture by suggestion, I have turned away to interest
myself in other matters, with an air of having forgotten all
about the subject. The latter would wait for a while, rather
embarrassed, as if he were expecting something more ; then
he, too, would seem to forget the contracture in which nobody
was now interested, and when, for any reason, he wanted to
move his arm, decontracture would take place, and the movements would be performed in a perfectly normal fashion.
Such a result is easy to explain. My suggestion had been
realised in the spirit in which the subject had understood it,
in the form merely of a tendency to assume the posture of a
person suffering from contracture *under special circumstances,
before a special individual ;* once that movement had passed,
other stimuli brought about the realisation of other tendencies,
and the attitude changed forthwith. When I was addressing
the Society of Neurology in such terms, Babinski declared that

he had been led to quite different conclusions. When he was house physician at Charcot's clinic, he induced paralysis by means of suggestion for demonstration purposes, and the paralysis would last for several weeks. I do not wish to appear too sceptical; I will merely say that Babinski's experiments were conducted in very special surroundings. Every one connected with the clinic had implicit faith in the importance of these experiments ; great deference was paid to the patient who was to take part in the master's demonstration classes ; his life was made very easy in spite of the paralysis of his arm, and, since suggestion was thus constantly kept up, the patient could maintain the symptom for a longer time, and his condition would appear more grave than it was in reality. When, some years later, I was working in the same clinic, I could not obtain such prolongations of suggested paralysis, etc., for the simple reason that the circumstances had altered.

But I am far from denying the existence of suggested paralyses or functional anaesthesias. I myself have published the record of a case of profound anaesthesia induced in a hysterical patient by means of suggestion. The anaesthesia in this case was so genuine and so lasting that a major operation was performed without the use of chloroform.[1] Segond, who performed the operation, was convinced that no amount of normal will could possibily have induced such a stoical demeanour. I am certain that among some of my patients I could by imprudent suggestion produce in them very serious conditions of paralysis. But I wish again to emphasise the fact that in these cases, too, I was dealing with quite peculiar subjects. Apropos of this I drew the attention of the Society of Neurology to a fact which I fear has not attracted sufficient notice : experimental suggestion can produce functional paralyses in those subjects only who have previously suffered from similar paralyses, and who have only recently been cured ; that is to say, in subjects who, owing to an advanced state of hysteria, are already in the special condition of dissociation peculiar to the production of these paralyses and functional anaesthesias. The marvels accompanying such transformations are nothing more than hysterical symptoms, and our suggestions play only a minor part in producing them.

[1] Cf. " Journal de Neurologie et d'Hypnologie," 1897, p. 22 ; Névroses et idées fixes, 1898, p. 481.

A final problem, one which will lead us to the same conclusion, is the problem of the time element in suggestion. The question of the persistence of suggested actions is extremely important, and here the importance concerns the practitioner, even more than the student of the theory of suggestion. The nature of such duration has been little studied, for we have been content to rely upon the old affirmations and have not even taken the trouble to find out if they are true. Most authors in the past have averred that a suggestion can last a very long time. Liébeault, at a modest estimate, reckoned the duration at 52 days.[1] Since his time, the persistence of suggestion has come to be calculated by years, and authors incline to believe that this is the case with all suggestions.

First of all, what precisely do we mean when we speak of the duration of a suggestion ? We must not apply the term to the simple persistence of a tendency in the latent form ; otherwise all our habits, all our faculties, would become '' persistent suggestions.'' Neither can we understand by the term those consequences, those more or less distant results, which a suggestion may entail. Bonjour was doubtless joking when, at the Psychotherapeutical Congress, he informed me that his suggestions lasted a lifetime seeing that his patients were cured for the rest of their mortal term. Suppose a patient should break his leg while carrying out a suggestion ; would it be correct to say that, because he was lame ever after, the suggestion lasted all his life ? Besides, in certain cases we have to recognise that the suggestion is transformed, and gives rise to habits, or even to fixed ideas, which have a completely different significance. Neither must we confound suggestion with a state of suggestibility. The latter, which in my view is a morbid state, may be very persistent, and may permit of the suggestion being made over and over again after long lapses of time ; but we must not look upon this as the persistence of the primary suggestion. We are only entitled to speak of a suggestion as perdurable when the induced action retains the characteristics of suggestion, when the action is prolonged, or is repeated, whenever there recurs a particular association of ideas.

A few years ago I tried to make some definite experiments

[1] Op. cit., p. 153

upon this matter, and I reported the results to the Psychological Society of Paris. Having selected thirty persons whom I regarded as extremely suggestible, to all of them I gave suggestions the carrying out of which could easily be verified, even without drawing the patient's attention to the fact that verification was being effected. I did not tell the subject that the suggestion was for a definite period, but made it as for an indefinite term ; then I verified the performance, or had the performance verified by some one else, without influencing the subject anew in any way. The attempt was repeated about a dozen times on the average in each subject, so as to obtain a fairly large number of instances.

To my great surprise, I found most of the suggestions made under such conditions had a very brief duration. The suggestion would be realised while I was present, and then once more a few moments after I had gone away ; after that, in most cases, its effect seemed to have completely disappeared. Such was the result in three-fourths of my experiments. It is easy to understand why the effective duration of suggestions should be thus brief. A suggestible individual remains accessible to all kinds of suggestions which speedily counteract the first suggestion.

In one-fourth of the instances there occurred interesting prolongations of suggestion, in some cases for several days, in one for sixty days, and in yet another for ninety days. As might have been foreseen, the suggestions whose effect was most obviously transient were those which conflicted with the subject's habits and tastes, those which were especially difficult to carry out, and those whose performance made the subject feel awkward or ridiculous. This is unfortunate from the therapeutic point of view, for therapeutic suggestions are the ones likely to encounter most resistance of these kinds. I was also able to note that a particular durability of suggestion would be characteristic of a particular subject. In some subjects, the durability was always very brief, whereas in other subjects the durability could always be measured by days ; here idiosyncrasy obviously played its part. The condition of the subject during the period for which the suggestion persists is worthy of careful study. Throughout this period there exist certain modifications of the mental condition which disappear rather suddenly when the realisation of the suggestion ceases. During the period of influence, the subject is, I think, in something akin to a secondary personality, in a quasi-hypnotic state. Thus the duration of the period is in part dependent upon the subject's habitual liability to pass into these secondary states; but it also depends upon the nature of his illness, upon the degree of his mental instability, and upon the form of hysteria by which he has been affected for a longer or shorter time. We shall have to return to these problems in the last chapter of this book, when we come to consider treatment by influence and guidance.

To sum up, most of the wonderful phenomena ascribed to suggestion seem to me to be dependent to a much greater extent upon the subject's illness, upon the neurosis, than upon suggestion itself. But, we shall be asked, is not hysteria endowed with a mechanism akin to that of suggestion? If we say that anything is due to hysteria, is it not due to suggestion? To some extent only are these implications true, but that is a minor question. The essential point is that such elemental and profound perturbations are the outcome of emotions and of natural suggestions deriving from the events of life, and we must not suppose that the power of our experimental and therapeutic suggestions can rival that of these natural influences. Art can only imitate them to a small extent and very imperfectly; our suggestions will never be as effective as natural suggestions. That is why I am unable to accept the view that medical suggestion can, unaided, produce the extensive visceral modifications and the motor or sensory dissociations which are ascribed to it. It cannot bring about actions or bodily and mental modifications of a higher grade than those which the normal will can ordinarily achieve. We shall have to approach the matter from a different outlook if we are in search of practical applications of suggestion.

2. PRACTICAL EFFICACY OF SUGGESTION AND HYPNOTISM.

We must cease to expect that hypnotic suggestion can lead to the performance of actions which are beyond the power of the normal human will. But is anything of this kind requisite ? Will it not be enough if we can induce actions which merely transcend the extant volitional powers of our patient ? The very persons in whom hypnotic suggestion is effective are neuropaths suffering from depression, exhibiting all kinds of disorders of the will, and, in a great many instances, affected by a powerlessness to act. They cannot begin an action ; or, having begun it, they are unable to continue it. That is the cause of their multiform paralyses, of their inability to walk, speak, eat, look, sleep, etc. If they try to perform these actions, they suffer from various disorders ; from emotions, anxieties, tics, agitations of manifold kinds ; and these disorders are nothing more than derivatives of their activity, which is incompetent to achieve the complete performance of the action they have begun. In other instances they cannot bring an action to a close, so that they are affected with impulses resulting from the involuntary development of tendencies which, having been once awakened, continue to operate in season and out of season, thus giving rise to convulsive paroxysms, crises, and various forms of delirium. We must not expect from such persons the performance of actions needing superhuman powers of the will. We shall have done a great deal if we can help them to perform actions which are well within the competence of the average human will, for that will suffice to relieve them of many of their sufferings.

Certainly, suggestion will not suffice to restore their lost powers of will. " Just as we cannot suggest to an individual to be suggestible when he is not suggestible, so we cannot suggest to a patient to cease to be suggestible when he is suggestible. If he displays a semblance of disobedience, he does so by automatic obedience, and not because he has reconquered the power of voluntary assent—any more than the non-suggestible healthy individual will lose that power through suggestion." [1] No doubt the actions thus induced will be impulsive actions, and not reflective voluntary actions ; they will have all the defects of direct assent, as contrasted with reflective assent. They will be less perfectly adapted to reality and to the extant situation ; above all, they will be less satisfactorily assimilated to the personality, they will leave little memory of what has been done, and will have

[1] L'automatisme psychologique, 1889, p. 169.

little tendency to promote the building up of the personality. All this is undeniable, and we may share the regrets of the medical moralisers that the subject cannot accomplish " true Actions " ; still, we must not forget that he is an invalid, and that these flaws in his activity are the outcome of his illness.

Furthermore, some of the defects of impulsive action can be greatly mitigated by medical suggestion. No doubt an impulsive action is ill adapted if it be made through the patient's unaided choice ; but, in the cases we are now considering, the choice of the action, the decision as to the movement to be made, is that of the medical adviser, who is a person capable of making a reflective decision. The suppression of the freedom of personal choice for a certain time during the illness and during the progress of the treatment, is not a serious matter, and may even be advantageous. The subjects themselves realise this. They are well aware of their incapacity to perform certain actions voluntarily ; or they know that the performance of their actions is disturbed by all sorts of scruples, useless efforts, and fixed ideas. They themselves want us to compel them to perform their actions under duress or automatically. " Have you made up your mind to feed me through a tube, if I refuse to take food ? "—"Certainly." —" In that case, you are forcing me, and the responsibility is yours. That suits me best." Thereupon the patient takes her food without further protest. " As soon as I try to eat," said another of my women patients, " I feel as if a voice were saying to me, ' Do not eat.' When this voice begins to speak, I feel stubborn, and I have to make terrible efforts to overcome my reluctance to eat. What I like best is to eat without thinking about the matter, without reflection."

These impulsive actions are, in fact, much easier than reflective actions, and that is why actions of the former type continue in persons whose tension is greatly lowered. In such patients, impulsive action, as we have seen, is still quite forcible ; whereas actions of the superior type, if still performed, are performed very feebly. It is precisely because suggested actions are non-reflective that they can be so useful in these cases.

Actions induced in this way entail a number of important advantages. First of all, some of these actions have physiological consequences which are, to a certain extent, independent of the way in which the action has been performed. There is not much difference in the way in which a man is nourished by his food if he has received it into his stomach through a tube instead of taking it in the ordinary way ; it does not matter very much whether he eats voluntarily, or involuntarily and unreflectingly. Similar considerations apply to other bodily functions, such as defaecation, urination, the functions of the genital organs, and even sleep and waking. My detailed account of Marceline shows that in certain cases we can artificially keep a patient alive by thus inducing the automatic performance of the functions.[1] Conversely, these suggested actions can have an inhibitive power, and can check other and dangerous automatic actions which the will is powerless to inhibit. The suggestion to eat and to retain what has been eaten can check vomiting, suggested movements can check chorea, and suggestion of normal breathing can check disorders of respiration. Guyau, in his book *Education et hérédité*, said that suggestion enabled us to create artificial instincts which would counterbalance preexistent undesirable tendencies. The statement is perhaps a little overdrawn, but it is true that many morbid troubles are the outcome of agitations and derivations. If we can restore normal activity, we shall relieve the patient of many such symptoms.

A tendency which is never realised, loses force, undergoes atrophy, so that less and less can it be activated by the will. Sometimes, the resulting changes are materially obvious. If a limb is inactive for a long time through paralysis, the muscles, even if they are not affected with a sort of active atrophy as a direct outcome of the nervous lesion, will certainly waste, and become obviously weaker ; the limb will exhibit the peripheral chilliness which I pointed out long ago, and of which other observers are now beginning to take note ; persistent contractures will give rise to deformity, and permanent adhesions may form. Regular movements, although automatically induced, can do much to prevent these disastrous changes. In certain cases we induce movements by electrical stimulation, but obviously it will be better if we can induce them by suggestion. Exercise will keep the function in good condition, so that its activation will

---

[1] Une Félida artificielle, L'état mental des hystériques, second edition, 1910, p. 545.

be much easier at a later stage when the will can get to work once more. On the other hand, we can do good by the automatic arrest of certain tendencies which have developed impulsively; we can check this development, and can thus make things easier for the will when, subsequently, it has to control the impulses in question.

I have said that the will derives advantage from the automatic exercise of tendencies, and, in fact, the will may soon be ready to intervene. Our study of the working of suggestion has shown that an action may at first be performed automatically, but that, at a certain grade of development, it will be adopted by the individual will. The same thing happens in the case of the functions which have been depressed below the level at which voluntary action is possible, and which seem to have been paralysed. Automatic functioning will gradually restore their integrity, until at length we are surprised by finding that the will has readopted them and can direct them once more. In cases of hysterical mutism, I have often had occasion to see how speech, which has at first been restored in automatic fashion during hypnosis or in periods of distraction, will, by degrees, become conscious and voluntary. Besides, into this automatic exercise of function there intrudes at a certain moment, as the subject is well aware, a factor which is preeminently competent to increase the psychological tension and to strengthen the will—I refer to the realisation of success. Those who endeavour to cure by moralisation are never weary of repeating that we must get out of the patient's mind the idea that he is paralysed, and that we must instil into him a conviction of power. To this end, they employ the most extraordinary arguments. But is there any sort of theoretical argument which can have so strong an effect upon the patient as his own personal perception of his ability to act ? In my book on automatism I recorded the remarkable case of V. (f., 30), who had long been bedridden, and was suffering from complete paraplegia.[1] While she was talking with Dr. Piazecki (who had taken me to see her), and was not therefore consciously attending to my words, I made her a number of " suggestions by distraction," and under the influence of these she got up and began to walk about. Then she became aware of what she was

[1] L'automatisme psychologique, 1889, p. 360.

doing, and, finding herself able to stand and walk, she delightfully exclaimed : " But I am cured ! " Her confidence being now restored, she went on walking voluntarily. Could any rational demonstration exercise so powerful an influence ?

The same considerations apply to all the tendencies which suggestion can activate. The mere automatic arrest of a number of anxieties and feelings of despair, the mere automatic development of a sense of confidence and hope, put the mind into the best possible conditions for the recovery of tranquillity and energy. A good many sermons would be requisite to produce a small fraction of these results. Of course suggestion has not worked a miracle in such cases. It has effected nothing which transcends ordinary human faculties. Still, it has achieved things which the debilitated will of the patient was no longer competent to achieve, thereby paving the way for a general reestablishment of the mental powers.

We may extend the same ideas to the hypnotic state. Even if we have now to abandon the notion that a development of wondrous and superhuman powers can be effected through hypnotism, is it not still possible that hypnotism may render us services of a comparatively humble kind ? Hypnosis, induced somnambulism, is a transformation of the mind, a change in the patient's mental state. By its very definition, it is a considerable change, for it is characterised by a breach in the subject's memory. Now, in neuropathic conditions, which tend to be indefinitely prolonged, and in which fixed and disastrous habits are apt to be formed, an extensive change of this character can hardly fail to be useful. This was so well known in former days that physicians used actually to try to induce hysterical attacks in order to modify a dangerous morbid equilibrium. Obviously, hypnotism can achieve the same result at less cost.

The modification we are considering has been turned to account in a number of different ways, and that is why hypnotism finds recurrent mention in so many chapters of the present work. It may be used as a means of repose, as a means of restoring lost memories, and as a procedure enabling us to increase tension by more liberal excitation. Our present concern with this modification in the state of mind is that it favours suggestion. Personal activity is sometimes lessened in hypnotism, and sometimes it is transformed. The subject no longer has the same disquietudes, and no longer makes the same efforts at supervision ; he does not remember what he does or hears while in the hypnotic state, and this is favourable to the influence of suggestion, which requires distraction and forgetfulness.

From another point of view, inasmuch as hypnosis differs from the waking state, certain tendencies which have been checked during the waking state, can manifest themselves anew during hypnosis. I recall the case of two patients who, through refusal of food and through persistent vomiting, had had their nutrition dangerously reduced. On being hypnotised, they could eat and digest perfectly. In like manner, paralysis, mutism, and amnesia, may temporarily disappear under hypnosis. Often the troubles will recur on awakening, but in the interim the lapsed function has been maintained and stimulated.

Another interesting peculiarity of hypnosis is that it is closely related to all the other secondary states, differing from the waking state into which these unstable hysterics are so apt to lapse. Such states are very numerous ; for instance, we have hysterical paroxysms, somnambulisms, deliriums, certain kinds of nightmare, and so on ; and in these various states there are manifested all sorts of symptoms over which we are able to exercise very little control during the patient's waking state. But during hypnosis we can revive the patient's memory of the symptoms of the somnambulist state, and this enables us to modify them far more easily. The fact has struck even those authorities who are reluctant, generally speaking, to use hypnotism. Paul Dubois, for instance, is willing to hypnotise his patients in order to cure nocturnal incontinence of urine occasioned by dreams. Bernheim, who has now broken the idols he used to worship, and who no longer regards hypnotism as of any value, is still prepared to admit that " in certain cases, when we have to do with psychoneuroses which manifest themselves during sleep itself, such as night terrors, obsessive dreams, nightmares, and nocturnal incontinence of urine, we may find it useful to induce sleep, to induce the very condition in which the psychoneurosis manifests itself." [1] Nay, more. I think that for the cure of the

---

[1] " Journal für Psychologie und Neurologie," 1911, Sonderabdruck, p. 477.

secondary state itself, for checking the onset of the paroxysm or the somnambulism, hypnotism may be of great value. Hypnosis is psychologically akin to these secondary states, and can readily be substituted for them. I pointed out in 1889 that a hypnotised hysteric no longer suffers from spontaneous paroxysms or spontaneous somnambulism. In 1891, Babinski made a similar remark when he wrote : " There is a sort of balance between hypnotism and the symptoms of hysteria. Hypnosis seems to function as an equivalent of some of these phenomena." [1] Gilles de la Tourette has said something of the same kind. The critic may contend that there is no obvious advantage in substituting artificial somnambulism for the crises of natural somnambulism. I do not agree. The spontaneous symptoms are irregular and undisciplined ; they begin when they please and stop when they please, and induce phenomena which cannot be foreseen. Hypnotic states, on the other hand, are at our own disposal. We can make the periods of hypnosis longer or shorter ; we can make the periods between the hypnosis brief or long ; and by the regulation of these states we can make them inoffensive and infrequent. There can be no doubt that one of the best ways of treating natural somnambulism is to transform it into the hypnotic state. Thus, from all these different outlooks, we see that hypnotism, like suggestion, may be of real service in the treatment of nervous diseases.

3. DANGERS OF THESE THERAPEUTIC METHODS.

Suggestion and hypnotism may do good service, but are we justified in using them ? Is it not possible that their drawbacks outweigh their advantages ? F. T. Simpson, discussing this matter a few years ago in the essay entitled *Hysteria, its Nature and Treatment* contributed by him to Parker's *Psychotherapy* (III, iii, p. 28), referred to various authors whose opinions upon this matter are conflicting. In one of my early works I made a detailed study of the alleged dangers of hypnotic suggestion, and must be content here with a summary of what I wrote on that occasion. Writing in 1860, Demarquay and Giraud Teulon said : " We must not assume that hypnotism is harmless because it does not intro-

---

[1] " Gazette Hebdomadaire," July 1891, p. 16.

duce any foreign element into the human body. A method which begins by shattering a nervous system can hardly inspire us with confidence." [1] There is gross exaggeration here. Hypnotism is not the sort of thunderbolt these authors describe; I even regard it as unfortunate that there is so little danger attaching to the use of hypnotism and suggestion. I say " unfortunate " for the reason that a medicament is not really potent unless it is able to be dangerous on occasions; and it is very difficult to think of any method of treatment which would be efficacious although it could never by any possibility do harm. The dangers attaching to the use of a poisonous drug make it necessary that we should study with great care how to administer it, and in what doses; but the fact that the drug is poisonous is the primary indication that it is powerful. We can hardly say as much of suggestion and of experimental hypnosis, for, even in bad hands, suggestion and hypnotism do not seem to have been able to do much harm.

If the methods are applied indiscriminately to all kinds of illnesses, they will usually have no effect whatever, and if they do harm, it will only be to the doctor. Charcot has written some admirable words on this point: " A miracle-monger can say to his patient: ' Take up thy bed and walk.' Why should we not play the thaumaturge, since it is for the good of our patients ? Well, gentlemen, I do not say categorically that you should never do anything of the kind. In certain cases, if you are quite sure of your diagnosis, perhaps you will do well to take the risk. You had better walk cautiously in such matters. Do not forget that, in practice, you have to deal with questions of taste, opportunity, and, let me add, medical dignity, for the importance of this last must never be overlooked. Do not forget that nothing can make you seem more absurd than to predict with great pomp and circumstance a result which will perhaps never be achieved. Suggestion is a difficult agent to handle; it is, if you will permit the metaphor, a drug whose accurate dosage is far from easy. The English, who are a preeminently practical people, have a saying, ' Don't prophesy unless you know.' I am in full agreement with their outlook upon this point, and I advise you to guide your own actions by so excellent a pre-

[1] Recherches sur l'hypnotisme ou sommeil nerveux, p. 8.

cept." [1] While the doctor risks his reputation, the patient is not risking very much. After unsuccessful attempts, he may feel tired, bored, disappointed—nothing more. In exceptional instances, when the attempt to hypnotise has been made publicly and dramatically, the subject may take fright, and may suffer from some of the disorders resulting from emotion. But in this case we must not blame hypnotism for the results. The patient has not been hypnotised! He is suffering from emotional disturbances which might have been induced by the failure of any other kind of treatment.

The problem grows more interesting when we have succeeded in inducing a genuine condition of hypnosis. Let us ask what are the immediate drawbacks which may accompany the use of suggestion or the induction of hypnosis. A suggestion may be misunderstood, or may be accepted in an exaggerated sense. I have known subjects who went on eating all day because they had received the suggestion to eat well at meal times ; and I have known others who suffered from insomnia at night because they had been forbidden to sleep during the daytime. These are trifling matters, and such troubles can readily be corrected by a more wisely directed education. Giddiness and nausea are occasional incidents, though rare. To avoid them, we shall do well not to have our sittings either just before or just after the subject's meal times. A commoner trouble is severe headache, which may be especially distressing after the first attempts to induce hypnosis, or when the sittings are resumed after a prolonged intermission. Even more violent paroxysms of headache may arise when, while, the subject is in the hypnotic state, we make war on his fixed ideas, and when we have succeeded in extensively transforming his amnesias and his anaesthesias ; but these headaches are not due to the hypnotism, and we may regard their significance as very favourable. Such headaches seldom last more than a few hours; they can be mitigated by suggestion, and by various precautions which we must take when we are awaking our subjects.

A more serious danger, which arises when we are hypnotising certain patients, is that we may induce a hysterical paroxysm. It is not merely that emotion can bring on the attack, for there is an intimate relationship between the psy-

[1] Leçons du Mardi, vol. i, p. 382.

chological condition during the hysterical paroxysm and that which is characteristic of somnambulism, so that the transition from one to the other is only too easy. Still, we have here to do with an annoying accident rather than a serious obstacle. A few precautions will enable us to diminish the danger, if not to avert it entirely. Besides, the hysterical paroxysm is not in itself very dangerous. Finally, in certain cases, when we have to do with symptoms which have lasted a long time, it may be a good thing to induce a paroxysm. We may thus change the orientation of the mind, may modify the state of sensibility and of memory. If we can guide the paroxysm, it may become the starting-point of a somnambulist state which can be of great use to us subsequently. In a word, there are certain cases in which I would rather bring on a hysterical paroxysm while trying to induce hypnosis than find myself unable to exercise any influence over my patient.

Greater difficulties are encountered when the time comes to awaken the subject. The magnetisers of old laid great emphasis upon the importance of this operation.[1] As a general rule the awakening should be made as complete as possible. We shall return to this question when we come to deal with the stimulant treatment of hysterics. Also, as a general rule the awakening should be postponed if a morbid symptom of any sort should intervene during the hypnotic state. Any such untoward symptom, such as a contracture or a delusion, must be relieved before the patient is awakened. Sometimes it is extremely difficult to put a term to such troubles and to bring the patient back to the waking state, for the reason that the hypnotic sleep has become transformed, quite independent of the hypnotist, into a hysterical sleep or into spontaneous somnambulism. These accidents, it must never be forgotten, are dependent upon the serious hysterical condition of the subject, and hypnotism, properly so called, is not responsible; they might have occurred during the waking state or during natural sleep, and they are not more serious because they happen to have developed in the course of the hypnotic sleep. They may usually be put an end to if the operator enters into closer rapport with the subject, and regains his influence over the current of the

[1] Cf. Baragnon, Etude du magnétisme animal sous le point de vue d'une exacte pratique, 1853, p. 210.

patient's ideas. If, all the same, his efforts are not successful, the morbid symptoms must be allowed to develop as though they were of an ordinary hysterical nature, and the patient will pass naturally into the waking state as though recovering from a crisis of the familiar type. In subsequent sittings, the hypnotist must gradually bring greater influence to bear upon the subject, so that such accidents may not recur.

It is a more serious matter when the attack or the sleep which have been induced by hypnotism is subsequently reproduced spontaneously. I think that, as a rule, it is best not to interrupt the course of treatment, but, rather, to continue it, and to induce a genuine state of somnambulism which will help to overcome these superadded attacks. I may also draw attention to the perturbations which somnambulism and suggestion introduce into the hysterical symptoms. For instance, the sudden suppression of one symptom often leads to its being replaced by another. I have insisted elsewhere on the alternations between hysterical vomiting and delirium. These are difficulties which are always liable to occur during the treatment of hysterics ; they are not dangers attaching to suggestion itself, but, in such cases, they render the use of suggestion a matter of infinite delicacy.

We see, therefore, that hypnotic and suggestive practice is not dangerous to any great degree, and that the dangers, which go to prove its potency in certain cases, are fairly easy to overcome. All the authors who have made use of these methods are convinced of this. Bonjour gives an excellent summary of many expert opinions in his *La suggestion hypnotique* (1908). Another summary may be found in the article by F. H. Gerrish published in Morton Prince's symposium.[1] C. Lloyd Tuckey sums up the matter in an amusing way : " Liébeault practised in Nancy for forty years, and a large proportion of the inhabitants must have submitted to suggestion at his hands. Since 1882 his most distinguished pupil, Professor Bernheim, has practised on an even larger scale, so that, as Professor Wood, of Philadelphia, said after his visit in 1889, ' the air of Nancy is heavy with suggestion.'

---

[1] The therapeutic Value of hypnotic Suggestion, Address delivered by the President of the American Therapeutic Society, May 6, 1909 ; reproduced in Psychotherapeutics, a Symposium, 1910, p. 47.

Yet we have no record of the health of Nancy—intellectual, physical, or moral—being inferior to that of other towns in France." [1]

If, then, there are very few dangers attaching to an isolated hypnotic séance, can the same thing be said as regards a long series of séances ? I do not think so, for now we are concerned with the extensive powers of education and habit, which may happily do a great deal of good, but may also do harm. There can be no doubt that a good many hypnotised subjects have, under bad guidance, acquired extremely undesirable habits. There is, unfortunately, a famous example of this in the hysterical states which were studied and cultivated in Charcot's clinic at the Salpêtrière during the decade of 1878 to 1888—the paroxysms that were so prolonged and had so regular a succession of phases, the contractures of a typical kind, the hypnosis occurring in three phases in all the subjects alike—these phenomena were largely manufactured by drill and, although they may not have been dangerous, they certainly cannot be regarded as having been wholesome. In a dozen or so of patients there was beyond question an undesirable development of neurosis, a fostered hysteria. This must now be frankly admitted. Still, we have to remember that similar dangerous possibilities arise whenever we exercise an educative influence over persons who are unduly docile. In the Nancy clinics, where the practice was to hypnotise 90 per cent. of the patients, where they were trained to feign sleep, and to exhibit the phenomena of " rotatory automatism " or to perform " horrible crimes " at the word of command, there was also a drilling process which cannot be regarded as harmless and which was applied to a very large number of persons. Those who are to-day treating such patients by persuasion, who keeps such patients in bed for an indefinite period until the unfortunates are compelled to pretend that they are cured in order to get permission to leave their beds and to use their tongues, certainly run the risk of inducing in neuropaths habits of idleness and hypocrisy. The doctor must never forget that suggestible patients are easily drilled, that they are influenced by the words, the attitudes, and the example of others, quite

[1] Cf. Parker's Psychotherapy, II, ii, p. 7.

as readily as by hypnotic suggestion. Aware of this power and this danger, he must be careful to use suggestion for good only. There is no danger in producing a powerful effect by suggestion and in producing it rapidly, if proper skill is employed.

Another criticism was made a good many years ago by Jolly.[1] He declared that hypnotism can induce a hysterical mental condition which remains latent for a time. I think this is true. Somnambulism with amnesia, and the dissociation of consciousness which attends it, are typical of the mental phenomena of hysteria, so typical that, as I have often pointed out, certain hysterics seem to be in a condition of persistent somnambulism. If we cultivate this condition, we are regularising, as it were, the patient's hysteria. This must certainly be dangerous in young persons who have only recently become hysterical, and in whom as yet the sub-conscious phenomena characteristic of the disease have only developed to a minor degree. In contradistinction to those authors who have repeatedly advised the use of hypnotism in the education of children, I consider that the practice of the hypnotic method where children are concerned should be restricted to cases of absolute necessity. Besides, when children fall ill, they can as a rule be readily cured by other methods. Jolly's criticsm provides us with an additional and weighty reason for prohibiting the non-medical practice of hypnotism, which was fashionable for a time. A good many persons who had previously been affected only by vague nervous disorders have acquired very definite hysterical troubles through being hypnotised by lay practitioners, who were sometimes persons of considerable renown.

Still, when well-marked hysteria already exists, I see no objection to inducing somnambulism. This will not cause depression, dissociation of consciousness, and the manifestation of subconscious phenomena, for these symptoms are already present ; it will only regularise them, and will enable us to guide and to suppress them. Finally, we must not hypnotise ourselves with the dread of the hysterical mental condition, which is perhaps the least dangerous among morbid mental states. If, in a patient suffering from one or other form of chronic mental confusion or of constitutional psychasthenia,

---

[1] " Archiv für Psychiatrie," xxv, 3, 1894.

we can substitute the hysterical mental state for this condition, we shall do good service.

From the medico-psychological outlook, the most formidable criticism of hypnotic suggestion is that, when used to excess, it accustoms the subject to perform automatic actions in which his will and his individual consciousness play no part. " Training in automatism," write Dejerine and Gauckler, " is a frequent if not an invariable result. Most of the hysterics who were drilled in former days became unfortunate beings unable to guide themselves through life in the absence of outside aid." [1] I think that this assertion is itself open to criticism. As a rule, the subjects drilled by hypnotists developed only a small number of partlal and definitely systematised automatisms, while retaining in other respects an independent, intractable, and arrogant temperament. If some of them were sorry specimens, we may presume that this was due to their disposition, which persisted unmodified, and not to their hypnotic training. Still, we will agree for the sake of argument that it is possible to accustom a subject to look to suggestion for guidance as concerns almost all the actions of life, and thus to lose the habit of individual initiative. But this danger can only arise from the abuse of suggestion. We must be forewarned, and must recognise that the employment of hypnotic suggestion must be restricted, that the dosage of the remedy must be regulated like that of any other. It must be utilised only to the degree in which it is required to modify the phenomena which the subject cannot control by the power of his individual will.

It is none the less true that, for a time at least, the hynotised subject will be dependent upon the doctor. Indeed, it has often been noticed that these subjects retain a remarkable need for somnambulism, and continue to exhibit undue obedience to the hypnotist. This is an important observation, for herein lies the danger, or at any rate the most essential characteristic, of hypnotic treatment, as I pointed out a good many years ago.[2] The influence of the hypnotist is the very thing that enables us to make these patients reasonable ; far from dreading it, we must encourage it to the utmost when the

[1] Op. cit., p. 401.
[2] L'influence somnambulique et le besoin de direction, Névroses et idées fixes, 1898, vol. i, p. 423.

illness is serious. If the subject could manage himself satisfactorily unaided, it would be a mistake to hold him in leading strings ; but if he be really ill, and if he present all the symptoms of hysterical automatism, we shall do him good service by exerting over his rebellious tendencies a control which he is unable to exert himself.

Since this excessive submission is the outcome of the subject's mental condition and not of the hypnotism, it plays its part in various other methods of treatment with which, to all appearance, hypnotic suggestion has no concern. You will find it in connexion with treatment by moralising persuasion, for here the subject is just as incapable of getting on without the doctor ; you will find it in the pseudo-religious methods of treatment ; and you will find it in the treatment by ordinary physical methods. Some patients continually haunt the waiting-room of the doctor who writes prescriptions for them, or dog the heels of the electrician or the masseur. One invalid of my acquaintance became the slave of an individual who pretended to analyse his urine several times a day. Some patients will squander their fortune and sacrifice their family for the sake of a miracle-working monk, or for that of a fortune-teller. When domination has become indispensable, I should prefer it to be manifest and avowed, for then it is more likely to be temperately used and turned to good account.

The best proof of the value of such guidance and domination is afforded by the success of the treatment in doing away with the need for guidance. The development of the rebellious tendencies has hampered and restricted the power of the will. Suggestion, by bringing these tendencies under control, enfranchises the will and facilitates the reconstitution of the personality. When the treatment is successful, suggestion, though requisite to begin with, soon becomes impossible, for the subject gradually loses his morbid suggestibility. We shall return to this matter in the chapter specially devoted to the problems of moral guidance. The only conclusion to be drawn at this stage is that the use of suggestion must not be frivolously undertaken ; that the practice must not be suddenly discontinued after the apparent cure of a single symptom ; and that the patient and his family must be warned that, underlying this symptom, there is a faulty mental condition which cannot be transformed all in a moment. A complete system of education is requisite, involving various kinds of treatment in addition to suggestion, and the general aim of treatment must be to achieve the reconstitution of the personality.

If we adopt the medical point of view, we see that the dangers or drawbacks of hypnotic suggestion are not very serious. These dangers and drawbacks, such as they are, can be diminished, if not entirely done away with, by a better knowledge of the disease and its treatment. They certainly do not outbalance the advantages that can be derived from this method of treatment in special instances.

4. ETHICAL OBJECTIONS TO HYPNOTISM AND SUGGESTION.

Although it may seem strange, and even a trifle ridiculous, I must, nevertheless, say a few words concerning objections which have been raised against hypnotic suggestion on purely moral grounds. Certain doctors, suddenly returning to a state of grace, have followed the example of Paul Dubois, and have declared that the method of treatment, even though it may be useful at times, should not be employed because it is humiliating and degrading for patient and doctor alike. I do not think it will be difficult to allay these scruples.

Some of the critics belong to the category I have already dealt with. Their objection is that hypnotic suggestion entails certain risks. Dejerine adds that hypnotic suggestion is too potent, and might be used for evil purposes by an unscrupulous doctor, seeing that it is possible to induce the commission of crimes by means of suggestion. Even supposing this to be true, I would ask what medical treatment or surgical operation would be free from reproach ? Must we exclude arsenic from the pharmacopoeia because of Lacenaire's crime, or blunt the surgeon's bistoury lest he should cut his patient's throat ? J. R. Angell of Chicago is dubious about the use of suggestion because of the obvious opportunity which mental healing offers to the quack.[1] An excellent sentiment, but what would remain of medical and surgical practice were we to endorse it ? Do not let us blame a method of treatment because it is potent, and might be misused in unscrupulous hands ; for this very reason it may, in good hands, be beneficial.

[1] Cf. Parker's Psychotherapy, I, i, 68.

Other criticisms are aimed more directly at the morality of the method ; they are based upon general principles. It is true that, in the practice of suggestive therapy, we do make use of rather dubious forces, or forces which have but little moral worth. Most of these authors stress the fact that the hypnotic sleep and suggestibility are hysterical symptoms, and they draw the inference that a doctor misdemeans himself when he turns such morbid symptoms to account. I find it somewhat difficult to understand why we should not draw good out of evil, and wherefore one should not take advantage of a peculiarity of the disease in order to bring about a cure. We might just as well be forbidden to make use of a symptom for diagnostic purpose. J. J. Putnam remarks, apropos of this, that morphine and chloroform, like all drugs, cause symptoms which are in certain cases of a morbid nature. And yet these drugs are used for therapeutical purposes.[1]

Dejerine and Gauckler go even further. For them, suggestion is not worthy of serious consideration because it acts upon the surface of the mind but does not penetrate into the depths of the soul ; it can only modify symptoms, and does not radically transform the patient's psyche.[2] Even if this were true, are we to be forbidden to have recourse to symptomatic treatment ? Besides, is not the healing of all other diseases fraught with the same difficulty ? Shall we not be allowed to open a local abscess when treating a tuberculous patient, and would not the purely local treatment of such an abscess have a beneficial effect on the general condition of the patient ? " What advantage is there," exclaim these authors, " in suppressing a symptom if the cause remain ? "[3] Sometimes the advantage is very great, as, for instance, when the symptom is in itself both painful and dangerous, and is preventing the rebuilding of the forces which can overcome it. If a hysterical patient is suffering from anorexia, and refuses to touch a morsel of food, it is well to insist on his eating, even if his mental state remains hysterical ; such coercion will contribute to the successful treatment of the primary mental disorder.

Another group of critics, who are more frequently quoted against us, are those who hold that hypnotic suggestion appeals

---

[1] Putnam, Considerations concerning Mental Therapeutics, 1906, p. 14.
[2] Dejerine and Gauckler, Les manifestations fonctionnelles des psychonévroses et leur traitement, 1911, p. vii. [3] Ibid., p. 402.

to the automatic tendencies of the patient, and not to his reason, his will, and to the " participation of his ego." Now it would appear that, according to the psychological deductions of certain physicians, the automatic tendencies of our mind are something inferior, base, far lower than the reason, the will, and the " participation of the ego." It is concluded from this, that a treatment which appeals to these purlieus of the mind must itself become despicable and degrading. After speaking of my books with a kindliness for which I am truly grateful, Paul Dubois deplores the fact that I still, all too frequently, make use of suggestion in the treatment of my patients. He then sadly remarks : " How can Monsieur Janet consent to enter the mind of his patient by this back door ? " I might answer that I am a person of a humble disposition, and that, in order to make my way into the mind of a sufferer, I would willingly avail myself of the tradesmen's entrance ! But what is the use of such metaphors, and of so much disdain for psychological phenomena which are little understood and hardly as yet differentiated one from the other ? " There is nothing base in Jupiter's temple " ; and I should like to know why deeply ingrained instincts, the legacy of a long line of ancestors, should be more contemptible than are the whims and caprices of the moment. What they regard as logical reasoning, is in high favour among these doctors ; but nowadays logic is a little discredited among philosophers. The latter declare that we falsify our knowledge by over-intellectualisation. They prefer intuition, which springs from the deeply buried instincts. Whom are we to believe ?

Besides, are we in a position to make a choice ? Can we only appeal to the mental faculty which happens to please us ? All these people discuss the matter as though the patient were not ill at all, and as though he could exercise any function he liked at pleasure. If he were in possession of such perfect powers of reasoning and such an ideal force of will, he would not come to consult us. In reality he comes to the doctor for the very reason that he is incapable of behaving like a complete man, the master of himself. " You can only pretend to reason with him, and you have nothing to plume yourself about when you do so," says Bonjour in the " Revue de l'Hypnotisme " (1906, p. 59). It will be best not to allow ourselves any illusions in the matter, but frankly to recognise that we have to make a direct appeal to the inferior functions which are still at the patient's disposal. Is not this our method in all medical treatment ? Such treatment never addresses itself exclusively to the pure reason. " It is difficult to see why it is any more a suspension of judgment to let a physician you have decided to trust lodge a helpful idea in your mind, than to let him lodge an ominous-looking capsule in your body." [1]

But these inferior functions, we are told, cannot give such happy results as the operations of the rational faculties would bring about. " The cure is not a voluntary one ; the patient does not feed himself, he is fed ; to eat by means of hypnotic suggestion is not to eat at all." What childishness ! You think it better to feed an anorexic patient through a tube ? He puts on flesh, you say ? So does the patient whom we induce to take food by suggestion. I agree that they are not ideal ways of receiving nourishment ; still, they are ways of making the patient partake of food, and are certainly preferable to starvation. When the patient is stronger, and can rise to a higher level, you will soon see whether he is capable of obtaining nourishment by methods which are on a higher moral plane. But meanwhile, I repeat, we have to deal with an invalid, and you must, without delay, provide him with what he stands most in need of. Live first ; then you can philosophise.

Other moralist critics adopt a somewhat different viewpoint. They do not talk about the degradation of the patient by suggestive treatment ; what they complain of is that the doctor loses caste morally when he uses so base a method. Dubois is indignant with the suggesters, describing them as miracle-mongers. He actually blushes when he finds it necessary to use suggestion in his own practice. R. C. Cabot has an uneasy conscience about the matter. He asks whether the prescription of bread pills and other placebos ought not to be regarded as a subtle form of falsehood. Not even to save a man s life would he assure the patient that the pill contains a drug which is not actually there.[2]

[1] Max Eastman, The New Art of Healing, " The Atlantic Monthly," 1908, , p. 645.
[2] Cabot, Veracity and Psychotherapy, in Parker's Psychotherapy, I, iii, 23.

I am sorry that I cannot share these exalted and beautiful scruples. While I must admit that my own judgment is formed on a much lower plane, my belief is that the patient wants a doctor who will cure; that the doctor's professional duty is to give any remedy that will be useful, and to prescribe it in the way in which it will do most good. Now, I think that bread pills are medically indicated in certain cases, and that they will act far more powerfully if I deck them out with impressive names. When I prescribe such a formidable placebo, I believe that I am fulfilling my professional duty, and that I am keeping my real though tacit undertaking with my patient; and I am quite sure that if he gets well he will not bear me any grudge. But you believe, says the objector, that the action of the remedy is psychological, and yet you allow the patient to believe that its action is chemical; you are infringing the general obligation to be absolutely sincere! Perhaps I am. We are faced here with one of those conflicts between duties which are continually arising in practical life; and, for my part, I believe that the duty of curing my patient preponderates enormously over the trivial duty of giving him a scientific lecture which he would not understand and would have no use for. Cabot, who in some of his other essays shows admirable discernment, is well aware that such white lies are often indispensable. In practice he accepts these compromises, but with regret; he keeps on repeating that, in theory at least, it would be better if the doctor were to make it a rule to hide nothing from the patient, to say nothing that is not absolutely true.[1] Can we be sure that this is a good rule? I knew a woman who went mad because the doctor told her bluntly that her husband's case was hopeless, and that he would be buried before the fortnight was out. The statement was perfectly true, but would not the doctor have done better to veil the truth a little? If truth be a virtue, must we not also recognise that discretion and tact are virtues? Did not our forefathers speak of " medical tact? " That is what we are concerned with here. There are some patients to whom we must tell the whole truth; there are some to whom we must tell part of the truth; and there are some to whom, as a matter of strict moral obligation, we must lie. I know

[1] Cabot, Suggestion, Authority, and Command, Parker's Psychotherapy, II, iii, 25.

perfectly well that this leads us along far more difficult and far more intricate paths than that on which we should walk if we made it a rule to speak truth everywhere and at all times. I am sorry, but " true morality laughs at morality."

The most fanatical opponents of suggestion have to make use of the method themselves. Bonjour, of Lausanne, finds it amusing to point out how large a part suggestion plays in the practice of Paul Dubois, and he adds : " It would be better, when he uses suggestion, to admit the fact frankly. . . . What does it avail to run atilt against suggestion, to cover it with abuse and ridicule, if you end by saying that human beings ought to be accessible to reasonable suggestions only ? Are we to suppose that suggestions are never reasonable unless Monsieur Dubois utters them, and that they invariably become crude and absurd in the mouths of other practitioners ? " [1] Similar remarks might be made anent Dejerine and Gauckler's book. When, referring to the treatment of the obsession of fatigue, they advise that the patient should be made to walk while his attention is distracted from what he is doing, so that he cannot fix his mind upon the thought that he is getting tired,[2] is not this a way of humbugging him ? A study of the writings of R. C. Cabot would lead us to a similar conclusion. Indeed, Cabot admits the fact.[3]

It is needless to dwell on these considerations. In all discussions of the kind there is a misunderstanding. Such objections are never raised where other illnesses and other methods of treatment are concerned. If a man with a Hunterian chancre comes to consult a doctor, the latter does not ask himself whether a sermon would be a more exalted and more moral method of treatment than a mercurial injection. The practitioner does not put on a veil to hide his blushes before making a digital examination of the anus, and he does not make much ado when he has to put a mirror into the patient's mouth. The invalid is an invalid, and our most exalted duty is to cure the sufferer in the best possible way. The only reason why these scruples intrude into psychotherapeutics is that people have not yet succeeded in ridding their minds of the notion that neuropaths and the insane are,

---

[1] La suggestion hypnotique, " Revue de l'Hypnotisme," 1908, pp. 32 and 40.   [2] Dejerine and Gauckler, op. cit., pp. 508 and 510.
[3] Parker's Psychotherapy, II, iii, 23.

as it were, ignorant disciples, or penitents who must be taught the truth and the morality that happen to be in fashion. When we learn to regard them simply as invalids, and when the psychotherapeutists have become doctors and nothing more, we shall have heard the last of such imaginary problems.

The most that can be conceded to these moral critics is that the conscientious medical practitioner must exercise due caution in the application of suggestion and hypnotism. He must avoid suggestioning or hypnotising a patient without the patient's consent, or, rather, without the consent of the persons entitled to exercise moral authority over the patient. The question arises whether witnesses ought to be present at the sittings, and I have myself discussed the problem at considerable length.[1] I abide by the conclusion to which I came in that essay, namely that in treatment by suggestion and hypnotism the doctor ought to be alone with the patient. Then only will the treatment be really effective, and in no other way can we avoid a good many dangers which are apt to be overlooked. We need not try to excogitate a special science of medical ethics where suggestion is concerned ; it will be enough to adopt in this particular case the general rules that govern psychiatric treatment. The relationship of a hypnotisable patient to the hypnotist does not differ in any essential way from the relationship of a lunatic to the superintendent of an asylum. By accepting this outlook, those who practice suggestion and hypnotism would escape a good many moral difficulties—difficulties which never trouble alienists.

5. RESULTS OF THESE METHODS OF TREATMENT.

The foregoing discussions are obviously futile. The only thing that really matters is that we should know whether hypnotism is practically effective. Have notable cures been achieved through hypnotic suggestion, employed in a definite fashion and to the exclusion of other methods ? Generally speaking, the answer is in the affirmative. Of course, a good many of the published records of cures by hypnotism are open to criticism. The earlier reports often contained errors

---

[1] Traitement psychologique de l'hystérie, in Albert Robin's Traité de thérapeutique, 1898 ; L'état mental des hystériques, second edition, 1910, p. 650.

of diagnosis, and were apt to be invalidated by vagueness in the description of symptoms. More recent reports are still at fault for lack of a really accurate definition of suggestion, so that the use of the suggestive method is complicated by the employment of various other kinds of treatment. But these numberless observations are none the less valuable. Even if it could be proved that some of the illnesses described as chronic rheumatism, or as disease of the spinal cord, were really hysterical contractures, the fact would remain that very serious hysterical contractures were cured by psychological methods of treatment in which suggestion played a great part.

In order to verify once more the curative power of suggestion, and in order to clear up my own opinion on the matter, I have reviewed and analysed from this special outlook my own case-notes during the last thirty years. I do not now wish to approach the matter either from the psychological or from the clinical standpoint ; I am only concerned to ascertain to what extent the patients were benefited by treatment. We then have to make a separate category of the cases in which hypnotic suggestion, as an exclusive and accurately defined method of treatment, gave curative results of practical importance.

The cases which come within this category manifested all sorts of neuropathic symptoms, and they exhibited a moderate depression of the level of mental energy. In addition, by a sort of defensive reaction characteristic of persons of a particular age and temperament, the subject showed symptoms of distraction, and of restriction of the field of consciousness. Here we had an assemblage of the factors essential to suggestion, so that treatment by an appeal to the patient's automatism was practicable. A few simple experiments enabled me, in such cases, to confirm the opinion that there was a predisposition to impulsive exercise of the faculties of will and credence. I would tell the patient that his finger would remain stiff after I had touched it or after I had made him slip on a magnetised ring ; or I would tell him that my arm had magnetic properties, and could attract his arm towards itself. Such little experiments are almost invariably successful when a correct psychological diagnosis has been made. The skilled observer soon becomes able to recognise beforehand the patients in whom these experiments will always be successful, and to distinguish them from the patients in whom the same experiments will invariably fail.   Here we have the fundamental psychological distinction between hysterics and psychasthenics properly so called.

We can easily cultivate the disposition to suggestion, either by leaving the patient in the state in which he first presents himself, or by modifying this condition, should it seem desirable to do so, by the use of a certain amount of hypnotism. Then we proceed to make suggestions bearing upon the particular form of action which is disordered in the patient. In many instances it will suffice to suggest the immediate performance of this action.   The subject, who is no longer capable of willing the act reflectively and with full awareness, is still perfectly competent to perform it impulsively.   But in other instances we shall find it advantageous to begin by instilling impulsive beliefs, and thus modifying the obstacles to the performance of the action.   The patient's conviction that there is pain or paralysis will vanish " because certain manipulations have replaced a dislocated tendon, because the doctor's hand contains a fluid which reawakens the spinal cord, because we succeed in modifying the subconscious phenomena," and so on.   The formula will vary with the subject's age and education, the essential point being that it shall not conflict unduly with his extant knowledge.   The experience of the early magnetisers showed that certain material symbols could help to maintain impulsive faith. The magnetised water of former days can be replaced by pills of marvellous strength, by a taraxacum draught, or a cachet of methylene blue.   I need not go into details upon this matter. The methods are familiar, but will vary from case to case. I merely speak of them in general terms, as a prelude to my account of successful results.

In a first group I shall consider cases in which the effect of suggestive treatment was so complete and so speedy that the cures were akin to what are usually termed miraculous cures.   They were cases of serious illness, which had existed for at least a month.   Treatment was begun at the first visit, without any detailed psychological analysis.   The method used was simple suggestion, in the sense already defined, sometimes in the waking state and sometimes after the rapid induction of hypnosis. Cure ensued after one or a few sittings (four at most). The cure was permanent, for I have not included in this group any patients who were not free from relapse for at least a year after treatment. There was no return either of the disorder actually cured or of a kindred disorder. I can only find in my case-books the record of a few cases able to satisfy these stringent conditions, but those that I do find have definite evidential value.

I have already mentioned one of my early cases, that of V. (f., 30), who for three months had been affected with flaccid paraplegia attended by anaesthesia of the lower limbs, and who was cured in one sitting through suggestion by distraction.[1] Orders given in low tones while she was talking to some one else led her, first of all to make subconscious movements of the legs, and then to get up and walk. I was surprised to find that the cure was maintained after this one sitting. I had news of the patient's condition for several years thereafter, and she had no relapse. Similar to this instance were other cases of functional paralysis in which suggestion began to take effect by awakening in an automatic form the tendency which could not consciously be set to work.—Two such cases were those of a girl of sixteen and a little girl of eleven, both of whom were suffering from complete paraplegia which had arisen as a sequel of emotion and convulsive paroxysms. The paralysis, grave though it seemed, disappeared after two sittings.—Sev. (f., 48) became affected with left hemiplegia because some one had fired a pistol close to her left ear; she recovered completely after four sittings.—Zrs. (f., 16), having fallen down the stairs, suffered from complete paraplegia for two months; she was enabled to walk at the first sitting, and had no relapse. I should mention that this patient had had similar symptoms two years earlier, and had been cured by immersion in the Lourdes piscina; but I think I am entitled to congratulate myself for having done the patient as much good as Lourdes would have done, while saving her the expense of the journey.

Zke. (m., 30) had been suffering from complete mutism for six weeks as a sequel of an emotional disturbance; the suggestion that examination by X-rays would have a mar-

[1] Cf. L'automatisme psychologique, 1889, p. 359.

vellously beneficial effect upon his larynx was promptly and fully successful.—Another patient Mkm. (f., 34), suffering from mutism of the same kind, recovered the power of speech after two sittings.—Nye. (f., 25), another sufferer from mutism, in whom however the trouble had lasted only a fortnight, had her powers of speech fully restored after a single sitting of hypnotism and suggestion.

Nofy., a girl of twelve, sustained a slight blow upon the left eye, and a few days later began to complain that she could no longer see clearly with this eye. When she came under my observation a month later, there was complete unilateral amaurosis. An examination by means of Flees' box showed that vision still persisted in the subconscious. A few suggestions made while using the box quickly brought back conscious sight which did not again disappear.

Hysterical contractures of long standing can likewise be made to disappear after a single sitting, though I believe this to be of rare occurrence seeing that the affection is peculiarly stubborn. A woman of twenty-three, after a fight with her husband, had a complete contracture of the right arm, which had lasted a month when she came under my care. The application of a large magnet brought about, by suggestion, the transference of this contracture to the left arm, and then induced the return of the trouble to the right arm. After a few oscillations of the kind, a complete cure ensued, and there was no further neuropathic trouble during the next eighteen months.—Qkd. (f., 40), having accidentally run a needle beneath a finger-nail, had had a contracture of the arm for six months. The trouble was easily cured by a little mobilisation of the limb and by suggestion under hypnotism, hypnosis having been induced at the very first visit.—Xof. (f., 21), suffering from contracture of the left wrist, was cured at the first sitting.—Wox. (f., 15), was brought on a stretcher, both her legs having been contractured for a week after a hysterical paroxysm ; she was able to walk after a single sitting, and no further treatment was requisite.—Lqu. (f., 27), whose case has already been quoted as an example of accidental suggestion, had had her head drawn back for months through contracture of the muscles at the back of the neck which came on after she had seen in the hospital mortuary the body of a man who had died of tetanus. She was cured after three sittings.

In a number of cases it was possible to stop disorders and automatic functionings of tendencies which had got out of hand.—Lec. (f., 25) became affected with chorea while looking at a child suffering from this disease, and while thinking that she would be very sorry to have such a trouble herself. When she had been affected by irregular movements of the limbs and face for several weeks, she came to seek advice. She was easily hypnotised, and was promptly cured of her grimaces. I should mention that two years later she began to suffer from major hysteria, and that I had then to treat her for a considerable time. But as far as the original trouble was concerned, it was cured at the first sitting, and there was no relapse for two years.—I had a similar experience in dealing with two other cases of hysterical chorea. In one of these patients, the disorder of movement had lasted six months, and in the other, for two months; both were cured by a single sitting. —Only two or three sittings were required to cure Ze. (f., 24), and Pea. (f., 30), suffering from chorea limited to the left side. —Equally successful was the treatment of Chp. and Nic., girls of nineteen, suffering from tremor of the right hand; and of T. (f., 22), who had an occupational chorea, and persistently made ironing movements.—Boi., a girl of ten suffering from rhythmical chorea, was cured in a quarter of an hour by the pretence of a surgical operation.—Bz. applied for treatment when fifteen years old, suffering from habit-spasms of the foot which made it almost impossible for her to walk, from habit-spasms of the face, and from hysterical anorexia; she was easily hypnotised, and all the symptoms vanished after the first sitting. Two years later, this girl became affected with major hysteria, and had to be treated for quite a long time; but for at least eighteen months after her first visit at the age of fifteen, she remained free from neurotic symptoms, and had no occasion to come to the clinic during this period.— Other cases cured by a very few suggestive sittings were the following: Hg. (m., 22), suffering from rotatory spasm of the head; Vel. (m., 25), suffering from a tic of the nose; Merc. (f., 22) and Qkv. (f., 27), affected with spasmodic cough; Eg. (m., 35), who had suffered from persistent hiccough for several weeks; Xs. (f., 11), Et. (f., 10), Pba. (f., 21), Zoa. (f., 23), Of. (f., 38), and Lovo. (f., 43), suffering from vomiting and respiratory tics; cure was no less easy in the case of Es. (f., 25), suffering from various forms of disaesthesia.

The tendency to utter cries of terror with which two girls, Cn., aged fifteen, and Ov., aged seventeen, were affected, was relieved in two sittings.—Keb. (f., 20), had been suffering for three months from almost daily attacks of convulsions, the paroxysm lasting about an hour ; she was cured by a single sitting of hypnotism and suggestion.—I find among my notes the account of at least seven other cases in which severe hysterical paroxysms were definitively checked after two or three sittings.

Next I come to somnolent crises which were no less easily cured. Such were the cases of Qkv. (f., 27), Lv. (f., 17), and Pba. (f., 21) ; such was the case of Di. (f., 27), who, upon the slightest emotion, and especially when she began to laugh, would fall to the ground and would remain asleep for several hours.—In the same category come cases of typically hysterical nocturnal sleepwalking, such as that of Zv. (f., 43) and Voz. (f., 22) ; the latter, after the death of her child, used to call him when she had gone to sleep, and would then spend the whole night playing with him in imagination ; both these cases were easy to cure.—It is true that some of the patients I have mentioned, as for instance Vel., Qkv., and Bz., had occasion to consult me later for other nervous symptoms, but they can be included in the present list because they were easily cured of the original trouble and thenceforward remained well for at least a year.

I have enumerated fifty-four cases in which the cure was so plain and so speedy that it seems hardly possible to suppose that any other factor than simple suggestion was at work ; and they were all cases in which the effects of the initial treatment remained favourable for at least a year. I think that these cases, and similar ones which can be culled at large from the works of other writers, justify the contention of the hypnotists that in hypnotism we have at our disposal a force which is endowed with a really remarkable curative efficacy, and which often takes effect in a very striking manner.

I shall class in a second category the more numerous cases in which the cure, though apparently complete, and persistent for at least a year, could not be effected so speedily.

The result was not immediate and quasi-miraculous. The patients in this group generally came for treatment twice or thrice a week for a period ranging from one to three months. I exclude from consideration here the patients who were treated for longer periods, seeing that, when this happened, the influence of other psychotherapeutic methods was usually superadded.

Under these specifications, I am entitled to include fourteen cases of functional paralysis. For instance, Bk., a girl of sixteen, was brought to the hospital on a stretcher, and was not even able to sit up. She was affected with flaccid paraplegia which had come on slowly after various sexual emotions and had already lasted five months. She was easily hypnotised, and by various suggestions it was possible to induce movements of the legs ; she was fully cured in a fortnight, during which there had been eight sittings. I was able to follow up her history, and I know that she remained free from any relapse of nervous disorder for at least eighteen months. She then became affected with other hysterical symptoms, which were relieved in the same way, though less speedily. Many of the cases of hysterical mutism which I have assigned to this category were cured within a month.

Cases of hysterical contracture, to the number of twenty-one, were cured in like manner.—For instance, one of the patients, a woman named Bz., whose case has already been quoted as an illustration of a rapid and to all appearance miraculous cure, had, three years afterwards, a remarkable experience which reminds us of one quoted on p. 152 from the famous seventeenth-century philosopher Malebranche. She saw her mother fall down the stairs, and sustain a bad sprain of the left ankle. The sight was all the more distressing to her because it reminded her of the trouble in the left foot from which she herself had suffered three years earlier. The consequence was that, while she was caring for her mother, she began to suffer from pains in the left groin and thigh. A few days later she became affected with contractures of the whole of the left thigh and left leg, fixing the limb in a position of extension. The same treatment was applied as in the earlier trouble—the induction of a moderate degree of hypnosis and the suggestion of various movements of the limb. This time the cure was less speedy, but in three weeks, after seven sittings, the contracture had completely disappeared. Eighteen months later, after some love episodes, she had a hysterical relapse. Menstruation was suppressed, her breasts swelled a little, and the abdomen became rapidly and enormously distended ; there were also severe pains in the belly and shaking movements of the abdominal walls ; in a word, she presented almost all the symptoms of spurious pregnancy. The same suggestive treatment as before relieved her of these troubles in a few weeks.—Another case I should mention in this connexion is one of a remarkable contracture of the arm and of the left hand in Vox., a girl of thirteen. Having been overtired by excessively long violin practice, her left hand became affected with involuntary twitchings, passing on into cramps, and then into a contracture which systematically reproduced the position of the hand holding the neck of the violin. Two months' treatment, with two sittings every week, were needed to bring about a cure.

In another category may be classed twenty-five cases in which there were involuntary actions of various kinds, such as tics, spasms, and choreic movements, coughing fits, screaming fits, paroxysms of hiccough, vomiting, palpitation, meteorism, etc. The notes of many of these cases have already been published. The only ones I need specially mention here are three cases in which there was excessive masturbation ; two cases in which girls aged respectively fifteen and seventeen suffered from incontinence of urine ; and the cases of two young women who had been married eighteen months and who suffered from vaginismus, so that any attempts at sexual intercourse induced spasms and hysterical paroxysms. In all these patients, a few suggestions under hypnosis effected a complete cure in a few weeks.

Among cases of mental disorders, such as fixed ideas, hallucinations, disorders of sensation, the refusal of food, an impulsive tendency to drink, or an impulse to strike people, I must include seventeen cases in which the cure (permanent for a least a year) seemed to me directly dependent upon hypnotic suggestions.—Nel. (f., 30) had fixed ideas of jealousy with hallucinations, she was very suggestible and easily hypnotisable, and was completely transformed in three months. I have elsewhere described the hallucinations of Cam. (f., 26), who imagined that she was constantly witnessing the burial of her children. Suggestion dispelled these hallucinations.—I must also mention the case of Dr. (f., 33), a dipsomaniac, who for a considerable period had the habit of getting drunk in an almost automatic way. In this patient, the dipsomania appeared to have the hysterical form, which is rare, but which I described a good many years ago in the case of Maria. Dr. was suggestible and hypnotisable ; four months' treatment sufficed to cure her impulse to drink ; several years later there had been no relapse.

Among disorders of perception, the case of Qo. (f., 26) is worth mentioning. When she first applied for relief, she seemed to be suffering from a rather peculiar form of ophthalmic migraine, for she persistently complained of pain in the eyes, of inability to see clearly, and of being constantly dazzled by a powerful but tremulous light. She had been working long hours by artificial light when preparing for an examination, the light being the flickering flame of an inefficient gas burner. Having failed in her examination, she felt that her sight was impaired, and she had a persistent hallucination of the tremulous gas flame. The visual troubles, in connexion with which a sort of fixed idea played a considerable part, were cured by a few sittings.

In the same group there may be included some cases in which suggestion overcame intense pain, and in especial the pain of surgical operations. Elsewhere I have described the performance of a number of dental operations in which the patients were saved from pain by suggestion, but there is another case which is worth reiterating here.[1] A woman of twenty-four had to have the neck of the uterus artificially dilated and the interior of the uterus curetted. The operation was performed by Segond under simple hypnosis induced by myself. During the operation, the patient apparently felt no pain whatever. When she had been awakened from the hypnosis it was not easy to persuade her that the operation had been performed, for she had no memory of what had been done, and no painful sensations of any kind. The insensibility was induced at the last moment in a single sitting, but the patient had been trained for the purposes in a number of previous sittings.

Cf. Névroses et idées fixes, 1898, vol. i, p. 481.

Suggestion and hypnotism have brought me the best results in cases of hysteria, particularly when accompanied by somnambulism with delirium. It is fashionable to-day to be sceptical as to the existence and the importance of such symptoms. They are, however, of fairly frequent occurrence, and are often very serious. I have had to deal with a considerable number of them. I can point to sixty-four cases in which the cure was quite clearly the result of suggestion and hypnosis. The hysterical seizure can readily be replaced by hypnosis, which, after it has served its turn, can easily be dispelled. The whilom magnetisers were already aware of such facts. Dupau, in his *Lettres sur le magnétisme animal* (1826, p. 178), writes: " The crises can easily be made to disappear by replacing them by somnambulism, . . . but as soon as one ceases to induce the somnambulistic state the crises recur with fresh energy." The latter contention is only too true, as we shall see later ; we have then to resort to other methods of treatment. But such relapses are far from being a general phenomenon, and in most cases the hypnotic state may be easily suppressed as soon as the delirium has disappeared. Hypnotists have made kindred observations. Gilles de la Tourette, in *L'hypnotisme* (1887, p. 173), tells us : " Far from manufacturing somnambulists by the gross, as Calmeil believed, magnetism cures those who suffer from this neurosis. The extraordinary thing is that induced somnambulism causes natural somnambulism to disappear, so that we may be almost certain of curing a sleepwalker of his nightly perambulations by means of hypnotism." This observation seems to me to be specially easy of corroboration. Patients who are suffering from accesses of delirium and from spontaneous somnambulism are peculiarly responsive to genuine hypnotisation, and are the ones who benefit most from such treatment.

First let us consider simple convulsive seizures, such as I have elsewhere described as " emotional attacks." If they be not too ingrained, if the fixed ideas which are responsible for their presence do not occupy too much space in the mind of the patient, then one is able, even in the midst of an attack, to transform such symptoms into induced somnambulism, in which state the subject comes to be in rapport with the hypnotist. By reproducing the state of hypnosis we can prevent the fit from occurring. In many of my cases the seizures were of recent date, having been present for no more than one or two months. But in about a dozen cases the attacks were of a serious character, and had persistently recurred for six months or a year. Even in the latter event I was successful in putting a stop to them in a few sittings, for the most part without having had to make the patients enter the hospital wards for treatment.

As I have often pointed out, hysterical sleep is not so different as people are apt to imagine from the delirious crises in which the patient talks sixteen to the dozen. The main difference is that in the hysterical sleep the delirium is hidden, but it continues as an inward chattering. In four of my cases, hypnotism sufficed within a few weeks to check serious crises of sleep. In one case, that of Zk., a young woman of twenty-two who was found fast asleep in a railway compartment at the Gare d'Orléans, and who was brought to the hospital because it was impossible to awaken her, I learned that for more than two years she had been subject to such crises of sleep lasting from two to ten days. After two months' treatment, she was freed from the trouble for six months. Then there was a relapse. Six weeks' further treatment cured her for another year. What happened after that I do not know.

I wish to lay special stress upon attacks that take the form of somnambulism, for it is easy, as a rule, to transform them into hypnotic states, and then we can make an effective use of suggestion. These interesting cases are primarily characterised by marked depression, which makes the patient incapable of adaptation to reality, incapable of self-control, and which intensifies the disposition to play-acting, the tendency to self-deception, which is so typical of mental lethargy. He leads an imaginary life filled with efforts to adapt himself to a past situation, to which he is " attached " (accroché) because he has not been able to liquidate it. That is why the somnambulist has persistent impulses to repeat some particular action, as may be noticed in those cases of hysterical dipsomania which are so remarkable and so little understood. Or the subject goes on trying to begin life over again in association with some greatly loved person, because there has been a failure to " realise " that this person is dead, or has broken away. In Nep. (f., 28), the somnambulist state was full of disquietude concerning the future ; almost every day, during the afternoon, she passed for several hours into a secondary state which was obstinately persistent.—In Ny. (f., 18), distress concerning the loss of a purse and dread of being accused of theft brought on frequent attacks of somnambulism.—In a girl of fourteen, whose case I have described at length elsewhere, similar attacks were induced by a scolding received at school and by the deprivation of the coveted violet sash.—In six patients, crises taking a somnambulistic form were reproductions of scenes of rape, and in two of these patients the reminiscence concerned the patient's father.—The basis of the illness is always the automatic activation of a tendency arising out of an effort to begin over again an action that has been imperfectly finished.

We shall study in subsequent chapters various methods of treatment suitable for such cases ; but I may say here that when the trouble takes the form of hysterical somnambulism, treatment is exceptionally easy. Hypnotism enables us to control these states of dissociation ; and suggestion, by the impulses it induces, brings about the arrest of the tendencies whose activation filled the mind of the somnambulist.—In the case of Nofs. (f., 25), who used to leave her bed every night in order to do something which had been imperfectly done during the day, a few sittings of hypnotic suggestion effected a cure.—In cases of more serious disorder it was not difficult to originate counteracting tendencies which could make headway against the impulses. " I wanted to drink," said Maria, " but my arm was no longer strong enough to raise the glass to my lips. My arm seemed dead, and I heard a voice laughing at me and forbidding me to drink."

In the cases frequently encountered in which the somnambulism is only the expression of a regret or of an unhappy love experience, I have availed myself of the power of suggestion to modify the face of the well-beloved, the face which the subject was continually calling up in imagination. I have equipped this image with carroty hair, with an absurdly misshapen nose, or with some other characteristic repulsive to the subject ; and I have often been surprised to find how powerful was the effect of such transformations upon these persons whose minds are simple and credulous.—Ap. (f., 26), with a history of having had somnambulist crises eight years earlier, had been abandoned by her lover. For eight months she had been subject to almost daily attacks of delirium in which she saw this lost lover, talked to him, and caressed him for several hours. She was amazed at the transformations I effected in the dream image, became rather indignant, and wanted to go on loving it ; but she could not succeed, and was completely cured in six weeks.—I could quote a dozen instances of the same kind. In other cases, the trouble took the form of remorse or terror, but could be similarly transformed.—Dz., a young woman of twenty-three, had been terribly frightened, on opening the door of a cupboard, to see within a mounted skeleton. She began to suffer from somnambulist crises in which she saw the skeleton, was greatly alarmed by it, talked to it, fancied she was struggling with it, and so on. I was able to rid her of her skeleton in three sittings.

I might include here a special study of hysterical fugues and their treatment, for the use of hypnotism is definitely indicated in this syndrome. But I have already written at so much length on the topic that I cannot venture to summarise my former studies here. Suffice it to recall the fact that if the diagnosis of hysterical fugue is correct, hypnotism will usually render prompt service. First of all, under hypnosis, we can rediscover the memory of the fugue and of the acts which comprised it, and this is in many cases important from the medico-legal aspect as well as from the therapeutic aspect. Next it enables us to discover the more or less subconscious fixed idea, the latent tendency, which leads to the persistent renewal of these fugues. Finally, it provides us with a really efficacious means of acting on the fixed idea.

I am speaking here only of simple cases, those in which suggestion is effective ; and I shall reserve for later chapters an account of the more complicated methods of treatment which may be necessary in certain instances. I shall be content to add only one case which is not included in my previous writings upon hysterical fugues. Ao., a young woman of twenty, a country girl, came to Paris as a servant. She vanished from the house where she was employed, and was found two days later at a police station. The police had taken charge of her because she was wandering along the banks of the Seine and could give no account of herself. She fell asleep as soon as she arrived at the police station. When she woke up, she was asked whether she had not intended to throw herself into the river, but she indignantly declared that she had never left the house, that she had never been on the banks of the Seine, and that she could not understand why, on awakening, she found herself at the police station. This behaviour was repeated three times, at a few days' interval, under precisely the same conditions, until her employers, wearying of the escapades, brought her to the hospital. Under hypnosis, it was easy to revive the girl's memories, and we learned that there was no warrant for the police inspector's theory that she had contemplated suicide. We found that she was simply suffering from a sort of home-sickness, from a fixed and somewhat infantile idea of going for a country walk. She wanted to be among trees, and by the water-side. A few suggestions and a little regulation of the girl's life brought about a speedy cure, which was stable. We can hardly overrate the importance of hypnotism both for the elucidation and for the treatment of all such cases of somnambulism.

There are certain cases in which hypnotic treatment is even more strongly indicated. I refer to those in which the somnambulist disorders have actually been induced by hypnotism, which has been unskilfully applied or suddenly broken off. Here is a very remarkable instance of the kind. Zyd., a woman of forty-four, came to consult me on account of very strange symptoms from which she had suffered for six months. She had fainting fits ; was liable to sudden accesses of sleep in the middle of the day ; performed actions which were apparently subconscious ; was affected with hallucinations of smell and vision, and with feelings of automatism. I tried to hypnotise her, and was surprised to find that in spite of her age she promptly passed into a secondary state with garrulity and consecutive amnesia. I then learned a fact which she had wanted to keep to herself, namely that for ten years she had been a professional somnambulist. Hypnotised by some one who kept out of sight, she held consultations and foretold the future to simpletons. Having accumulated a modest fortune, she retired into private life. But the poor woman was unable to enjoy her repose, for soon after the sittings had been discontinued she began to suffer day after day from the various troubles I have already mentioned. I had with her a few hypnotic sittings, which were really interesting, seeing that in them she related to me the incidents of her career. In these sittings, I was able to relieve her of the troublesome symptoms. I should add that the good woman, becoming aware that she had a quasi-physiological need for hypnosis, would not allow me to rid her of this need by degrees, as I proposed. She preferred to resume her former profession, which kept her well and improved her fortunes.

In other cases, where a habit of induced somnambulism had been acquired, and where fixed ideas thereanent had been instilled into the subject's mind, I was able to work a real cure by gradually reducing the length of the sittings, and by increasing the intervals between them. These happy results were secured in five cases. The most notable was that of Von., a girl of twenty-two. She had become seriously ill as a sequel of ill-advised attempts at hypnotism practised on her by a cousin. Whenever she saw this man, heard his name mentioned, or thought of him, she would lose consciousness, and would fall into a deep sleep from which nothing could awake her. The same thing would happen when she looked any one in the eyes. But in this case, as in the others, hypnotism speedily repaired the damage it had done.

I need hardly say that the morbid symptoms resulting from spiritualistic practices belong to the same category. I may refer in this connexion to my earlier writings on the topic, and in especial to the cases of My. (f., 40), and Meb. (f., 30), in whose cure hypnotism played a considerable part.[1]

I could quote many additional instances to show how suggestion and hypnotism, sometimes speedily and sometimes after being practised for several months, have sufficed to bring about a complete and permanent cure in patients suffering from all kinds of neuropathic symptoms, many of which were serious.

In a third category I shall class the cases in which hypnotic suggestion had no more than a temporary influence, and in which it did not bring about a cure even when the treatment had been persisted in for at least a year. Always, in these cases, the original nervous troubles, or kindred ones, obstinately recurred after a longer or shorter interval. I have

---

[1] Névroses et idées fixes, 1898, vol. ii, p. 338; L'état mental des hystériques, second edition, 1911, p. 505.

records of several hundred cases of this kind. I need not dwell on them here, for they are much less interesting than those I have hitherto recorded.

Still, we must not be too ready to suppose that treatment by hypnotic suggestion was of no value to any of the patients in this group. In some of the cases, although it did not bring about a permanent cure, it certainly did a great deal of good. Consider the following remarkable instance. The case is one I have had under observation for many years, that of No. I treated her for the first time in 1894, when she was twenty-six years of age, and I published her clinical history in 1898, apropos of hysterical contractures of the muscles of the trunk.[1] After a surgical operation on one of the ovaries, this woman, who had been markedly neuropathic even before the operation, suffered from spasms and contractures of the muscles of the abdominal wall, so that she was forced to adopt persistently a posture in which the body was strongly bent forward. At this early stage, I hypnotised her, and made various suggestions. The abdominal contracture disappeared. When she left the hospital she was, to all appearance, completely cured, and I saw nothing more of her for some time. But seven months later she turned up again, bent forward as of old. The abdominal contracture had recurred after a quarrel with her husband. There was no difficulty in hypnotising her again, and in relieving her at the first sitting. Once more, apparently, she was cured. But from 1894 down to the time of writing, 1915, for twenty-one years, she has been persistently liable to relapses.

From time to time—the frequency varies, but the average is twice a year—No., after some fatigue or emotion, which has usually been in the form of a quarrel with her husband or with some other member of the family, feels uneasy, benumbed, and unfit for work ; she lies down, and passes into a troubled sleep. During this sleep, her body grows stiff and is curved forward, so that when she wakes up she can no longer straighten herself. The contracture always affects the same muscles, the abdominal muscles and the flexors of the thighs. But there has been a remarkable evolution in the disease. By degrees the contracture has become more extreme, so as to necessitate the most exaggerated and absurd

[1] Névroses et idées fixes, p. 297.

postures. At first, as may be seen in the photographs published in my initial account of the case, she could stand almost upright, having merely to lean forward a little. But, as time passed, in the successive attacks she found it necessary to lean forward more and more, so that, in order to keep her balance, she had to bend her knees. The knees came closer and closer to the chest, until at length they actually touched it, so that the patient was positively doubled up. But since the feet and the legs were practically unaffected, she was still able to walk, or, rather, to drag herself about in a crouching posture. The photographs I have taken at successive dates give a clear demonstration of this gradual advance in the flexion of the body during a dozen years. In this condition she has herself carried to the Salpêtrière, and then drags herself along to my room. There, notwithstanding the apparent advance of the disease, the sequence of events is always the same. I do not trouble to ask any questions, for I know the whole story already. I have merely to lay my hand upon her forehead. Thereupon she shuts her eyes, and remains motionless as if asleep. I then say to her sharply that she is standing before me in a ridiculous posture, and that she must immediately straighten herself. At the same time I give a few little taps upon her abdomen, making a pretence of massage. No. groans, trembles, weeps, and writhes convulsively, as if in intense pain. She raises her head, straightens her body, stretches her legs, and stands upright, trembling, and swaying a little. Now I blow in her face. She shakes herself, opens her eyes, and, without saying a word, walks rather unsteadily out of my room, holding herself quite erect. She sits down on a chair, and spends a few minutes in trembling and groaning; then, almost always, she has a fit of convulsive laughter. But these symptoms soon pass. She gets up and walks home, perfectly straight, to the great amazement of those who saw her come in quite doubled up. The whole business, if I am pressed for time and do not want to talk to her, does not take more than a quarter of an hour. She feels rather tired for a day or two, but is fully relieved of her symptoms by a single sitting, and has no need to consult me again for the nonce. I hear nothing more of her for a few months. Then comes some fresh domestic quarrel and the whole sequence is repeated da capo.

We have to do, in this case, with a hysterical disorder of a very remarkable kind. For twenty years, the symptoms were unchanged, for precisely the same contracture of the abdominal muscles reappeared in all the relapses. This furnishes an interesting example of psychological automatism. But the treatment is no less worthy of attention. Is is of a purely mental or moral order. I merely say a few words and make a few signs, for the massage is entirely fictitious. I therefore regard the treatment as wholly suggestive. We have to do with a series of movements and actions which are easily and automatically carried out as a sequel of my words and gestures, although the patient does not understand how the cure takes place, and although she is unable to reproduce it at will. If a relapse occurs while I am away on holiday, No. makes all possible efforts to straighten herself, but cannot succeed. On one occasion she remained thus doubled up for six weeks, but on my return I was able to " put her to rights " quite as easily as usual. There is an automatic habit in the treatment just as in the disease. The treatment is not genuinely curative ; No. has never had a whole year without a relapse. Still, we cannot say that the treatment has been useless or that it has been difficult. For twenty years it has enabled No. to go on living at home and to work hard without ever being troubled by her infirmity for longer than a few days at a time. When we think how hysterical contractures can incapacitate people for years and even for a whole lifetime, we are compelled to admit that in No.'s case suggestive treatment has been really serviceable.

Side by side with this remarkable case I should like the reader to consider some other cases in which hypnotic suggestion has likewise been useful. Kz., with whom I first became acquainted in 1895 when she was seventeen years old, suffered from crises of sleep after having sustained a fright. Each crisis began quite suddenly with a fainting fit. At first it lasted for half an hour, but later for several hours. The attacks occurred about once a week, except during menstruation, when she might have as many as four or five daily. Although Kz. is hypnotisable and very suggestible, I have never been able to rid her of her trouble, for she is still subject to these crises of sleep. Still, a single sitting of hypnotic suggestion will always check them for weeks or even for months.

In other cases, the advantages of treatment by hypnotic suggestion have not been so obvious. I have notes concerning about one hundred patients who needed to be subjected to hypnosis or suggestion for hours every day in order to prevent the continual recurrence of crises, contractures, or accesses of delirium. Although suggestion could ward off the symptoms for a few hours, they would then recur, and the treatment would have to be resumed. In other, and yet more numerous cases, the patient would be relieved of a troublesome symptom, but in a few days some other manifestation of the neurosis would crop up. When this had been dealt with, a third symptom would appear, and so things would go on for an indefinite time. Charcot was fond of telling an illustrative anecdote. A young doctor was called to see a woman suffering from hysterical mutism. He hypnotised the patient, and, after a few suggestions, he was able to restore her powers of speech. A wonderful, a miraculous success ! A week later, the thaumaturge was again summoned, for the patient had once more become speechless. The cure was repeated, but did not this time arouse so much enthusiasm. Two days later, he had to begin over again. Then he had to pay daily visits. Before long he was called in every two hours. In the end, the young practitioner besought Charcot to deliver him from this hysteric.

I have myself had similar misadventures fairly often. Pkp. (f., 19) suffered from attacks of delirium. My presence seemed necessary to stop them, for they always recurred two hours after I had gone away.—Dye. had various symptoms which could be checked by a long sitting—for an hour or two.— I had under my care a hysteric who had been admirably drilled by earlier advisers, a woman of twenty-six, Mrb. Any conventional signal could relieve her of most of her nervous troubles for a time. She used to carry about with her a scrap of paper inscribed with directions as to what was to be done to her in an emergency : " If you find this young woman asleep on a bench, you will be able to awaken her by pulling her left ear ; pressure on the right breast will restore her powers of speech ; downward passes will overcome the contracture of her muscles." But all this could not prevent constant attacks of illness. I am afraid that these cases in which hypnotic suggestion does little good are very common.

We have reached the boundary beyond which suggestive therapeutics cannot help us. Even though we have recognised that suggestion is of great value in many instances, we have to admit its limitations. Still, in these refractory cases suggestive treatment is not entirely useless. For the time being it can remove serious symptoms, and it may prevent the symptoms from becoming fixed, chronic, and hard to modify. Suggestion can thus be a useful accessory to other and indispensable methods of treatment ; but it is obviously not all-sufficing in cases of this kind, and it is quite impracticable if it has to be continuously applied for an indefinite period.

We see, in fact, that it would be absurd to persist in the use of a treatment that is doing no good, and to declare that hypnotic suggestion is a panacea. It is nothing of the kind. But the cases I have recorded in this chapter show that in many instances it can do excellent service.

6. Recourse to the Patient's Automatism.

I shall conclude this long chapter with some brief deductions concerning the practical value and the significance of suggestive treatment.

The foregoing observations enable us to decide that hypnotic suggestion, understood in a definite sense and utilised as the sole remedial factor, can lead to real and permanent cures. If we exclude the patients in the third category (for whom suggestion was by no means useless), we find that the first two groups comprise 195 persons in whom the treatment relieved the symptoms for at least a year, and sometimes for a much longer period ; and we note that the relief was often achieved by a single sitting, and always with remarkable speed. I do not think that these facts can be disputed and they are confirmed by the writings of various investigators whose work has been too harshly criticised and too speedily forgotten.

Captious critics may deny the importance of such cures, on the ground that the sufferers were neuropaths, whose maladies, say the critics, are of little gravity, and who often get well of themselves, without any treatment at all. I think such objections are superficial. They do not apply to the well-marked neuropathic disorders I have been describing. These are illnesses of an extremely serious character which may render life a burden for many years. I have just seen a woman named Keg. who began to suffer at the age of seventeen from hysterical paroxysms and contractures brought on by the emotions she suffered when witnessing an anarchist outrage. She is now forty years of age, and her legs are still contractured, with the feet in the equino-varus position, and with incurable shortenings of the tendons. Beyond question, she would have been greatly benefited had these contractures been dispelled in her youth by a few suggestive sittings. It is a grave mistake, in such cases, to refrain from treatment on the ground that " the nervous troubles of young girls undergo a spontaneous cure." Many of the cures described by practitioners of suggestion have been definite and important.

But when we have made this concession to the early hypnotists, we find it necessary to insist that some of their assertions were too ambitious. Think of the palmy days of hypnotism! Wetterstrand and Forel declared that they could cure 97 per cent. of patients taken at random. Liébeault and Bernheim were content to claim 90 per cent. of cures. But the important thing to note is that these authors applied the treatment to all diseases. Suggestion was used for the cure of every kind of mental disorder ; of epilepsy, locomotor ataxia, and organic hemeplegia ; of rheumatism and gastritis. The blind were made to see ; deaf-mutes were made to speak ; migraine was instantaneously cured. Liébeault wrote quite seriously of using hypnotic suggestion in the treatment of cancer.

I suppose I must be a bungler, but, since I am putting in as evidence my own observations during several decades, I have to admit that my conclusions are far more modest. Looking through my case-books, I have been able to select 200 interesting cases of cure ; and I am perhaps entitled to add to these another 50 cases belonging to the third category, cases in which suggestive treatment, though it did not bring about a positive or permanent cure, nevertheless did unquestionable good. We will place these 250 cases to the credit side of the account of suggestion as an exclusive method of treatment. But these cases have been drawn from a huge collection. All my life I have been recording and classifying cases with the enthusiasm of a collector, and I have now more than 3,500 case-notes. Hypnotic treatment was tried in nearly all of these ; and in the exceptional instances in which no attempt was made to hypnotise the patient, it was because I was convinced from the first that hypnotism would be useless and impracticable. Thus the proportion of cures ascribable to suggestion is no more than a pitiful seven per cent.

A still more serious matter is that, while attempts at cure by suggestion were made in the most varied types of disorder, the only successes were in a particular kind of patient. For instance, notwithstanding prolonged endeavours, I have never been able to induce a satisfactory hypnotic state in one who was epileptic and nothing more. The few epileptics I have been able to hypnotise and to influence by suggestion, suffered from hysterical paroxysms as a complication. For a long time I used to try to influence by hypnotic methods the patients to whom I have given the name of psychasthenics ; I mean the patients who are affected with obsessions, doubts, and phobias ; they must not be confounded with subjects who have fixed ideas of a hysterical type, for the mental condition of these is quite different. I could never get definite results in psychasthenics, and I believe such patients to be very little accessible to suggestion. Nor had I any notable success with lunatics, persons suffering from melancholia with depression, and persons affected with systematised delusions. I must confess that I find myself unable to understand the case-records in which so many authorities declare that they have hypnotised persons suffering from doubt, obsession, or melancholia.[1] In fine, I have to repeat what I found it necessary to say as the outcome of my early studies, namely that treatment by hypnotism and suggestion gives practical results almost exclusively in cases of hysterical neurosis. The word " hysteria " has fallen into disfavour nowadays. No matter whether it denotes a special form of disease ; or a malady of the character ; or, as I think, a special form of mental depression. Anyhow, there is a peculiar psychological state which is met with in certain persons and not in all, and which gives typical characteristics to mental depression and to the symptoms that result therefrom. The doctors who are so much troubled and divided as regards the definition of hysteria, have no difficulty in agreeing with one

[1] Cf. Milne Bramwell, Obsessions and their Treatment, Parker's Psychotherapy, II, iii, 31.

another when it is only a question of diagnosing this disease. Now, the great majority of the 250 patients in whom I found that hypnotic suggestion did unmistakable service, belonged to the category of what every physician would have agreed to call hysterical neurotics.

I think it might be proper to restrict the application of this method of treatment within even narrower bounds. The Myers formulated an axiom which seems to me rather ambitious. They said : " Whatever hysteria can cause, suggestion can cure." [1] This is certainly an exaggeration. We are not yet sufficiently well informed concerning the psychological mechanism of hypnotism and suggestion to be able to use it with the certainty of good results in every case of hysteria. I have just pointed out how often, in such cases, hypnotic suggestion gave nothing more than temporary relief. In a good many other instances, hysterics were entirely refractory to hypnotic suggestion. A careful study of my successful cases shows that all these patients had certain special characteristics. Most of them were quite young. In the first category, comprising the patients who were cured by one sitting or by a very few sittings, the majority were children or very youthful persons. Thirty-eight out of the fifty-four were under twenty-five years of age. The majority of those belonging to the second group were of an age ranging from fifteen to thirty. With few exceptions, older patients could not readily be benefited by suggestion. I have even had occasion to note that when relapses occurred after some years in patients who to begin with had been cured quite easily, such relapses were apt to prove obstinate.

Next we have to note that in these patients the illness was of fairly recent date. It had not continued more than a few months, and had therefore not induced a profound and lasting depression. In one who had been a neuropath for years, the same symptom would usually run a different course, and its disappearance under the influence of suggestion was no more than temporary. We may phrase the matter differently. The troubles cured by suggestion were localised affections of this or that psychological tendency, but were attended by little if any general depression of the mind as a whole. The subjects, though incapable of walking or of recalling a lapsed memory,

[1] Proceedings of the S.P.R., 1893, p. 202.

showed hardly any signs of generalised psychological asthenia. They were not affected by the abulias, the doubts, the sentiments of incompleteness, which are so typical of cases of well-marked depression. The restriction of the field of consciousness characteristic of hysteria is a sort of defensive reaction which lessens the general depression. It gives a peculiar stamp to the patients belonging to this category.

I think that these observations harmonise with what we know of the nature of suggestion. The essential characteristic of suggestion is that it artificially induces, in the form of an impulse, the functioning of a tendency which the subject's personal will cannot activate. We simply substitute direct assent for reflective assent; we make an appeal to lower-grade activities, to the subject's automatism. If this appeal is to be heard, if it is to cause activation, the subject must have (despite the ostensible paralyses) a reserve of tendencies that are well organised and sufficiently charged with energy. In short, he must have a vigorous automatism. Suggestion serves merely to awaken and to guide these latent activities, whose existence is presupposed. Suggestive treatment is not concerned with the strengthening of mental and nervous activity, with the creation of new resources; suggestion aims merely at the better utilisation of the mental resources that already exist. We can perhaps most effectively illustrate the role of suggestion by a comparison which I have often found useful in psychiatric studies. We may compare human behaviour and the utilisation of the mental powers with pecuniary expenditure and the organisation of a budget. One who falls sick may be likened to one who is unable to balance his budget, so that bankruptcy is imminent; he has become incapable of meeting the cost of certain indispensable activities. The doctor is called in to liquidate the situation and to reorganise the budget. Suggestive treatment does not modify the general tenor of the life of the household, it does not provide the steward with any new resources; it merely shows him that he possesses important resources which he has not been utilising, it opens drawers where precious rouleaux of gold pieces had been stored away and forgotten, and it puts these overlooked resources at the disposal of a poor wretch who had quite mistakenly fancied himself to be ruined.

Obviously we have here a very simple way of reorganising our jeopardised finances, but the unfortunate thing is that the method is not applicable in all cases. If we are to be able to make use of it, the imminence of ruin must be more apparent than real, and the accountants who have been enquiring into out financial state must have been so ill informed as to cry bankruptcy when as yet there was nothing worse than disorder. As a rule, financiers know better. Still, the mistake is sometimes made, for the existence of hysteria proves it. The liquidator who is competent to recognise the real character of the situation, and who, by pointing out the existence of a drawer full of gold which has been overlooked, enables the whole household to resume normal activities, is one who does excellent service. But for him, the threatened bankruptcy would have come, and the drawer would not have been discovered until too late. The doctor must be competent, when occasion demands, to play this beneficent and easy part, to practise this simplest of all psychotherapeutic methods. That it is an interesting method is undeniable, but we must not be surprised to find that it is often inadequate, and that in most instances we have to search out other and more complicated ways for the reestablishment of fortunes that are seriously compromised. We have already learned that certain very special psychological conditions are requisite for the success of suggestive treatment. We now have to realise that the method is applicable only in certain forms and certain grades of the diseases in which those conditions are fulfilled. For these reasons, the possibilities of its application are restricted.

Is this a reason for condemning it? Shall we despise the use of inunctions of sulphur because the only disease they can cure is the itch; and because they will do a great deal of harm if the patient is suffering from eczema? Are we to think the administration of injections of emetin an absurd measure because, though they will cure amoebic dysentery, they are useless in bacterial dysentery? Every one would be amazed at such questions in the domain of general medicine. It is only in the field of psychiatry that any one ventures to ask them. The reason why they are asked in the latter case, is that psychiatry is in so backward a state that medical practitioners are still surprised at having to make a psychological diagnosis, and at having to ascertain the precise conditions under which a method of treatment must be applied.

These reflections concerning the medical value of hypnotic suggestion in the strict sense of the term, enable us to understand better the general significance of treatment by suggestion and the place of the method in the history of psychotherapeutics. Like medical moralisation, which we studied in the third chapter, suggestive treatment is obviously a form of psychological treatment, and it is one of a comparatively advanced type. We are not concerned here with an involuntary and unconscious appeal to the powers of thought, as in the case of miraculous healing and in that of Christian Science ; we are concerned with a conscious and fully deliberate utilisation of psychological laws. But suggestive treatment differs from moralisation, and may I think even be regarded as superior to moralisation, in virtue of the fact that it is based upon a more precise view of psychological laws, and also for the very reason that its use is restricted.

The great defect of moralisation is that it is a theriac, a remedy that can be administered in any kind of disease which can be vaguely classed as neuropathic, that it has recourse to any kind of activity which can be vaguely classed as psychological. That is what makes it so difficult to satisfy ourselves as to the cures claimed by the moralisers, to verify their experiments and their teaching. Suggestion, though by no means free from difficulties, is a phenomenon of a very different kind ; it is a sufficiently precise psychological phenomenon, a particular way of performing actions which is differentiated from other ways. The operator who is trying to induce actions by suggestion is not content with the production of an undifferentiated psychological phenomenon ; he is in search of a particular phenomenon whose occurrence or non-occurrence may be difficult to prove, but one whose nature is definable, and distinct from the nature of other psychological phenomena. This investigation cannot be carried out on all comers. It is only too obvious that experimental suggestions do not succeed in every patient. Consequently, the method of treatment is not applicable to all patients, whatever the diseases from which they are suffering. We have to make a diagnosis, to ascertain the nature of the disease we propose to treat by suggestion, and to study the mental condition of the sufferer. No doubt there are still difficulties attaching to the conception of hysteria, but investigators are at length agreed that hysterics constitute a particular category of neuropaths, and the name " hysteria " is not applied indiscriminately to all kinds of psychoneurosis. Although the psychological notion of hysteria may still be open to discussion, the diagnosis of the disease is now a part of regular medical study, and the students of any particular school apply the name of " hysteric " to the same patients. Consequently, hypnotic suggestion is no longer a vague theriac about which we cannot argue. It is a definite treatment, one whose application is restricted, one which we can commend or condemn, one which we can advise more or less frequently, one whose results can be ascertained.

If I mistake not, these characteristics are of the utmost importance. They enable us to emerge from the religious and moral epoch of psychotherapeutics and to enter the genuinely scientific epoch. Hypnotic suggestion may develop in days to come. On the other hand, further experience may be unfavourable to it, so that it will perhaps disappear from the medical arsenal. But the fact will remain that hypnotic suggestion was the first precisely formulated psychological method of treatment ; and that, by freeing us from the yoke of vague moralisations, it paved the way for the discovery of other, and more precisely formulated, methods. We must give credit where it is due. The efforts of all these investigators, continued for more than a century, have contributed to the progress of medical science.

PART THREE

PSYCHOLOGICAL ECONOMIES

INTRODUCTION

THE failures and inadequacies of treatment by suggestion and hypnotism have naturally led to the inauguration of a great many researches and to the application of a great many other methods of treatment. Some of these are new. Others, already well established, have acquired an important place in medical education and medical practice. These, like hypnotism and suggestion, are definite methods to fulfil particular indications, and are therefore entitled to be enumerated among the special varieties of psychotherapeutics. In this third part of my book I shall consider the methods of psychological treatment whose common characteristic seems to me to be that they are methods of mental economy, methods which aim at reducing the work of the mind and at promoting the storage of its energies. Under this head come treatment by rest properly so called, treatment by isolation, and treatment by the dissociation of fixed ideas or by moral disinfection. Apropos of these methods of treatment, I think it important to examine the psychological problems raised by the study of the fatigue induced by arduous efforts and actions, by the study of the exhaustion that is caused by social relationships, and the study of the expenditure entailed by traumatic memories and by imperfectly liquidated situations. Summaries of case-histories will enable us to appreciate the effects of the respective methods in specific instances. The fact that all the methods discussed in Part Three have common characteristics will become more apparent after they have all been described, and when the features of the various methods can be considered in a concluding summary.

CHAPTER NINE

TREATMENT BY REST

THE most typical among the methods of psychological economy is the treatment of nervous disorders by systematic rest, which came into vogue first in the United States and subsequently in Europe, contemporaneously with the later researches concerning hypnotism.

A fundamental instinct teaches animals and human beings to overcome some of the disturbances that result from action by a special kind of action, known as rest. Just as the tendency which leads to the taking of food is first manifested under the form of hunger, so the tendency which leads to repose, in its initial stage of activation, manifests itself as fatigue, and this fatigue is speedily dispelled by absolute rest. Now, seeing that a great many pathological disorders resemble those induced by fatigue, would it not be proper to apply in their case a treatment akin to that we instinctively use for the relief of fatigue, to apply the method of repose ? Ostensibly, rest or repose is nothing more than motionlessness, the simple cessation of movement, the discontinuance of the actions which have induced fatigue. For a long time it has been customary to treat certain diseases by rest of the affected organ. Diseases of the stomach were cured by abstaining from food for a time ; diseases of the heart were relieved by abstaining from active exercise, by staying in bed.

Similar considerations would seem to apply to neuropathic disorders. These patients have a very definite feeling of fatigue and exhaustion. In some of them this feeling is pushed to an extreme, and becomes an obsession. They persistently have, or assume, the aspect of persons overwhelmed by fatigue ; they tell us that they are utterly exhausted as soon as they have walked a few steps. Should we not do well to take them at their word, and to apply the treatment for which they instinctively clamour, while making this treatment at once intelligent and comprehensive ?

1. History of Treatment by Rest.

Certain American physicians endeavoured during the latter half of the nineteenth century to formulate the treatment by rest the need for which can be deduced from the foregoing considerations. Samuel J. Jackson advocated a method of treatment which was taken up once more and rendered more precise by S. Weir Mitchell in 1875, and by Playfair in 1877.[1] Substantially, this treatment was simple. The patients were put in the position which all healthy persons adopt when they are resting. They had to stay in bed, and while in bed they had to be as motionless as possible. Weir Mitchell went so far as to forbid spontaneous activities in the performance of the elementary actions of daily life, such as those of food-taking and the toilet. Everything was done for the invalid by the nurses, who were to speak to the patient as little as possible. The latter was fed like a little child, was washed and cared for like a little child. Since the muscular inaction might have been followed by atrophy, a general daily massage was prescribed. In addition to rest and massage, Weir Mitchell insisted upon superfeeding ; his system was not only a " rest-cure," but also a " mast cure." The dietetic regimen of these patients, the number and size of the meals they had to take, the amount of milk they consumed in the twenty-four hours— these details are really rather amazing. In some cases, the patient would within six weeks gain in weight by as much as from 50 to 70 lbs. For the better carrying out of the treatment, the patient was removed from his home surroundings to an institution under the immediate supervision of the physician.

The method soon became famous, and was popularised by various writers who were impressed by its psychological characteristics. William James and Annie Payson Call, with their numerous imitators and followers, extol the effects of the relaxation and repose which form an indispensable part of the labours of life. " The boat's crew that wins the race is said to be the crew that learns to rest between every stroke and thus to postpone the accumulations of fatigue

[1] Cf. Waterman, Treatment of Fatigue States, in Psychotherapeutics, a Symposium, 1910, p. 97.

which exhaust." [1] In the midst of an active and restless life, we must leave room for periods of complete repose of body and mind. In the United States, the inference was speedily drawn that the best way of curing a psychosis would be to take refuge in a sanatorium, and " to call in Dr. Diet and Dr. Quiet." Numerous sanatoria sprang up for the practice of the Weir Mitchell treatment, and for a long time it was the fashion in the United States to spend a few months, now and again, undergoing a rest cure with superalimentation in order to recuperate the energies needed for the battle of life.

Though rather slowly, these ideas made their way into Britain and France. Charcot adopted them to some extent, and helped to spread them.[2] After a time, there came into existence on the Continent sanatoria similar to those which had had so striking a success in the United States. I do not think, however, that in these institutions the Weir Mitchell treatment was often applied strictly in all its details. Lagrange, in his admirable works upon movement and fatigue, demonstrated the essential function of repose, and supplied a physiological justification for these therapeutic methods. When we put an organ at rest, we supply the conditions necessary for the rest of various associated organs ; now, the locomotor apparatus affects all the other organs, and muscular rest is essential to the repose of the organism as a whole. Rest in bed brings about complete muscular relaxation. " The therapeutic mechanism of the rest cure," writes Lagrange, " is to be found in the dynamic results of an economising of nervous energy."

Somewhat later, a kindred treatment was applied to the mental disorders of the insane. As long ago as 1852, Guislain wrote : " It will hardly be imagined how powerfully, in the insane, prolonged rest in bed contributes to the restoration of tranquillity." Conolly and Falret tried to apply this method to the treatment of mania, but did not generalise its use. In 1897, Magnan brought the " no-restraint " method to its climax, and gave the final quietus to the idea of cellular confinement, by the treatment of acute and sub-acute cases

---

[1] Cabot, The Use and Abuse of Rest in the Treatment of Disease, Parker's Psychotherapy, II, ii, 23.

[2] Cf. Levillain, Traitement de la neurasthénie, 1891, p. 237 ; Philip Coombs Knapp, Traumatic Neurasthenia, " Brain," 1897.

of mental disorder by rest in bed.[1] Paul Sérieux, in his study of Magnan's work, writes : " Rest in bed gives results of undeniable value in the mitigation of the most distressing symptoms ; it frees the patient from bodily and mental complications. . . . In especial, it entails a consequence which to Magnan seemed of supreme importance. I refer to the complete change which the adoption of this method effects in the physiognomy of the lunatic asylum. This ceases to be a place in which the insane are watched by keepers, and becomes a hospital where the invalids under treatment happen to be suffering from mental disorder."[2] In 1898 Kéraval, in 1899 Pochon, in 1899 Toulouse and Marchand, and in 1902 d'Anglade, stressed the value of this method of treatment.[3] They gave numerous examples to show that sufferers from melancholia, and even sufferers from mania, are more easily cared for and get well more quickly if they are kept in bed during the greater part of the illness. More recently, at the Amsterdam Congress of Neurology in 1907, Ley, Basterbrook, and W. Mabon, demonstrated the great advantages of this method of treatment in asylums.

I think that there are good reasons for classing in the same category as the Weir Mitchell treatment a remarkable method which has never become widely known, one based upon the induction of prolonged hypnotic sleep. It is a familiar experience that in a certain proportion of cases the hysterics who are liable to spontaneous crises of sleep lasting for several days, will awaken from these slumbers in a condition that has notably improved. They are less benumbed, suffer less from anaesthesia, and have fewer morbid symptoms. In especial I recall the case of a female patient who was suffering from maniacal delirium, contractures, and widespread anaesthesias. Her condition was a very serious one, and for several months we were unable to do her any good. Then, spontaneously, she passed into a lethargic condition which lasted about ten

[1] Magnan, De l'alitement, clinothérapie dans le service central d'admission des aliénés de la ville de Paris, " Bulletin de l'Académie de Médecine," July 23, 1912.
[2] Sérieux, V. Magnan, sa vie et ses oeuvres, " Annales Médico-Psychologiques," 1917, p. 504.
[3] Cf. Trénel, Traitement de l'agitation et de l'insomnie dans les maladies mentales et nerveuses, Congrès de Bruxelles, 1903, p. 371.

days. When she awoke, she was free from delirium, contracture, and anaesthesia. The same sequence of events was witnessed in this patient on several occasions. In her case, relief from the greater manifestations of hysteria always came by way of a prolonged sleep.

Long ago, the magnetisers noticed that hypnotic sleep, when it lasted for a considerable time, had a tranquillising and restorative influence. Charles Despine used to say of his subjects : " Magnetic sleep calms their nerves." [1] J. P. Durand spoke of a calmative and somniferous hypotaxia which sometimes lasted for a good while.[2] Noizet alluded to the good effects of a hypnotic sleep lasting three days.[3] Liébeault, too, writes of " the restoration of energy during this sleep, when it lasts for a considerable time." [4] I myself devoted attention at one time to these prolonged slumbers, and in 1889 I recorded the case of a hysteric suffering from a paraplegia of old date which, after proving refractory to other methods of treatment, disappeared after a hypnotic sleep lasting four days.[5]

Wetterstrand, a Swedish physician, realising the interest of these observations and experiments, formulated a systematic method of treatment based upon them.[6] He applied the method to patients suffering from various forms of nervous and mental disorder—to epileptics and to sufferers from obsession or melancholia as well as to hysterics. Having induced hypnosis, he suggested rest and sleep, and would leave the patient asleep for a long time, even for three weeks or more.

Such prolonged somnambulism can be induced more readily than might be supposed, and is not attended by any inconvenience. In the hypnotic state, the subject will at stated intervals do whatever has been suggested ; eating and drinking at fixed hours quite as well as or better than in the waking state ; passing urine and going to stool as directed by the hypnotist. When not engaged in the performance of these

[1] Op. cit., pp. 149, 151, and 183.   [2] Cours de braidisme, 1860.
[3] Op. cit., 1854, p. 316.   [4] Du sommeil, etc., 1866, pp. 199 and 200.
[5] L'automatisme psychologique, 1889, p. 134.
[6] Wetterstrand, Ueber den künstlichverlängerten Schlaf besonders bei der Behandlung der Hysterie, " Zeitschrift für Hypnotismus," 1892, p. 17 ; Hypnosis and its Application to Practical Medicine, New York, 1897.

suggested actions, the subject remains motionless, and plunged in profound sleep. As a rule, there is no difficulty about awaking the patient when the time has come. We may note a moderate degree of bewilderment, which speedily passes off ; and it can then be perceived that there has been a striking reestablishment of sensibility, and that all the cerebral functions have been favourably influenced.

The results of the method are said to have been extra-ordinarily good. Hysterical paroxysms, contractures, delirium, and even fits of major epilepsy, vanish never to return. Not-withstanding these extensive claims for the treatment, few other investigators [1] have taken any interest in the matter, and hardly any attempts have been made to repeat Wetter-strand's experiments. I shall subsequently have to speak of my own experiments along this line, an account of which I published in 1896. Here it may suffice to say that the epoch was not propitious, for the medical fashion had changed. Doctors were disgusted with hysteria, hypnotism, and sugges-tion when they found that these matters could not be under-stood without a little study of psychology ; and they therefore preferred to ignore the whole subject. Thus, the method of treatment by prolonged sleep passed unnoticed.

Among comparatively recent books upon treatment by rest, the most interesting, a work guided by ideas which are in the direct line of succession from Weir Mitchell, is that by Deschamps published in 1909 and entitled *Les maladies de l'énergie, thérapeutique générale*. By its very exaggerations this work, which is remarkable alike from the theoretical and from the practical point of view, gives us a better under-standing of the rest treatment of the neuroses. I shall, there-fore, devote a few pages to the discussion of the author's explanation of these diseases, and to an account of the treat-ment he advises.

Deschamps unhesitatingly adopts, in the case of quite a number of sufferers, the interpretation which they themselves put forward to account for their condition. They are over-worked persons, sufferers from constitutional fatigue ; their

[1] J. Bonjour is an exception. Cf. his article Emploi du sommeil prolongé dans un cas de somnambulisme hystéro-épileptique, " Revue de l'Hypno-tisme," 1895, p. 347.

fundamental clinical symptom is an undue liability to fatigue, a predisposition to experience readily and speedily the noxious subjective and objective effects of fatigue. Every subject who fails to recover from fatigue after a normal period of rest and thanks to the ordinary enjoyment of food and sleep, is a " fatiguable " (p. 89). In these patients, exhaustion ensues very early during work, and can only be overcome very slowly by rest, which in them must last, not for hours merely, but for weeks.

This essential symptom is not, according to Deschamps, a simple psychological phenomenon ; it is related to various physiological troubles. The reflexes are at first exaggerated and subsequently diminished ; in like manner, the nitrogenous excretions are at first increased and subsequently diminished ; we can detect arterial hypotension, a decline in the number of red blood corpuscles, vascular spasms which cause a fall of the surface temperature and sensations of chilliness ; etc. (pp. 132 and 175). Deschamps thinks that all these phenomena are dependent upon extensive modifications in the functions of the central nervous system. In the nervous system there is a " sthenogenic function," guided by the vago-sympathetic apparatus (p. 21) ; the medulla oblongata and the cerebellum are accumulators of energy (p. 36). The asthenia from which these patients suffer is a variable trouble of the sthenogenic function, a defective organisation of the reservoir of energy, a trouble whose invariable clinical expression is the loss of energy, " fatiguability." When the supply of available energy is slightly in excess of the demand, there is sthenia ; but when the energy cannot cope with the demand, there is asthenia (p. 47). In the latter case, the energy applied by the nervous system is too enfeebled to acquire a reasonably high tension ; it is promptly expended without any possibility of storing reserves. Deschamps' theory enables us to connect with this debility the lowering of psychological tension, the psychological hypotony which in 1903 I myself described as the essential characteristic of these patients.

These fundamental disorders are the cause of all the other symptoms. One of the most interesting among such symptoms is the incapacity for being trained (in the athletic sense), or " aphoria," as Deschamps terms it (p. 96). The subjects are absolutely incapable of being trained as we can train one who is in good health or one who is convalescent from illness. There may not seem to be much amiss with them ; but they are constitutionally incapable of increasing their stores of energy by regular exercise, as really healthy people can do. If a patient takes five or ten years in learning how to walk for five minutes longer, can we call that training ? (pp. 96, 101, and 103). The same fundamental disorder is responsible for the amyosthenia, or diminution of motor activity, and for the amyotony, or decline in automatic muscular tøne. This amyosthenia is one of the main factors of the sensation of fatigue, for it compels the patient to make at each step an exhausting expenditure of energy. The hypotony manifests itself in numerous symptoms, such as : inadequate extension of the fingers ; a drooping of the shoulder-blades ; a certain amount of scoliosis ; the slowness and hesitancy of the gait ; the difficulty of standing upright for any considerable time ; the impossibility of rising on tip-toe (for the asthenic is incapable of supplying motor energy to a large number of muscles at once—pp. 113 and 114) ; the difficulty of squatting on the hams and of kneeling ; the various disorders of coordinated movement (p. 118) ; etc. The same considerations apply to all the symptoms which are specially regarded as mental. The reaction times are modified, becoming either shorter or longer, the subject not having the requisite amount of energy to make the rapid synthesis which constitutes attention (p. 93). He cannot feel or do several things at once ; he cannot read or write more than ten or twelve lines without a pause for rest ; he can only do mental work when recumbent, and the psychological debility may be so extreme as to amount to absolute cerebral impotence for years (p. 126) This reduced vitality in conjunction with an excessive individualism gives rise in all these enfeebled subjects to a very high degree of attachment to their own personality, together with a persistent dread of death (p. 312). In a word, all the symptoms are dependent upon the primary asthenia of the nervous system which is manifested by the excessive liability to fatigue. This exhaustion is due to an inadequate production of nervous energy and to the consequent lack of nervous tension.

The therapeutic indications deducible from this theory may be summarised in a single word—rest. " In the treatment of these primary asthenias, rest is not everything, but nothing can be achieved without rest " (p. 316). " There is nothing equal to rest ; it is the art of husbanding our energies, the art of life." When a man is up and dressed, he cannot always regulate the amount of his activities, and circumstances often compel him to do more than he would like ; only when he is in bed can he be kept perfectly quiet (p. 322). That is why the nature and situation of the bed are so important. Too soft a bed is heating ; to hard a bed is tiring. The invalid should sleep alone ; undue solicitude for his welfare is no less enervating and disturbing to him than selfish indifference or loud snoring. Besides, the double bed is a persistent encouragement to sexual relationships, which are always injurious in these cases, being a frequently renewed cause of exhaustion (p. 191). The patient must be kept warm, and should wear woollen bedsocks. The room must be guarded against noise, whether from within the house or from without, for the asthenic has an urgent need for silence. The patient should remain quite still in bed, making no movements that can possibly be avoided. Everything must, therefore, be done for him ; his attendants must add or remove blankets as may be needed, must feed him, must bring the necessary utensils. The same precautions must be taken to ensure mental rest, for to read is no less tiring than to walk. The author tells us of a patient who " for three years read nothing, said not a word more than was absolutely indispensable, and accepted this life of immobility ; he deserved to get well " (p. 329). But when is this period of complete rest to come to an end ? " Who can tell ? Time does not really exist ; it is an invention of the philosophers."

Still, when physical changes arise, when the invalid is excited or impatient, he can get out of his ordinary bed for a little while to pass a few hours, not in the open air, not upon a long chair, which would be tiring, but on a folding bed. Care must be taken as to the situation of this bed ; it must not be in a summerhouse, or in the corner of a room. " I was sent for one day to see one of my patients who was feeling rather weak—to find her in the corner of the room ! ! ! She was breathing a confined air ! ! ! " (p. 347). Later, much later, the patient may be allowed to walk for a few minutes. " If he can walk for two minutes, let him walk for two minutes every day, and not increase the time until he has stored up a larger capital of energy. At any given time, the asthenic has a certain amount of capitalised energy. For the nonce this capital is stable, and will provide a fixed amount of interest in the way of work, but the slightest excess will lead to bankruptcy, to overwork (p. 325). If the patient persist in walking farther, the asthenic symptoms will return to the acute stage : directly an effort is made, illness begins ; in these patients there is no such thing as pleasant fatigue, exhaustion comes on abruptly. As an asthenic improves, the duration of possible expenditure increases, and the period of rest can be reduced. Still, these patients will never get very far, for we cannot remake a nervous system " (p. 325).

I do not think it would be possible to find a more extreme statement of the explanation that nervous diseases are due to fatigue, or of the contention that the proper way to treat them is by rest. Deschamps' book is the climax we reach when Weir Mitchell's notion is pushed to its utmost verge.

2. Disdain for Fatigue.

Confronting this interpretation and this method of treatment, we find a very different doctrine which we may place under the aegis of Paul Dubois, for he is its best exponent, and other writers who have expressed the same view are, as a rule, merely repeating his theories.

When Dubois has to do with one of these patients who say they are utterly exhausted and who have stayed in bed for years, Dubois' attitude is the precise opposite of Deschamps'. He will not take the invalid seriously. He does not deny that his patient talks about fatigue, and he may even admit that the latter has a certain feeling of fatigue ; but he denies that the patient's assertions are justified by a genuine fatigue, or at any rate by the physiological disturbances which correspond to genuine fatigue. " We have no right to speak about fatigue," he says, " when no work has been done. . . . If you analyse this fatigue you will find that there is a barely perceptible nucleus of fatigue hidden away in voluminous wrappings of the autosuggestion of fatigue."   In the behaviour of these patients it is easy to detect all sorts of contradictions which betray how illusory their feeling of fatigue is. A man will tell us that he is tired out if he walks a hundred yards on the high road, while he will potter about his park for hours in succession. A woman will declare that she is unable to teach her children for an hour, but will spend the whole day reading novels. " The real trouble is a conviction of impotence which ensues upon some trifling though real sensation magnified by one whose frame of mind is pessimistic. We should ignore such fatigue, just as we have to ignore the complaints of hypochondriacs."

A good many writers express opinions akin to Dubois'. Waterman of Boston, U.S.A., thinks that these patients who seem exhausted have abandoned work and the normal activities of life while suffering for a moment from real fatigue, but that they have been relieved of this fatigue by rest long since, and that they are simply afraid of resuming work. They imagine that they will be fatigued anew; they attend so closely to the most insignificant feeling of fatigue, and in fancy they magnify it to such an extent, that they promptly believe they are tired out, and go on believing it for days to come.[1]

Münsterberg pours forth his scorn upon the contemporary talk about overwork. He declares that our forefathers had much more reason than we have to suffer from exhaustion, and he concludes by showing that there is a vast amount of exaggeration in the language of neuropaths who describe themselves as overworked and exhausted.[2] Grasset, while he admits that harm can be done by excess of work and even by excessive devotion to sport, declares that there is a great deal of exaggeration in the current talk of overwork. In every one, he says, there exists an automatic tendency to idleness, a power of abstraction and distraction, which is an excellent means of defence against overwork. This latter, he concludes, can hardly be said to exist even in persons who describe themselves as utterly exhausted.

Dejerine is especially enthusiastic in his adoption of Dubois' views. No doubt he goes so far as to admit that certain neuropaths who have been ill for a long time, and who have been uneasily keeping watch upon their symptoms, drugging

[1] Waterman, The Treatment of Fatigue States, in Psychotherapeutics, a Symposium, 1910, p. 96.
[2] Münsterberg, Psychotherapy, 1909, p. 194.

themselves, and unduly restricting their diet, may become exhausted in the long run; [1] they are " past masters in the art of neurasthenia." Such exceptional cases are quite different from Deschamps' patients, young people whose primary asthenia is not due to malnutrition or to the late onset of cachexia, but is a fundamental disorder of the nervous system. Dejerine, like other neurologists, is aware that some neuropaths of this kind are perpetually complaining of a terrible sensation of fatigue, that they are fatiguable in the sense that after the most trifling effort they declare themselves to be exhausted. This is a matter of clinical observation, but he will not admit that there is an underlying physiological reality. " We are concerned only with a psychic phenomenon, with an auto-suggestion, with a memory of fatigue called up over and over again." [2] It is true that the patient seems incapable of being trained (in the athletic sense); he is affected by what Deschamps terms aphoria. But this is to be explained in the same way. The patient has a fixed idea. He is convinced that he cannot walk for more than ten minutes without fatigue, and he anxiously looks forward to the end of these ten minutes. Directly he is made aware, in any one of a hundred ways, that he has exceeded what he regards as the limits of his powers of training, the old troubles recur as automatically as symptoms will appear in one to whom suggestions have been made by a hypnotist, and he seems to be utterly exhausted. Some of the patients declare that the exhaustion may come on quite suddenly, taking them by surprise when they were not thinking about it at all. This is only because, through distraction, they had forgotten for a moment their fixed idea of fatigue. Then, being suddenly reminded of their condition by some almost imperceptible sign, they are overwhelmed in an instant by all the accumulated fatigue which they ought to have been feeling (p. 168). The argument is invariably the same. We must not accept as a physiological truth a patient's obsessions concerning his own condition.

Turning to examine the symptoms exhibited by the patient in his behaviour, Dejerine makes the same remark as Dubois, saying that this behaviour does not prove much, for it is

---

[1] Dejerine and Gauckler, Les manifestations fonctionnelles des psycho-névroses, 1911, pp. 170 and 176.   [2] Op. cit., p. 160.

packed with contradictions. The patient will declare that he is incapable of doing some particular action, but will perform a thousand times some other action which, objectively considered, is just as fatiguing. A woman who cannot lift her arm when we ask her to do so, will, morning after morning, spend a whole hour doing her hair (p. 169). A man who declares that he is unable to walk for five minutes on end, will walk for hours if he finds himself in pleasant company which takes him out of himself. This alleged asthenia is always variable and illogical (p. 170).

It is none the less true that we can observe a great many disorders when we study the behaviour of these patients. Some of them make exaggerated movements which are not requisite for the action they are performing. They walk too quickly without sparing their breath ; they make violent movements and disproportionate efforts ; they cannot sit still, and are continually wriggling about in their chairs (pp. 172 and 179). Others, and these are even more numerous, exhibit signs of muscular rigidity, partial contractures ; they hold their breath, and stand as stiff as a post. The exaggerated movements and the muscular rigidity are real causes of fatigue ; they give the patient a persistent feeling of effort, and arouse in him the notion of fatigue. A very common symptom in these cases is the rapid onset of eye-strain. This is because they fixate too stiffly, and thus grow tired just as a healthy person would who should fixate too long upon the same point, or who should induce conjunctivitis by rubbing his eyes for a long time (p. 231). All their actions are characterised by disharmonies which disorder these actions and make them difficult, and induce a fatigue which is more or less real.

But what is the cause of such disharmonies ? This is a matter on which Dejerine has little to say, but we can divine his thought. The disharmonies are usually the outcome of the fact that the patient pays undue attention to all his actions ; he is continually watching himself, and can never act automatically and simply, can never let himelf go. The conviction of difficulty inhibits effort, and the intervention of psychic phenomena checks an action which cannot be performed satisfactorily unless it is performed automatically (p. 173). The patient interferes with the working of his intellectual functions by the way in which he keeps them under observation (p. 281). He is still thinking of the previous word when the next word comes, and this makes him believe that he cannot understand, that he cannot follow a train of thought (p. 282). If we carry the enquiry a stage further, and ask the reason for such excessive and restless attention, we shall not find a definite answer in this particular book upon the psychoneuroses, but our knowledge of Dejerine's other writings enables us to foresee what his answer would be. The cause, he would say, is simply restlessness and emotion. He is fond of declaring that work does not induce the disorders characteristic of fatigue unless it is accompanied by emotion, and he seems inclined to conclude that the essential trouble of the neuropath is not excessive fatigue but emotivity. Such an idea is, moreover, commonly held. R. C. Cabot, voicing the thoughts of most of the American authors who have discussed this subject, writes that what causes disturbance is not overwork in the strict sense of the term, but excess of emotion. The neurasthenic suffers from undue fatigue, not because he has done so much work, but because his mental and moral machinery revolves with so much internal friction of part upon part." If a man is troubled by a nail thrusting up inside the heel of his shoe, it is true that he can get some relief by modifying his gait and by occasional rests; but the essential remedy is to take out or hammer down the nail.[1]

Of course the authorities who deny the importance of fatigue in the pathogenesis of the neuroses will not admit the need for the rest cure which was excogitated as a deduction from the fatigue theory. They all emphasise the dangers of rest. As long ago as 1898, Morton Prince was criticising the exaggerations implicit in Weir Mitchell's method. The increase of fat and blood does not, he declared, induce a normal condition of the nervous system, and does not suffice to dispel the feeling of fatigue. There are many neuropaths whose symptoms will not be alleviated by a rest cure. On the contrary, by this method of treatment we shall foster their neurosis; we shall give them a morbid habit of thinking too much about their bodily health. Although they may appear to be cured as long as they remain in the artificial environment of the sanatorium,

<hr>

[1] Cabot, The Use and Abuse of Rest, etc., Parker's Psychotherapy, II, ii, 32–33.

they will speedily relapse and become worse than ever when they resume their customary life.[1]

" Even when rest is an indispensable element in the treatment of a disease, as, for example, when we bind a broken arm to a splint, or fix a broken leg in rigid plaster of Paris, it is also distinctly harmful. . . . The rest is indeed necessary to ensure the healing of the broken bone, but when that is accomplished we have still to cure the patient of the disease (the degeneration and loss of power) which our treatment has itself produced. . . . Bind a healthy, unbroken arm to a splint, and in a few weeks it will be reduced to the same pitiful wreck of its former self that we see when a broken arm comes out of splints. It is the rest, not the fracture, that makes the bone and muscle begin to die on their splints."[2] A good many other writers, such as Lloyd Tuckey, Milne Bramwell, Münsterberg,[3] and Waterman,[4] advocate similar ideas. Treatment by rest is dangerous even in sufferers from tuberculosis ; all the more, then, must it be dangerous in neuropaths. They speak of patients who had been on their backs for years and had grown fat, only to become more abulic and more phobic than ever. Münsterberg, in this connexion, makes an interesting psychological observation. He says that these patients find it very difficult to bear extensive changes in their behaviour. If we prescribe absolute rest to some one who is normally a hard worker, we shall impose upon him a change in his mode of life which he will be likely to bear badly.[5] Dejerine, who appears to favour absolute rest, seeing that he condemns his unfortunate patients to immobilisation for months, to isolation in their curtained beds, nevertheless does not attach any theoretical importance to this practice. He only considers such rest useful for the cachectics of whom we have spoken, and even in them he only advises it until they have recovered their normal weight. Then, just like the beforementioned authors, he insists that the patient shall begin to walk about, shall practice other exercises, shall undertake a rational education of activity which will banish fears. He

---

[1] Morton Prince, The Educational Treatment of Neurasthenia and Certain Hysterical States, " Boston Medical and Surgical Journal," October 6, 1898.
[2] Cabot, The Use and Abuse of Rest, etc., Parker's Psychotherapy, II, ii, 29.
[3] Münsterberg, Psychotherapy, 1909, p. 192.
[4] The Treatment of Fatigue States, in Psychotherapeutics, a Symposium, 1910, p. 99.   [5] Münsterberg, op. cit., p. 196.

reiterates the sermons of Paul Dubois concerning the advantages of a Spartan discipline.

We thus find ourselves faced by two conflicting theories, Weir Mitchell's to the effect that the fatigue of these patients is real and essential, and that of Paul Dubois to the effect that their fatigue is illusory and insignificant. How are we to choose? Deschamps, who sees that there is a difficulty, suggests a simple way of conciliation. It will be enough to admit that the patients are not all alike. Some of the neuropaths suffer from an essential and primary asthenia; these are Deschamps' patients, and we are to speak of them as asthenics. The others have fixed ideas of fatigue, and their actions are interfered with by phobias; these are Dubois' patients, and we must speak of them as "intercalated or inhibited psychopaths." Thus, both the contending parties will be right, and every one will be well pleased.

This position is extremely courteous, but I fear it is untenable. How did it come about that there were so many real asthenics in Deschamps practice, and that so few real asthenics went to consult Dubois or Dejerine? No doubt Dubois (p. 519) and Dejerine, as we have just seen, admit that a certain number of genuinely exhausted patients came under their notice, but these were cachectics, suffering from various organic disorders and exhibiting symptoms of malnutrition; they were not Deschamps' asthenics. I am certain that the same patient, successively examined by practitioners of the rival schools, would have had his case differently diagnosed.

The crux of the conciliatory method is, in fact, this matter of diagnosis. If we are to agree that there are two categories of patients, there must be no possibility of mistake about the differential diagnosis, and it does not seem to me that Deschamps has been successful here. In his attempts at differential diagnosis, he appeals to the argument as to contradictory behaviour which Dubois and Dejerine use in the very opposite way. He refers (pp. 110 and 111) to the case of a man suffering from agoraphobia, who when in the street declares himself to be utterly exhausted after taking three or four steps, whereas he can walk for miles within a private enclosure. Deschamps will not admit that this man is really an exhausted asthenic. He must be sent to listen to Dubois' sermons. A summary conviction ! How can we tell that more careful observation would not have enabled us to discover similar contradictions in the behaviour of all Deschamps' asthenics ? That is precisely what Dubois and Dejerine believed they were able to do in every such case, and indeed it is not difficult to detect these contradictions in the behaviour of our own asthenic patients. Lydia (f., 40) appears at first sight to be a typical asthenic of the Deschamps pattern, and as such I have always regarded her ; she has been bedridden for ten years and I find it very difficult to make her get up even for a short time. Recently I wanted to study in her some interesting disorders of movement of the kind described by Deschamps. I asked her to crouch on her hams, to shuffle along in that crouching attitude, and then to rise from this posture and stand on tip-toe. I found, as Deschamps had led me to expect, that she could not perform any of these actions, that she could not stand on tip-toe even for an instant without swaying and falling. " It is very odd," she remarked, when she became aware of her own powerlessness. " Sometimes I have to stand on tip-toe when my sister wants me to hand her down some things from the upper shelf of the wardrobe, and then I can stand on tip-toe for quite a long time." There are, then, contradictions in Lydia's behaviour, and I must classify her as an " intercalated psychopath " instead of as an asthenic.

In reality, if we wish to apply these contradictions of behaviour when we are formulating our diagnosis, we must take a precaution which is overlooked by the before-mentioned writers. We must take steps to ensure that the two actions we are comparing are really upon the same level, that they are equally difficult psychologically speaking, and that they do not differ in respect of the addition of the idea of fatigue by the subject in one case, and not in the other. But such a determination is extremely difficult, and I doubt if it be possible in the types of behaviour which are stigmatised as contradictory. Dubois has told us that the behaviour of one of his female patients is contradictory because she can read novels all day and yet declares herself incapable of teaching her children for an hour. I cannot see any contradiction here, for it seems to me that the teaching of children is a complex action for which a high tension is requisite, whereas to sit quietly in an arm-chair and read a novel is a very simple action and one for which only a low tension is requisite. For a psychasthenic, walking in the street is a very different kind of action from walking in a private enclosure. When I ask Lydia to stand on tip-toe, the action I demand is one of obedience to the physician, one of those actions which are to enable me to verify a point of medical observation. Now, I have known for a long time that Lydia is incapable of such actions ; they require too high a tension, and the attempt to perform them induces an emotional derivation. She has never been able to hold out her wrist properly when I want to feel her pulse. She tries to do so, but her arm shakes all the time, so that it is very difficult to count the beats. To stand on tip-toe at the word of command, and to stand on tip-toe without thinking about it because she wishes to get for her sister something that is on the top shelf of the wardrobe, are very different kinds of action, and only those who have not learned how to analyse the doings of their patients can regard them as strictly comparable. My inference is that, without any contradiction in behaviour, a patient may be too much exhausted to perform one of these actions, and not too much exhausted to perform the other. How is it possible to base on so superficial an observation a diagnosis upon which so much turns ?

Deschamps finds it necessary to admit that, under the influence of strong emotion, an asthenic can perform actions which are beyond his powers at ordinary times. If the house is on fire, the patient will save his life by running out, and will not say a word about fatigue. I have reported hundreds of instances of the kind, and I have recently had occasion to observe a good many more in Lydia's behaviour. When caring for her sister, to whom she is devoted, she can display wonderful energy and heroic powers of resistance. Deschamps can, of course, explain away the contradiction. " The patient uses up his stores of energy in a moment ; when the moment has passed, when the stores of energy have been dissipated, he slips back to a lower level than before " (p. 111). Is this always true ? Dejerine does not believe it (p. 174), neither do I. I have often had occasion to note that a great shock has been the starting-point of remarkable improvement ; this is a matter to which we shall have to return when we come to study excitations. Are we to exclude from the group of asthenics all the patients in whom excitation can induce such reactions, just as we have already excluded all the patients who can perform easy actions ? I am afraid we shall not have any asthenics left !

In actual fact, no doctor ever makes diagnoses of the kind for which Deschamps asks. He himself regards almost all his patients as asthenics, whereas Dubois finds that every one whom he treats by his method is an " intercalated psychasthenic." Substantially, the respective authorities are right to apply a single name to all the cases which seem to them to be pretty much of the same kind. There is no reason why either Deschamps or Dubois should try to subdivide the group upon the supposition that some of the patients are affected by a real and others by an imaginary debility. But if no such diagnostic subdivision is possible, we cannot take refuge in the conciliation suggested by Deschamps, and we are still faced by the embarrassing contradiction. We are compelled to recognise that the contradiction really exists, and that it is impossible for the views of both schools to be sound. There must be a mistake on one side or the other, perhaps on both. If we want to discover the mistake or mistakes, we shall have to examine somewhat more carefully the arguments put forward by the rival schools.

3. ROLE OF FATIGUE.

Even though we admit the justice of Paul Dubois' criticisms, even though we agree that what these patients say about their fatigue is exaggerated, and that it may be the outcome of delusion, we still have to ask whether there are not real disorders underlying such delusions—disorders which must, up to a certain point, be compared to fatigue and treated in the same way.

The patients who complain of terrible fatigue, who continually declare that they were born tired, who stay in bed for years, are suffering from obsessions and phobias, and their behaviour is obviously the outcome of their hypochondriacal obsessions of fatigue. In this connexion I have already referred to the case of Lydia. I now come to the case of Kx., which is even more characteristic. She is a young woman of twenty-six, who, at the age of fifteen, began to be affected by prolonged crises of over-scrupulousness in which she was afraid that she was about to commit or had committed horrible crimes, and during which she was continually wanting to go to confession. Subsequently she suffered from claustro-phobia, from a phobia of water and of boats, and above all, from a phobia of carriages. This last was so extreme that she once threw herself out of a moving carriage because she could no longer bear the sight of the ground running away under the wheels. She was treated by Weir Mitchell's method, spending seven months in bed. The result was interesting. The treatment appeared to diminish the earlier phobias, inas-much as it suppressed the opportunity for their manifestation ; but it gave rise to a far more serious obsession and phobia, the obsession and the phobia of walking and fatigue. The patient was willing to get out of bed and to take a few steps in the room in order to reach an arm-chair ; but she would not go out, would not walk in the street, would not take any kind of exercise, for she was certain that this would instantly bring on the most distressing symptoms, due to fatigue. If those in charge of her insisted upon her going out, she im-mediately began to suffer from all sorts of spasms of the facial muscles ; she became excited, wrung her hands and twisted her arms, shed tears, and uttered piercing cries. This happened, she said, because everything had become strange and sinister, because she felt a sense of vacancy in the head and had a horrible feeling of " goneness." She was afraid of losing her memory, of forgetting her very name, of losing her personality, and of losing the power of sensation. She would pinch herself, and would prick her arms until the blood came, in order to make sure that she could still feel. " I am trying to find myself ; it seems to me that I am dying, that I am disappearing utterly, for everything is so far away and so unreal." To check this paroxysm, she had to sit down, or to lie down on the ground wherever she might happen to be, and it was necessary to bring her home upon a stretcher. After a few hours' absolute rest in a perfectly quiet room, the distressing symptoms would gradually subside. Such a crisis would ensue after any kind of activity requiring an expenditure of energy ; after a few minutes reading or conversation (especi-ally a conversation with more than one person), just as much as after a walk. That was why Kx. obstinately refused to get up, to take her meals with other persons, to engage in any kind of activity. Matters have been going on like this for five years, in a young woman who sleeps well ; who eats a great deal, perhaps more than is good for her ; who digests well, and who seems fat and strong. When we have to do with such a case, how can we help thinking that an obsession with fatigue, an obsession which is tantamount to a delusion, must be a notable factor ?

In some instances, it is even more obvious that the notion of fatigue is a delusion.—Ry. (m., 37), who appears to be in the best of health, took to his bed seven years ago and suffered all the afflictions of intense poverty without trying to stir, on the ground that eight years ago he had been tired out by his work as hotel manager, and that he would need years upon years of rest to recover from his fatigue.—Aq. (f., 57) extends the notion of her fatigue to the inanimate objects in her environment. She has terrible obsessive crises concerning " the water which flows, the sea which rolls, the pendulum which never stops swinging, the two poor old fowling pieces which have been hanging on the wall for years, the unhappy department of Seine-et-Oise which surrounds the department of Seine and can never get rid of it. Why is it that nothing in the world can stop and rest for a little ? "

When a sufferer from obsession shudderingly tell us of his remorse for unnamable crimes, are we to regard him as a criminal, and to have him sent to gaol ? There can be no doubt that those who consider fatigue the fundamental factor of the neuroses, are paying far too much attention to what the patients say, and that the doctor has come to share his patient's delusions. We ought not to take the utterances of such invalids so seriously.

All the same, we must avoid exaggeration. I agree that an obsession of fatigue does not prove that fatigue is really present ; but the fact that the patient has an obsession of fatigue does not justify us in concluding that he has no real fatigue. Many of those who are obsessed with the idea of syphilis have never been infected with this disease ; but some of those who are obsessed with the idea of syphilis, are at the same time really suffering from syphilis. A real disorder may underlie an obsession. The foregoing considerations, therefore, do not solve our problem, but serve merely to show us that there is need to walk warily. If we want to study fatigue in neuropaths, we must avoid selecting patients who are obsessed with the idea of fatigue. We must choose patients who have other obsessions, other phobias, or other symptoms, no matter what ; and we must endeavour to ascertain whether, without their being aware of it, or at any rate without their paying much attention to the matter, they are suffering from real disorders of activity independently of what they may think about these disorders. Then we have to enquire whether such disorders can be assimilated to those which arise from fatigue.

For a long time I have tried to show that, in the clinical examination of neuropaths and the insane, we must not be content with ascertaining the existence of the obvious delusions, obsessions, phobias, and algias, of which the patient complains. Our aim must be to look beyond these superficial symptoms, and to discover the fundamental disorders that affect the performance of actions. Sometimes the patient shows himself vaguely aware of these disorders, for he suffers from sentiments of incompleteness ; but sometimes he ignores them, as happens in those who bear the genuine brand of psychasthenia. In many instances, the disorders of movement are so conspicuous that they make themselves obvious during the simple performance of movements.

Arnaud, likewise, has drawn attention to this. He speaks of the disorders of movement that can be observed in abulics ; and he tells us that their gait and their gestures are stiff, strange, jerky, and so on. I am delighted to find that the neurologists who, to all appearance, reject the idea that neuropaths really suffer from fatigue or exhaustion, such neurologists as Dubois and Dejerine, are to-day pointing out (though in a very imperfect manner) the disorders of action which I myself used to demonstrate in neuropaths. At present they speak only of stiffness and of contortions, terming these " disharmonies." Still, this is a good beginning, and after a while the fact that neuropaths exhibit all kinds of disorders of action will be generally admitted.

Let us consider an additional example of such phenomena, a case in which disorders of action are conspicuous. Emile, a lad of sixteen, is a typical sufferer from major psychasthenia. He is obsessed with bodily shame, is erythrophobic, has a dread of being seen, a terror that people will divine his thoughts, and so on. He has no ideas relating to fatigue and exhaustion, he does not complain of such symptoms at all, and finds it difficult to understand that he is an invalid. When he thinks he is alone in his room, and when we watch him without his being aware of it, his movements are calm and easy. But if he has to speak to any one, or if he has to go out into the street, he becomes quite stiff, as if his muscles were partially contractured. He presses his arms forcibly against his sides, holds his head stiffly stretched forward, and keeps his eyes convulsively closed or stares skyward. From time to time he shakes himself violently. He taps his feet on the ground, or he drags them, or exhibits some other peculiarity of gait. He pants instead of breathing quietly; and, within a few minutes, he is dripping with perspiration. Here we have a patient who exhibits the most extensive disharmonies of movement, and yet he never says a word about feeling tired. Obviously, then, such disharmonies are not invariably connected with a fixed idea of fatigue.

Dejerine, when he describes disharmonies of this kind, is inclined to explain them as the outcome of a sort of voluntary action. The patient, says Dejerine, pays too much attention to what he is doing, keeps perpetual watch upon all his actions and thereby transforms them. I agree that there is a certain amount of truth in this explanation as regards the patients who have a fixed idea of watching their own doings, just as other patients have a fixed idea of fatigue ; but the explanation will not explain all cases. Emile has only recently begun to suffer from obsessions of bodily shame competent to induce a craze for watching his own doings. But it is several years since his elders had their attention drawn to the peculiar stiffness of his gait, before he became aware of it himself. The trouble was indicated by the curious way in which he wore out his shoes. At this time he had no obsessions ; and he was very much surprised when he first noticed that he became stiff, held himself badly, and sweated profusely, whenever he was walking. His own account of the matter is that his obsessions and his longing to hide were brought about through others having pointed out to him that his attitudes were grotesque. Nevertheless, we shall find a similar stiffness and similar sweats in persons who have no obsession about

their postures, and do not spend their time in watching whatever they are doing and in taking stock of their own bodies.—
In the early stages of his illness, X. would become rigid, would
be drenched with perspiration, and would even have an erection,
when he was seated at his desk and was trying to study a
mathematical theorem.   If at this time he thought of anything
at all, it was only about the imminent examination and about
the difficulty of a career.—We may make another observation
in this connexion, namely that attention to the body and its
postures does not necessarily induce stiffness and absurd
attitudes.   An actor or a lecturer who desires to produce a
certain effect in the audience, watches his own attitude and
deliberately modifies it far more than Emile did, but does not
for this reason make any contortions.   Emile himself, when
I had been able to improve his condition a little, and to raise
his psychological tension, learned to watch his own postures
to advantage.   I helped the poor lad to pass his examinations,
and actually advised him to keep constant watch upon himself so as to avoid adopting any ridiculous postures.   He thus
became able to move and to hold himself quite naturally.
We see, then, that it was not merely self-observation which
made him so ridiculously stiff and awkward.   If self-observation was to blame, it was self-observation of a morbid kind,
and what has to be explained as a pathogenic factor is not the
self-observation but the morbidity.

The fact is that the obvious disorders of movement are
the outcome of deep-seated disorders in the development and
the activation of the tendencies.   This is not the place for a
detailed discussion of the various factors ; of the different
forms of mental agitation ; of the unending repetitions ; of
the intoxication by a word, a phrase, or a question ; of the
mania of seeking ; of the dread of action.   Enough to point
out that these forms of agitation are always attended by inadequacies of function.   The patients can never complete an action,
and can never perform it pleasurably ; when the disease is
far advanced, they cannot even call up a mental picture of a
happy event, without having this picture promptly distorted,
so that it becomes tinted with gloom.   They cannot arrive
at a decision, form a conviction, or achieve a belief ; they can
come to no definite conclusion, and they cannot understand
anything clearly.   In bad cases, these disturbances are per

fectly plain; when the disorder is less grave, we are made aware of them only as concerns the more elevated tendencies and the more difficult kinds of action : but they invariably underlie the obsessions, the phobias, and even the delusions.

That is why I see little reason to modify the explanation I used to give of all these phenomena. I do not regard the stiffness and the disorders of movement as primary and quasi-voluntary phenomena ; I look upon them as secondary, and as the expression of a deep-seated malady. In Emile, there were no contortions when he believed he was alone, so that he did not need to activate any tendencies other than those which were purely self-regarding ; the disorders of movement manifested themselves when he had to undertake the far more difficult social activities of which he had gradually become incapable. We must not be satisfied with noting that he became stiff. It is essential also to note that the lad, though very intelligent, is unable, despite his best endeavours, to carry out the simplest kind of social action ; that he can no longer make himself understood, ask for anything, answer a question, or make his way through the streets. The symptoms are not only those of agitation, that is to say of the exaggerated and ineffective activation of lower-grade tendencies ; there is, in addition, an inadequate activation of higher-grade tendencies. The facts may be summarised in terms of the theory of the lowering of psychological tension. The superior tendencies can no longer achieve a high degree of realisation, and the inferior tendencies are agitated in consequence of a kind of derivation. The inference is that the phenomena which Dejerine speaks of as disharmonies are an outcome of the fundamental depression of neuropaths, the existence of this being a matter as to which there is now widespread agreement.

Such patients may suffer from many and very different kinds of depression. The depression of the melancholic, for instance, is very like that of the psychasthenic in respect of the inability to act and to believe, but it differs because the melancholic is affected with a particular kind of mental suffering which has hitherto been very inadequately analysed. It seems likely that we are concerned here with a type of depression which does not only inhibit the reflective powers, but also influences a lower grade of activation, that of desire. We find it difficult to grasp the nature of these different kinds of depression, and we feel that it is necessary to compare them to commoner kinds of psychological phenomena, to ones of which we have had personal experience. Now in health, as I have shown, there occur certain psychological phenomena which we believe we know something about, and which are analogous to oscillations of the mental level; these may be compared to depressions. I think particularly of sleep, emotion, and fatigue. We are tempted, therefore, to compare the depression of the neuropath to one or other of these normal phenomena, in the hope that this will render the nature of the depression more intelligible. Some writers maintain that hysteria is a form of sleep; others declare that it is a state of emotion; and yet others insist that it is a form of fatigue. The remarkable thing is that they are all equally cocksure, and that the one thing upon which they are agreed is that the rival theories are utterly wrong. In actual fact, all the theories are partly wrong and partly right. Hysterical depression obviously resembles sleep, emotion, and fatigue, for all these phenomena are varieties of depression. But the depression of hysterics differs in certain respects from the depression of sleep, emotion, and fatigue, seeing that it is a pathological modification of the psychological tension, and must, therefore, differ in certain essential respects from all the depressions which are classed as normal. Still, the comparisons we have been considering are not devoid of interest, provided that we recognise that their worth is merely relative, and provided that we never forget that they are nothing more than analogies. We shall do well, therefore, to ask which among these comparisons is the most interesting and the most fruitful.

If we return to the study of the before-mentioned disharmonies, and of the depression they disclose in neuropaths, we shall find that many writers, and especially Dubois and Dejerine, prefer to assimilate them to emotions, and declare that they have no resemblance to fatigue. " Overwork," writes Dejerine, " is accompanied by an emotional state, and it is with this associated emotional state that we are concerned in the disease " (pp. 350 and 356). " Overwork will not give rise to neurasthenia unless emotion is superadded " (p. 349). If we are to discuss this contention, we must know precisely what Dejerine means by " emotion " and " fatigue," and how he distinguishes between them. I cannot find that he has anything very definite to say about this matter. As regards emotion, he appears to accept the definition which I myself propounded to the Neurological Society; and he gives no definition of fatigue. But, when discussing emotion, I have endeavoured to show that from the symptomatic point of view there is scarcely any perceptible difference between emotion and fatigue. Both these phenomena are psychological states of depression in which there are inadequacies and agitations. The most we can say by way of distinction is that in current parlance we speak rather of fatigue when inadequacies predominate, and of emotion when derivative agitations predominate. We surprise our hearers a little when we show them that muscular, mental, or visceral agitations occur in fatigue; and we surprise them when we show them that emotions are always attented by inadequacies. Thus, from the symptomatic point of view the difference between the two conditions is trifling, if there be any real difference at all. It is difficult, therefore, to speak of a pure fatigue unattended by emotion, or of an emotion unattended by fatigue; such descriptions are more or less conventional. The symptoms of the two conditions run into one another, and mutually induce one another. An individual falls sick after taking part in a competition. "That is because he has been emotioned," says Dejerine; "because he is fatigued." Can we not say that he became emotioned because he began to feel fatigued? Would not the second description be quite as accurate as the first? The actual fact is that the subject came by degrees to exhibit the symptoms of both conditions, and we make a rather artificial distinction when we draw the symptoms of one group into the foreground and thrust the symptoms of the other group into the background.

Fortunately, however, there is another standpoint at which common sense ordinarily takes up its station so as to distinguish between emotion and fatigue. They are both more or less profound states of depression, and akin by their symptoms; but they appear to supervene under different conditions. Emotion is a disturbance which comes on at the moment when we perceive a situation, developing prior to action, and appearing even to inhibit action; fatigue is a disturbance tending to manifest itself at a later stage, after

intense and repeated action or even inaction. Ostensibly
this may seem a considerable difference ; in reality it is a small
one, but it suffices for the practical purposes of speech. If
we adopt this outlook, can we say that the depression of the
neuroses is more closely akin to that of emotion than to that
of fatigue ?

There can be no doubt that the morbid disturbances
which take the form of depression, have, in many cases, an
origin akin to that of emotions. They arise in connexion
with a perception which has been followed by inadequate and
ill-adapted actions. The disturbance seems to have existed
from the very outset, and to have prevented the proper performance of the action, this being, according to popular phraseology, the essential characteristic of emotion. The comparison
of morbid depression to an exaggerated emotion is therefore,
in many instances, both natural and legitimate.

But I think that the comparison to fatigue has even more
to be said in its favour. First of all, we can ascertain that
nervous disorders accompanied by depression arise under
conditions identical with those which produce fatigue ; that
is to say, after the performance of an action when the work
has lasted too long, has been too intense, or has been performed
with undue haste. This first attracted attention in the case of
bodily fatigue. Tissié, of Bordeaux, has published some
remarkable studies, which might almost have been laboratory
experiments, concerning the mental disorders that occurred
in the competitors in a six days' bicycle race. " The will
power is in abeyance, and the patient inclines to suffer from
obsessions and phobias."—" At the end of the six days' race,
these patients suffer from delusions of persecution." [1]

I have notes of a good many cases of the kind, in which
typical depressive disorders began, just like fatigue, after
strenuous or unduly prolonged activity. Young people who
leave the country for the town in order to become domestic
servants or to undertake factory work, have to make a difficult
adaptation to entirely new circumstances, and sometimes
have to do far too much work. This was the exciting cause of
neurosis in a dozen of my cases. To take one instance only,
a remarkable one, G. M. (f., 18), who was country-bred, had to

---

[1] Tissié, " Revue Scientifique," 1896, vol. ii, p. 642.

make a long railway journey every morning and every evening, and to work very hard throughout the day as a shop assistant. After eight months, though she had hitherto been perfectly normal, she began to suffer from tics, manias, and doubts. She took to lying habitually. What was even more strange, she wrote letters to herself, and had bouquets sent to herself. This inclination to lying, and especially to self-deception, is characteristic of the depression which takes the form of mental lethargy.

Long and arduous journeys were the cause of depression in ten of my cases. It was after riding about a hundred miles on a bicycle that Ax. (f., 42) became uneasy, and had a peculiar obsession regarding some splotches upon the skin of the thighs which she feared her servant might have caught sight of.—It was after spending two sleepless nights in the train that Aq. (f., 60) began to pay attention to the breathing of a lapdog, and developed a phobia concerning people's breathing. The terrible overwork enforced by the war, quite apart from emotional stresses, was the obvious cause of neuroses and psychoses in many cases. In my own practice there were a dozen such cases among soldiers and doctors who had never been to the front at all, and in whom the illness was due to nothing but fatigue.

Excessive mental work will induce like disturbances. Facts confirming this statement may be gleaned from Galton's investigation concerning overwork in schools; [1] from Lagrange's researches into the effects of the prolonged concentration of attention; from a great number of German writings, inspired especially by Kraepelin; from the observations of Tissié, Mosso, Féré, Binet, and Henry. " Fatigue," writes Féré,[2] " often engenders ideas of negation and of persecution; altruistic feelings yield place to egoism, which manifests its presence under very varied forms; the subject is incapable of reacting against obsessions and impulses, which may become irresistible." Disorders due to excessive mental labour are so numerous that it must suffice to adduce only a few examples. —Zov. (m., 45), on the death of his father, undertook the management of a large business without having had sufficient training or previous experience; a sense of responsibility

---

[1] " Revue Scientifique," 1889, vol. i, p. 102.
[2] " Médecine Moderne," November 1898.

leads him to expend an exaggerated amount of energy in running the concern. After a few months of hard work, during which his efforts are crowned with success, he becomes hesitating, cannot make up his mind, is incapable of issuing orders: "What used to be no more than child's play, has become a labour of Hercules," finally he is obsessed with scruples and overwhelmed with the fear of ruin.—In the case of Dh., we have a girl of twenty-two who has been made ill by too intense and too prolonged study. She suffers from heart disease, and desires to make up for her enforced physical inertia by a very great cerebral activity. She works day and night: "I read while walking, and even while getting tea ready. . . . I was horribly tired, but I would not heed such feelings, I wanted to overcome my nerves by my will." She soon lost her appetite, could not sleep, became run down, and suffered from obsessions.—Such cases are more especially to be met with among persons preparing for examinations, as in the case of Myes. (f., 20), who had been working up for a painting competition; in that of Qv. (f., 23), because of an entrance examination at the Conservatoire, in which she was successful; in that of eight young persons as the sequel of the preparation for an examination in advanced science, when hard study led to more or less grave crises of depression towards the close of the scholastic year, either at the time of the examination or soon after.—A foreign student, twenty-four years of age, endeavours, for eighteen months, to follow a course of study in a language she does not really understand. At all cost she is determined to embark upon an intellectual career, but she succumbs to doubts and to religious phobias.—These are but a few cases among a legion. It is no use telling me that such people have a predisposition. This may be true for some of them. But innumerable predisposed persons are able to keep their balance all through life; whereas those who succumb at a particular moment do so because of overwork.

Another group is formed by cases that are even more interesting. These comprise individuals who are constitutional neuropaths, have become neuropaths in consequence of previous misadventures, but have been able to attain to a state of relatively good health, have acquired a degree of psychological tension which, though it may not be very high, is at least sufficient for the needs of everyday life, and who do not actually suffer from any specific symptoms. Such persons, however, become seriously ill in circumstances which would simply cause fatigue in ordinary mortals. They have been named "fatiguables," because fatigue-states overtake them very rapidly, as soon as they exert themselves in a way which would entail no bad consequences in normal human beings ; and because, in them, fatigue immediately becomes a serious illness, and causes grave depression. Any action which is a trifle more difficult—which takes slightly longer to perform, though it may have apparently been performed correctly, that is to say without having been arrested or disturbed by emotional derivations—brings about relapses, and the reappearance and aggravation of the morbid symptoms.

Here are some examples to illustrate these important facts.—Pj. (m., 30), who, as the sequel of the explosion of a shell quite near him, develops a typical hysterical hemiplegia with persistent amnesia and retrograde amnesia, is completely cured at the end of two years ; if, however, he walks too far, or if he works too arduously, he again suffers from hemiplegia and amnesia, the attacks lasting twenty-four or forty-eight hours.—The scruples and remorse which had apparently disappeared in the case of Fp. (f., 29), reappear as soon as she agrees to perform some heavy work away from home.—For some time I was puzzled to find the reason for Vkp.'s relapses. She was a woman of 27, who, though she seemed cured of her troubles, would suddenly succumb to agoraphobia, to the obsession that she was not being treated with due respect, and to crises of enteritis. The patient was at a loss to explain these relapses. They were preluded by a visit from her mother, who could not refrain from criticising the daughter and finding fault with her for neglecting her household affairs. Vkp. was quick to realise that her mother was right, and made strenuous efforts to put things in order ; she insisted on doing everything herself so as to be free from self-reproach ; she became absolutely infatuated with her tasks, and would get so exhausted that she would relapse into her sickness, and would come along " to be told to rest."

Ws. (f., 31), if she takes a slightly longer walk than is customary, if she tries to tidy her flat, or if she pays a rather longer call than usual, complains that she has what she names one of her "lapses." These lapses are a kind of eclipse of consciousness, which I have often described in cases of psychasthenia. She cannot hear what is said to her, and she appears to herself to have ceased to live. If she tries, at such times, to continue to attend, to read, to listen, or to speak, she has a feeling of heat and of pain in the head, she is assailed by a desire to sleep, and cannot refrain from weeping. She is simultaneously exhausted and agitated ; she makes exaggerated efforts to perform the simplest act as if " I were constantly trying to arrange everything that was said to me in the pigeon-holes of my mind " ; she has a feeling of haste, as though everything must be finished at once and she must on no account be stopped. Unless these troubles can be speedily relieved, the fatigue becomes the starting-point of a serious relapse.

Eo. (f., 31) relapsed into grave depression, with abulia, moaning, and phobias of sleep and of insomnia, after a year and a half of perfect health, because, in the early months of pregnancy, she had to nurse her husband night and day for six weeks while he was suffering from bronchopneumonia. At the end of the six weeks, she showed signs of agitation ; she could not put an end to her work " because I feel that I have a superabundance, a surfeit, of life within me which will wear me out." And, indeed, at the end of two or three weeks she had a complete relapse into her depression. This interesting case brings up the problem of periodically recurring depression, a state which has been named the manic-depressive psychosis. Those who prefer to replace clinical observation by preconceived theories will maintain that the patient inevitably relapses in virtue of a periodic law, and that fatigue plays no part. I have already given my views concerning this interpretation, during the course of a discussion at the Neurological Society in Paris. The case was that of Vkm. (m., 60), a secondary school teacher, who relapsed regularly at the end of the second school term if the work of teaching had made larger demands than usual upon him, whereas, in favourable circumstances he had no relapse at that time.—The same may be said of Eo. During the whole course of her illness, the part played by exterior circumstances which call upon her to make an effort and which bring about exhaustion, is manifest. Though she may get better in a nursing home where she has nothing to do, she soon relapses when she is allowed to return to her familiar surroundings and endeavours to do a little housework. A few good days will be followed by a very bad period, because she had thought herself cured and had made an expenditure of energy which exceeded her capacity.

The same phenomenon may be observed in Lydia, whom I succeeded in getting out of bed and in reeducating. A great deal of caution is necessary, for, after an effort which appears to us minimal, she will collapse again, and the onset of sentiments of incompleteness warn us that we have reached the limit beyond which we must not force her to go. " It seems as though life were ebbing away ; I feel as if I were dying ; I am no longer myself ; I am no longer finished, completed, natural." She becomes inattentive ; we observe disorders of perception, which are the heralds of obsessions of being ugly and humiliated. When at the theatre, or when taking part in a conversation which is well within her powers of understanding, suddenly her mind " grows empty," she suffers from a feeling of intense gloom, begins to repeat the same phrases over and over again, and fails to understand what is said to her. Looking back, the other members of her family can now recognise that these symptoms really date from childhood. When she had been for rather a long walk, she would complain of intense drowsiness, and yet would not be able to sleep, precisely because sleep is an action for which a certain tension is requisite, and her mental tension had fallen below this level. When watching Lydia, we can detect the difficulty of an action, and how much it costs her to perform it. At ordinary times, she can receive visits from her mother and her brother, and can converse with them for a while without suffering in any way ; but when she has been greatly put out by the breaking off of her brother's engagement, she can no longer hear what they say, and cannot answer them without falling ill again. She now feels once more that her "human dignity has been mutilated and degraded " ; and she is again affected by disorders of the ratiocinative faculty. Conversation has become much more difficult ; she can no longer let her tongue run freely, but must keep watch on herself lest she should allude to her brother's former betrothed, of whom she is fond and for whom she is very sorry ; she has to simulate an interest in topics which seem to her quite unimportant. The act of conversation, which had been simple, has become difficult, and demands a great expenditure of energy; she is no longer equal to it.

Similar phenomena may be observed in many patients.—Wkg. (m., 19) will sometimes, when engaged in conversation, begin to stare fixedly at his interlocutor, and will at the same time cease to understand what is being said.—Zob. (f., 60), after having had a number of visitors, suffers from symptoms of digestive disorder, and becomes affected with obsessive doubts.—In a good many other patients, though they can play their part in conversation quite well for a short time, we can note signs of mental disturbance, and in some instances the onset of actual delirium, if the conversation should be continued for more than half an hour. Such symptoms of disorder become even more conspicuous when study is prolonged rather than conversation.—Nen. (m., 18) will write intelligently enough for a page, but on the second page he begins to pen absurdities. If we watch him at work, we shall see that when he reaches the second page he is becoming pale and that he has tears in his eyes. If we speak to him at this juncture, we find that he answers jerkily and uncomprehendingly.—Lkv. (m., 32), like so many other patients, becomes anxious and is affected by over-scrupulousness when he has been reading for half an hour or so.—Mba. (m., 36) has quite a changed expression of countenance in the afternoon; the tone of his voice has become dry and haughty; he finds it difficult to refrain from tears; he is afraid of everything, and especially he is "afraid of life." These changes have come about because he has been at his office in the morning, and has been trying to work there for a couple of hours.

We are much struck by the terms in which Madame Z. complains of her fatigue. "I am good for nothing now; I can no longer do any work. . . . Some friends have been to visit me, or my son has been talking to me for a little while, or I have been reading a magazine article which has interested me, or I have merely tried to dress myself unaided. Some such trifle is enough. I am done for; I collapse like a pricked air-balloon, or like a soufflé which has been allowed to get cold. Despite all my efforts, I cannot prevent this. An icy coldness descends upon my head, eyes, and nose; there is a roaring in my ears; I seem to see all sorts of absurdities. I grow stiff all over, and my whole body trembles. I can no longer recognise the things around me ; I fancy that I cannot be in my own room any more, and that I must be in some unfamiliar place. This fatigue is so intense as to be positively painful ; I feel as if I were going to die of fatigue."

I should like to dwell at some length upon the treatment of the case of Emile, the lad of fifteen, of whom I spoke a little while ago. Since he was suffering from various tics, his medical adviser had thought it well that the patient should undergo a course of gymnastic exercises and of the reeducation of movement, this advice being based upon the widely accredited theory that such tics are nothing more than disorders of movement. By making great efforts, the patient was able to do the exercises fairly well, but only by stiffening all his muscles, while looking fixedly in front of him and speaking in a jerky voice. Still, the gymnastic teacher was fairly well satisfied with the results. But now the patient began to suffer from serious mental agitation, with shamefacedness and delusions of persecution. Stranger still, he became affected with muco-membranous enteritis, a disease whose relationships with mental depression have not been adequately recognised. He was obviously overworked, becoming subject to attacks of delirium, and to febrile paroxysms in which the temperature rose to 104°. Any kind of therapeutic measure tending to increase the exhaustion became impossible for months. The same sort of thing has recurred repeatedly in this patient's clinical history. When he has been improving very nicely, he is, for instance, given some fencing lessons, which please him greatly ; but thereupon he promptly relapses into sentiments of imcompleteness, masturbates to excess, and has an attack of piles. Mental effort has similar results. If he converses with friends for a few minutes, he can manage well enough ; but if the talk is unduly prolonged, he relapses, and the tics and phobias reappear. In the treatment of this lad we have constantly to bear in mind his extreme sensitiveness to fatigue.

The same remark applies to the treatment of Sophie, whose case is one of great interest. She is now a woman of thirty-five, but I have had her under observation for more than ten years. When I first knew her, she was a psychasthenic, suffering from over-scrupulousness, an obsession that she was not being treated with due respect, an impulse towards asceticism and ridiculous acts of devotion, and various other symptoms of mental disorder. From time to time, the maniacal condition and the obsessions became aggravated, so that consciousness in the ordinary sense of the term would lapse. She would then be affected with irresistible impulses, and would present the characteristics of those delirious psychasthenics described by myself a good many years ago, and admirably portrayed by Arnaud as well. We shall find it interesting to study one of the ways which, in this patient, obsession would pass into delirium.

At a time when Sophie seemed quite well, she came to Paris with some friends. They tramped the streets, visited museums, and spent the evening at the theatre. Next day she was transformed; she could no longer pay attention to anything, or fix her mind upon any idea. But, to use the expression I am accustomed to employ when describing her condition, " her thought flitted about like a butterfly." One ridiculous idea after another would take possession of her mind from moment to moment. She would insist upon her need for independence that she might develop her will power; she must devote herself to her own education, or must spend all her life in acts of charity. She was obviously on the high road to relapse, to a recurrence of all her more preposterous types of behaviour, her maniacal efforts, and her contests with the members of her environment. If I had allowed her to repeat such visits to Paris, she would have been quite delirious in a day or two. I have no space here to record the innumerable incidents which have shown me that Sophie's obsessions are always the outcome of a lowering of psychological tension, and that delirium ensues when the lowering of tension is extreme. Always, in her, fatigue is the cause of the depression. Anything which necessitates a great expenditure of energy will induce delirium. This will be the effect of a long journey in a motor-car, of trying to help in harvest work, of paying too many visits to her parents, and so on. No doubt, fatigue is not the only cause of the lowering of psychological tension that occurs in Sophie, not the only cause of an increase in depression, but it is certainly one of the main causes. Moreover, it is one of the most dangerous causes, for from the first her obsessions have taken the form of over-scrupulousness, and have led her to make excessive efforts in order to retain her own self-respect. But these efforts serve only to increase her fatigue, and culminate in delirium unless suitable measures can be taken to prevent the working out of the cycle. The process resembles that of an avalanche. It is common in cases of mental disorder, and its nature must be understood if we are to guide such patients intelligently.

Beyond question, a great many difficulties arise in connexion with the explanation of these phenomena of fatigue. We must draw certain distinctions between such morbid kinds of fatigue, and the normal fatigue that occurs in a man who is in good health but has been working rather too long. This normal fatigue is, in reality, a particular form of behaviour, and not a disorder of the health. It is first of all characterised by the cessation of the actions which have induced the fatigue ; then comes the adoption of the special attitude known as the attitude of repose ; finally, we have the maintenance of this attitude for a considerable time. Substantially, fatigue is the behaviour of a man who is resting ; and the feeling of fatigue is nothing more than the desire to behave in this way. The phenomenon which forms the starting-point of the behaviour leading to the discharge of the appropriate tendency consists of a number of changes that occur in the performance of the actions that are arousing fatigue. These actions grow more difficult ; they are less rapidly and less accurately performed ; such changes awaken the tendency to repose, and then activate it to the stage of desire. The tendency in question belongs to a group of tendencies which are fairly numerous, and are known as controlling or regulating tendencies. Psychological consciousness belongs to the same category. They are not activated by an external stimulus, but are spontaneous reactions to the results of our own activities. Understood in this sense, fatigue is not a real disorder ; it must rather be looked upon as essentially a precaution, as a defensive reaction against the dangers that might ensue if activity were unduly prolonged.

When we have to do with persistent morbid disorders, we shall do well to speak of " exhaustion " rather than of " fatigue." Exhaustion denotes the totality of the disorders of behaviour that are entailed by the performance and the prolonged repetition of actions which ought to have been checked by fatigue but which fatigue has not succeeded in checking. Exhaustion differs from fatigue much as starvation differs from hunger, seeing that hunger is the desire for food arising in us as a safeguard against starvation. The patients whose cases I have just been describing have not suffered from fatigue, in the strict sense of that term, for they did not check their activities when they ought to have done. Some of them, like Madame Z. (who complained bitterly of fatigue), had a feeling of fatigue, but did not know how to activate this longing for repose. Those who tried to rest, did not succeed in resting satisfactorily ; for the tendency to rest was already disordered, so that their attempts were fruitless. Typical sufferers from exhaustion, in whom there occur disorders of the activation of tendencies, are especially prone to disorder in the working of the tendency to the particular form of behaviour known as repose. It is when they are beginning to get better, and when they are suffering less from depression, that they become capable of spontaneously performing the actions of repose. At this stage we are surprised to hear them talk of having a feeling of fatigue, although in the early stages of their illness, and when the symptoms were far more serious than they are now, these patients made no complaint of fatigue. The disappearance of " exhaustion " renders the appearance of " fatigue " possible.

These considerations show that we were not perfectly accurate in using the word fatigue in the course of the foregoing remarks. But we were adopting a special standpoint, and were trying to ascertain the cause of our patients' symptoms. Fatigue and exhaustion have the same starting-point. They both arise out of the performance and prolongation of actions, and from this point of view there is no inconvenience in confounding the two terms.

Additional difficulties face us if we enquire at what moment the symptoms of exhaustion can be said to begin. In the simpler cases, the symptoms arise rapidly after action, or after the activity has been prolonged for a certain time This has been manifest in a good many of the cases we have just been considering. Here are some additional instances, simple ones.—Wkm. (f., 18) begins some form of activity, a piece of needlework, for instance, with good will and satisfaction. But after she has been working for ten minutes, she is seized by an insurmountable dislike for what she is doing, and if she persists in the work she becomes affected with a crisis of self-analysis and doubts.—Hk. (m., 30) says naively : " My feelings never last. As soon as I fall in love with a woman, I begin to regard her with disgust and even hatred."—Every doctor is familiar with cases of the type described by Féré, in which a man is subject to intense depression immediately after sexual intercourse.—Wkx. (m., 29), in whom when he is depressed the feeling of reality is apt to be disordered, is greatly alarmed after coitus because his mistress " looks like a corpse, seems to be a body without a soul."—Under like conditions, Kv. (m., 36) and Neb. (m., 32) become affected with doubt and abulia, and find it necessary to stay in bed for a couple of days.

But in other cases, the results of exceptional activity may be entirely different, and the majority of these cases are ones in which the symptoms have been severe. I have been able to follow day by day the evolution of the disorders induced in Lydia by fatigue mingled with emotion. There was danger that a factory with which she was connected would be burned down. She had to stay up all night, awaiting news, and rendering minor services. I expected that she would be very ill next day, but, instead, she was perfectly well and quite calm ; this was one of those phenomena of excitation which we shall have to study in a subsequent chapter. It was not until a week later that she began to suffer from breathlessness and anxiety, complained of feeling very weak, and demanded champagne and an extra-liberal diet, these being the usual premonitory symptoms of her attacks of depression. Then she went on to complain that she no longer had any feelings, that waves were running down her spine, and so on. Not until a fortnight after the night spent at the factory did she declare that she was "completely submerged in nonentity and vacancy," and show the other signs of the great crisis of depression for which I had been waiting. Here the sequence of events was plain. In other cases, as in that of Lise, which I quote so frequently in *Les obsessions et la psychasthénie*, there were several weeks' interval between the exhausting occurrences and the subsequent depression. This intercalary period is of great interest ; it corresponds to the period of "rumination" described by Charcot as occurring in the course of the development of hysterical symptoms. Doctors used to suppose that throughout this period a process of autosuggestion was at work. A subsequent idea was that "rumination" was akin to the phenomena of anaphylaxis described by Charles Richet. It is probable that during this period of incubation the subject, who has from the first made strenuous efforts at adaptation, who has been unable to achieve a satisfactory reaction, and who feels unbalanced, continues energetic attempts to bring about a better adaptation. This leads to a steady increase of exhaustion, which must show itself ere long. It will be necessary to return to the study of the period of incubation in a later chapter of the present work, apropos of traumatic memories and imperfectly liquidated situations. Suffice it, for the present, to point out that such latent periods between the initial efforts and the manifestations of exhaustion are of frequent occurrence. Unless the observer is aware of this, he will be liable to misinterpret symptoms whose onset has merely been delayed.

Furthermore, in most of the foregoing cases, we have only been studying generalised fatigue, that is to say, exhaustion due to the activation of a single tendency, but very soon generalised to affect most of the other tendencies and especially the higher-grade tendencies. In other, and more remarkable cases, the symptoms seem to be more or less exclusively localised upon the tendency which has played the leading part in exciting them. I shall give a few examples. Cu. is a girl of fifteen, brought up in the country until the age of thirteen, practically without education. But at this age her education was taken in hand. She was sent to school and was taught her catechism; she was scolded for speaking badly and reading badly; and was unremittingly trained in speaking, reading, and recitation. School work is predominantly oral, and the faculty which was most vigorously exercised in this child was the faculty of speech. I am inclined to attribute to overwork of the linguistic tendencies the remarkable crises from which she suffers every month during menstruation. She has fits of agitation during which she chatters incessantly, reciting fragments of her lessons, and unmeaning phrases, for forty-eight hours at a stretch. The crisis of talkativeness is apt to be followed by complete mutism, which lasts for several days, although the intellectual faculties remain unimpaired. It would really seem that in her case the function of speech betrays its exhaustion, at first by agitation, and subsequently by paralysis.

Elsewhere I have given a long account of the unhappy history of Jean. In this youth we observe a remarkable exhaustion of the genital functions after masturbation. He is shamefaced, overwhelmed with remorse, and affected with a disgust for sex. " A woman's body is repulsive ; though she is fastidious, she passes excrement just like myself." In this connexion, he has a number of phobias and sexual obsessions.—Pya.'s case is a strange one. He is forty years of age. As a sequel of sexual excesses and a surfeit of emotions, he has been suffering from psychasthenia for a long while. The debility chiefly affects the sexual function. In the early stages of the illness, there was complete suppression of sexual activity, both physical and moral. But the sexual powers were restored by slow degrees. The first sign of recovery was the reappearance of automatic emissions. Then he became able to perform incomplete coitus, attended by disgust and phobia. After a time, coitus became fairly normal, except that it gave him very little pleasure. It was more than a year after the beginning of the illness before the power of sexual intercourse had become entirely normal once again. These variations in the genital function were accompanied by very remarkable mental manifestations.

In other patients, the symptoms are those of a disorder of the visual function. Asthenopia or photophobia may come on when the eyes have been tired, as happens in the case of Madame Z., and in that of Emma (f., 40). These patients can no longer fixate an object or follow a moving object with their eyes ; every act of vision demands a distressing effort. " I have to try very hard in order to see ; all the time I have to keep on thinking about seeing." They have strange feelings with regard to their eyes, akin to sentiments of incompleteness. " My eyes have changed, they are no longer attached to the orbits, they make me look like a Japanese. They make me look stupid ; they annoy me." In addition to such visual troubles, the patients often have severe pains in the nape of the neck or in the front of the neck. Some observers are inclined to regard these pains in the nape from which asthenopes suffer as dependent upon disturbances of the visual centre in the cortex, or (more plausibly) as due to a stagnation of blood in the lateral sinus. I think a simpler supposition is that they depend upon stiffness of the muscles of this region. We may recall, in this connexion, the intimate association of the movements of the neck and the nape of the neck with the movements of the eyes during fixation. The disturbance affects the whole system of the organs connected with the visual tendencies.

In many cases, such depressions appearing as localised affections of a certain group of tendencies manifest themselves after an excessive functioning of the tendencies in question. In Emma, asthenopia began to trouble her for the first time after she had been doing book-keeping for long hours by artificial light. But, sometimes, such localised depressions show themselves as a sequel of fatigues which have no special bearing upon the affected tendency. Thus, Emma was liable to suffer from a recurrence of asthenopia after a long journey, after a party, and so on. This fact is apt to make the diagnosis rather perplexing at times, for although some specific exhaustion may have been the original cause of the trouble, the real starting-point is not always obvious.

In none of the cases we have just been considering had the patient any obsession or any phobia of fatigue. Until the matter had been pointed out to them, they were quite unaware that fatigue had anything to do with their relapses. There is no warrant, therefore, for explaining their symptoms as due to a fixed idea of fatigue. It was the medical adviser, studying the attacks of depression and the circumstances under which they arose, who was able to realise that the essential trouble was an incapacity to activate certain tendencies, this incapacity having been induced by a too prolonged activation of the same tendencies. It was obvious that, mutatis mutandis, the symptoms were akin to the phenomena which generally pass by the name of fatigue.

Thus depression in neuropaths, if we consider its apparent causes, would seem to be quite as closely akin to fatigue as it is to emotion. Besides, have we any right to contrast the two mechanisms of fatigue and emotion ? It may be said that, in the case of fatigue, the symptoms appear to come on after the performance of the action ; whereas, in the case of emotion, they appear to arise at an earlier stage, and even to hinder the performance of the action. This formulation is not perfectly correct ; the subjects begin to react at the moment when the emotioning circumstance makes its appearance. The movements, the efforts, the disbursements of energy, are considerable, because we are concerned with a weighty circumstance which evokes potent tendencies. Owing to the nature of the initial event, that of the conditions under which it occurs, and that of the antecedent condition of the subject (lack of preparation, prior depression, etc.), the reactions are unsuccessful, and induce nothing more than derivations and agitations of all kinds. Even after the initial event is over and done with, the subject, discontented with the lack of equilibrium, continues his efforts throughout a certain period of incubation, with the result that ere long he becomes more or less completely exhausted. I have already had occasion to point out that the origin of the emotional disturbance is fundamentally akin to that of the disturbance known as fatigue.[1] In both cases alike, the depression arises as a sequel of an expenditure of force necessitated by action, whether correct or incorrect. We cannot deny the accuracy of the views of those who maintain that there is good ground for comparing the depression of neuropathic patients with phenomena akin to those of fatigue.

4. Exhausting Actions.

In our study of psychopathic disorders, we shall find it very useful to know exactly what kinds of action are exhausting. In a household budget, we are careful to ascertain what articles are cheap and what articles are dear, what kinds of work are expensive and what kinds of work are inexpensive ; this knowledge enables us to adapt expenditure to income. But we are unable to balance the budget of our mental activity because our ideas of the price we shall have to pay for this or that kind of action are so exceedingly vague. Ordinarily this does not matter much, for people in good health almost always have a superabundance of mental and moral energy to meet the expenditure they are called upon to make. But

[1] Cf. Rapport sur le problème psychologique de l'émotion, " Revue Neurologique," December 30, 1909.

invalids are impoverished persons, and to them, therefore, it is of vital importance that they should know what they are spending.   Dejerine is right when he says that the acts accompanied by emotion are the most depressing.   This is not because emotion is a cause of depression, but because emotion is itself depression.   Actions attended by emotion are difficult and costly.   In some persons they induce rapid depression during the very course of the action which passes by the name of emotion ; and in other cases they induce delayed depression, which appears when the action is over, and passes by the name of fatigue.   We always come back to the same question. What are the actions which, in the neuropath, induce exhaustion, and are therefore followed by profound depression ?

Generally speaking, this is difficult to ascertain, for we do not know enough about the mental condition of each patient, about the previous acquirements thanks to which custom has made this or that action comparatively easy, about the disposition in which he approaches one action or the other.   We can merely speak in general terms.   The first and most obvious point is that, in many respects, the circumstances of life remain the same from generation to generation, so that one generation after another is faced by the same problems, by a demand for the same difficult actions, which, in innumerable cases, lead to a break-down and to mental disorder.   There has been good reason for the classification sometimes adopted by those who have spoken of the malady of the first communion, the malady of the betrothal, the malady of the honeymoon, or the mother-in-law malady.   The doctor must not consider it beneath his dignity to study such environing circumstances.   Here I can only classify them crudely, but I am quite certain that in days to come they will be classified with extreme care.

The First Communion.—In a great many subjects, the first manifestations of neurosis occur between the ages of twelve and fourteen, when the puberal development is lowering the powers of resistance.   They are apt to take a mystical form because this is also the period of life at which children's attention is concentrated upon religious practices on the occasion of the first communion.   Now there arises a mania for repeating prayers, a mania for perfection, a phobia of hell, and, in precocious children, an obsession of sacrilege.   Girls of no more than fifteen think that they have conceived by the Holy Ghost, and will tremble as they turn round to look at what they have passed after straining a little at stool, " in terror that there may be a living being there." These disturbances may be restricted to religious actions, but in this form may persist indefinitely. Wyx., a woman of forty-nine, is still terrified when she has to prepare for communion. " It is just as it was when I was only fourteen. I cannot help thinking at this moment that the Eucharistic union merges into corporal union; I cannot hear any one speak of St. Joseph without thinking of the most horrible things; when I want to perform religious actions, I lapse into obscenity. It has been so all my life."

The Entry into Life.—Usually, neurotic and psychological troubles begin somewhat later, and the majority of neuroses and psychoses have started, almost unnoticed, between the ages of seventeen and nineteen. Here is an example. Cq. (m., 22) has had disorders of action since he was eighteen. By nature he is slow in his movements, but the slowness has become exaggerated; he can never perform an action at the suitable time; he never finishes an action, no matter how simple it may be; he does not complete his toilet, and if he cuts his nails he pares seven and leaves the other three untouched. Gradually he has dropped all the work in which he had previously been interested, has given up his studies, his music, and his reading. Finally, he has reached a stage when he cannot perform even the simplest actions; he demands that some one shall dress him, for he can no longer do so himself. His intellectual powers seem to be unaffected, and he gives an admirable explanation of all he feels. " The fact is that when I try to do anything I am troubled, ill at ease; the action appears to me to be ridiculous, repugnant, and above all, irreligious. I get morally fatigued; and the fatigue which comes over me is an ugly fatigue; it is accompanied by hatred, by mockery, by a longing to scoff at everything. . . . At such moments, no kindly thoughts ever enter my mind, I jeer at things that have a right to our respect; I loathe the things which I previously loved and admired; I seem to be possessed by a demon of revolt. . . . When I am putting on my necktie I feel as if I were doing a criminal act, as though

God did not wish me to put on my necktie, and as if I were doing so in order to provoke him. . . . I cannot perform actions so long as I have a feeling of hostility to the commandments of God. . . . Of course all this must sound absurd; but these feelings are very hard to bear. . . ."

In this case we have to do with a typical state of depression accompanied by a feeling of falling into sin; the state arises as soon as any prolonged effort is made, and it bears in its train obsessions of sacrilege. Similar exhaustion occurred in a young man of a timorous disposition. "My fatigue," he said, "began while I was trying to do something difficult; it started while I was hesitating as to whether certain religious and moral beliefs were to be retained or thrown aside. It is so tiring to cogitate about life, about one's career, about the world which one cannot avoid seeing and which one hates. . . . I am so afraid of thinking!"—Another sufferer, Céline (f., 32), said to me: "At the age of seventeen, I noticed for the first time that I could think; this was such a painful discovery that I could have wished never to do so again."—Myvc. (m., 26) told me that it was because at the age of seventeen he had come to realise that he had to live and to think, that he became "so clumsy" and did "such silly things."—The transition from childhood to youth not only makes extensive demands upon our physical organism, because of the bodily changes that occur at puberty in connexion with the development of the reproductive functions; the transition likewise necessitates important and difficult moral adaptations. At that time we are simultaneously faced by all the problems of life, of love, and of religion, etc., they often press harshly upon us; as a result of trying to solve them we are assailed by that "fear of life" which is so frequently observed in the early stage of mental diseases in young people.

Social Functions, College life, Examinations.—Later on, when the young people have to attend social functions, and when they go to college, fresh causes for trouble arise. Illnesses due to shyness and timidity are well known to be occasioned by difficulty of adaptation to social claims. Myvc., in especial, a characteristically shy person of twenty-three, dares go nowhere, and cogitates about the world "which is not as it should be"; he muses upon the "indefiniteness of life," a life he would gladly escape from. " I am at one and the same time too young and too old, I have not got the interests which ordinary young men have. . . . Oh, if only I could go and live in a desert island, like Robinson Crusoe ! "

Others are depressed by scholastic work, they are frightened of college and examinations.—Wkq. (m., 19) falls ill while he is attending college ; a task to perform, a lesson to learn, an essay to write, and he is overwhelmed ; as soon as he endeavours to fix his attention, he is stopped by all sorts of queer tics, by mental ruminations concerning religious scruples ; each attempt to accomplish the task leaves him more depressed and more abulic.—Ned. (m., 19) is an extraordinary example of the " retrogression " so characteristic of psychasthenics. He is unable to attend the lectures on philosophy because he feels as though he had not properly completed his course of rhetoric ; he now wishes to read the books which should have been read during the previous course, saying : " I cannot enter upon a new task before having completed the preceding one."—Lba. (m., 22) suffers from discouragement, from crises of fear, from erythrophobia. The reason is that he has not adapted himself to university life, though he distinguished himself at his matriculation. He dreads speaking to the professors or to his fellow-students ; he cannot order his work or prepare for his examinations ; above all he cannot follow the lectures. He thinks too deeply and too slowly ; he stops to master a phrase, and cannot then understand the following phrase ; he is at a loss if the professor passes from one subject to another ; he is inordinately alarmed by short lapses of attention, by momentary periods of mental confusion : " I must understand instantly or never, of this I am convinced." Such initial troubles, which are due to his work, lead to phobias and obsessions.

Rest, Holidays.—It is amazing to find that holidays give rise to numerous troubles : many of these young people are more ill after a month's holiday than during term time. The reason is not far to seek. Rest itself, and amusement, do not entail an absence of action ; on the contrary they are specific actions, and necessitate special adaptations. Many persons are less capable of resting than of working. They complain of not being able to put up with having nothing to do ; they do not know what to be at ; they are bored ; and they become depressed because they are incompetent to perform the special actions which go by the name of "inaction." Dupuis, in an article entitled *Le moindre effort en psychologie*, which appeared in the " Revue Philosophique " (1911, vol. ii, p. 164), writes most interestingly upon this matter. " She cannot bear leisure. Reverie, in which her thoughts wander at haphazard, is a veritable torture to her. A task to perform, a precise object upon which to rivet attention, serve her as a defence against the inner void. She is not strong enough to live without having something to do." Our observation of Noémi (f., 30) confirms Dupuis' remarks. This patient suffers from frequent crises of depression, which she herself says are heralded by an inability to rest : " I cannot relax, even for a moment relax ; I cannot loaf."

Holidays nowadays are, besides, the occasion of an upheaval in our lives : they entail a journey, and a change of dwelling-place for parents and children alike. Travel, which used to be considered a cure for neuroses, must be looked at askance ; very often it makes matters worse, for the change of place and of people, the feeling of aloofness from familiar surroundings, makes claims on the powers of adaptation to a new environment, and demands an expenditure of courage which fatigues those suffering from psychasthenia. How often have I been told by such patients, that a journey is only pleasant after the return home, and in retrospect : " While I was travelling, I was anxious, and seemed only half alive." These patients are alarmed even before the start. " Oh dear," moans Pepita every year when July comes round, " I shall have to go to the country to visit Mother, take the children to see her, meet my brother-in-law. What a lot of trouble to put up with. Besides, what on earth can I find to do there ? I'm sure to eat too much and make myself ill." She seizes the opportunity to make herself ill beforehand !

Jean wishes to travel during the holidays ; he is not particularly keen, but wants to do what every one else does. It is obvious that the lad is incapable of making any journey by himself ; he does not even know which countries it would be suitable for him to visit ; he does not know what luggage to take ; he cannot buy a railway ticket ; and so on. He fails at the very start, for the so-called preparations for the journey bring about a recrudescence of his manias and his anxiety. His failure to carry out the plan aggravates his illness, and every year, in July, he has a serious relapse on account of this famous holiday journey.

Nervous symptoms engendered by travelling are legion. Many a person who has been in perfect health while remaining at home has become a prey to serious depression because he has been sent on " a pleasure trip." Gt. (m., 30) complains : " As soon as I am away from home, I become sad and doleful ; everything seems to be crumbling to pieces ; I feel as though I were wandering amid ruins and graveyards." Anna (f., 26) tells me : " When I go on my travels I can no longer understand the things around me ; I find them queer, unreal, they don't stand out in relief. It is dreadful not to know whether things exist or not, not even to know whether I myself exist." I have notes concerning ten foreigners who had been sent to Paris to rid themselves of gloomy thoughts. They were so depressed by the journey that I had to consign them to a sanatorium to undergo a rest cure. The attacks of mucomembranous enteritis which so frequently occur in these cases are closely connected with the condition of nervous exhaustion. Other sufferers cannot even bear that the children should go away while they themselves stay quietly at home : " The house is never the same when the children are away. It is very disturbing not to see the customary faces round the table at meal-times. I feel quite poorly in consequence. Oh, what terrible things holidays are, to be sure ! " In many families the month of July spells relapse—but we must not be too ready to speak of periodic disorders.

The Occupation, the Household.—The profession or trade by which an individual earns a livelihood is responsible for so many mental disorders that such troubles have come to be known as " occupational psychoses." I need not dwell on the obsessions and phobias to which lawyers, doctors, dressmakers, or barbers, are liable to succumb. But the disorders are not always as specific as these ; they may be quite commonplace, and yet they arise out of the particular occupation of the patient. —Mca. (f., 24), when suffering from one of her crises of sadness and despair, has the strange mania of pulling out her hair and eating it ; her illness is due to her having been taken from her country home and placed in service in Paris.[1]—Nebo. (m., 40) becomes a prey to a mania of doubt, and to a craze for making good resolutions, because he has to manage his parents' business.—Ej. (f., 21) becomes abulic and full of doubts, cannot perform any action without beginning it anew an indefinite number of times, nor is she able to take a step forward without taking one backward as well ; she has a mania for looking at herself in the glass (a very frequent trouble among those suffering from depression). This mania she explains in the following way : " All the time I feel as though I were disappearing, getting lost ; I look at myself just once more so that I may find myself still there." Her troubles were due to the fact that her father had given her the situation of cashier in his shop.—Wkx. (m., 29), whenever he has a rush of work, feels that his hands are becoming queer, " as if they do not belong to me. . . . Anguish of soul overwhelms me, an interior anxiety, poignant scruples of conscience, a weight like lead which crushes the soul, and spreads all over the world, which seems to suffer and to die. . . . The men walking about in the street no longer appear to be alive ; they are shades, mannikins, and one is surprised to find that they have a nose and eyes."—Lbf. (m., 33) has tried his hand at all kinds of trades : commerce, soldiering, medicine ; " but nothing succeeds, I am filled with despair."—Francis (m., 25) goes one better. Having been made a corporal while serving in the army, he is distracted at the idea of having to issue commands ; he deliberately absents himself without leave and does not return for four days in order that he may be degraded ; he has a fixed idea that he must have his stripes removed ; finally he is court-martialled. Subsequently, in spite of his talents, he is unable to remain more than a few weeks in any of the commercial houses in which he finds a situation for himself. He is shy and proud ; he fancies at every turn that he is being slighted ; he commits a host of blunders ; he ends by running away, and knows not whither he is going.

The ordering and guiding of home affairs is, for many, and especially for women, a serious avocation. It gives rise to all kinds of troubles. I have often described women who fall into profound depression because they have to look for a new maid, or because they have to arrange the daily bill of fare.

[1] Cf. Les obsessions et la psychasthénie, 1903, vol. ii, p. 232.

Family life, reciprocal adaptation of the persons who compose a household, resembles the adaptations which have to be made in the occupations by which people earn their livelihood. I am of opinion that such adaptation and failure of adaptation are of deep significance to mental medicine. But the difficulties arising from a clash of character among persons living together in the same house, and the mental troubles resulting therefrom, will be studied in the next chapter when we are considering treatment by isolation. Let it suffice for the present to say that a serious and difficult mental labour is requisite to enable persons to become adapted to those who form the family circle. To be able to live on satisfactory terms with the persons constituting the home, with parents, friends, etc., is a fine art. Failures in this respect are responsible for most mental disorders.

Changes in Environment.—The difficulties arising out of the profession, trade, or domestic life, are as nothing, however, to those engendered by a change in the way the patients earn a livelihood or by a change in the home surroundings. I could write a whole treatise on the pathology of house-moving, so amazing and serious are the illnesses brought on by such an upheaval of the home. I will content myself with recording a few cases in which disorders were due to such changes in environment.

A man of sixty, who has, it is true, always been abulic and a sufferer from obsessive doubts, became very seriously ill as a sequel to a change of domicile ; he fell into a state of depression which lasted two years, and which transformed his obsessions into delusions.—A woman, forty-six years of age, has a fit of depression simply because her flat has been redecorated and the furniture arranged somewhat differently. She explains the matter thus : " I was frightened about it even before the painters set to work, and that made me feel quite ill. First of all I was agitated, and then I became a prey to sadness and dread."

In three cases I have observed such symptoms as claustrophobia and obsessive ideas of sacrilege, following upon a removal ; either a transference of the home from Paris to the country, or merely a change of district in the town where the patient resides. One will regret his comfortable bachelor life in Paris and the easy access to recreations of all sorts in the metropolis, which are not to be had in the provinces ; another is furious because he has to take a tram in order to reach " the pleasant and really live part of the town where I can enjoy myself." Such persons have always been slow to adapt themselves to their environment, tardy in acquiring new habits. " Exile has uprooted me," they will grumble ; " a change like this is bad at my age." The disruption of the life they had got accustomed to, the fruitless endeavours to acquire new habits both of behaviour and in the manner of taking their pleasures, cause repeated depressions and colour their whole life with sadness and shame. Add to this the association of ideas, the memory of the sorrowful days when they could not satisfy their desires, the repressions, symbolic manias, and declamatory manias—and the picture is complete. " How miserable I felt : I could not have a really fine emotion even in the church at Lourdes ; in spite of myself, I had an impulse to defile an old priest and to rape a descendant of Bernadette. Oh, it was disgusting ! To feel one was both foul and mad ! "

A change of profession, or, indeed, even a slight modification in the way of carrying on the profession, demands a change in behaviour, and inevitably leads to troubles in these persons whose powers of action are impaired.[1]—The headmistress in a girl's boarding-school is changed : why should this affect the porter's wife, a woman of thirty-one, whose position is no whit altered by the change of head ? " Oh, but I shall be seeing a new headmistress, who will not be so friendly with me : I shall have to greet her differently . . . ; perhaps she will draw up new rules ; perhaps she will go by my lodge at a different hour. . . . It's dreadful ! " The unhappy woman can no longer sweep the yard, does not know when to get up in the morning, suffers from anxiety, has delusions of persecution, and is finally reduced to spending three months in hospital.—Then there is the case of Lvy., a man who had worked as head clerk in a bank until he had turned forty, and had fulfilled his duties admirably. The bank manager died and my patient got a rise, which naturally entailed greater responsibility. He could not bear the change and became affected with severe melancholic depression, no trace of any

[1] Cf. Les obsessions et la psychasthénie, vol. i, p. 517.

symptom of the sort having been observed in him before.—
Even in sanatoria where life is, or should be, monotonous, the
patients have serious relapses sometimes simply because they
are moved to another ward, or because they are given a new
nurse.

During the war there were frequent and terrible changes of
situation and of profession, and these changes often became
the starting-point of very serious neuroses. " I am uprooted,"
says the unhappy victim ; " I have been hurled too suddenly
into a life which is completely different from that to which I
am accustomed."—Rkb. (m., 33) is distraught at the idea that
he will have to present himself again for medical examination,
that he may be roughly dragged from his present occupation
and put to do absolutely different work : his symptoms are,
great anxiety, with crises of suffocation and polypnoea.—
Daniel (m., 41), who has for three months carried out his
duties as officer with courage and distinction, is distracted,
not by the risks he is running (which he faces without emotion),
not by his work, but by the difficulty he finds in adapting himself to a social environment so different from the one he is
accustomed to. " I am bewildered, off my orbit, ' unwedged '
so to speak, because I am away from home, because I pine
unless I am in familiar surroundings, unless I am in places
which are peopled with memories. Otherwise I seem to be
off my balance. . . ." He is perpetually assailed with scruples
and doubts. " They expect me always to display presence of
mind. I cannot understand a command ; I am haunted by
the fear of not being able to carry it out, and by the thought of
the terrible consequences which my incapacity may entail for
others and for myself. . . . The dread of not being able to
keep cool-headed, the dread that all my faculties might suddenly and simultaneously fail me, overwhelm me with distress
and despair. . . . I tremble and shudder before a superior
officer : to be subject to an authority which is blind and deaf,
a poor will-less creature like myself to be at the tender mercy
of persons who expect us to act to the very limit of human
capacity, who can demand what they like and for as long as
they like ; . . . and I have always been so weak and so sensitive ! This situation is a veritable martyrdom ; it is a deep
and poignant anguish which is becoming more acute day by
day. I am like a dog which has lost its master. . . . And

this ghastly illness is understood by no one, and excites no pity." The total lack of intelligence which is part of all rigid discipline, and failure to adapt himself to military life, have played havoc with a man who knows neither how to command nor how to obey, and yet has been placed in an environment where one must always command or obey. He exhausts himself by excessive enthusiasm for his work ; he does not know how to get others to help him, nor does he wish that others should help him ; he dreads the rapid changes to which he may not be able to adapt himself quickly enough ; he cannot live peacefully from day to day because of the perpetual alarms of active service : " Nothing is ever settled in the profession of arms ! "

Quarrels, Dangers.—Quarrels in the family circle or in the occupational circle, fights, litigation, all are responsible for serious upheavals. Ub. (m., 44) appears to be suffering from a very simple form of obsession and phobia. " I am afraid of contracting an illness which will prevent me from passing water easily and when I please." He has a dread that he will get a stricture, which will necessitate the use of a catheter : " This would be the acme of torture." There is absolutely no reason to think that such an illness is likely to afflict him ; we have merely to do with a hypochondriacal obsession. The patient's condition, however, was sufficiently serious to necessitate his staying in a sanatorium, and his illness lasted two years. Who could have believed that all this was the outcome of a family quarrel ? He had had to go to law with his brother who was his partner in business. The worry, the long waiting, the insomnia caused by the law-suit, resulted in depression followed by a mania of pollakiuria. These symptoms gradually became localised on to a deep-rooted fear which had arisen during childhood.

If I had not already done so elsewhere, I might enumerate all the cases in which the patient has been upset by a quarrel with a friend, or by an unpleasantness with a servant or the house porter. " I cannot live if I feel that there is some one in my evironment who does not care for me ! " Most hypochondriacal neuroses develop because of the dread of an illness, real or imagined, against which it will be necessary to fight.

The Death of near Kin.—I need not adduce here any new instances of disorders arising in consequence of the death of near kin. Such cases are numberless, and I have myself already analysed a great many of them. It will be well, however, in this connexion, to draw attention once more to a basic psychological fact. The disorders vaguely described as being due to the emotion caused by moral suffering, are really induced by the same mechanism as the disorders we have just been considering. The death of a near relative modifies the subject's environment, renders many of his extant tendencies futile and checks their activity, introduces him into a new situation which imperiously demands new adaptations. What we call " emotions due to the death of near kin " are really disorders in this work of adaptation. I made this analysis elsewhere in Irène's case ; [1] I could easily repeat it in the case of a great many other patients. I shall content myself with one example of a very different kind.

Zoé (f., 26), who has inherited from her father an infirmity of will, and has always been restless and undecided, suddenly loses her mother. At first she behaves well and bravely, but in reality she is already abnormal. She does not feel any distress, is very restless, receives and pays too many calls, neglects her child, and so on. After five or six weeks, she becomes affected with rather severe depression, and has all kinds of obsessions. She suffers markedly from a peculiar phenomenon to which I may give the name of " attachment." In connexion with minor happenings she will try to perform some particular action, and will not succeed very well. Thereupon, her mind will become attached, so to say, upon this happening, and upon regret for her failure to perform the action properly. She will not be able to get away from the idea. " This morning I wanted something, and I asked some one to give it me. It was a great step that I should have had a definite wish, for I am now indifferent to everything. If only what I wanted had been brought to me at once, I should have been greatly moved, I should have been able to shed tears, and I should have been instantly cured. What a pity that no one would listen to me this morning ! " She will go

---

[1] L'amnésie et la dissociation des souvenirs par l'émotion, " Journal de Psychologie Normale et Pathologique," September 1904 ; L'état mental des hystériques, second edition, 1911, p. 507.

on repeating this phrase in various tones hundreds of times every hour all through the day. She can do nothing else, and does not know what is going on around her, for her mind has been attached firmly upon this incident of the morning, and she cannot get beyond it. The same thing will happen in the case of all kinds of trifling occurrences. Once, Zoé's mind was attached by such a futile regret for as long as six weeks. Herein we see one of the ways in which an obsession may arise, for there are various mechanisms competent to produce obsessions. For two years this patient remained in a condition of serious depression due to the exhaustion that ensued after her mother's death.

Betrothal, Marriage.—The disorders arising out of the various incidents of the sexual life are just as common and just as serious as those we have been considering. In my other writings I have frequently described the disorders brought about, towards the age of seventeen or eighteen, by the mental changes that occur as a sequel to the puberal development—by the appearance of new desires, by the revelation of sex, by seduction, sexual excess, etc. I must stress once more the illnesses that arise in connexion with betrothal and with marriage, for here the part played by disorders of action is extremely characteristic. In all the psychoses which may occur in connexion with betrothal, we see, on the one hand, secondary or derivative phenomena, such as obsessions, physical or moral agitation, and anxiety ; and, on the other, hesitation, indecision, vacillation, as regards the contemplated action. The patients and the members of their families are almost always inclined to explain the phenomena of the second order by the phenomena of the first order, and to say that the illness and the obsessions are the cause of the hesitancy. I have tried to show that this view is erroneous, and that vacillation is the primary trouble.—Lym. (m., 27) passes all his time in breaking off relationships with the mistress of whom he has to rid himself before he marries, and then lapsing into the old relationship.—Cht. (f., 22) will alternately write love letters to her affianced, and letters breaking off the engagement.—In most cases, this vacillation expresses itself in the form of an inward conversation. X. is continually repeating to himself that his betrothed is perfect and that he

adores her ; and then that she has a harsh expression of countenance which he will never be able to put up with.—A few
years before her mother's death, Zoé (f., 22) had suffered for
more than a year from a serious crisis of mental depression,
accompanied by extreme emaciation and various other
symptoms, the exciting cause having been that she had been
asked in marriage by a young man with whom she was in love
and whose proposal she had long been expecting. " The proposal has come too late, has come at a bad time, when I no
longer know whether I care for him or not." Sometimes she
was sure that she was devoted to him, and that he suited her
in every respect ; sometimes she was sure that she loathed
him and might feel inclined to stab him.—The vacillations of
these patients disclose the insufficiency of some particular
form of action, betray the slowness or the lack of a specific
kind of reaction that is demanded by circumstances. Here,
again, we have to do with depression through exhaustion. If
the act of the betrothal has been properly carried out, the
marriage will be effected without much difficulty. This is
what happened in Zoé who, having at first been very ill at the
time of her engagement, got better, and then married without
any disturbance. But it is well to know that, as a rule,
marriage may be brought to pass by the pressure of the
families concerned rather than by the action of the two prin-
cipals, and that in the latter case these have really remained
inactive. That explains how it is that in certain subjects
there has been very little disturbance during the period of
betrothal, or the disturbance during this period has been
mastered, and yet serious illness may arise after marriage, and
occasionally a long while after.—In one woman, this crisis of
indecision was deferred for six years. She had already had
three children when she finally acknowledged that she was still
hesitating to accept her husband for good and all. " I must
really make up my mind if he is the man whom I am marrying
for good and all. The decision has been so difficult for me, and
I have continually been putting it off. I was simply passive
in my engagement, in the civil marriage, and in the religious
marriage. When living with him, I have been hesitant and
uneasy, saying to myself that I would make up my mind later.
This has always made me unhappy and ill ; now I can bear the
uncertainty no longer."

Furthermore, marriage renders indispensable the performance of specific actions which are superadded to the actions which have preceded the marriage, and these may entail special disorders. First of all, in marriage, comes the bodily sexual act. Now, this is not an undifferentiated sexual act, but a sexual act under specific conditions with a particular person, and we must not suppose that these details are matters of indifference. A man who has been fully equal to the occasion with his mistress, will not necessarily be equal to the occasion with his wife. On the other hand, there are married women who suffer from incurable vaginismus when the husband attempts intercourse, while there is no trouble of the kind when they have intercourse with a lover. Thus it is that in connexion with a specific sexual relationship, both in men and in women, there may occur spasms, contractures, anxieties, phobias, scruples, delusions of all kinds. Think, for instance, of the strange feelings and remarkable scruples that occur in men and women who believe that they are abnormal, and who reproach themselves bitterly because they have married without love. Think, too, of those who, instead of blaming themselves, blame the sexual partner.—" My wife is too cold ; she makes me so nervous that I'm no good."—" I might as well have a dead woman in my arms ; she terrifies me."—" She must be badly formed, must be abnormal in some way."—Such a man will make his wife consult doctor after doctor in the hope that an abnormality may be discovered and rectified.

In many instances, such delusions may become very serious, and the doctor must on no account ignore them. The case of a young married woman aged twenty-six was characteristic in this respect. Lo. had long been psychasthenic, complaining that she lived perpetually in a dream state and that she suffered from a dread of life. Her relatives, influenced by the absurd notion that marriage is a cure for neurosis, were imprudent enough to arrange a marriage for her. During the period of betrothal she passed through a phase of excitation, and was believed to have been thoroughly cured. But just before the marriage, she grew uneasy once more. On the wedding night, she became affected with fears and anxieties, and, finally, almost crazy, she ran away to her parents' home. A serious condition of depression ensued, with crises of obsessions, and this lasted for months. It is probable that any further attempts at sexual relationships would have had even more disastrous results, but fortunately for her a divorce was arranged. In three cases I have seen these matrimonial phobias grow worse owing to persistence of the exciting cause, so that grave delusions have ensued, and the patients have had to be put under restraint.

In all cases of this kind the inadequacy of the sexual act is obvious. There has either been complete impotence ; or coitus has been incomplete, unattended by pleasure, and not terminated by a relaxation of tension. These cases afford good examples for the study of the mechanism of the disorders that ensue when action is inadequate. But in other instances, matters seem less simple, for the physical act of intercourse appears to have been correctly performed, and nevertheless kindred disturbances ensue. In this case we have to do with inadequacy of another kind of action, with an imperfect mental adaptation to the new type of domestic life. This maladaptation, which is just as important in its consequences as inadequacy of the physical sexual act, has seldom received sufficient attention. I have in my notebooks the reports of a score of remarkable cases in which young men or young women became affected with serious psychasthenic disorders within a few months of marriage. The symptoms from which these patients suffered were very varied. Some of them were affected with morbid doubts : " I cannot make up my mind whether I love him or hate him." Others had phobias, like the strange case in which a man had a terror of his wife's eyes. Others, again, were afflicted by obsessions. A wife was obsessed with jealousy " of the blond mistresses whom my husband must certainly have had before marriage." A husband was obsessed with the thought " of my father-in-law's political opinions, so different from those which have always been cherished in our family." A wife was obsessed with the idea that her marriage was a disgrace to her because, before marriage, her husband had made " a sacrilegious communion." These cases are not so different as they may seem at first sight. In all alike, the basic disorder is the depression caused by a struggle with a difficult moral situation. The effort of adaptation to the partner's character, the organisation of a certain amount of intimacy, and the resultant exhaustion, are, I think, the starting-point of all these disturbances, which are as common as they are strange.

Such moral difficulties are further complicated by the material, pecuniary, and social difficulties with which young married people have to contend. Dm. (f., 30) had for years to defend her husband against his own parents, help him to get on in his profession, and organise the household under difficult conditions. Not until success was assured, not until she was no longer sustained by the excitation of the struggle, did she succumb to fatigue. Then she became sluggish, indifferent, incapable alike of rest and of activity, and crazed by the thought of all that she had to do. Depression and obsession supervened upon the exhaustion induced by prolonged struggle and effort.

These examples, which I have rapidly summarised, may enable the reader to understand how the moral and material organisation of a household must be regarded as a very difficult and extremely exhausting form of activity, and will account for the fact that it plays a considerable part as an exciting cause of neuroses.

Separations.—Whilst marriage may be a cause of illness, it must not be supposed that the closure of marital relationships is an indifferent matter. The death of one member of a married pair may cause disorders akin to those which we have described as occurring after the death of near kin. Every one must have seen instances of the kind. " I have spent fifteen years in getting used to my wife, and now, when it has become impossible for me to get on without her for a moment, she takes it into her head to die and to leave me alone. I do call it a shame ! " Acts of infidelity, the sharing of affection, secret amours, entail numerous complications, difficulties, and vacillations, resulting in all sorts of disorders. " How am I to choose between my husband and my lover ? My husband is an idler, a good-for-nothing, a fool, and a brute ; my lover is a splendid fellow, and one who would commit any crime for my sake. But my husband is useful to me ; he is well off ; I should miss him, should not know how to get on without him, for he has always arranged everything for me. Yet how can I break with my lover, who will very likely kill himself if I do so ? And what am I to do about my little girl ; how can I leave her ? "

What intense despair, how much illness of a depressive character, ensues when liaisons are broken off. " All my religious sentiments had become centred in him ; he was my god. Our very souls were intertwined, and we shared all our ideals. I have always needed to combine veneration with my love, and to feel that I was myself the object of passionate desire. What on earth am I to do now ? How can I go on living without marks of tenderness without ecstasy, without having some one to whom I can say, ' You are my ivory Christ ' ? " After such ruptures, it is necessary to relearn how to live alone, and for this a difficult process of adaptation is requisite ; or else a new intimacy must be established, and this may be an arduous task. A divorced woman of great intelligence was well aware that hard work would be necessary if she were to escape from her depression. " To construct a new life, to build up new loves—how easy to talk about, and how difficult to achieve ! People hardly seem to realise that love involves effort. To please, to effect a conquest, to keep what one has conquered, to act in a love relationship, need effort, need the overcoming of scruples, doubts, weariness, disheartenment. If this effort is to be clad in pleasure, if happiness is to convert effort into additional joy, the excitation must be greater than the effort. If I remain solitary although I have so keen a longing for affection, it is because the recognition of this effort of which I have spoken deters me from action."

The Education of Children, Old Age.—Hardly has the new household been established, when fresh difficulties arise. Even when sexual relationships are legalised, the first signs of pregnancy may entail multifarious troubles and all kinds of anxiety. " I find this pregnancy most annoying. My husband's relatives are delighted, and it humiliates me so to please people whom I loathe." And when pregnancy is clandestine, when a pretence must be kept up that it does not exist, or when secret attempts to procure abortion have to be made, neuroses are very apt to ensue. But pregnancy is a cause of vital excitation which counteracts the before-mentioned depressing influences, and for that reason neurosis is comparatively rare in the later months of pregnancy. Moreover, in this situation as in others, time works wonders. As the months pass and pregnancy advances, the relatives have time to accept the situation, which means that they learn to adapt themselves to it.

Childbirth and lactation may give rise to exhaustion, and may thus induce a number of neuropathic symptoms. Then, as children grow up, other causes of depression come into play, for the upbringing of children is a difficult and responsible matter. Many young mothers are almost crazy at the thought that they have injured or may injure the baby ; they are tormented by the fancy that they may drown the baby in its bath or may drop it into the copper. Side by side with these ridiculous fancies, we may find either in the father or in the mother symptoms of mental disorder of a more serious kind, likewise due to the exhaustion resulting from the responsibilities of parenthood.—" I have always been timid on my own account," says Zbs. (m., 42). " Now I have transferred my terrors to my unhappy children, and find myself imagining that they will be buried alive. . . . Sometimes I cannot perform the simplest action, such as going to have my hair cut, without thinking that this may have a ghastly repercussion upon those whom I love."—Daniel (m., 40) pushes this to an extreme. He is persistently tortured by the thought of his responsibilities as a parent. He is alarmed by the least stroke of good fortune, for he thinks that he may have to pay for this by a death in the family ; he dares not make any plans, for these may irritate some occult power and bring ill luck upon his children. The craze checks his activities in all sorts of ways. " I had ordered some shirts, and then, absurd as it was, I had to countermand them, being troubled by the thought that I should be wearing them some day when I should have an accident. I can't even read any more. Directly I open a book, the thought seizes me that something dreadful may happen to my children, and I am overwhelmed with sadness. I try to make a fresh start in my reading, and to sustain my mind with ideas of confidence and hope. Thus I may spend a whole evening, trying vainly, again and again, to get past the two or three lines which have turned my thoughts in an unhappy direction. How shall I possibly be able to keep my household together and to bring up my children ? "

It is obvious that all the phases in the lives of children,—illness, puberty, the first communion—can readily remind parents of the problems which they themselves had to face under identical conditions ; a good many women have a crisis of over-scrupulousness at the time of their children's first communion. A still more serious incident is the marriage of the young people. I have notes of five cases in which a woman has become seriously ill on the occasion of her daughter's marriage, has become affected with a grave crisis of doubt and over-scrupulousness, this being a repetition of the illness she had had twenty years earlier on the occasion of her own marriage. I have seen the same sort of illness in men. For instance, Mce. (m., 50) had a grave crisis of depression when his daughter was married.

When the young folk set up house for themselves, fresh difficulties arise for the parents. Lox. (f., 50) is dissatisfied with her daughter-in-law and with the latter's domestic surroundings. Above all she is uneasy as to her own attitude, and as to the way in which she ought to play the part of mother-in-law. " I wish I were not so cold with her, but I can't help it. She is a stranger who has intruded into the family and has upset everything. Besides, I have to put up with visits from her parents, wearisome people whom I never knew before. What a nuisance it all is ! " In fact she is well aware that she lives in a world which is too complicated for her. She cannot understand its jokes. She hates the rapid exchange of ideas, which give her a sense of inferiority. When she has anything to say, it can only be by way of criticism, for in no other manner can she show her interest. The result has been that her son's marriage has resuscitated her fixed idea of the injustice of society, her obsession that the world is out of joint and that she must set it right.

But when the children are safely married, it does not follow that tranquillity will be restored. The parents are now isolated, and adaptation to the new conditions may be painful. Retirement from active work presents us with similar problems. Finally we have to consider all the depressions of old age. There are various causes of such depressions, but more often than people are apt to realise they depend upon the difficulties of life and action. " I can make no better job of being old than I could make of being young," said a good old fellow who had suffered all his life from timidity and mental depression.

Thus we find that in all the stages on the road of life there are steep hills to climb. On every one of these the carriage may prove too heavy for the horses.

5. EXPENDITURE DURING EXHAUSTING ACTIVITY.

This enumeration of circumstances and actions which are apt to induce exhaustion, ought to facilitate general conclusions as to the characteristics of these exhausting actions, so that it will become possible to recognise and avoid them.

No doubt the best solution of the problem would be a physiological one. What we should like to be able to do is to measure the expenditure of nervous energy, or, if the term be permissible, of " nervous fluid," in the various actions, so that the latter could be characterised quantitatively in terms of such expenditure. The authorities who follow Weir Mitchell are inclined to envisage the problem from this outlook. They speak of the exhaustion of the nerve cells, and try to formulate an anatomical and physiological theory of such exhaustion. Unfortunately, since we have no relevant anatomical and histological knowledge, and since physiological experiments bearing on the matter are entirely lacking, the theories in question are, as I have often pointed out, merely translations of psychological observations into a pseudo-scientific terminology.

Since all we are entitled to do is to describe the clinical phenomena as they present themselves, to describe them in psychological terms, our business is simply to discover characteristics common to all the actions that have been followed by exhaustion. The authors who propose to treat neuropaths by absolute rest in bed, would seem to act on the theory that the expenditure of energy in muscular movement is the essential cause of depression, and they declare that certain kinds of activity are dangerous precisely because of the enormous expenditure of motor energy which they necessitate. There is, of course, an element of truth in such a contention. I have myself pointed out how depression may arise after excessive motor activity, and I have referred to Tissié's description of depression in the competitors in long-distance bicycle races,

When we consider the actions considered in the foregoing pages, we may agree that undue activity, inducing excessive fatigue, contributes to the causation of a certain number of occupational depressions, and that this factor plays its part in the illness of women who exhaust themselves in their zeal for housework. In one case of depression which came under my notice, the cause seemed to have been an occupation in which the patient had to stand for several hours a day. The same sort of physical fatigue is sometimes witnessed in society life, at school, during journeys, in contests, as an outcome of sexual excess, in connexion with childbirth, in the management of young children. It is true, therefore, that bodily fatigue sometimes plays its part as a factor of disease ; it is true that the quantity, the force, and the duration of movements may contribute to exhaustion and depression.

But I do not think that such an explanation can take us very far. In 1903, I discussed a kindred hypothesis when I was trying to understand the significance of the idea of lowering of the psychological tension.[1] I asked myself whether this lowering of tension found expression in a diminution of sensation, or in a diminution of movement in the strict sense of the term. Depressed persons, apart of course from those who were suffering from cachexia, did not seem to me to have lost the physical energy of their movements simply because they were depressed. I need hardly say that it is futile to attempt a precise estimate of the energy of such patients by means of dynamometric experiments, or by ordering them to make certain movements for which an effort is requisite. Patients suffering from depression carry out such orders badly. It is futile, likewise, to record the force of their defensive movements and of their resistances. We must content ourselves with easy observations which can be made without the patient's becoming aware of what we are doing. A depressed patient whose arm will tremble when we ask him to stretch out his hand, will strike his attendants violently, or will break up the furniture, if we try to force him to eat or to put on his clothes. He will prowl about for days like a wild beast in a cage, or will shriek unceasingly for long periods. Dubois and Dejerine are fond of pointing to the contradictions in the behaviour of such patients, and make criticisms which are not always valid when

[1] Les obsessions et la psychasthénie, vol. i, p. 499.

applied to the actions of the patient, but are valid enough when applied to their movements in the restricted sense of the term.

On the other hand, it is easy to ascertain that only in quite exceptional instances does great motor expenditure, great muscular exhaustion, induce psychological depression. Numerous observations upon normal persons prove this. Simple and elementary movements will, when frequently repeated, induce fatigue ; but this fatigue comes on slowly, and it is not serious. Speaking of long-distance bicycle racers, de Fleury points out that Terront, when he had ridden a thousand kilometres in forty-two consecutive hours, must have made more than three hundred thousand thrusts with the foot. Yet there was very little sign of fatigue, for only the muscles and the spinal cord had been seriously at work. The term fatigue, says de Fleury, should be reserved for the description of cerebral and psychical phenomena.[1]

Finally, it is obvious that in a great many of the cases we have been considering there has been no sign of such exhaustion due to excessive movement. Religious exercises, society life, quarrels arising out of litigation, doubts and hesitations connected with an engagement to marry, adaptations to conjugal life—none of these things entail excessive physical fatigue. Many of my patients were exhausted by preparation for a holiday or a journey, rather than by the actual exercise on these occasions. Many of them were depressed by attempts to rest and to loaf, whereas prolonged walking was a delight to them. Change of scene and change of associates will often have more to do with the onset of depression than the real fatigues of a journey. Gt. (m., 30), who is bored to death when he sits quietly in a hotel far from Paris, is quite in his element when driving a motor car all day through the streets of the capital. The material labours of Ej. (f., 21) when acting as cashier, or those of Wkx. (m., 29) when writing a newspaper article, are not extensive. Francis was not exhausted by his work as a ranker, but the mere thought of having to issue orders to subordinates was utterly exhausting to him. The burden of responsibility is the main factor of the depression that may affect those who have charge of children, and any talk of muscular exhaustion in such cases is merely metaphorical. In a word, while we have to recognise that the quantity of move-

[1] De Fleury, Introduction à la médecine de l'esprit, 1897, p. 232.

ment may play an important part as a cause of exhaustion, it
is plain that the quality, the psychological nature, of actions,
is of even greater significance in this connexion.

The starting-point of exhaustion will be more readily
discovered from another outlook. We have to concentrate
attention upon the work of adaptation, and upon the nature
of the actions demanded of the subject by the particular
circumstances in which he is placed. When enumerating the
conditions which have led to serious disorder, it became obvious
to us that changes of environment were of considerable importance. The beginning of school life or university life,
house-moving, marriage, separations, the death of near ones
and dear ones, and the like, invariably demand adaptation to
a new situation. This adaptation necessitates the organisation
and activation of a certain number of habits. New tendencies
have to be created.

This would seem to be a stumbling-block to our patients.
They are overwhelmed by such changes, and are exhausted by
their efforts at adaptation. Even if they succeed, in the end,
in adapting themselves to the new conditions, the process takes
a very long time. Their sufferings are always the outcome of
the inadequacy of the new kinds of action requisite in the
changed environment. When a new occupation has to be
undertaken, an occupational incapacity will be manifested.—
Mca. is unable to learn her work as a servant.—Nebo., who
becomes head of a commercial concern when his father dies,
cannot acquire the habits suitable to his new occupation.
" The least among my employees is more capable than I am,
and can do well in five minutes a thing which it takes me hours
to do badly. I make unending verifications, and still fail to
be accurate. This is what wears me out."—Ej., a cashier,
hesitates indefinitely before writing a word, and keeps on
forming the letters over and over again.—Wkx. is far too timid
and conscientious to do his journalistic work with the necessary speed. He is himself aware that he cannot work as well
as his colleagues, and that the result of his trying to do better
work than they do is that he achieves nothing at all.

Incapacity to effect the necessary adaptations is likewise
the explanation of the various troubles that arise in connexion
with the organisation of new households. In some cases we

have to do with a sort of psychological impotence that arises in persons who are incapable of adapting the sexual function to a particular circumstance, to the presence of some specific person. In other cases, the trouble arises because one who has become a confirmed old bachelor or old maid marries too late in life. Kvo. married when he was sixty, and could not adapt himself to family existence.

The following case is of great psychological interest. Vy. (m., 25) became affected by severe depression with obsessions a few months after his marriage. He was tormented by the thought that his wife and his wife's relatives held political opinions differing from those which had been traditional in his own family. This worried him by day and by night, made him unable to sleep, brought on emaciation, and reduced him to the last stage of weakness and despair. " How dreadful, how disastrous, to have married a woman who holds such opinions." Though in theory he recognised that his wife's family was just as good as his own, this obsessive thought made him feel that he had dishonoured himself by marrying into it.

If we wish to understand the nature of the mental disorder in this case, we must go back a little, and must analyse the young man's character. He was intelligent, but was lethargic and infirm of will. He had always exhibited the qualities characteristic of psychasthenia. He lacked self-confidence and was continually in need of guidance and support. Like all these patients, he was ever on the look out for some one whose affection and devotion would save him the trouble of making any efforts on his own account. " I want things to be settled once for all ; I want to find some one whose affection shall be above proof, so that I can depend upon it for all time." Unfortunately, although he was an amiable fellow, he never succeeded in finding the object of his quest. Beneath a mask of boldness, he was shy, and did not know how to express his feelings or how to make himself loved. He could easily enter into social relationships of a superficial character, but took a very long time in plumbing the depths. " It takes me years and years to get used to a new acquaintance, and I never seem to become intimate with any one. Some of my friends take me into their confidence, and this is always a fresh surprise to me for I can never reciprocate." Persons of this type of character are common enough, and most doctors must be familiar with them. Vy. did not suffer much from the lack of intimacy, for he was able to console himself by an illusion. He was continually repeating to himself that some day he would marry, and that in marriage he would easily and promptly discover the complete and intimate affection of which he was in search.

He married, and his reason told him that his marriage was an excellent one ; but what a cruel disappointment was in store for him—the desired intimacy was not achieved. It must, indeed, be admitted that the wife's disposition was serious and cold, so that intimacy with her was difficult to achieve. Such difficulties are readily overcome by a person accustomed to social relationships, by one who combines a facility for the expression of his feelings with a fair amount of patience, by one who is able to understand that intimacy between two persons who, though they may love one another, know very little of one another, is a fruit which must ripen slowly. But Vy. was amazed to find that he was less intimate with his wife than with the friends of his childhood's days. He made titanic efforts to achieve intimacy, and was surprised to discover how much these efforts exhausted him. " How absurd it is ! I am positively worn out if I have a private conversation with my wife. When we spend our Sundays together alone in the country, I find the days detestable. How strange it is that I am only at my ease if I go without her to dine with my parents." The efforts and the consequent exhaustion increased his depression, intensified the need for affection and guidance, and magnified the sense of disillusionment induced by the lack of intimacy. " I suffer terribly, for I know that we are playing a comedy of love, the perpetual comedy of a non-existent gaiety and intimacy. We are living together, we are materially united, but that is all. Something essential is lacking, something which I cannot communicate to her and which she cannot communicate to me. I dreamed of a woman upon whom I should act and who would act upon me ; a woman I could console if she were sad, or a woman whose lightness of heart could comfort me if I were sad ; one between whose heart and mine there would be no barriers. But there is an insuperable barrier between us, and neither of us can influence the other. She is stiff ; she does not understand me ; she can't bear me to be playful with her. Far from being at ease with her, I have to keep watch upon my words and actions just as if I were with a stranger. It is plain to me that I cannot be guided or comforted by my wife. I shall have to go on trying to be self-sufficient and to decide everything for myself. When I have children, this will only mean that I have more decisions to make. Marriage is merely bringing burdens to me, and yet I was convinced it would free me from burdens. How wretched it makes me that we cannot lean upon one another."

The mind wants to explain itself to itself. We need, if you like to phrase it thus, an intelligible explanation of the troubles from which we suffer. Delusions, in many cases, are merely formulas, are merely symbols which give expression to an underlying disorder of activity. The more intelligent a person, the greater may be his need for delusion. No doubt a moralist would have found a simple way of describing this young man's troubles. The moralist would have said that he was timid, that he was awkward in expressing his own feelings and in inducing others to express their feelings towards him. Above all, the moralist would have said that my young friend was in too great a hurry, was too sedulously analysing a commonplace situation which time would gradually modify. But Vy. was not a trained psychologist, and he jumped to a conclusion. " I know what the trouble is. There is a radical difference between my wife and myself, a difference which will always keep us apart." His pride led him to believe that the difference was ascribable rather to some defect in his wife's family than to any inadequacy on his own part. That was the origin of his fixed idea about the political opinions of his wife and her relatives, and of the obsession that he had married beneath him.

In the cases we have just been considering, the troubles arose in connexion with the attempts to organise intimacy and to ensure new adaptations to a joint existence. In other cases, when separations, ruptures, or deaths have occurred, the problem is of an opposite kind. The subject has to learn how to live alone when a familiar companion has been removed. Lydia, as I have said, had a twin sister, from whom she had been inseparable. The two girls had always been dressed alike. Lydia had always done exactly what her sister did, so that she had become incapable of acting alone, and had never

even tried to act alone. Without taking any kind of precautions, the family arranged a marriage for the twin sister.
This came as a terrible blow to Lydia, but she tried to conceal
her distress and to accustom herself to live alone. Now the
art of living alone, of acting alone, of taking the initiative in
isolation, is an art of a very special kind, one which stands at
a high level, one which has developed slowly, and which has
played an important psychological part by becoming the
starting-point of ideas of unity and freedom. Lydia was
quite incompetent to practise this art. She had not even
learned how to sleep by herself, and she spent the whole night
rolling on the floor or sobbing in bed. Lydia did not know
how to eat unless her sister was there. She could not perform
any kind of action properly unless her sister was there, for now
her attempts at action were checked by tears, scruples, tics,
and anxieties. She speedily became affected by serious
psychasthenia, which lasted for years.

We have already learned that Zoé (f., 26) suffered from
serious disorders of the will after her mother's death. The
starting-point of her disturbances was an infirmity of action
produced by the mother's death. The patient was well aware
of what was amiss, and could herself explain it satisfactorily.
Always weakly and vacillating, she was entirely under her
mother's sway. The mother, being somewhat domineering,
had favoured the development of this tendency, and had been
in the habit of guiding all the daughter's activities. When in
good health, Zoé was able to act independently in matters of
little importance ; but she always knew that her mother was
in the background to assist her in case of need, and this gave
her confidence. She was like one of those people who have
just learned to swim, and who can keep afloat well enough for
a few strokes, provided that the pole or the boat of the swimming instructor is within easy reach. If the place of refuge
is too far away, they become frightened, and forget how to
swim. When the mother died, Zoé no longer had this permanent support, and found it necessary to organise her
behaviour along new lines. Either she must win self-
confidence, and learn to awim unaided, or else must put her
trust in some one else—must learn, for instance, to depend
upon her husband, must swim towards another boat. Either
course was difficult, and both of them were beyond her powers.

She began to splash about wildly, and was in danger of drowning. These emotional disorders, too, are illnesses due to imperfect adaptation.

This supposition is confirmed by a study of details, by the examination of special difficulties that arise in the course of an attempt at new adaptations. The *complexity of the situation* is a factor in a good many instances. In a rigidly Catholic circle, where the indissolubility of marriage is an article of faith, the position of a divorced woman is a ticklish one in any case. Now, if this woman wants, not only to maintain her respectability and to preserve the affections of her respectable intimates, but also to enjoy the fruits of illicit adventures (which, she says, are the only things that make her feel truly alive), we need not be surprised if inextricable entanglements arise, and exhaustion ensues. The case of Héloïse offers an interesting example.

Vok. (m., 27) lives with his parents and, unknown to them, has brought his mistress to a little flat quite close to his home. He wishes her to be happy, and hopes some day to make an honest woman of her. He is filled with the idea of " raising a fallen angel " ; at the same time he borrows money on all hands wherewith to pay for her caprices. His intelligence is not very strong, and all this is far too difficult for him. He worries continually, becomes incapable of action, and succumbs to a peculiar form of sub-maniac agitation which terrifies his parents and leads them to discover everything.— Similar is the case of Wkv., a girl of good family, twenty-two years of age. She has been seduced, and, unknown to her relatives, is continually going to visit her lover. Since she spends a great deal of money, she tries to tap a new source of supply by secretly acting as a nude model for a sculptor. The life is too complicated for her. Very soon she begins to suffer from exhaustion, complaining that her head feels quite empty and that everything around her has become unfamiliar. Various phobias supervene.

When we have to do with patients who are already enfeebled, trifling complications will render action dangerous. —Patients prone to enteroptosis will suffer from any form of activity which keeps them standing for hours at a time.— Daniel (m., 41) can play his part in a conversation well if he is alone with his interlocutor ; but when several persons **are** talking at once, he cannot follow the conversation properly, becomes troubled in his mind, and soon feels quite ill. I think this circumstance, trifling at first sight, has definite practical importance. I have seen the same symptom in a good many patients, and we must take it into account when we have occasion to talk to depressed persons.—Analogous is the case of Madame Z. She has to take her meals alone, for she cannot simultaneously eat and listen to some one ; she is quite upset if any one has lunch with her.—Lydia, as soon as she grows tired, can only do one thing at a time, and no longer wants any one to speak to her while she is walking.—Sophie cannot bear it when several visitors come to the house at once.—In like manner, Fn. (f., 36) dreads the happening of anything unusual at home. I am not speaking here of the manias and obsessions of such patients. We can often notice that their troubles are aggravated by some little change in the environment, even though the change is accordant with their desires, and they do not expect it will make them ill. For instance, Fn. wants her mother to pay her a visit, and feels certain the visit will do her good. But I notice that she immediately becomes affected once more by the feeling of haste, the feeling that she is wasting time, and the feeling that she makes herself a nuisance to every one ; and I know that these feelings are the prelude to one of her crises. The disturbances produced by the complexity of life are real enough, and are independent of the subject's fixed ideas.

An important factor in these cases is the *rapidity of the reaction*. In my studies of the essential symptoms of psychasthenia, I have repeatedly had occasion to insist upon the slowness with which these patients act, and I have been led to formulate the hypothesis that one of their fundamental disorders is the slowing down of the reactions by which adaptations are effected.[1] One case, in particular, taught me that the main troubles supervene when circumstances demand a rapid adaptation such as these depressed patients are incompetent to make. Wo. suffered from depression for several weeks because a pianoforte she had bought had arrived sooner than she had expected. I was surprised at the great effect produced by so slight a cause. Her own explanation of the

[1] Les obsessions et la pyschasthénie, 1903, vol. i, pp. 478 and 497.

matter was interesting. " If I had only been looking out of the window so that I could have seen the cart which was bringing the piano, if I had been able to foresee that the instrument was about to arrive, if I had only had a few moments in which to prepare for the pleasure of its coming, I should not have fallen sick. . . . If I am forewarned, when any sort of emotion is to affect me, I prepare my mind for this or that feeling, saying to myself : ' Keep quiet ; don't get into a whirl ; don't get flustered ; keep your mind fixed on what is going to happen.' . . . But when things happen unexpectedly, when they come too quickly, it makes me ill." [1] My comment on this case was that such patients are slow-minded. They need time to make a decision, time before they can fix their attention, time for the realisation of emotion ; and especially do they need this when the incident is comparatively unimportant, and one which does not arouse stimulant tendencies. If the requisite time be not forthcoming, the emotion that ensues is more or less frustrate. It is an emotion in which lower-grade phenomena predominate, and consequently depression results.[2]

These observations have recently been confirmed by L. Dupuis, who has made an interesting study of the psychology of shyness and timidity.[3] Dupuis sets out from my own idea that the emotion of timidity is a derivative of abulia, of a real social apraxia ; but he endeavours to analyse this social apraxia, and to discover what, in these persons, accounts for their essential incapacity for social activity, for their inability to perform actions when they are under observation. Owing to the extreme complexity of human behaviour, and owing to the suddenness with which changes occur, we are obliged, when one or more other persons are present, to react promptly, and we must be ready to react in all possible directions. " It is essential that the mental organism should be prepared to react rapidly. We have to find a way out at a moment's notice. The demands of self-preservation do not allow us to temporise. . . . Measures that will safeguard us cannot be put off till the next day. . . . Now, a defensive reaction can only be organised if the individual concerned is both supple

[1] Les obsessions et la psychasthénie, 1903, vol. i, p. 540. [2] Ibid., p. 541.
[3] Les stigmates fondamentaux de la timidité, " Revue Philosophique," 1915, pp. 332 and 423.

and energetic, so that he is competent to follow promptly through all their metamorphoses the spontaneity and the essential mobility of the person with whom he has to do." [1] We see, then, that the urgency which is characteristic of social reactions will be a stumbling-block in the way of those whose energies cannot be efficiently actualised, so that one whose motor elaborations are unduly slow will inevitably be a social apraxic and a timid person. To verify these hypotheses, the author illustrates by his enquiries and by the report of numerous cases " the slowness with which motor reactions are elaborated in timid persons " ; and he concludes that slowness is one of the fundamental stigmata of constitutional timidity. The symptoms of timidity are nothing more than derivative phenomena, being dependent upon the inadequacy of reaction when circumstances demand speedy reaction and the subject is incompetent to react promptly.

I think that Dupuis' inferences are perfectly sound, and that it will be well to extend them to a wider sphere than that of timidity. A great many of the disorders I have been describing have arisen because circumstances have demanded a rapid reaction of which the subject was incapable. They would not have arisen if the difficulty had presented itself less suddenly. This becomes obvious when we reexamine some of our cases in the new light.—Cq., the young man of twenty-two who became affected with strange feelings of sacrilege when he was called upon to act, was much less disturbed when there was no hurry. " It is when I am hustled that I feel that I must be provoking God."—Lba. (m., 23) is quite intelligent, and would be able to understand his lectures " if the professor did not get on so fast, and if he did not jump from one subject to another. That is what makes me ill."—In the case of journeys, it is the rapid change of locality, of dwelling, of associates, which induces fatigue and depression. In occupational work, it is the rapid adaptations which neuropaths find most difficult and most injurious.—" The least of my employees," says Nebo, " can do in five minutes what I need hours to do. It is when I am hustled that everything goes wrong."—What terrorises Daniel in his work as a soldier is that orders come so suddenly and are changed at a moment's

[1] Les stigmates fondamentaux de la timidité, "Revue Philosophique," 1915, pp. 432 and 434.

notice. " I am expected to have perpetual presence of mind. That is asking too much."

House-movings, monetary losses, changes of situation, are dangerous in proportion as they are sudden and unexpected.— We have seen how Lvy. fell ill because he was promoted owing to the sudden death of his chief.—The symptoms induced by the death of an intimate are always more serious when the death occurs suddenly. Zoé's case was a characteristic instance.—In five of my cases, crises of depression occurred in young people upon whom a sudden decision was forced in connexion with a proposal of marriage.—In the remarkable case of Vy., one of the causes of the mental disorder from which he suffered was that marriage had compelled him to attempt the rapid achievement of intimacy with his wife, whereas he was never able to enter into an intimacy at short notice.—We see the same thing in the case of ruptures of relationships, when parents are affected by their children falling ill, or by the marriage of their children, when old people retire, and so on. Always it has been the suddenness of the occurrence, the demand for prompt adaptation to new circumstances, which has played a predominant part in causing the trouble. The patients themselves are well aware of the fact. —" Even in the simplest matters, like eating or dressing," said Vkp., " I must not be hurried. If I try to get on too fast, things go wrong. I have spasms of all kinds, especially in the stomach and the abdomen. I can only act without disturbance if I am given time to act slowly and in the way to which I am accustomed."

Still, I find it hard to understand how agitation induced by the pressure of circumstances and by the demand for a prompt reaction can explain the multifarious symptoms of depression. The explanation can account for certain depressive symptoms that supervene very soon after the event which has given rise to emotional disturbance ; but it does not account for the far more numerous instances in which depression ensues slowly, and in which there has been a period of incubation after the emotional disturbance. We have to recognise that other characteristics of the action besides its complexity and its rapidity must entail difficulty and danger.

My own belief is that the *duration*, the prolongation, *of an action* is the main factor of exhaustion. I need not recapitulate all the instances which show how symptoms of depression have ensued upon the performance of prolonged and repeated actions. I have stressed the fact that depression arises under the conditions which induce fatigue. One fact may be usefully recalled here, namely that in many instances the symptoms have manifested themselves after prolonged expectation—as of an appointment to a post, a serious decision, a cure, etc.—Zoé became affected with a serious crisis when she had been asked in marriage, and felt herself unable to give an answer. She said that she had been in love with the young man for a long time, and had been expecting his proposal. The prolonged expectation had exhausted her, and had made it impossible for her to say Yes when the proposal at length came.—Noémi, who had always needed her husband's guidance and encouragement, was left alone when he was called up for military service. For two months she bravely looked forward to the end of the war and to her husband's return, making great efforts to behave well. Then, all of a sudden, she once more had the feeling of being " wrapped in cottonwool, as if the world were a long way off." Once more she had " the horrible, the hateful impression " of watching herself living and thinking, of listening to herself as she talked. Once more she had a jealous horror of happy persons. Since the state of expectation was prolonged, exhaustion and depression speedily ensued.—Some patients, like Sophie, are so susceptible to expectation that we can, if we choose, aggravate their symptoms almost experimentally by merely making them await something.—Expectation, in fact, is a prolonged action. One who is expecting anything must keep a particular tendency in a state of preparedness or erection, but must nevertheless simultaneously inhibit the development of this tendency, for the action cannot yet be carried to fruition. This involves complicated and difficult activities, especially if the expectation be prolonged.

The various characteristics of the circumstances which have proved dangerous to the persons concerned, their novelty, complexity, rapidity, duration, and so on, modify the psychological nature of the ensuing actions. It does not suffice to say that the actions must be stronger, more numerous, more rapid, more prolonged ; what must be recognised is that such actions need to be transformed in order to adapt them to the circumstances.

The transformation is easy to perceive when there is a question of rapidity involved. Walking cannot be speeded up without transforming it into running ; writing cannot be accelerated without having recourse to shorthand. A journey which necessitates the use of a motor car or an express train is not identical with a walk ; such a journey demands different preparations, different arrangements, different kinds of outlay. To be able to speak is not enough to enable us to make a proper use of telephone and telegraph, nor does a knowledge of simple arithmetic suffice when rapid reckoning is needed in a factory or in a big business firm.

Even a simple act which seems to change its nature to a very slight extent during performance, will obviously become more difficult and exacting if it has to be performed quickly. I have to catch a train at a terminus, and there is plenty of time ; I may take a tram there or I may walk ; in either case the expenditure is slight. But let us suppose that I am delayed and become worried lest I miss the train ; I may have to take a taxi and promise a handsome tip to the driver ; in such a case the same distance will cost a great deal more. Suppose that in my anxiety I disconcert the driver by excessive promises of reward if he gets me to the station in time, that, in order to encourage him, I constantly pop my head out of the window to speak to him, I may distract him so much that he will collide with another vehicle, and may cause damage for which I shall have to pay ; in these circumstances, catching the train becomes positively ruinous. Similar phenomena occur in mental life, and may be understood by analogy. When we are faced by a situation which we are accustomed to respond to slowly, and which on this occasion suddenly demands a speedy response, the habitual tendency cannot be made use of ; we must have recourse to exceptional measures, that is to say to tendencies less well organised ; in the latter event, the expenditure of energy will be greatly increased. The unusual and more speedy reaction will probably call for greater tension, which is always most costly, especially at the outset. It may happen, however, that there is not yet organised within us a reaction suitable to the new situation, or speedy enough to respond. We shall then have to fall back on improvisation, have recourse to the primitive tendency, rely upon the agitation which makes trial of movements in all directions so as by a lucky chance to hit upon a suitable expedient. Hence the emotion, the dismay, the disorder, which arise when we are unduly hurried.

An action which responds to a complex situation is not simply an action made up of numerous movements, an action which necessitates the putting into play of a larger number of muscles ; it is a unique action, sometimes a very simple one, but belonging to a higher stratum of the hierarchy of tendencies, and demanding greater psychological tension. The action of eating in company is a particular action necessitated by social life : it is not only a more complex action, but a more recently acquired action, less of a habit, less automatic, and differing very greatly from the primitive action which simply consists of eating to satisfy hunger.[1] Conversation with a considerable number of persons when there are cross currents of talk is not the same action as that exchange of views which constitutes a colloquy between two individuals. The former is another way of talking, it requires shorter speeches, quicker adaptations to changes of thought, and sudden leaps from one subject to another. The command of an army is not a simple multiple of the command of a squad ; it is an absolutely different psychological operation, and one performed on a higher plane.

Psychoanalysts, followers of Freud, have laid much stress on the importance of mental conflicts, and they consider such conflicts (not without exaggeration) to lie at the foundation of neurotic disorders. Doubtless the mental agitation of certain patients, their constant vacillations, are often the results of depression, and they must not always be looked upon as the starting-point of exhaustion. Nevertheless, it is true that a complex situation, instead of arousing a unique tendency (as might be done by a perception), nearly always arouses in the mind the idea of several sorts of behaviour, and gives birth to conflicts ; in such circumstances a person can only respond after deliberation, after making a choice, after coming to a decision.

Religious exercises, study, occupations, betrothals, create problems for the will and for the beliefs. There is always a

[1] Les névroses, 1909, p. 384.

question to decide ; whether we are concerned with business, or with marriage, or with the management of men. The circumstances in which an individual is forced to choose between two opposing kinds of behaviour, either performance or abstention, the yea or the nay of a betrothal, the choice between the lover and the husband—all these are typical cases. The feeling of responsibility is nothing else than a lively representation of motives when the latter entail serious consequences in the field of action. The operations of deliberation and decision entirely alter the behaviour. Instead of the appetitive tendencies corresponding to the stage of desire in the activation of tendencies, we have to do with reflective behaviour, which corresponds to the stage of reflection and control of the desires. The psychological tension at once becomes higher. This being so, need we be surprised that many individuals are incapable of performing such actions correctly, and that mental conflicts arising out of complex circumstances may give rise to great exhaustion ?

In other cases we see persons who are able to make decisions, who know, in theory, what it is suitable to believe and to do, but who fail as soon as the moment for action arrives. Mba. (m., 36) is indignant if any one accuses him of infirmity of will ; he holds, not without good reason, that he can form prompt and accurate decisions. He is fully aware that it is incumbent on him to do this or that, that he ought to begin the study of such and such a question. But, having got thus far, he is assailed by scruples, he enters upon interminable psychological analyses: he is overpowered with vexation as soon as he is obliged to fix his attention, " to absorb something " ; that is to say, as soon as he has to put his resolve into execution. Many persons find the performance of actions which have to be repeated regularly and for a long time intolerable. In especial when such actions cannot be performed at the time and in the manner the subject likes, we find that they entail much suffering to the patient. " I could work all right if only I had the feeling that I could stop work and get away when I liked ; it is simply awful to think that, come what may, I am forced to work till noon." The numerous disorders induced by the continuation of an action after a check are of the same character.

Here, once more, we see that behaviour is transformed.

In the carrying out of resolutions, in the continuance of actions, we are no longer concerned, as a rule, with reflective tendencies, but with tendencies of a lower grade for which I have proposed the name of " ergetic," for they are characterised by effort and work. As has often been pointed out, work is only performed by persons belonging to the higher races ; it needs a peculiar collaboration of the whole mind ; it gives rise to extremely complex ideas, such as those of production, aim, means, and cause ; it constitutes a highly specialised and exalted form of activity. The transformation of behaviour, even of reflective behaviour, into behaviour characterised by effort and work, is far from being insignificant, for it implies the transition to a much higher degree of psychological tension. That is why, when we demand an action of long duration, or demand a period of expectation, we are requiring an action of an exalted kind, and one that necessitates considerable expenditure.

Finally, let us consider adaptation to a new situation, and the creation of new tendencies. We are usually told that habits and tendencies are created by action. Speaking generally, the statement is true, but it is far too vague. The inferior types of activity, the lower grades of activation, have no more than a very slight power of creating and strengthening tendencies ; they possess this power only in the germ. We have within us special forms of activity whose precise purpose it is to constitute new tendencies competent to function in the future. Thus the realist tendencies which comprise will and belief, organise tendencies to action. To take a decision is to organise a particular grouping of actions and words, to organise it so strongly that it becomes capable of functioning regularly for years to come. To believe something is nothing else than to form the decision that we shall act in a certain way when certain circumstances arise. No doubt our earlier habits, our tendencies to obedience or to loyalty, render this action possible ; but it is none the less difficult, and it demands high tension. The conative or ergetic tendencies which organise the work, give precision and force to these new groupings of action. Finally, the ultimate degree of activation, that which brings in its train what we term the " triumph " of the action (which makes the action a joyful one, and which is the mainspring of all artistic creation), this ultimate degree is the starting-point of all the great changes in the individual, of the artistic creation of a new personality. When we find that so many disturbances arise in connexion with such adaptations, we are naturally inclined to attribute the exhaustion to a difficult functioning of these higher tendencies.

My earlier studies had already prepared me for drawing such an inference. When analysing agitation, I was led to consider the phenomenon of *psychological derivation*. I wrote : " Derivation occurs whenever the production of a superior phenomenon, one characterised by high tension, has begun, but when the production of the phenomenon has been checked by a lowering of mental tension which has rendered the appearance of phenomena of high tension impossible." When this happens, instead of the complete activation which culminates in decision, effort, and triumph, there occur convulsive paroxysms, tics, questionings, interminable debates, multifarious visceral agitations. " How does it come to pass that in place of the suppressed phenomenon, which seemed unique and inconsiderable, there should occur an enormous quantity of other phenomena which last for a very long time ? The answer may be found by developing our hypothesis anent the psychological hierarchy and the grades of psychological tension. When one psychological phenomenon is superior to another, the force requisite for its production may be adequate to produce a lower-grade phenomenon a hundred times over." [1] In a word, an act of high tension is a costly one, and needs an expenditure far in excess of that requisite for an action of inferior type. This conception has been verified by our recent studies, for we are able to note that a decision, a work, or a triumph, will exhaust our patients infinitely more than the most violent and prolonged lower-grade agitations.

None the less, it is very strange to see how actions which are good in themselves, these decisions, these labours, can induce exhaustion. Actions of high tension are not usually exhausting actions. On the contrary, their aim is to reduce expenditure and bring us advantage. A definitive decision simplifies future behaviour, and enables us henceforward to act at less cost. One who by hard work wins a fortune or learns a science does much to facilitate profitable behaviour in the future.

---

[1] Les obsessions et la psychasthénie, 1903, vol. i, p. 559.

The validity of these considerations is indisputable, but the advantages accruing from such actions will accrue in the future. For the moment, expenditure is greatly increased. It is as if we were buying a costly machine, or were spending a large sum in the purchase of valuable shares. We expect to gain by it in the end, to husband our energies or to receive dividends, but here and now we have to pay. Some purses are so light that they are emptied before the necessary immediate expenditure can be met. In like manner, there are minds which are not strong enough to sustain an action good in itself and likely to be beneficial in the future. The immediate expenditure cannot be met.

Another point has to be considered. Such patients cannot *fully* accomplish actions demanding high tension. They begin the action, but stop acting before it is finished. They begin it again and again, but remain perpetually faced by the same problem. The action which is dangerous for them is not merely a difficult action, but an action which " misses fire," which does not solve the difficulty, which does not make an end of the need for adaptation. When a check has been sustained, the individual is once more in a peculiar situation demanding a fresh adaptation. He has then to choose between three possibilities. He may begin the action over again, without any modification ; or he can begin it over again while modifying the strength, the duration, or the combination of the necessary movements ; or he may abandon the attempt, and may renounce the satisfaction which the completed action would have brought.

The third of these solutions is an extermely important one. It takes the form of resignation, with a feeling of necessity and impossibility. Here we have action of a new kind, an action occupying a lofty position in the hierarchy, and one which in my lectures I have associated with the tendencies relating to work and causality. Very few of our patients are capable of this kind of resignation. In my study of the characteristics of depressed persons, I have been especially struck with their inability to recognise the impossible and to resign themselves to circumstances. They can never be content, like the fox in the fable, to say " the grapes are sour." In the grounds of an asylum, one day, I saw Sophie jumping up again and again trying to reach something. On drawing near, I perceived that

this something was the branch of a tree about ten feet above
her head. The absurdity of what she was doing did not strike
her, and I had to distract her attention before she would give
up the attempt.   I have seen women take incredible pains
for years in the hope of curing a poor wretch suffering from
paralytic dementia, for they were incapable of realising that
the malady was incurable.

While our patients are thus unable to resign themselves to
circumstances, they are hardly less incompetent to adopt the
second type of behaviour. They cannot modify their activities,
since for this they would need invention and initiative.
They are thus almost invariably reduced to the adoption of
the first alternative, to the adoption of the simplest and most
time-honoured form of behaviour, the one which demands a
minimum of tension. They begin the action over again. The
mania of recommencement is familiar in the case of the petty
movements of the subjects who are continually opening and
shutting a door, who undress and dress over and over again,
who continually repeat their prayers and their penances. The
same need for recommencement plays a great part in certain
more complicated actions, although here it is less obviously at
work. Young people will persist in essaying a task or in
reading a passage in a book, without ever arriving at the goal
of understanding. Léa and Lydia persisted for years in their
attempts to make the two households live together, in their
endeavours to educate their respective husbands. Zoé, after
her mother's death, tried to go on behaving as if the mother
were still alive, and she was always on the look out for her
mother. Emma, when her relationship with her lover had
been broken off, was continually trying to get back to the old
footing. " I simply cannot realise that all is over. I go on
believing that we can make a fresh start."   This sort of
behaviour is a commonplace whenever the mind is enfeebled,
and we may say that the majority of such invalids spend their
lives in kicking against the pricks. We shall soon have to
return to this matter, when we come to study traumatic
fixed ideas. Suffice it here to say that, by their inability to
complete an action, the patients are led to prolong their
activities indefinitely, and that the danger to their health
ensues because the undue duration of activity induces
exhaustion.

In the cases which usually come under our notice, the advantage of the action is nil, and the expenditure involved is enormous. Nothing can be nore costly than the perpetual mobilisations of capital with a view to purchases which are never made. The ineffective investor thus squanders his substance, and will ruin himself in the end. The exhaustion from which the patient suffers is due, in most cases, to the perpetual recommencement of higher-grade operations which never reach their term.

In days to come, the problem of psychological expenditure, the problem of the mental cost of activity, will be one of the cardinal problems of psychology and psychiatry ; but at the present time few people seem to suspect that such a problem exists. It will suffice, in this connexion, to adduce a few practical notions. There can be no doubt that certain kinds of activity are, psychologically speaking, more expensive than other kinds, and have a more marked tendency to use up our energies. This accounts for the origin of quite a number of nervous symptoms. It is, however, difficult to say precisely what are the costly types of activity, to specify the characteristics whereby these types of activity are distinguished from other and less dangerous types.

Ordinarily, when this question is raised, a ready answer is forthcoming. People speak of the psychological quantity of the actions concerned, of the force of the movements, of their complexity, their speed, and their duration. We are told that actions which require energetic, numerous, rapid, and prolonged movements, are fatiguing kinds of action. This may be to some extent true when we are dealing with normal fatigue, but the statement is quite inadequate when we have to do with pathological exhaustion, and with depression. In the latter case we have to take into account, not merely psychological quantity, but also the psychological tension of actions, to consider the characteristics dependent upon the hierarchical elevation of the actions. We have to realise that the performance of higher-grade activities, those which belong to the domains of reflection, work, and triumph, is far more likely than the performance of lower-grade activities to induce exhaustion and depression.

6. ABSOLUTE REST.

These studies of exhaustion in the neuroses can, of course, be verified by an examination of the results of treatment by rest. If it be true that the depression of neuropaths is increased by activity, if in them there is no such thing as a pleasant and healthy fatigue, if, when they try to work, complete exhaustion ensues without transition, then we shall do well, when we treat their illness, to suppress their activities to the utmost, and to give them a chance of restoring their energies by rest. According to Lagrange, rest may be defined as the physiological state in which the activity of the living organs is temporarily suspended or abnormally lowered. The most perfect rest is secured by lying down, for then the activity of all the organs is reduced to the utmost   The antidote to motor fatigue is to combine the taking of food with muscular repose, with rest in bed. If you have been for too long a walk, eat a hearty dinner, and go to bed early ;   by next day, all your losses will have been made good.   If the disturbances that occur in neuropaths and psychopaths are due to a depression identical with fatigue, let them rest in bed and they will be cured.   That is the theory upon which are based all the methods of treatment by hyperalimentation and rest, the methods which have culminated in the remarkable exaggerations already described.   I propose now to analyse the results of these methods of treatment, making a careful study of the numerous cases I have recorded.

The value of treatment by rest in bed is well shown by the results of Wetterstrand's method. As previously explained, the essence of this method is to induce deep sleep by hypnotism and suggestion, and to leave the patients in the artificial sleep for days or weeks.   I have myself tried the method in a good many cases. In certain subjects, it is easy to prolong the hypnotic sleep for a considerable time, and in these cases we can, by suggestion, ensure a very effective rest. My own experience has been that the method ensures excellent results in hysterics affected with delirious crises, and in certain patients in whom choreiform agitations are the most conspicuous symptoms. Five hours' hypnosis has led to the disappearance of obstinate contractures. In a case of persistent hiccough which had been resistent to other methods of treatment, twenty-four hours' hypnosis effected a complete cure. In Berthe, who had been having an interminable series of crises, three days' sleep broke the sequence. Similar results were secured in another patient who was suffering from delirious paroxysms with refusal of food. An especially interesting case was that of Pauline. She was a girl of seventeen with anaesthesia of the left side and hysterical coxalgia. In addition, she had so marked a mania of contrariety that in the waking state it was impossible to get her to obey the most trifling orders or to make the slightest effort of attention. She ate very little, digested badly, was extremely constipated, and passed during the twenty-four hours only 300 grammes of urine containing no more than 5 grammes of urea. I was able to induce profound hypnosis, and to leave her in this artificial sleep. After the sleep had lasted a few hours, she had already become more obedient, so that I could regulate her behaviour to some extent. I ordered her to remain asleep, and not to move at all except when her food was brought, or when she needed to relieve the calls of nature. During the first twenty-four hours, she took more food than before, but there was no other conspicuous change. On the second day, the anuria gave place to polyuria, for she now passed 3 litres of extremely limpid urine containing 27 grammes of urea. On the third day she passed $1\frac{1}{2}$ litres of urine containing 21 grammes of urea, and the bowels acted normally. On the fourth day, she awoke spontaneously in a perfectly natural way, free from coxalgia and other hysterical symptoms. She had no relapse for two months.[1]

I am, therefore, inclined to think that the method may be useful in special cases. By Wetterstrand's treatment we can carry the patients through the periods in which they are suffering from attacks, we can break their morbid habits; and, above all, we can get the better of the resistances, the false notions and fixed ideas, which are so apt to accompany contractures. I cannot here study the methods by which such artificial sleep can be induced and prolonged, the watchfulness it demands, or the possible duration of the hypnosis. It has been enough to make a brief allusion to the matter, but I think

[1] Traitement psychologique de l'hystérie, in Albert Robin's Traité de thérapeutique, 1908, vol. xv; cf. also L'état mental des hystériques, second edition, 1911, p. 667.

that in the future Wetterstrand's method will be found valuable
in the treatment of certain hysterical symptoms.

But the great defect of the method is that it is only
applicable to suggestible and hypnotisable hysterics, to patients
who can be subjected to a vigorous hypnotic drill. We may ask,
therefore, whether the results achieved are not exclusively
due to suggestion and education. For my part, I do not think
so, for, especially in Pauline's case, I have secured, by this
prolonged sleep, results which I had long and vainly endeavoured to bring about in other ways. Still, the phenomena
with which we are concerned here are complicated and exceptional. The practitioners who tell us that they have made a
routine use of Wetterstrand's method, and that they have
turned it to account in hundreds of cases, have probably failed
to make an accurate diagnosis of hypnotic sleep and of suggestion. I think it likely that they have given the name of
hypnotic sleep to a vague condition of tranquillity. Their
method was nothing more than an application of rest in bed,
the method we have now to consider.

Indubitably, in a great number of nervous and mental
disorders the results of simple rest in bed are excellent. Let us
consider first of all the most straightforward cases, those in
which we have to do with patients who have been definitely
exhausted by a bodily illness or by excessive physical toil ;
patients who have been considerably emaciated, who show
signs of exhaustion of the organic functions, and who are more
or less cachectic.

Nex. was a sickly girl of seventeen, ill nourished, and worn
out by hard work. She began to suffer from hysterical
paroxysms and various other hysterical symptoms. She was
taken to hospital and was completely cured in three months,
rest and good feeding being obviously the main factors in the
cure. When she first came to the hospital she was suffering
from well-marked left hemi-anaesthesia, with the usual psychological accompaniments of hysterical anaesthesia. Since at
that particular date it was the fashion to be sceptical as to the
existence of hysterical anaesthesia, I demonstrated the case to
a good many people. Unfortunately, however, the tactile
sensibility of this patient became an object of undue curiosity,
and was examined far too often by the students. According

to the theories of the day, these repeated demonstrations ought to have increased and fixed the anaesthesia. Nothing of the kind happened, and under the influence of careful dieting and rest in bed the hemi-anaesthesia gradually disappeared, together with the other hysterical symptoms.

In sixteen of my cases, hysteria has been cured by rest in a period ranging from one to three months. Kz., who had become subject to frequent crises of hysterical sleep, was cured by two months' rest in bed ; and the same thing happened in two other cases of the kind. Ten cases of tremor, paralysis, and other motor troubles, were successfully treated in the same way. Finally, hysterical anorexia, which is apt to be a very obstinate disease, was cured in three instances by two month's rest in bed. I have recently had under my care Jui., a young woman, twenty-eight years of age, a domestic servant who had come to Paris from the country and had been overworked. She became affected with disorders of the will, obsessions, and mental confusion. I kept her in hospital for two months, in bed nearly all the time. In this case it is not surprising that rest should have worked a cure, which for the time being at any rate was complete.

Vkp. (f., 32), when I first saw her, was not only suffering from a severe crisis of psychasthenic depression with obsessions concerning humiliation and death, for in addition she was extremely emaciated, having been exhausted by a sharp attack of enteritis, by very low diet, and by hard work in the home. Absolute rest in bed for two months was of great help in the treatment.—Ch. (f., 21) had had a very difficult labour in which it had been necessary to use the cephalotribe, with severe intrauterine infection as a sequel. The neuropathic symptoms, though grave, were no more than secondary, and were readily dispelled by five months' treatment, which was mainly physical, and of which one of the most important factors was rest in bed.—A woman aged twenty-nine had been exhausted by a distressing pregnancy which she had attempted to conceal, by a difficult labour, and by uterine infection, to say nothing of the emotional distress due to the death of the child and to financial difficulties. She became affected with phobias of various kinds, which culminated in persistent mental alienation. She was cured by suitable treatment, three months' rest in bed having obviously been the most important among the remedial measures.

In cases of this kind, rest in bed has moral effects as well as physical. Obviously, it is in line with the various physical methods of treating the neuroses, the methods we shall discuss in a subsequent chapter. When the patient is kept in bed, the circulation of the blood is facilitated, and the digestion often improves. From the moral point of view likewise, the patient is more readily kept under supervision, and this is often a matter of importance ; he is better enabled to realise that he is an invalid ; he is tranquillised by rest in bed and becomes inclined to sleep a good deal ; finally, he is placed in the best conditions for the economising of his energies. Thus treatment by rest in bed is definitely indicated in all cases in which there are marked symptoms of organic enfeeblement.

But the use of this method must not be restricted to such cases. Many neuropaths in whom there are no conspicuous signs of physical disorder can be greatly benefited by complete rest. First of all I will refer to cases in which neuropathic disorders affecting a particular function, and apparently due to excessive use of this function, have been much relieved by rest. Emma and Ty. were suffering from photophobia, which had obviously been brought on by excessive use of the eyes. In both cases, rest in bed in a darkened room gave speedy relief.

But rest in bed will dispel more generalised disorders.— Boia. (f., 35), suffering from agoraphobia, and obsessed with the thought of death, was kept in bed almost continuously for three months. She was greatly tranquillised by the treatment, so that she even became able to go out into the streets alone.— Fn. (f., 32), the patient to whom I have already referred as suffering from over-scrupulousness and agitation, was obviously benefited by two months' rest in bed, or on a long chair. She herself had noticed that she invariably felt a good deal better when anything happened to keep her in bed for a while. For instance, three weeks' complete rest after childbirth had always induced marked moral tranquillity, and had strengthened her powers of will. " The strange thing is that at such times I am better able to make my children and my servants do what I tell them, and everything in the household goes on more smoothly than when I am up and about, and am busying myself with these matters."—I have notes of eight equally striking cases of the same kind.

A patient of whom I specially wish to speak in this connexion is Sophie, whose remarkable case Monsieur Arnaud and I made the basis of our study of psychasthenic delusions. This young woman, who is now thirty-five years of age, had already had two very serious attacks of psychasthenic mental disorder, having on each occasion been kept under restraint for eighteen months. After the second of these attacks she had been in good health, both physical and mental, for two years. Then, after a number of fatiguing incidents, a tour in a motor car, too many parties, etc., the characteristic symptoms returned. Since by this time I was well acquainted with her troubles, it was easy to detect all the signs of a relapse which threatened to be exactly like the previous attacks of illness. She had the same passion for self-sacrifice ; the same regret that she was not caring for the sick, was not repopulating France, was not commanding the armies ; the same exaggerated sense of obligation ; and so on. At the outset of the previous attacks, complete rest had never been tried, but I now decided to keep the patient in bed under conditions of perfect tranquillity. A month later, all the alarming symptoms had disappeared, and she was able to return home, having been saved from an attack which would probably have been as serious and as long as the previous ones.

Phenomena of this kind would seem to justify the extraordinary precautions which certain patients take in order to avoid the slightest expenditure of energy ; they seem to explain the phobia of fatigue.—At. (m., 55) is a very tiresome patient, one who at first appears positively ridiculous. To outward seeming he is perfectly well, and is a man of great intelligence ; but for fifteen years he has not merely given up all the work which used to interest him, but has practically renounced every kind of activity. He sedulously calculates every movement, and never walks more than from 500 to 750 yards a day. He knows the exact length of his room and of the passages in his flat, and has carefully paced the neighbouring. streets. One flight of stairs counts for 100 yards. He keeps careful check whenever he is afoot, so that he shall not exceed his allowance. When he feels exceptionally well, he will permit himself five

minutes' reading and ten minutes' conversation per diem ;
while he is talking to any one, he has his watch in his hand all
the time. He spends the rest of the day lying down, not in a
long chair, for this would be too tiring, but in bed, and trying
not to think. He declares that a slight pinching sensation in
the temples warns him when his strength is almost exhausted,
and nothing will ever induce him to step out of bounds. " I
am like a boiler in which there is too little water. We should
ruin the boiler if, in these conditions, we were to stoke the fire."
—An officer, aged forty, had received a bullet wound in the
occipital region, and the bullet could not be extracted. For
the last eighteen months he has suffered from very remarkable
mental symptoms, which are worthy of a detailed description.
But for my present purpose it is enough to say that his behaviour
has become exactly like At.'s. He calculates every movement,
rationing his reading and his thoughts. " I do this to avoid
relapsing into cloudiness and darkness of mind."

These patients resemble those described in the early part
of the present chapter, the persons who are obsessed with the
thought of fatigue, and at whom Paul Dubois levels the shafts
of his criticism. But there is one marked difference, inasmuch
as, apart from the almost incredible precautions they take, they
are extremely intelligent, and their behaviour is all that can be
desired. During the brief moments in which he deigns to give
his mind to worldly affairs, At. amazes me by his prompt
decisions, his successful calculations, and even his states of
satisfaction. I cannot note in him any of the inadequacies
of the higher-grade tendencies, any of the sentiments of
incompleteness, which are so characteristic of psychological
depression. Are we to suppose that so extreme an obsession
or delusion of fatigue, one which has transformed the patient's
whole life for fifteen years, can have developed to such an
intensity without the existence of any underlying additional
symptom of depression ? Such an idea would seem to conflict
with all our observations. Is it possible that these patients
have been enabled to avoid the depression and the other
disorders characteristic of psychasthenia precisely because
they spend nearly all their time in bed ? The disciples of Weir
Mitchell, and Deschamps in especial, would not hesitate to
answer this question in the affirmative.

In fact the Weir Mitchell treatment presents itself to us

as exceedingly simple. The patient has been exhausted by undue activity. Very well, then, let us prescribe rest. Let us, as far as possible, suppress every form of activity. The subject is not rich enough to bear the cost of the life he is leading. We need not trouble to enquire which items in his expenditure are excessive and ruinous ; it will suffice if we simply prohibit every kind of expenditure, for then we shall be quite certain that the patient will have to economise his energies. There is nothing inherently absurd about such a prescription. Obviously, it is more likely to help the invalid than the opposite method, that of those who would have him disdain fatigue and pay no heed to imprudent expenditure. Most neuropaths, whether obsessed with fatigue or not, are suffering from exhaustion, and are on the verge of bankruptcy. We shall seldom fail to do them a good turn by insisting upon rest and upon the economising of energy. I will go so far as to say that when we are consulted for the first time by one who is plainly suffering from serious illness, in whom we have not yet been able to make an adequate psychological analysis, and in whom the mechanism of the exhaustion from which he is suffering is not yet ascertainable, we shall always do well to prescribe rest in bed for a time. This will give us a better chance of grasping the situation, and in a great many instances we shall find that the initial rest is directly beneficial to the patient.

In sanatoria for the treatment of nervous disorders, the view is apt to prevail that rest in bed is a sort of universal panacea for such cases, and that it can be suitably applied for an indefinite time ; and the same idea is sometimes voiced elsewhere. It is, however, only too easy to point out the difficulties, dangers, and inadequacies of treatment by absolute rest. No doubt in certain patients, for instance in the case of rich and idle women, there is little inconvenience attached to the prescription of several weeks or even several months in bed. But, often enough, such a suspension of all activities would be a very serious matter. Uk., who in youth had been affected by rather a severe mental crisis characterised by obsessions, became at the age of forty the managing owner of a large factory where he had worked in a subordinate position all his life. For fifteen years he had aspired to become the head of the concern. Unfortunately, he was now overwhelmed by the thought of his new responsibilities, and began to manifest various symptoms of mental disorder. There was marked motor and verbal agitation. When at home, he was continually uttering despairing harangues anent his own incapacity and the dangers of the situation. Painful scenes were of frequent occurrence. He attempted suicide again and again, though the attempts may be regarded as spurious. His digestion was disordered ; he suffered from sleeplessness, sexual excitement, etc. Translating these facts into our own technical terminology, we may say that the tendencies connected with the management and the ownership of the factory, exhausted by unduly prolonged expectation, and thereby fatigued, had had their tension so greatly lowered as to have become unable to secure complete realisation. To some extent they were activated, for the patient continued to manage the factory ; but they were unable to bring about the full realisation of decisive, confident, and satisfactory action. Hence there occurred various derivations affecting the elementary functions, such as the sexual functions ; hence the agitations and obsessions. From one point of view, no doubt, the best treatment for Uk. would have been to prescribe rest in bed for several months. But the factory could not have been left to run by itself ; and a substitute manager would probably have wanted to feather his own nest, so that that prescription would have been likely to entail the patient's financial ruin. Moreover, it was perfectly clear that Uk. only gave his disorders free rein after his return home in the evenings. During the day, while at the factory, he worked hard and managed his affairs quite well. Should we have been right, in these circumstances, to make him lie up ?

We are often faced with similar problems. One such case under my care was that of Vkm., a man of fifty. He was a teacher by profession who had had disorders of the same kind as those with which Uk. was affected. Having been promoted to a higher teaching post, he became depressed, was obsessed by thoughts of humiliation, and entertained ideas of suicide. Ought I to have advised a course of treatment which would have involved an open avowal that he was suffering from mental disorder, and which would have ruined his career by making him ask for leave at so inopportune a time ?

Even if the patient is prepared to resign himself to an indefinite stay in a sanatorium, does not this involve serious risks ? He may take a liking for such a life of absolute idleness, and may hesitate to get well when the time comes for a return to normal existence. Ns., a man of thirty-five, who has spent two years at rest in a sanatorium, will not hear a word of leaving the place, although his family is being ruined by the cost of maintaining him there. " General practitioners do not understand my trouble. All that they can prescribe may be summed up in a few words—calmness of mind, equability ; anybody can give good advice of this sort. But it is life itself that troubles me, the things one has to do in ordinary life. I want to stay where I am, for the doctors here understand my case, and prescribe the absolute physical and moral rest which is so essential to me." Is that a cure ?

If the requisite sacrifices are to be made, if the patient is to be exposed to the dangers thus outlined, the doctor must be thoroughly convinced of the sovereign value of the remedy. But it is an unfortunate fact that the cases in which treatment by absolute rest seems to have had good results can be counterbalanced by cases which bear a very different interpretation. The method utterly fails, sometimes, even when pushed to an extreme. I cannot in my own notebooks find the record of any cases in which treatment by rest in bed was applied in its full rigour for a long time without any good result, the reason being that I have never had the patience to continue such treatment for an indefinite period without endeavouring to help on the cure by the superaddition of more active remedies. But I have frequently had occasion to note facts of the kind in the history of patients who have given me a detailed account of the various remedial measures which have been fruitlessly attempted for their relief. Such stories are especially frequent in the mouths of American and English patients, for in Britain and the United States the doctors seem peculiarly fond of consigning their patients to sanatoria for interminable periods.— I recently alluded to the case of Kx. (f., 26) as a typical instance of a sufferer from obsessions and phobias of fatigue. It is well to recall the fact that in the early stages of her illness, when she was suffering from obsessions of over-scrupulousness, she was kept in bed for seven months. As a result, she was much worse than before the treatment, having become unable to walk, speak, or write for a few moments without a feeling that she was about to faint. Such was her condition for seven years.

It may be that we are not entitled to regard these additional symptoms as the direct consequence of prolonged rest in bed. The undue continuation of the rest served only to give a special trend to the hypochondriacal depression and obsessions that already existed. But this much is clear, that seven months' rest did her no good ; and that, during and after the period of rest, the illness continued to develop.—Lema (f., 37), another patient of the same kind, who, since the age of twenty, has always collapsed when she has made a few steps or moved her limbs a little, has tried multifarious systems of treatment. On several occasions she has stayed in bed for months at a time (on one occasion for eighteen months consecutively), and her illness has always been aggravated by such treatment. —A like story was told me by twelve other patients.—Should not such facts give us pause ? I know that they will not disturb Deschamps for a moment. " If the patient is not cured after the lapse of eighteen months, this is because he has not yet had a long enough rest. Let him stay in bed a few years longer, and move his limbs even less than before. Time does not really exist ; it is an invention of the philosophers." A pretty phrase, no doubt, but the patients who have some important occupation, and those who need to earn their livelihood, and cannot afford to pay for months of sanatorium treatment, will hardly share Deschamps' enthusiasm for prolonged rest.

How are we to explain the failures of the rest cure in view of the importance of fatigue and of rest as shown by the foregoing studies ? First of all, people are under illusions concerning rest. It is looked upon as being purely negative, as comprising merely a suppression of objective and conspicuous activity. If that were all, it would be perfectly easy to ensure rest by sending the patient to bed. But we make a great mistake if we suppose the matter to be so simple. A neuropathic patient is not necessarily at rest because we keep him between the sheets. Long ago I had occasion to point out that such invalids do not know how to assume the attitude of repose ; they do not know how to lie down, or how to sit comfortably in an armchair ; they sit crookedly, they twist about, have all their bodily stresses wrongly applied, and they continue to keep their muscles tense. I said of Lise that her muscles remained so taut all night that they were quite stiff in the morning. Vkp. tells us: " My will makes me do everything stiffly, so that I am stiff even when I am asleep. When I am dosing, my very toes are in a cramped position ; I can never lie easily in my bed, with all my muscles relaxed ; I simply don't know how to rest." Dejerine draws attention to the same phenomenon. " It is stupid to be content with advising a patient to rest, for there is no remedy which is more hopelessly misapplied. Rest in bed is absolutely valueless if the patient wearies himself by adopting unharmonious postures, if while motionless in bed he assumes vicious attitudes which make his limbs numb and his head congested." [1] A patient of mine was even more awkward in his attempts to rest. We discovered one day that he had extensive bruises on the inner and hinder surfaces of the left calf, the left knee, the left thigh, and on the front of the right leg. These bruises had been caused by the vigour with which he pressed his legs against one another.

What has just been said concerning movements is even more applicable to thoughts and moral efforts. Dubois gives his patients admirable advice : " Rid yourself of all your worries ; don't let anything distress you ; keep your mind fixed upon pleasant thoughts." Delightful, but is there not an element of irony in the advice when we have to do with persons who lack the power of guiding their thoughts and of fixing their attention where they please ? When they are in bed, motionless and idle, they are continually excogitating new chimeras. They wear themselves out by calculations, by pondering difficult combinations ; they make an immense effort to achieve difficult resolutions. Of course they fail, and their efforts merely lead to new and injurious motor or mental derivations.—This is what happens in the case of Vom. (m., 19), in whom treatment by rest has to be discontinued after a fortnight, for he has become much more restless and agitated than he was before.—Rel. (f., 40) becomes sexually excited when kept in bed, and is continually masturbating, though she has not done this before.—Gj. (m., 49) grows more agitated if he is forbidden to leave his bed. He feels a need to be constantly walking about, for he fancies that some one wants him.—When a patient has really important business to do, the effects of enforced rest in bed may be even more serious. I am quite certain I should have done Uk. harm if I had kept

[1] Op. cit., p. 461.

him away from his factory, and had completely cut him off from the possibility of keeping an eye on his business. Every alienist knows that agitation must as far as possible be allowed to find vent. We do not ensure rest by compelling the patient to undergo a new kind of agitation.

When studying treatment by rest, we encounter another difficulty, which illustrates a strange fact familiar to alienists, though I do not think enough attention has hitherto been paid to it. It is not always true that neuropaths will be found to have made moral progress when they have been rested and physically fortified. Moreau de Tours noticed long ago that some patients had violent delirium after a good night's sleep, whereas they were perfectly calm if they had not slept at all.[1] Zs. (f., 65), affected with melancholia, anxiety, and delusions, will have a good night from time to time. After these good nights, she is always much worse, with a recrudescence of agitation, violence, and delirium. After bad nights, when she seems very tired, she is better and more tranquil.—Madame Z. makes " desperate efforts to rest and sleep," and sometimes she succeeds. After sleeping quietly for a few hours, she wakes up with some difficulty, and is then in a strange condition. She shakes all over, and feels extremely anxious. Her tics, her pains, her complaints, have been greatly intensified. " It's too bad ! " she says. " Sleeping makes me ill, and I am fit for nothing after I have been asleep. I hear myself groaning as if I were having a baby, and I feel as if I wanted to scream. I am better when I have had a bad night, and when I am positively worn out." In this connexion she recalls the fact that she used to feel much better after she had a great crisis of agitation which had left her utterly exhausted.—The same phenomenon can often be noticed in melancholics. They will be subjected to a roborant treatment, will be given strengthening diet and dosed with tonics. They put on flesh and their physical health is obviously improved ; and yet they suffer more, their obsessions and delusions are worse. Gn., for instance, cannot endure hydrotherapeutic treatment, which has a tonic effect upon her body but makes her mind worse.

We cannot go into this question fully at this stage, for it would have to be assimilated to another remarkable phenomenon, namely that neuropathic symptoms are sometimes

[1] De haschisch et de l'aliénation mentale, 1845, p. 270.

relieved in the course of debilitating bodily diseases and after an exhausting expenditure of energy. We shall find it better to return to the matter in connexion with the study of excitations and discharges, enough here to say that the phenomenon is connected with an important psychological law. Under normal conditions, and in well-balanced individuals, a definite relationship must be maintained between the available energies and the psychological tension. It is not wholesome to acquire much energy when the psychological tension is low, for this will give rise to agitation and disorder.

The foregoing theories of fatigue and repose are concerned only with psychological weakness and psychological strength ; they are interested only in the acquirement of energy conceived as the power, the rapidity, and the duration of movement ; they disregard the problem of tension, that is to say the degree of activation of the higher tendencies. This is a grave error, for nervous or mental disease, though often accompanied by bodily weakness, is something different from simple organic or muscular enfeeblement. Organic weakness, profound anaemia, the cachexia that ensues in tuberculosis or cancer, are not psychasthenia or melancholia. No doubt those who hold the theories we have been discussing, entertain the hope, are animated by the unexpressed supposition, that an increase in the patient's energy will suffice, unaided, to restore his psychological tension. Such a sequence may occur, but it is neither general nor inevitable ; and when the effect of rest and hyper-alimentation is merely to restore energy without raising psychological tension, we only pave the way for agitation and disorder.

This train of reasoning confirms the facts of observation, and shows that the ideas of disease and treatment upon which the rest cure is based, are far too simple. It is almost chimerical to attempt the suppression of all the expenditure of a living being, to aim at the discontinuance of all disbursements of energy. The economies we try to realise in this way are apt to be illusory. If they are really effected, they leave the patient equipped with ill-regulated resources which he is incompetent to turn to good account.

Our conclusion is that in many cases there is no reason for suppressing all movement and for enforcing absolute rest ; it will be enough to insist upon prudence in the expenditure of physical energy. We shall find that one patient is quickly exhausted by prolonged standing, that another cannot take a long walk without suffering for it; here we have obvious indications. A great many women have been restored to tranquillity of mind simply by reducing the amount of housework they have to do.—The cases of Vkp. and Fn. were interesting from this outlook. It was not necessary to keep them in bed for more than a few days. After that, they were told to get up rather late in the morning, and to rest for a couple of hours after meals. But the main requisite was the careful regulation of the bodily activities. Vkp. was quick to understand that she had to avoid undue effort, undue concern with her household affairs. She agreed to run things on a smaller scale, to have a lower standard, and not to bother much about her mother's ideas on the subject. " You have been able to make me realise that my life activities must be restricted. I must simplify my life. If I enter into too many relationships, if my existence is too complicated, I can no longer keep watch over myself, and I lose my self-control. Strict economy of energy is essential to me." In this way, for some years, she has been able to ward off her crises of depression, which used to recur very frequently, and for which it had more than once been necessary to place her under restraint.—Dm. (f., 31) is in like manner exhausted by her domestic acitivities, and becomes crazed by overwork. It is enough to forbid her receiving or paying visits, and to make her have a general servant who looks after her household and her children. Her peace of mind is restored. " Everything at home is quite different. The articles of furniture which seemed to me both unreal and dirty, now look quite solid and have got clean."—Doctors find it difficult to grasp the fundamental truth that in some cases their main duty is to regulate the domestic life of their neuropathic patients.

From the same standpoint, we may consider the disciplining of sexual acitivities, for these activities may lead to great expenditure of energy. I agree with the psychoanalysts that in certain cases a restoration of sexual activity is essential to a cure. But it is easy to exaggerate here, and in many cases we shall find it necessary to forbid or to ration sexual activity, when the patient performs sexual actions incompletely, and is much exhausted by them.—In the case of Ea., a man of forty, the complete discontinuance of sexual intercourse for a time, and the subsequent careful regulation of sexual activity, played a great part in the treatment.—Masturbation often passes unnoticed, especially in young women, who sometimes practise it without realising its significance. Céline (f., 28) naively complained of a vibration in the abdomen, and of shocks in the pelvis. She did not realise that these symptoms were the outcome of the masturbation in which she indulged whenever she was sitting down. In some subjects, as in this one, explanations and a little education will put matters right. In others, we have to exercise perpetual watchfulness, or to take certain familiar precautions.

But when we proceed to regulate domestic life and sexual activities, we are not prescribing rest as that term is ordinarily understood ; we are not recommending simple motionlessness, but an economy of expenditure.

7. RATIONAL ECONOMIES AND THE SIMPLIFICATION OF LIFE.

More often than might be imagined, the patients give us a clue to their treatment. Some of the symptoms of a disease are not direct manifestations of the malady, but are the outcome of the resistance of the organism ; they are defensive symptoms. In the pathology of bodily disease, the fact is familiar ; fever and congestion are protective reactions. The same thing happens in mental pathology, and doctors have to recognise that a nervous patient's behaviour is not always as absurd as it may seem.

There is a tendency to regard diseases, and especially diseases of the mind, as inevitable, as maladies of which the patient has carried about the germ within him. But I am confident that mental disorders are largely dependent upon the life which has been led by the sufferer, and upon the situation in which he is placed. We rub shoulders every day with persons whom we regard as thoroughly sensible and normal, but who have inherited an extremely debile mental constitution. These people would certainly have found their way into lunatic asylums were it not that circumstances have made their lives quiet and easy. We have to distinguish between persons of a psychasthenic temperament, and persons in whom the typical symptoms of psychasthenia have actually developed. The former may be regarded as hot-house plants, which flourish under glass, but will die if exposed to cold. Among our associates there are a great many excellent folk who have inherited a modest competence, who live in an uncomplicated environment, whose education has not been dangerous, has not been such as to arouse ambition. But though they are extremely susceptible, they reach the end of their days without manifesting any signs of mental disorder. As J. J. Putnam said in his lectures on Certain Prevalent Nervous Derangements (lectures delivered at the Lowell Institute in 1905), " these individuals owe the unity of their mind to its limitation."

Nay more, some persons of this type are fairly well aware of their own weakness, and are ingenious in the organisation of an environment which suits them. They manage to find unassuming occupations, which do not necessitate much effort or demand dangerous initiative. The public offices are often cities of refuge for persons whose lives have to be regulated by superiors, who must have neither shocks nor responsibilities. They do not marry, have no mistresses, no children ; they have a minimum acquaintance, and are extremely careful in the choice of the very few persons with whom they enter into relationships ; they live alone, as far as it is possible to do so, in order that they may not need to make concessions. Even if they are well-to-do, they spend very little money ; they never interfere in other people's affairs, never attack any one, never compete with any one. Owing to their precautions and their silence (for they know how to hold their tongues), they are rarely exposed to attack. Besides, they feign blindness, pretend not to feel hurt, and bury their heads like the ostrich. If needs must, they bear the brunt of an attack. Anything rather than fight ; when it begins to rain they pull up their coat collars and turn their backs on the shower. They are shrewd in evading orders and claims. When a frontal attack is made on them, they grow stubborn, draw in their horns, or escape in some way, so that no one can have any effect upon them. They are generally regarded as egoists and poltroons, but perhaps they are wise in their generation.

These patients whose psychological tension is low have learned what kinds of action are dangerous to them. All the phobias of fatigue we studied in the beginning of the present chapter arise out of the realisation that effort is dangerous, and that the activation of the ergetic tendencies entails suffering. Numerous other phobias are connected with the fear of the decision which would have to be taken after reflection, with an eagerness to avoid the activation of the reflective tendencies.

A great many psychasthenics who have been tormented by religious scruples will spontaneously renounce every kind of religion. I could quote a score of illustrations, strange though the fact may seem. " Religion does not suit me at all."—" I cannot go to church in the proper frame of mind, so it seems to me better not to go."—Others will abandon the practice of the arts, or will relinquish serious study. But in many cases these renunciations are temporary.—Cq. told us that he had given up playing the violin, because he was always troubled with sacrilegious thoughts when he was playing. A year later, he began to play again. Quite recently, he has put the instrument aside once more, perhaps for a long time. —The women whose torments we have witnessed when they were hunting for love and intimacy, have been able to find tranquillity by a more or less genuine renouncement of all ardent feeling.—" I shall get on better if I can make up my mind to do without happiness."—" When anything has come to distress me too much, I thrust it out of my thoughts, and then nothing can disturb me. . . . I put my feelings in a glass case. . . . One is nicer to one's husband when one is not too fond of him, so I'm going to cool off towards mine."—These are various ways of economising energy, when the patient has become definitely aware of the cause of his troubles. L. Dupuis, in his essay upon the law of least effort in psychology, writes : " Man has only a limited quantity of energy at his disposal, and he therefore has an instinctive desire to husband his expenditure. While it is true that persons of an extremely active temperament, who are true geniuses in their own fashion, squander their energies without counting the cost, enfeebled subjects, persons of lymphatic temperament, elderly folk, and psychasthenics, shun effort and are disinclined towards any action that demands a considerable expenditure of energy." [1]

These precautions, these economies of effort, give rise to strange morbid symptoms. In this connexion I may refer

[1] Le moindre effort en psychologie, " Revue Philosophique," 1911, vol. ii, p. 164.

to a type of behaviour which has often interested me. In its lesser degrees I speak of it as the "mania for liquidation," and when it is more intense I term it the "impulse to liquidation." Irène's case is an illustration. She is extremely affectionate and devoted, and suffers cruelly at any separation from her intimates. A cousin of hers, a woman of whom she was very fond, found fault with her one day for no good reason, and broke with her, presumably without any intention that the estrangement should be permanent. Irène was greatly distressed. She was ill for several months, obsessed by the thought of the lost affection. Then, when she began to get better, she suddenly gave up speaking about her cousin, and would no longer think about the quarrel. If any one referred to the possibility of making it up, she received the advances with indifference. "People like that have gone out of my life. Let us turn over the page." Studying this patient, I perceive that she has a way of "turning over the page" in the case of all the persons and all the things giving rise to disagreeables.

Such a trait is fairly common, and in a good many instances it may become definitely morbid. Yd. (m., 33) is prone to be terrified and driven almost crazy by the difficulties of a situation in which he finds himself, not infrequently because of his own imprudence. When this happens, the only thing he can think of is how to get out of the coil at any cost. He must dissolve his business partnership. Being engaged to marry, he must instantly break off the engagement, and from his point of view he has already broken it off, although he has not said a word of the matter to the person chiefly concerned. He is on a journey, but must return home at once, before reaching his destination. He will not wait, will not manoeuvre, will not try the effect of a few simple precautions, so that he can get out of his obligations with a minimal sacrifice. He has no regard for anything or anybody. The whole matter must be liquidated on the spot, at all hazards ; and the most trifling delay racks him with anxiety. In the mental and moral sphere, this phenomenon is equivalent to the "fugue" which is so common in neuropaths when they are seized with an urge "to get away without a moment's pause, to go anywhere as long as it is not here."

As I have said, these processes of liquidation can readily

take the form of manias and impulses. Efforts to escape from
difficult situations are apt, in neuropaths, to find expression
in absurd actions and to become phobias. The patient will
begin by avoiding actions which are too complicated, too
rapid, or too prolonged, to be suitable to the low level of their
psychological tension. At the outset, this renunciation may
be reasonable. But, little by little, the bounds of reason are
overstepped. A young man will shun social entertainments
of every kind ; a lawyer will be sick of his law-books ; a priest
will loathe the sight of the confessional ; a doctor will hate
the thought of seeing a patient and writing a prescription.
Thus anxieties and phobias are superadded to the patient's
troubles.—Cq. does not only give up playing the violin, but
gives up dressing himself. He stands motionless in the hall,
umbrella in hand, and says : " I will put my umbrella in the
stand as soon as my head is rested ; the essential thing is that
I should not do anything when my head is tired."—Claire
began by making up her mind that she would not marry,
as she did not feel equal to it. In the later stages of her illness,
she had a phobia of all elongated objects ; she could not bring
herself to touch a bottle because it called up the thought of
the penis.—The invalid begins with reasonable precautions
and appropriate defensive reactions, but ends with ludicrous
phobias and with delusions.

It is incumbent upon the doctor that he should understand
these defensive reactions, restrain them when necessary,
guide them and utilise them. Obviously, he must try to
counteract phobias when they become exaggerated and
dangerous. That is why I doubt the wisdom of the Weir
Mitchell treatment, the wisdom of prescribing absolute rest,
for, in this way, as I have shown by several instances, we
may encourage the phobia of fatigue. If we discover a phobia
in a patient who refuses to leave the sick room, in one who
suffers from dreadful anxiety when he hears the sexual act
mentioned, or in one who cannot carry on his professional
work without being terrified, we must make a psychological
analysis. We must ascertain whether we have to do with
anxiety brought about by the association of ideas, or by interpretation, or by the mania for liquidation, or the like ; or
whether, on the other hand, the anxiety is precautionary and

reasonable, a means of avoiding the performance of a difficult action which would have dangerous derivations. Such differential diagnoses are difficult. No general rules can be given, for each case requires special consideration. Moreover, the problem will face us once more, with fresh difficulties superadded, when we come to study treatment by excitation. In any case, when the doctor is convinced that his patient's phobia is exaggerated and absurd, he must do all that can be done to hinder its development, and must make the patient practise the dreaded activities. This is a method of treatment to which we shall return. But the doctor must never forget that in certain instances the patient's fears have a serious foundation. More frequent, however, than the cases in which the patient has a dread of performing certain actions, are those in which no such dread exists, and in which it is the doctor's business to recognise that particular forms of activity are difficult and dangerous, and that the repetition of these actions must be prevented or minimised. From this outlook, treatment by rest assumes a new aspect. It takes the form of a treatment which is indispensable in neuropaths, treatment by the *simplification of life.*

In this connexion, our first aim must be to put an end to the unceasing efforts occasioned by " attachments." We must " disattach " the patients ; we must unravel, as far as may be, the complicated situations in which they find themselves, and in which they have become enmeshed. In some cases of a comparatively simple type, we must ourselves perform actions which will modify the environing conditions, and will achieve a solution for the patient. We must take responsibilities, formulate decisions, make the requisite efforts, and vicariously solve the patient's problem. In this way we can put an end to false situations, and we shall be surprised to find how many mental disorders, serious to outward seeming, and christened by the doctors with fine-sounding names of an exotic flavour, will vanish as soon as it has been possible to get the patient out of a delicate and difficult situation.—When Vok. (m., 27) had made his confession, it was easy, without consulting him further, to compound with his mistress and to rid him of her. Thereupon, an amazingly rapid cure of his agitation ensued.—In like manner, it was necessary to liquidate the complicated intrigues of Wkv. (f., 22). This was not an easy matter, because the poor girl begged me not to breathe a word to her parents. She recovered tranquillity as soon as she was out of the toils.—I grieve to say that no less than eight times I have had to help in the breaking off of engagements to marry. X. was being driven crazy because his affianced had a harsh expression. " I am terrified by any one who has a harsh expression." He lived a life of sexual restraint, being afraid of women ; and suffered from various forms of mental agitation, and also from rather grave disorders of perception. He was unable to fix his attention upon anything, for his thoughts were continually " fluttering " as a butterfly flutters from flower to flower. Being afraid that even more serious mental disorder would ensue, I found it necessary to convince the family and the patient himself that the engagement was having a disastrous effect and must be broken off. After this had been arranged, X. was completely restored to health in about six weeks.

In other cases the " disattachment " is more difficult, because we are not ourselves in a position to perform all the actions requisite for the solution of the problem. Some of them have to be done by the patient himself. Take, for instance, the case of a young man who has become ill because a proposal of marriage has been made for him, and because he is suffering from nervous exhaustion after having tried vainly for months to say " yes " or " no." The doctor has to examine the situation, but is not competent to come to a decision unaided ; the patient must accept the decision, must himself clinch the matter. Or, if we have to do with a marriage which has actually taken place, we may advise that the alliance shall be continued or that it shall be dissolved, but it remains for the principal to take action accordingly. Here the alienist has himself a problem to solve, for he has to induce his patient to do something important and useful. That is a problem which requires separate consideration, and we shall return to it in the chapter on treatment by excitation. For the moment we are thinking of only one aspect of these activities, we are solely concerned with the economy they will facilitate. When the patient has been " disattached," he will resume his journey through life, and we shall often be amazed by the ease with which he will advance after the removal of the obstacle against which his energies have been beating in vain.

It does not suffice to rid the patient of an attachment. We must take care that the wheels of his carriage shall not become locked once more within a few paces, and if we are to guard against this possibility we must guide him into a road which is free from ruts and loose stones. In my initial studies upon the treatment of hysteria, published in 1894, I pointed out that the simplification of life was essential to a neuropath. " ' The true remedy for hysteria is happiness,' wrote Briquet in 1859.[1] The statement is perfectly true, but it remains to ask what sort of happiness is suitable for a hysteric. I think we can sum up the requisites in a word or two. The patient needs an easy life ; a life in which the problems of the family, love, and religion, have been reduced to a minimum ; a life from which renewed daily struggles, anxieties concerning the future, entanglements of all sorts, have been sedulously removed. No doubt, abundant private means can greatly facilitate the provision of such a mode of existence ; I have seen hysterical patients cured by a comfortable legacy, but the remedy is not at every one's command. Still, the choice of a suitable career and of a favourable environment, in conjunction with the renunciation of unduly exalted ambitions, can certainly contribute to the bringing of the kind of happiness with which we are now concerned." [2] These general recommendations may be supplemented to-day by particular applications.

Many doctors have recognised the importance of this simplification of life. Grasset put the matter well when he said that to prevent the aggravation of the symptoms of nervous disease " we must forbid predisposed persons to engage in struggles, rivalries, and competitions ; must keep them out of the professions in which emulation is keen ; must help them to avoid those dangerous occupations in which brain-work is not restricted to the ordinary working hours of the day." [3] Those who come under our care as patients are persons who have not known how to cut their coats according to their cloth, and who have been so rash as to attempt " to

[1] Op. cit., pp. 365 and 615.
[2] Traitement psychologique de l'hystérie, in Albert Robin's Traité de thérapeutique, 1898, vol. xv, p. 140 ; L'état mental des hystériques, second edition, 1911, p. 677.
[3] Défense sociale contre les maladies nerveuses. " Revue des Idées," 1906, p. 173.

live just like every one else." Quite a number of doctors, and Grancher in especial, tell their tuberculous patients that it will be necessary for them to resign themselves to leading for many years a life which differs from that of ordinary persons. We have to make neuropaths understand that similar considerations apply to them, and that they will avoid disastrous bankruptcy if they will only learn to husband their psychological resources day by day, and always to " save the pennies." What we have to find out is, which kinds of activity are especially dangerous. Though there are, of course, many individual variations, we can learn a good deal from the study we have just been undertaking anent the higher-grade and more costly types of activity.

Difficult as it may seem at the outset, we must do all in our power to enable the patient to avoid work and effort. Unduly prolonged labour is dangerous, not merely because of the big expenditure it necessitates, but also for the very important reason that it entails a liability to checks. When a failure occurs, there is something to be liquidated ; but the patient does not know how to achieve this liquidation, and therefore begins the task over and over again. Apart from this, failure is depressing per se. Psychological depression is not directly proportional to the exhaustion consequent upon excessive and prolonged activity ; in certain conditions, it manifests itself primarily, or as a sort of reflex effect. Human beings are equipped with a mechanism whereby their tension is increased or diminished as circumstances may demand. Just now, we are concerned only with the lowering of tension, and it will therefore be enough to remember that we all know how to reduce our tension enormously by sleep, rest, or relaxation. One of the conditions in which a marked lowering of tension occurs is the condition of check to an action. Disappointment, the feeling of having made a mistake, the expectation of punishment, the idea that energy has been expended in vain, the thought of the efforts that have still to be made, will one and all induce depression ; and such depression is especially conspicuous in neuropaths, who are always prone to discouragement, self-criticism, a feeling of incapacity. It will be much wiser for them to abandon a particular form of activity, rather than expose themselves to the danger of a reverse. One of the difficulties we are apt to meet in these cases is that the patients are so often over-scrupulous, and believe themselves to be under a moral obligation to work, as, for instance, "to do their bit during the war." Whenever possible, we shall find it expedient to arrange for them some form of occupation in which the work is fictitious because the really hard part is done by some one else. Thus the patient's conscience can be eased while real fatigue is avoided. But our main object must be to make the patient realise that his first duty is to keep sane, and that he must therefore avoid efforts that will be useless and injurious.

Finally, in such patients, it is necessary to reduce to a minimum the interpolation of reflective tendencies, and to make voluntary decisions and reasoned acts of belief as infrequent as possible. We must be careful to make the patient avoid changes which will necessitate such adaptations. A cardinal principle in the management of neuropaths is to render their lives exceedingly monotonous and regular. The doctor must be on his guard against the tendency of anxious parents who, with the best intentions, will perpetually try to make the patient change his mode of life. For every neuropath, even the best of changes is a disaster, seeing that it will be almost certain to retard recovery for several months.

When a change involving action on the part of the patient has become inevitable, a good way of preventing reflection is to avoid giving the patient time to think. If he has to take a step of some sort, do not warn him about it, for if you do he will begin to weigh up the pros and cons, and to weary his thinking apparatus. Wait until the last moment, and then tell him that the thing has to be done here and now. Take his assent by storm. The relatives of a patient of mine were greatly alarmed because a change of room had become necessary for the patient, and any change of this kind used to put her mind out of gear for a long time. By my advice, the change took place while she was out for a walk, and when she came back she was conducted to her new room without any explanation. Thus the disturbance was reduced to a minimum.—Under my directions, Clarisse's nurses organised her whole life with extreme care. Every minute was arranged for and no modifications in the routine were permitted. When any new kinds of action became essential, she was not told about the matter until the last moment, and was then made to act promptly. Under this regime, her abulic crises became much less frequent.

The cases summarised at the beginning of the chapter offer numerous instances of this method of simplification and renouncement. When we have to do with young people whose minds are disturbed by the first communion, or by the religious problems of the days of " mental puberty," we must suppress religious practices more or less completely. We forbid going to confession and communion, saying, " I assume all the moral responsibility." This relieves the patient of a feeling of responsibility, enables him to think of his problem less often, to postpone it, to forget it. When the reasons are carefully explained, such a prohibition is in most cases well accepted, even though the family be very religious. If consciences are exceptionally tender, you will probably be able to find an intelligent priest to lend you the weight of his authority. I have notes of quite a number of cases in which a prohibition of the kind bore excellent fruit. Must the prohibition be permanent ? Sometimes it must. I know three women who for the space of twenty years have always suffered a relapse when they have attempted to resume religious exercises. In most cases, however, the prohibition need be no more than temporary. As we shall see later, it is often advantageous, in due time, to advise the resumption of religious mental activity. But, in any case, the suspension must be continued until the nervous crisis has been definitely surpassed.

The prohibition of mental work is a comparatively familiar method of treatment, being a usual prescription at the outset of nervous disorders. I think that circumspection is requisite here : first of all, because study may have an important bearing upon the patient's future ; and, secondly, because mental work is not necessarily injurious to a neuropath, and may be positively beneficial. The prohibition of study must not, therefore, take place simply " in order to give the patient rest," though the prescription is usually made in this routine fashion ; it is only justified when a psychological analysis shows that, in the particular case, mental work is a morbific factor, that it is giving rise to exhaustion. In three cases I have seen a cure speedily ensue in women who had rashly entered upon higher studies, and had worked for examinations which were too difficult for them. In five other cases, the

prohibition of study in young people was promptly followed
by favourable results.

It is well to stress the importance of simplifying holidays,
which are often taken in such a fashion as to be more fatiguing
than study. We must also remember the need for simplification when we prescribe travel for a neuropath " in order to
distract the patient's thoughts." I showed above that travel
can be an extremely complicated affair, and can be very
fatiguing to the mind. In a good many cases, I have found it
possible to check the development of serious nervous disorder
by cutting short ridiculous voyages round the world which
had been ordered as remedial measures. An exhausted
neuropath should not be heedlessly ordered change of scene,
and sent upon a journey, but should be kept for a considerable
period in an unchanging environment. Few people seem to
realise what a long time a neurotic person needs in order to
become accustomed to a locality and to accommodate his
motor habits to its peculiarities.

But if the analysis shows that occupational work is a
preponderant factor of the disease, the work must, of course,
be discontinued. I have known many cases in which servants
have been cured by being sent back from town to their homes
in the country, and many in which lawyers or doctors were
cured by abandoning their professional work.—We must not
be outraged to find that a man like Daniel cannot endure
active service at the front, and we must help him to secure a
post in which he can continue to do good work without going
off his head.—The history of Lvy. is no less demonstrative.
The reader will remember that this man of forty had become
affected with melancholia because he had been promoted in
the bank where he worked. When I was able to arrange for
him to take up his earlier post once more, he recovered with
marvellous rapidity.—It was not so easy to smooth matters for
Uk. in his factory ; but by advising him to restrict his business
for a time and to engage more helpers, I was able to mask
his responsibilities from him.—When we have to do with
patients who are even more debilitated, we must render every
kind of action easier for them. Thus, I arranged that Madame
Z. should always take her meals alone, and that Emile should
never converse with more than one person at a time.—In all
cases alike, we aim at simplification, at reducing activity and

expenditure. Even when the patient seems to be cured, when the crisis of depression has passed, we shall best guard against relapse by safeguarding him against ambitions and adventures, by teaching him to restrict his activities and to live a life of modest retirement.

Such a simplification of life is, to my way of thinking, a sounder and more practical method than the ostensibly simpler plan of ordering absolute rest in bed. No doubt in certain cases, when the patient is emaciated or cachectic, absolute rest is useful for a time, but it entails many inconveniences and must never be unduly prolonged. It is extremely apt to leave traces in the patient's mind, to leave at work causes of exhaustion far more serious than could be any movements made by a patient who is up and about. We should not be so childish as to attempt to rest our patient by suppressing all his actions indifferently ; we must bestir ourselves until we find out precisely what action it is that is causing the exhaustion, and must deal specifically with that one and that only.

It is none the less true that all these methods of treatment by restriction derive from the fundamental notion of the treatment of neuropaths by rest, by economising action. As we shall see even more clearly in the sequel, this is a specific and an extremely valuable method of treatment. Morton Prince told me that Weir Mitchell, in later days, had disavowed the " Weir Mitchell treatment." He had come to the conclusion that absolute rest in bed was of no use per se ; and that its only value was that it afforded a pretext for the doctor's conversations, and for a sort of moralising treatment. If this be true, Weir Mitchell must also have been infected by the epidemic of moralisation ; he must have shown the same weakness as Bernheim who, as we have learned, repudiated hypnotism when he was converted to the fashionable moralisation. These abdications are signs of moral weakness, and they are mistakes. The treatment of neuropaths by repose, and their treatment by hypnotic suggestion, are different methods from the commonplace treatment by moralisation. They are better methods, for they are far more precise and can be applied in a much more definite way. Still, they cannot be turned to full account until we have made a psychological analysis of the patient, and a far more accurate diagnosis than is usually made in such cases.

CHAPTER TEN

TREATMENT BY ISOLATION

THE chief difficulties in life arise in connexion with social relationships, and it has long been felt that social activities are more exhausting than any other kind. On this recognition has been based a method of treatment which is often associated with the rest cure of nervous diseases, namely, treatment by isolation.

I. HISTORY OF TREATMENT BY ISOLATION.

The word " isolation " signifies separation from the social environment, the utmost possible severance of the ties which unite us with our fellows. To people who are in good health, this seems the climax of wretchedness alike from the material and from the moral point of view. It would thus appear that isolation from human society must be a great evil. The tragedians of ancient Greece exemplify the despair of isolation in the lamentations of Philoctetes; modern writers tell us of the sufferings of shipwrecked solitaries like Robinson Crusoe on his desert island, and those of prisoners in solitary confinement.

Nevertheless, there must be some good in isolation, must be a certain charm in the practice, for we find that it is advocated in one form or another by all the great religions,[1] for in this respect, as in others, religion has taken the initiative in the matter of the various methods of psychotherapy. In the religions of India and of ancient Egypt, and above all in the Christian religion, there were men who withdrew from the society of their kind in order to live alone in the desert, in the forest, or in a cave. Such a solitary was called a " monk " (μοναχός, from μόνος, alone). Some of them, the hermits,

[1] An interesting historical account of the practice of isolation will be found in the already quoted work by Camus and Pagniez, Isolement et psychothérapie, 1904, pp. 8 et seq.

the recluses, the anchorites, lived quite alone in grottoes or cells ; but in most instances the isolation was not complete, being so modified as to maintain its advantages while mitigating its drawbacks. The men who desired isolation would combine in order to secure the benefits of the division of labour, and in order that they might suppress only those elements in social life which they regarded as undesirable. Thus, notwithstanding the contradiction in terms, there came into being a society of solitaries. In ancient India, there were innumerable monasteries of this kind ; some of them were hollowed out of mountain rock, and their walls were adorned with numberless sculptures. In the third century of the Christian era, the love of solitude assumed an epidemic form, and the names of some of the early anchorites have become famous. We think of St. Benedict (480–543), the founder of the order of Benedictines, of which the Cistercians and the Trappists were later offshoots ; of St. Anthony, St. Pachomius, Cassianus. Monasteries sprang to life everywhere, and many of these early foundations have persisted on into our own times. Men took refuge there from the brutality and strife of their day, seeking the rest and the tranquillity favourable to exalted meditations. The monasteries were already an asylum for weaklings, for persons unfitted to play their part in the struggle of life, for those whom life had conquered.

At a much later date, laymen sought the advantages of this isolation. In the seventeenth century, the solitaries of Port-Royal were persons who had left the world in order to lead a life of comparative isolation. Several of these recluses wrote enthusiastically of the charms of their retirement, one of the most noted among such writings being Arnauld d'Andilly's ode, La Solitude. At this period, isolation may almost be said to have become a fashion ; and a description of the solitaries of the day will be found in Mlle. de Scudéry's novel Clélie (ten vols. 1654–1661). We find that to-day the adepts of religion still advise a retreat, still recommend that the individual should from time to time withdraw from his customary environment and live for a while in a religious house where he will pray, meditate, practise self-examination, and undergo moral improvement.[1] " Solitude is to the mind what dieting is to the body." [2] Not until a comparatively recent date

---

[1] Camus and Pagniez, op. cit., p. 9. [2] Vauvenargues.

did medicine follow the example of religion, in this matter as in so many others. But at length medical practitioners began to advise isolation as a method of treatment for certain cases. As long ago as 1579, Johann Weier recognised the utility of isolation for keeping the " possessed " apart one from the other. Joseph Raulin the Elder, in 1758, and Zimmermann at about the same time, recommended the identical method for the treatment of nervous and mental disorders. Even before this, Cullen and Willis had made use of isolation in the treatment of the mental malady of King George III. Philippe Pinel (1745–1826) made a systematic use of treatment by isolation as part of his famous reform in the care of the insane. " The patient," he said, " must be isolated from his family and his friends. We must eliminate from his environment all those whose injudicious kindliness might help to maintain persistent agitation or might even aggravate the danger. In other words, we must change the moral atmosphere in which the insane person has to live." Simultaneously with the work of Pinel in France, a kindred reform in the treatment of the insane was going on in England, the initial step in this development having been the foundation of the asylum known as the Retreat at York, which henceforward became a model for English asylums. The founder of the Retreat was William Tuke (1732–1822). He projected the York Retreat in 1792, and in 1796 the place was actually opened, under the management of the Society of Friends, its financial basis being entirely provided by voluntary contributions. It was not until ten years later that the managers of the Retreat had cognisance of the reforms carried out by Pinel at Bicêtre. Samuel Tuke (1784–1857), grandson of William, was superintendent of York Retreat for forty years. In 1813, he published a history of the asylum, entitled *Description of the Retreat near York*. The most celebrated member of this distinguished family was Daniel Hack Tuke (1827–1895), younger son of Samuel Tuke, who for a time was visiting physician at the York Retreat. Daniel Tuke was author of *Illustrations of the Influence of the Mind upon the Body in Health and Disease* (1862), *History of the Insane in the British Isles* (1882), and other important books. In France, Esquirol (1772–1840) continued Pinel's work ; in 1822, he recommended isolation for all the insane, on the ground that in this way they could be saved a great deal of suffering, and could be advantageously treated by methods that were impossible while they remained in their families. At this time there were founded in France numerous fine asylums with extensive grounds. These institutions have earned a well-deserved fame.[1]

To begin with, this treatment by isolation was only applied to persons who could definitely be regarded as insane, although Briquet had already referred to the fact that a moral revulsion and a change of environment were valuable assets in the treatment of hysteria.[2] Weir Mitchell in the United States, W. S. Playfair in England, Charcot in France, and Burkart in Germany, taught that it was well to give others besides the insane the advantages of isolation treatment.[3] The isolation which had proved so serviceable to the insane was turned to account by these authorities in the treatment of various neuroses, such as hysteria and neurasthenia. " I can hardly speak too emphatically," said Charcot, " of the cardinal importance of isolation in the treatment of hysteria. Beyond question, in this disease, the mental factor is largely influential in a majority of cases, and in some instances it is predominant. I became convinced of this nearly fifteen years ago, and my whole experience since then has served merely to confirm my opinion in this respect." [4]

The process was extremely simple. The patient was merely withdrawn from the family environment, and was suddenly removed to unfamiliar surroundings. Hydrotherapeutics was then fashionable for the treatment of neuroses, and this was a convenient pretext for a change of domicile. Charcot usually insisted that the patient should not be visited by any members of the family, and should have neither messages nor letters from them. He was fond of saying that an inappropriate letter could completely arrest progress, and that a young woman who had hitherto been perfectly tractable would become unmanageable if her mother passed beneath the window often. Charcot's pupils, and especially Gilles de la Tourette, did their

[1] Cf. René Semelaigne, Les grands aliénistes français, 1894.
[2] Briquet, Traité clinique et thérapeutique de l'hystérie, 1859, p. 622.
[3] Cf. J. Planques, De l'isolement dans le traitement de l'hystérie et de quelques autres maladies, Paris, 1895.
[4] Charcot, Oeuvres, vol. iii, p. 238. Cf. also " Progrès Médical," February 28, 1885 ; Oeuvres, vol. iii, pp. 235 and 244 ; Leçons du Mardi, vol. i, p. 117.

utmost to promote the widespread adoption of this method of treating the neuroses. " We must break the charmed circle in which the patient is prisoned ; we must forcibly remove the victim from the excessive and harmful sympathy of the onlookers ; we must rid the sufferer of the longing to play an unending comedy, and we can only do this by ensuring the absence of the audience whose complaisance is a perpetual encouragement to play-acting." Thus there simultaneously came into existence in various countries " asylums " of a new kind, " sanatoria " no longer designed for the reception of the insane as the term is ordinarily understood, but for the " borderland cases," for those patients euphemistically described as " neuropaths."

A remarkable variety of Charcot's isolation treatment was inaugurated at the Salpêtrière by Dejerine in the year 1895. It occurred to this authority that his patients might be isolated yet more effectually by keeping them in a sort of solitary confinement for an indefinite term, in beds with the curtains drawn. I have already described, in the chapter on Medical Moralisation, this ward in which all the beds were surrounded by carefully closed white curtains. Dejerine's method was a quaint combination of Weir Mitchell's rest cure, Charcot's isolation cure, and Paul Dubois' moralisation cure.[1]

I do not think that this exaggerated form of isolation has secured a wide vogue. Deschamps, although as we have seen he pushes to an extreme the theory of fatigue as a cause of nervous disorder, and the method of treatment by rest, does not in the matter of treatment go so far as Dejerine. He does not wish to keep his patients for an indefinite time in curtained beds ; but he insists that they shall live in a sanatorium where they will be completely cut off from the life of the outer world. He writes : " The patient cannot, in his bed, bear the burden of a busy life all round him ; not even if we considerably reduce the intensity of that life. Noises from without and noises in the sick-room, necessary conversation, family interests in which he must perforce share, the giving of orders, undue sympathy with his troubles, the inevitable criticism of his utterances and his actions—all these things are a persistent

---

[1] Cf. Manto, Traitement de l'hystérie à l'hôpital par l'isolement, 1899 ; Camus and Pagniez, Isolement et psychothérapie (with a preface by Dejerine), 1904.

and unavoidable source of fatigue. . . . But how rarely do
the members of the entourage understand the patient's difficulties in this respect ; what tragi-comedies are played around
the sick-bed of an asthenic ! . . . The family is simultaneously
the best thing in the world and the worst, and in these cases
it is apt to be the worst. . . The patient should always be
removed to a sanatorium where his only visitor will be the
doctor." [1]

As a rule, however, the isolation of a sanatorium patient
is not rigorous. The invalid is removed from the family, but
continues to see his relatives from time to time ; he associates
more or less freely with the other patients, and with the staff
of the establishment. All that is achieved is a transference
from the habitual environment to an artificial one. But the
fact remains that these different forms of treatment by isolation
are coming to be applied more and more both to neuropaths
and to the insane.

2. Obvious Effects of Isolation.

The treatment of the insane and of neuropaths by isolation
in a special institution is not a panacea. It is attended by
certain drawbacks, and is therefore subject to criticism. Still,
the strictures have been less numerous and less precise than
those passed on the rest cure.

One of the most manifest objections, and the one which
parents are most apt to put forward when sanatorium treatment
is proposed, is that in these establishments there is usually
an aggregation of a large number of patients suffering from the
very same mental troubles for which this particular patient is
to be sent to a sanatorium. Thus our invalid will not merely
be exposed to fresh sources of disorder or emotion ; but will
be actually presented with undesirable examples, so that his
own symptoms will be apt to be intensified through imitation
and suggestion. Elsewhere I have myself described the cases
of five young women who in their own homes had presented
heterogeneous symptoms, but who, when assembled in the
same ward, all became subject to similar paroxysms and
delusions. Charcot's clinic, say the objectors (though there is
some exaggeration in the charge), was a forcing-house for the

---

[1] Deschamps, op. cit., p. 336.

artificial culture of grave forms of hysteria. What happens in the case of hysterical symptoms, must also occur as regards phobias, hypochondriacal ideas, and delusions. In sanatorium and asylum patients we can from time to time note the existence of morbid ideas and fragments of delusional explanation which have obviously been borrowed by one patient from another. Surely it must be a pity to amplify a patient's illness by superadding the symptoms of a wardmate?

This is what Dejerine hoped to avoid by the complete separation of his patients one from another, by curtaining off the beds for weeks or months. The method has been sharply criticised, one of the harshest critics being Sollier. My own opinion is that it can do good in the early stages of treatment, when it is applied for a few days only ; but it is obviously unsuitable for a protracted course of treatment. The sufferer grows impatient, or may pretend to be cured in the hope of being released from duress, or may make a " row " in order to be sent away. Many have boasted to me of having behaved in this way. The organisers of the treatment safeguard themselves, like Paul Dubois, by declaring that they will only treat neuropaths, and will have nothing to do with the insane. This leaves the door ajar for an escape from any difficulty. A patient who obstinately refuses to get well is simply classified as a lunatic. Perhaps the method of treatment by isolation might be yet further perfected by confining each patient in a real cell like that of a prison, where the isolation could be continued even longer. Joly has published an interesting account of certain Belgian prisoners sentenced to complete isolation. He tells us that the prisoners' intelligence does not suffer as much as might have been expected, and that ameliorations and mental evolutions occur.[1] I doubt whether the matter has been adequately studied, and I do not think that persons whose minds were disordered would endure such solitary confinement so well as the prisoners described by Joly. When we have to deal with wealthy patients, a way out is provided by certain high-class institutions like the famous Falret asylum. Here, each patient has his own bungalow, his own garden, and his own attendants, and does not come into contact with any of the other invalids. But this method can only be applied in special circumstances, and it can rarely be carried into full

[1] Henri Joly, Problèmes de science criminelle, 1910, p. 192.

effect. Almost inevitably, in actual practice, the patients in these institutions see one another and talk to one another.

The drawback we are considering is, in reality, less important than appears at first sight. It is obvious that the symptoms of the other patients seen in a sanatorium or an asylum will have much less effect upon the mind of the individual in whom we are specially interested than would have the reaction of his own symptoms upon his kindred if he were at home. In the hospital, the subject is well aware that such symptoms are morbid manifestations, and they are therefore less alarming to him and less strange than they were at home where so much ado was made about them. The danger is not so much in the patient's witnessing a fit of hysterics or an attack of delirium, as in the excitement or in the superstitious terror which such a paroxysm can induce in the onlookers. There is little danger of imitation or suggestion when we have to do with patients suffering from various psychoses or from psychasthenic depression. If, from time to time, one of the patients should adopt the delusional explanations of a neighbour, this is of little importance, for the explanations are merely formulas ; and if our patient had not adopted that particular formula, he would have found some other expression of the morbid state which is fundamental. Generally speaking, however, these patients pay little attention to one another, and are little, if at all, affected by the sight of one another's disorders. Only in special cases is suggestion of much importance. A few simple precautions will usually enable us to spare our patients undesirable sights, and to reduce the danger of noxious suggestion to a minimum.

Some of the objections are more serious. The sanatorium environment is an artificial one, and does not prepare the patient in any way for real life. The symptoms are only suppressed for the time being, and will reappear as soon as the invalid leaves the institution. Unfortunately, this criticism is often justified by experience. A young woman of nineteen, after being admitted to hospital, ceased to suffer from anorexia and took her food perfectly well. As soon as she returned home she began to refuse her food once more, and in a fortnight she was as bad as ever. Another young woman, twenty-four years of age, was suffering from incontinence of urine, obviously hysterical. The trouble disappeared as soon as she was sent to a sanatorium, and during the two months of her stay in the institution she was quite free from it, but it recurred as soon as she went home. A similar sequence will be all the more likely to occur in cases of hypochondriacal obsession, and in connexion with the various disorders dependent upon psychasthenic depression. Many of these patients, who have been relieved by isolation, relapse as soon as they return home. This method of treatment has produced a race of neuropaths who move on perpetually from one sanatorium to another, and spend most of their days excluded from the real life of human society.

There is a yet weightier objection, and it is one which makes even more manifest the weakness of treatment by isolation. The objection is that what should be a hospital for mental disorders tends in general to become a lunatic asylum, a receptacle for the permanent care of unfortunates whose cases are regarded as incurable. Of course, we shall be told that the permanent inmates of these institutions were incurable from the first, that at the very outset the prognosis of their illness was hopeless, and that the doctor should have unhesitatingly admitted that there was no prospect of cure. To-day, a good many authorities maintain this theory as regards cases of dementia praecox in the confusional or paranoiac form. I cannot agree with such a view. The patients classed under this name constitute a very confused group. It is possible that the group comprises certain patients who were from the very start suffering from incurable lesions of the brain, but no one has as yet described any symptoms by which these can be distinguished from the others, who are, to begin with, identical with the neuropaths commonly designated hysterics or psychasthenics. The illness of a paranoiac often begins with psychasthenic delusion. Many sufferers from dementia praecox have been persons affected with severe psychasthenia in whom the lowering of psychological tension has continued to increase despite rest and confinement in an asylum. There are, then, a great many neuropaths whom isolation fails to cure. The fact is so obvious, and instances are unfortunately so easy to find, that I need not stress the point.

We are even entitled to ask whether, sometimes, unduly strict isolation and too monotonous a life may not have a disastrous influence. Long ago, Leuret was opposed to very strict isolation. " Ideas and passions are essential to the human intelligence, and if we suppress them we contribute to the annihilation of that intelligence." [1]   In certain " open " asylums, like the Gheel asylum in Belgium, experience has shown that even dements can improve when made to live in families and to engage in minor occupations.   Of course, there is no great danger in enforcing isolation for a few months.   The worst we need fear is that, when the patient is discharged, a little reeducation will be needed to effect the readaptation to social life.   But if isolation is continued for years, the patient soon grows accustomed to an easy life in which there are no relationships and no social difficulties, and he may become incapable of ever resuming a more complicated existence. We saw that the abuse of treatment by rest in bed might lead to bad results, and the same is true of the abuse of treatment by isolation.

In opposition to these criticisms, a good many authorities have dwelt on the advantages of isolation.   Charcot's arguments, in especial, are now classical.   Certain persons, he said, become ill because, in their environment, they have before their eyes unfortunate examples of neuropathic disorder. The environment is unwholesome, for many nervous disorders are disseminated by the contagion of example.   This was the cause of the sometime epidemics of convulsive seizures, St. Vitus's dance, barking, and so on ; this was the cause of multiple instances of demoniacal frenzy in convents or schools.   Certain fixed ideas are continually being awakened by the conversation that go on in the environment where these ideas first originated. We see conspicuous instances of the kind in the family with a craze for spiritualism to which Charcot was fond of referring in his lectures.[2]

The patient's neuropathic symptoms were often fostered by the wonder, the dread, or the undue sympathy with which they were regarded by the members of the patient's environment.   That was why it was so useful to transfer the invalid to a circle whose members were accustomed to such symptoms, and who therefore took a comparatively light view of them. " Nil admirari," Charcot was fond of saying ; " this dictum is just as needful in the treatment as in the study of neuropathic disorders."

[1] Leuret, Essais psychologiques sur la folie, 1848, p. 168.
[2] Charcot, Oeuvres, vol. iii, p. 236.

A change of environment and of condition facilitates changes of behaviour. In all the neuroses, habit and automatism encouraged by the environment play their part. No doubt the patient will bring his fixed ideas with him into a new environment, but he will pay less heed to them when the old associations have been broken off ; and, in favourable cases, he will end by forgetting them. In many instances, the patient will be able to rid himself of bad habits if he will only make a small effort. A change of environment will give a stimulus to such an effort and will facilitate it.

Isolation can also have this stimulant effect in the production of effort. We can indeed represent it to the patient, not crudely as a punishment, but at any rate as a disagreeable measure necessitated by the state of his health, and as one that will become superfluous as soon as he begins to get better. Mathieu and Roux insist upon this outlook in their study of gastric hysteria.[1] In the new environment, the patient does not feel so free as he did at home, but recognises that he is more under the thumb of the doctor. A woman who, while still at home, has made it a point of honour to resist medical orders, will be only too delighted to listen to the doctor and to obey him when she has been isolated. In this connexion, Charcot quotes a remarkable letter from a patient who said that she had given way and had taken her food because she felt that he was the master.[2] Many a patient has told me that nothing would have induced her to give way in the presence of her husband. One young woman said : " Nothing in the world could have made me willing to walk if Mother could have seen me." A girl of twenty, while at home, had every few minutes been affected with an attack of delirium accompanied by shrieks. The trouble vanished directly she came into the hospital. " Now that I am here, I take a little trouble to stop the attacks when I feel them coming on."

Finally, it is not difficult to show that isolation facilitates the hygienic and medical treatment of the patient. Obviously, it is not easy to enforce a strict alimentary regimen upon a neuropath who takes his meals with the family, whereas it is easy to see that our prescriptions are observed when the patient feeds apart. This remark applies especially to sufferers

---

[1] Mathieu and Roux, Hystérie gastrique, " Gazette des Hôpitaux," February 1, 1906.   [2] Oeuvres, vol. iii, p. 243.

from bulimia, who eat too much, and to sufferers from anorexia, who eat too little. Isolation is also a help in the enforcement of absolute rest, and assists us in the application of various other kinds of treatment. These attendant advantages have been obvious from the first, and they explain why treatment by isolation has been so successful in institutions for the cure of nervous disorders.

3. Social Behaviour of the Neuropath.

For the better understanding of the therapeutic value of isolation, and in order that we may be able to apply the method more accurately while maintaining its advantages and minimising its drawbacks, we must gain a better understanding of an important psychological problem, namely that of the expenditure demanded by social activity, and of the costly efforts requisite for social life. We must gain more precise notions concerning the action exercised by human beings one upon the other, concerning what Tarde used to call " inter psychology," which has never been adequately studied. People do not make sufficient allowance for the way in which one person may affect the psychological tension of another, of the serious extent to which one person's doings may lower the tension of another, thus producing a real crisis of psycholepsy. If we had a better knowledge of these matters, we should know what kinds of society and what individuals a patient ought to avoid. Instead of prescribing isolation in an absolute fashion without understanding its conditions, we should be able to regulate the method in a far more practical manner.

I cannot here undertake a general examination of this problem, but can at least discuss some of its details. I propose to summarise our knowledge of an important aspect of the neuropath's behaviour, his behaviour in social relationships. I shall describe how he behaves towards the members of his family, towards those who form his immediate entourage. This summary will enable us to enquire what influence the neuropath's behaviour can have upon the persons with whom he comes in contact. As a result of such a discussion, we shall be able to understand better why isolation, or at any rate the separation of certain persons one from another, is at times so important and so useful.

Lethargy and Social Abulia.—We know that neuropaths have no liking for work of any kind ; that they do not know how to begin an action, especially if it be unfamiliar ; that if they do begin an action, they tire of it quickly ; and yet that they do not know how to leave off.   The upshot is that they never achieve anything practical, that they fail to adapt themselves to a situation, and that they seldom or very slowly acquire the habits which result from the satisfactory performance and repetition of an action.—" I never feel at home anywhere, I never feel that there is anything for me to do at home ; I have no ambitions in the domain of material reality." —" I detest everything that is materially and practically useful in the way of household work ; I loathe making collections, taking photographs, going on journeys ; I hate whatever entails my doing something."—" I don't form habits, I have an objection to being tied by custom, I have always been like that."—A man of fifty declares that having to send a registered letter is " an abomination, like having to pay a bill."—Ya. (f., 40) will not even try to take her own ticket at the station and to make a little journey by herself.   " I've never done anything so silly as that in my life, and I hope I shall never have to do it."   At most she can put up with " intellectual activities."   She says :   " I want to have everlasting sensations and ideas.   When I think that a sensation or an action may be transient, I am disgusted with it, and I will not have anything to do with these fugitive matters.   I care only for great and enduring concerns, such as honour, my country, and religion.   Nature, which is always beginning the same thing over and over again, is immoral, and we ought to pay no attention to it whatever."

When such persons are compelled by circumstances to begin the performance of one of these actions which they find so repugnant, agitation ensues.   A lower-grade and disorderly activity takes the place of the useful activity.   Some of the sufferers from major hysteria will sit quietly in their chairs or lie at ease in their beds as long as they are not asked to do anything ; but when the time comes for getting up, dressing, or taking a meal, they at once grow agitated, shriek, become abusive, strike their attendants, break something.   Even in patients whose illness is less advanced, when we insist upon making them talk or making them do something, we often find that they become angry, make ugly faces, burst out laughing again and again, or betray one kind of obsession or another. "Directly you make me sit down to eat, I become filled with remorse, I am afraid that I lack kindliness, everything seems queer and false."

These fundamental disorders of action are, of course, reproduced in all forms of social activity. Under the head of social activity I include all the actions in which consideration for others must play a part, even a remote part ; and I think of others' action upon us as well as of our action upon others. Let us consider, in especial, two important types of social activity, acts of command and acts of affection. Psychasthenics are amazingly awkward and impotent in respect of both these fundamental types of action.

They can neither command nor obey. A great many such patients never open their mouths to give an order to their servants ; they would rather do what they want themselves than ask any one to help them. Wkx. tries to avoid his servant even in the passage. An effective order involves insistence upon the formula, a repetition of the formula until the order is carried out, preparation for a struggle, the continued training of subordinates ; it involves, that is to say, the maintenance of a fairly high tension for a definite period of time, and psychasthenics are incapable of this effort. Obedience, although in certain respects it is easier than command, likewise needs the paying of attention to the order, the checking of counteractive tendencies, and the activation of the tendency that has been awakened until the action has been effectively performed. Consequently, these patients are as unfitted to obey as to command. When we ask them or order them to do something, they fail to do it. Instead, as we have seen, they become angry or agitated. In many cases, the agitation is systematised in the form of a stubborn resistance. The patient will not simply refrain from making the movements requisite for the performance of the action, but will make movements of an opposite kind, will draw away from the person who has given the order, will tear off the garments that are being put on, and the like. This is one of the forms of the syndrome which has been termed "negativism." It is often described as characteristic of dementia praecox. As an actual fact, it is present to a greater or less degree in all sufferers from depression ; but in psychasthenic dements it manifests itself more quickly, and in connexion with comparatively simple actions.   We may be astonished to find that a patient who lacks strength for action, is nevertheless able, when the question is one of resistance, to expend an amount of energy which seems far greater than that which would have been requisite for the action.   The paradox is only apparent.   Agitation and resistance are very simple actions.   An extremely low tension is requisite for their performance, and therefore the depressed patient finds it much easier to resist than to obey.

Such patients are constantly talking about their feelings and their affections, and in many cases they even have a mania for loving, but we must not allow ourselves to be deceived by appearances.   They do not really know how to love.   They cannot render apt service, cannot save another person trouble, for they are never ready at the desired moment, they are alarmed at the complexity of any action which might be superadded to their petty routine ; they are unwilling to sacrifice one of their whims, one of their perpetual claims.   Although they use high-sounding terms for the description of their feelings of affection, the feelings are merely skin-deep, and the fondness vanishes when there has been the most insignificant misunderstanding, or merely as the outcome of a brief separation.—" I must see people constantly if I am to love them.   With me, out of sight is out of mind.   I should not care for you at all if I only saw you once a fortnight."—Many of the patients realise that they are incapable of loving.—" Children are tiresome little beasts, and there's nothing of the mother-hen about me."—" I only cared for my husband for a very short time."—" I used to have a faculty for loving, but it vanished when I began to menstruate."—" All my life I should have liked to have my heart full of love, for life is worthless without that ; but God would not vouchsafe me the faculty of loving." —" I cannot love because I am in such poor health.   Since I lack health, how can I have a feeling which is only possible for those who are strong and well."—" As soon as I want to do anything, it becomes impossible ; I wanted to love my daughter, but thereupon I hated her."—The patients are incapable of organising the tendencies which constitute the foundation of family life.   " I have been married for twenty years, and I still need to make an effort in order to remember that I am married. I wish I was still called Miss instead of Mrs. I have remained a pure-minded girl, and have never lived the life of a married woman. I grow confused and humiliated when I recall the fact that I have lost my maidenhood."—" My husband did not succeed in animating me ; he missed a fine chance of playing the part of Pygmalion."—" I doubt if I should notice it if my husband and my six children were to vanish."

What is even more surprising is that such patients appear to be no less incapable of hating than of loving. Though they will often utter expressions of hatred, they are disinclined to take any trouble, to throw off their inertia, to sacrifice their tranquillity, even in order to gratify a grudge. Hatred which does not stimulate an effort to satisfy the feeling is not very deep. The fact is that, in psychasthenics, the tendencies both to love and to hatred are unstable ; either tendency is speedily exhausted, so that room is left for the temporary manifestation of the opposite tendency.—" I never know on what terms I am with her. For a few days she seems passionately fond of me, and then I suddenly find that she detests me."—Simone (f., 26) is herself aware that she cannot love several people at once. For a fortnight she will be devoted to her mother, and will loathe her nurse ; then comes a period in which she cannot endure her mother, and lavishes affection on the nurse.

As we shall see, psychasthenics have an inordinate desire to be loved ; unfortunately they are unable to attract affection to themselves. Not only are they incapable of performing any service for others, but they cannot be amiable, cannot please people by the manner of their greeting or by their conversation.—" My parents," said Plo. (with some reason), " are both snobbish and untidy. They are always talking about keeping up appearances, and cutting a dash, but they lack the energy to be orderly and clean. There are always pots of jam on the arm-chairs in the drawing-room, and Father's socks lying about in the dining-room. They say they want to receive company, but they never want to tidy things up. . . . When any one does come, they say, ' What a nuisance,' tell the visitor they are engaged, and of course he never calls again. . . . Then they complain that their friends neglect them."—The patients do not know how to make the effort necessary, either to listen to what others say or to express their own ideas. They never know what has been said to them, and will not take the trouble to make themselves comprehensible. —" I don't say anything, for I find it so tiring to think clearly enough in order to speak."—It is seldom that they are as self-critical as this. They are content to express a half-formed thought in an unfinished phrase ; or else they will be tedious and involved ; " one feels as if one would like to shake them to get some sense out of them." Yet they are furious if their hearers do not understand them ; that is to say, they are furious because the auditor does not himself do the work of disentanglement which they ought to have done in order to make themselves comprehensible.—Tt. (m., 30) is disturbed when he has to speak in company. For him this is a very grave affair, and he is greatly alarmed at the thought of the effort requisite for polite conversation. This makes him irritable, brusque, choleric, and rude. " It's absurd ; I am like a child ; I can no longer behave as befits my education and my class in society ; I have lapsed to a lower level, and am full of false ideas and false sensibilities."—The majority of such patients shun social effort. Wkx. will receive no visitors, and compels his wife to break with all their friends. Dl. (m., 55), always restless and agitated, bolts when any one calls. When out of doors he goes through back streets in order to avoid meeting any one he knows, and would have no friends left were it not that his wife spends most of her time in patching things up. These comprise the totality of the inadequacies in social life which pass by the name of shyness, though this name implies undue insistence upon emotional derivations which are secondary, and overlooks the social lethargy which is the main factor. The neuropaths who are continually lamenting the isolation of their lives, are persons who have no friends because they are incapable of friendship.

Mania for Secretiveness, Mania for Lying, and Mania for Hindering.—In place of these normal and difficult actions which they are unable to do, neuropaths perform other actions peculiar to themselves. First of all, I may point out that they take numerous precautions against having to act, against becoming involved in action which they find so costly. They restrain their desires ; they avoid having special tastes ; in almost all cases they cultivate a kind of asceticism which is only a form of lethargy.[1] The pleasures of luxury, and even the pleasures of dress, never seem to them worth the pains. Another very frequent characteristic of such persons, which is also an outcome of lethargy, is their passion for secretiveness. " Hide your life," said the Sage; and the precept is one after their own hearts. Just as they want to make a secret of their fortune and their family life, so, too, they never wish to say where they are going, what they are doing, what they are thinking about. " I should like to be a mystery to every one." Though they pretend to long for affection, in reality they dread intimacy, and they are in terror lest their face, their eyes, or their smile, may betray them, and may enable others to enter into their thoughts. This is the explanation of a great many of the classical obsessions and phobias. Why they dread to be known is that their weak point would then be disclosed, they would be more open to attack and could readily be compelled to make additional surrenders ; people could take liberties with them, could demand services from them, levy contributions from them, involve them in expenditure or rather in action. But this last is what they especially want to avoid. A very simple way of eluding activity is by lying. Our actions are in many cases demanded, not simply by circumstances, but by the persons who are in contact with us and who have seen the circumstances. If we are able to change the idea of the circumstances in the minds of our parents, our superiors, the people who are entitled to order us about, we shall thereby rid ourselves of a great many orders, a great many claims, a great many reproaches. Thus we shall free ourselves from the need for performing a great many actions. That is why lying makes its appearance as soon as depression gets beyond the first degree, that of sadness, to reach the second degree, that of lethargy. It becomes habitual, and takes the form of a mania for lying, when the depression grows more or less chronic. In a young man, a mania for lying may be regarded as a pathognomonic symptom enabling us to forecast the development of psychasthenic disorders.

The mania for lying imparts a particular hue to the social behaviour of these persons ; their behaviour becomes different

[1] Les obsessions et la psychasthénie, 1903, vol. i, p. 436 ; vol. ii, pp. 23 and 346.

from that of other people.   All they say is transformed, their actions are accounted for by false deductions, they accustom themselves to describe things falsely.   In the end, they can neither understand nor believe that other persons are sincere; they continually suspect their friends to be liars like themselves ; they distrust whatever is said to them, and will clumsily try to verify it.   At the same time, they have a strange feeling whose presence I have had occasion to note in several of the patients described in this book.   They are astonished when people speak frankly to them, and they seem to feel that this frankness is a sort of rudeness, is the expression of a hostile attitude which they deplore.   A possible explanation of such a feeling is that they dislike to see in others a virtue which they themselves do not possess, so that the frankness of others becomes for them an implied reproach.   I think a more plausible explanation is that they do not wish to see the naked truth, and that they regard as unseemly the bluntness of those who wish to present truth unveiled.

When the members of the patient's circle catch the offender in the act of lying, and draw attention to the falsehood, the liar is not abashed.   He makes a smoke-screen, denies the evidence, and supplements the lie told to others by lying to himself.   There is nothing unusual about this form of reaction, for people have a way of behaving towards themselves as they behave towards others.   We know how often neurotic girls will send themselves bouquets, and will even post love letters to themselves, and be much gratified by the reception of these spurious missives.   The mania for self-deception plays an important part in the organisation of beliefs and delusions. It gives a peculiar complexion to the reverie of the lethargic patient, which becomes a comedy, half believed to be fiction and half accepted as true.   We shall fail to understand the somnambulisms and many of the other symptoms of hysterical patients unless we have grasped the existence of this state of mind.   But, quite apart from these extreme forms of the phenomenon, lying is a factor in the daily life of such debilitated persons.   It enables them to transform reality, to replace it by an imaginary and easy world, to avoid seeing imminent dangers, to be blind to circumstances which make a claim for effort, and to be deaf to calls to action.

When they at length realise that, despite their mystifications and their lies, they are about to be affected by the actions of others and that they are likely to be compelled to join in the actions of others, they resign themselves to action, but their action takes a form which seems to them the most simple and the most prudent. They refuse to participate in others' actions; they resist these actions; they oppose whatever is done.

We may, perhaps, regard this as a variety of the negativism which was described above. But instead of simply resisting orders by refusing to perform the action which is commanded, the action which they dread, these patients try to check the activities of the persons with whom they come into contact, even when the latter ask nothing of them.—Bkf. (m., 55) plays a remarkable part in the business house of which his son is the real manager. He tries to interfere with all the activities of his son and his employees. " He is so uneasy and so obstinate that he hinders everything."—Di. (f., 55) has for many years made the life of her family very difficult. She contradicts everything that is said; she angrily objects to whatever is done, opposing the action in every possible way and declaring that it is absurd; she is constantly trying to interfere with the carrying out of her husband's business appointments, and to disorganise her sons' work. In a word, she hampers every one's activities.—Xob. (m., 45) hates that his wife should spend any money, for he is miserly. When she brings forward any scheme, he seems to accept it at first, but he adds that it has been suggested at a rather inconvenient time, for his business is not going well. Next day, he says he has had bad news; and before long he declares that he is almost ruined. If his wife takes alarm and gives up her scheme, he is tranquillised, and nothing more is said about the imminence of bankruptcy until the next proposal to spend money crops up. Being himself an ascetic, like other persons suffering from depression, he has no wants, and does his utmost to prevent his wife from having any. " He has ended by depriving us of all our friends, and by taking the savour out of life."—Zso. (m., 50) has a different tactic. He monopolises his wife, wants her for himself alone. He is full of kindness, but also brimming over with claims. To outward seeming, he is greatly concerned about his wife's health; he is always talking about this, and will not let her stir a finger without telling her that she will make herself ill. In this way he has completely isolated her, and has shut the door upon all the friends of the family. She cannot open her mouth without being contradicted; and whenever she begins to do anything, he raises objections. " He does all this out of affection, for he is devoted to me. He does not want me to read, not even when he is dosing in his arm-chair. The real reason is that he wants me always to be thinking about him. If I were reading, I should be thinking of something else, and should not be ready to answer in a moment if he were to wake up and say something. Thus he is on the watch although his eyes are closed, and he wakes up if he hears me turn over a page. Nothing will make him understand that he is selfish. His view of the matter is that I shall make my head ache if 'I read. There is nothing I can do without his declaring that it is bad for my health."—Aj. (f., 37) has all her life suffered from marked abulia, being incapable of coming to any decision regarding household affairs. " At first," said her unfortunate husband, "'I had always to make up her mind for her, to buy the cooking utensils, choose the plate, arrange about the house-moving, and so on. I even had to choose her dresses and her hats. You can't imagine what a lot of work it means when one has to live for two people at once. . . . Still, I could carry on as long as she allowed me to do so. But of late she has taken it into her head that it is wrong to let me act for her, and she wants to make up her mind for herself. Her system is very simple. She puts down her foot whenever I suggest anything, vetoes all my proposals, and continues a stubborn resistance. Sometimes I succeed in making her do something really indispensable by proposing the exact opposite, but this is rather a complicated way of getting things done. . . . If I make no suggestions at all, she is at a loose end. Since she has no longer anything to contradict, she is in despair, and weeps all night, lamenting that I no longer love her. Life has become impossible ! " The actual fact is that the woman is now more seriously ill than she was at first. She is no longer competent to perform even the minor grades of action which her husband had left for her to do, and that is why she has adopted the new method of persistent opposition. " I can't think or act as quickly as my husband," she said with a groan. " It's too complicated, I can't keep up with him and never shall be able to. . . . I am always running after time, always short of time ; my husband goes too fast ; I stop to examine a difficulty which he never sees ; I come back again and again to the same thing, with ever-renewed irritation ; I am like a piano key which has got stuck. I cannot bear for him to run on ahead of me, I cannot bear that he should leave me alone where I am."

This inclination to hinder others' actions may become a positive mania. Here is the description one of my patients gave me of the way her mother behaved. " She never stops forbidding our doing whatever we may happen to be doing, however trifling it may be.—' You are walking up and down the room. Can't you see that you are making a draught ? '—' Don't stand there like a stuck pig, you look absurd and it annoys me.'—' Don't stand there swinging your arms.'—' Why are you not talking ? I suppose it is because I am here.'—' Do stop chattering, you are making my head ache. Can't you make those birds stop singing ? '—She diffuses a sort of restlessness around her, which acts as a kind of badly lubricated brake to check all the activities of others ; and she watches these activities narrowly that she may ever be ready to interfere with them."

In some cases the resistance of these abulics is so effective that it completely inhibits all activity on the part of others. The family of Cy. (f., 28) has a very difficult time of it. She will not permit any kind of " luxuriousness " in the household or the kitchen, and even objects to having the kitchen fire lighted. Occasionally the mother will light the fire on the sly, but the appearance of a cooked meal leads the young woman to keep better watch in future. There are tears, supplications, scenes. The family has had to resign itself to a diet of bread and cheese. This resistance to others' doings is one of the most remarkable among the social acitivities of the neuropath !

4. THE IMPULSE TO DOMINATE.

The Mania for Helping and being Helped.—In other cases, which are perhaps commoner, the neuropath does not definitely oppose another person's action, but wants rather to participate, to have a finger in the pie. To begin with, he watches what is going on, always hoping either to stop the action or to turn it to his own advantage, his main desire certainly being to get the maximum advantage at the minimum of cost. No doubt the action is useful to him by its material results : but a more important point, and one which is apt to be overlooked, is that action is stimulating per se and helps to raise the psychological tension ; this is a matter we shall have to study in a subsequent chapter. Our patient is well aware of the fact. Being incapable of acting on his own initiative, he wants to be made to act. The urge to participate in others' activities is so natural and so general that we are continually seeing instances of it in everyday life. Who can fail to have noticed how a crowd forms round a workman who is knocking nails into a post, or round one who is building a wall, simply because of the longing to see another at work ? Persons who are themselves incapable of vigorous bodily exercise will spend hours in watching runners or wrestlers, or in reading newspapers which describe these sports. The same taste is even more strongly developed in our patients.—" My dream is to sit watching a man at work especially a man who is writing. Do let me watch you writing the whole evening ! "—More often, however, there is a desire for an active collaboration. The patient wishes us to work with him. We are to do all the difficult part, start the operation, overcome the obstacles, and so on ; but we are to pretend that his assistance is of the utmost value, and, besides thanking him for his precious contribution to the work, we are to let him take all the profit.—Bs. (m., 41) had a mistress who played this part perfectly. She was always fussing round him, keeping him at work, making him write a little. When she forsook him, he was utterly at a loss, and became affected with serious depression.—Lydia could do nothing without her twin sister. " I need to have the same sensation as she, and to perform the same action. I can't do anything unless she does it with me. My life is merely a reflexion of hers, and, though we are twins, she is really my elder sister."—Bkn.'s mother wears him out by continually asking him to work for her, to help her in doing something.—" I always need," said Aj., " to have some one with me who distracts my thoughts, makes me talk, helps me to tidy my drawers and tidy my thoughts."—Ye. (m., 28) says : " I cannot settle down to work unless I have a companion who, like myself, is studying for his doctor's degree, who is reading the same subjects, and is just as far on as I am."—When Sophie first fell ill, she wanted to help all her associates in their work. I learned from these associates that she believed she would be of the utmost service, would help them to do splendid things and to have lofty thoughts.

Thus, the mania we are considering exhibits various forms. Sometimes the patient's chief desire is to be helped, and it then resembles the mania for asking questions ; sometimes the patient wants to render help, to participate in other people's activities, this being akin to the disposition manifested in the mania for devotion.

The Mania for Command : Authoritarianism.—The best collaboration, that which (in appearance, at any rate) demands the least expenditure of work, is the giving of orders. No doubt command in the full sense of the term, when it implies initiative and guidance, is very difficult ; and we have seen that a great many patients are incapable of commanding in this sense. But there is an elementary factor of command which consists in formulating an action without undertaking the action oneself, in insisting upon this formula until some one else takes the requisite action, while the person who issues the order is regardless of the worth or usefulness or interest of what is done. Command in this sense is an easy matter, and brings much satisfaction to the weak. They need make no personal effort, and yet they can enjoy the feeling of participation in action ; and they can modify the behaviour of their associates so as to avoid dreaded changes in the environment. When such orders, or most of them, are obeyed, the individual who has acquired a habit of giving orders has a feeling of security and comfort inspired by the recognition that a great many persons are at his disposal and are his subordinates. This reassures and stimulates him. That is why there are so many domineering persons in whom the habit of giving orders has become a veritable mania.

We are apt to think that the habit of domination, and a passion for command, are appropriate to persons of energetic temperament, to those whose will is active and powerful. We therefore feel surprised to find that authoritarianism is one of the symptoms of psychological depression. But the feeling that there is something paradoxical here can be dispelled by drawing a distinction between the genuine domination exercised by the strong, and the authoritarianism of the weak, which is but a parody of true domination. A strong and ambitious man pursues a great aim, hopes to achieve an important result. For him, the domination of others is no more than a means to his end. He does not enjoy the exercise of power for its own sake ; and domination is to him merely an instrument whereby he can intensify his activity. In a word, the wish to dominate, like true command, has an ulterior aim. The authoritarianism of depressed persons has no ulterior aim. These weaklings, who can hardly be said to have schemes or wishes, do not entertain any thought of having particular things done by others, and they have very little interests in the results of the actions they command. They only verify the results in order to ascertain that they have been obeyed. They want obedience for its own sake; they want to dominate merely in order to dominate. The feeling that they dominate is what gives them a sense of security and comfort. The behaviour of one who is really a chief is a manifestation of high tension. Even in weaklings, the imitation of such behaviour gives rise, by a sort of reflexion, to a moderate elevation of tension.

Elsewhere I have recorded numerous examples of this moral disposition, which plays an important part in family life.[1] I have already pointed out that authoritarian persons fall into two natural groups : the tender authoritarians, who never use force, but try to ensure obedience by tears and supplications ; and the tough authoritarians, who attack and threaten their associates, when these display a yielding disposition, in order to reduce them to slavery.

In the first group, I shall mention about a dozen cases. —Bkf. (m., 50) is continually declaring that he will die if people go on causing him intense suffering by disregarding his wishes. Though a person of low-grade intelligence, he is sly as a fox, and he is able to keep his household entirely under his thumb.—Lkc. (m., 55) never gives any one a moment's rest, and incites all the members of his entourage to febrile activities, for he is so devoted, so good, and would be so terribly unhappy unless every one obeyed his orders.—Zby. (m., 60), an exacting busy-body, continually expecting that he is about to achieve wonders, gets his own way in everything by fawning, and by holding out ingenious promises.—Lkd. (m., 45), perpetually nervous, uneasy about trifles which for

---

[1] Les obsessions et la psychasthénie, 1903, vol. i, p. 393 ; vol. ii, pp. 153, 175, 360, 370, and 403.

him bulk enormously, is convinced that he can only act if he and his wife are absolutely one. " I have an affection for her." He wants to teach her how to guide all her actions by reason ; he makes her study questions of hygiene and domestic economy ; by gentle and unflagging insistence, he makes her spend her evenings in writing detailed accounts of all she has done during the day, accounts which have to be presented to him every week-end. " All I want," he says, " is to make her perfect." He is good, virtuous, austere, doctrinaire, and absolutely intolerable.—Byc., whose essential trouble is extreme abulia, can find energy for one thing only, for dominating his wife. He treats her as a child while pretending to help her. Indeed, he has really helped her now and then, and in return he demands absolute submission.—Cj., a boy of fourteen, belongs to the same category. He is tied to his mother's apron-strings, and never allows a moment to herself.—Another of these tender authoritarians is Byd., a lad of eighteen, continually obsessed with the fear of what people will think. This makes him tremble before strangers. But towards his mother and his sister he is proud and exacting, and, though plaintive and gentle, he makes their lives a perfect martyrdom.

I have notes of fifteen cases belonging to the second group. Cx. (m., 50), authoritarian and hard, keeps a tight grip upon the fate of the whole family, and exercises a domination over all the members of his household, so that they hardly dare to speak or move.—Lsx. (m., 50) cannot bear that his wife should have any ideas of her own, or undertake any action except at his instigation. Whatever is done in the house, however trifling, must be done upon his orders. He issues these orders brutally and aggressively. He cannot endure to have any one near him except inferiors who are paid by him, and whom he believes for that reason to be thoroughly cowed. —The case of Ew. (f., 45) is extremely interesting. She has always been bad-tempered and almost impossible to live with. She has a daughter whom she is constantly " rowing " to make the girl afraid and thoroughly subservient. She is terribly jealous and suspicious of any one who comes near the daughter and to whom the latter might become attached. She keeps watch on all the doors of the flat, and if any one goes near the door of the daughter's room, she goes there too. She is critical

of everything she hears that other people have done, and she
attacks every one who comes near her, for she always fancies
they are encroaching. In the end, she drives her son and
daughter out of the house, saying : " If they were to stay,
I should no longer be chief in my own household, and should
not be able to control the servants." She is continually
repeating : " This is my house. It is for me to give orders
here. Nothing ought to be done in my house without my
orders." All the same, she is just as much inclined to give
orders in other people's houses, and to interfere in other
people's business.—Fv. (f., 70) is also of a very remarkable
type, and has adopted an extraordinary mode of life. She
never goes to bed, but sleeps in her chair ; she eats at odd
times and has no regular meals ; her room is like a pig-sty.
Rich and miserly, she is always in terror of poverty, and has
spent her whole life in dominating and robbing her children.
Since her fear was that they would outgrow her influence,
become stronger than herself, and dominate her, she guarded
herself against this danger by keeping a very tight hand on
them pecuniarily.—Guh. (m., 50) is a terrible authoritarian
who makes his associates' lives a calvary. There is no end to
his exactions, many of which are absurd. " If he tells you
that the table is round when it is square, you must echo his
words. You will do it in order to have peace and lest worse
befall."

In a complete study of authoritarianism it would be
necessary to take into account the persons over whom sway is
exercised. Some people are authoritarian with all comers,
but this is exceptional. It is more usual for neuropaths to
reserve such behaviour for the members of their own family.
A peculiar form of family authoritarianism consists in the
desire to gather together and to keep together all the members
of the family, and never to allow any to escape, to go out, to
act independently.—In Lox.'s family, the mother insists that
her husband and even her grown-up children shall always be
gathered round her, remain with her, and never leave her.
She will not allow any one of them to go for a journey alone,
or to visit a friend, or, for a moment, to leave the family group.
This insistence is all the more amazing seeing that, once all
the members of the family are assembled, she has no further
use for them and cannot even talk to them. No matter ;

she wants to have her court around her, to guard her, or to serve her in case of need. " The whole lot of us must be bored in company."

In many instances, this mania for domination is systematised or concentrated upon one particular individual. The neuropath, indifferent to all others, tries to exert authority over one special person, who is to become a slave.—Il. (f., 55) seems to have little will power and to make few claims ; any one can manage her. But she has a ruling passion, to dominate her daughter aged thirty. The younger woman has to do everything, however insignificant, under the mother's direction ; she must be told when to go out, when to come in, when to change her dress, and so on. The daughter is treated as if she were still a child, and as if from moment to moment the mother wanted to make quite sure that the role was still acceptable. I need hardly say that the least sign of refractoriness arouses an outburst of fury and even delirium.—In some instances a woman tries to exercise this exclusive authority over a sister, but the husband is perhaps the most frequent victim. I have had occasion to note that authoritarian persons have sometimes a penchant for dominating individuals of a particular type. Just as certain women who excel in beauty or charm may find these qualities a positive nuisance because of the number of lovers they attract, so there are persons whose quality it is to arouse in others the passion for domination. —Jsa., a woman of thirty-six, is, quaintly enough, surrounded by a group of persons who are all equally domineering, and each of whom, jealous of his rivals, tries to put the grappling-irons upon her. She is rather a bright-looking woman with a specious air of energy, and she arouses in the minds of authoritarian persons the idea of an easy and delightful conquest.

Another form of systematisation of authoritarianism is to concentrate the orders, not upon certain types of person, but upon certain types of activity. We see neuropaths whose fancy it is to demand from their associates the frequent performance of special kinds of action. They will begin by demanding peculiar precautions. They will make rules about the way in which people must behave and speak in their presence, for an infringement of these rules will arouse disquietude or induce anxiety.—In the case of Kr. (m., 65) the demand is for the most precise punctuality. The poor man cannot wait a minute, and every one must keep time by his watch.—A good many patients insist that every one shall speak to them very slowly, and that no one shall do anything quickly in their presence, for they are themselves slow, and the sight of rapid action makes them uneasy. " It takes him an hour to understand the most elementary joke, and he is in a fury if any one seems to have grasped it sooner."—With other people, there must not be even the most trifling disorder upon the tables or in the arrangement of the furniture ; and no noise must be made in walking, eating, sleeping, etc.— Lq. (m., 35) cannot look any one in the face, and is afraid of his wife's eyes. When they are at table together, she must always turn her profile to him, looking constantly to the left so that he shall not have to meet her gaze.—Some demand incessant precautions. They are so terribly afraid of draughts that no one must even open a drawer while they are in the room. Others insist upon moral precautions, so that nothing may be said which might imply criticism, raillery, or a distant allusion to what they have done or said.—" You must never utter a surname in my presence, for if you do I shall be kept awake all night trying to think of the Christian name and the address. All those who live with me have learned never to mention any one by name."—" How could you contradict yourself in this way before me ? First you said ' I am sure ' ; and then you said ' I think.' They are not the same thing at all, and you were warned that I can't endure people to contradict themselves, that it makes me quite ill."—In a word, such patients insist upon numberless precautions, numberless special observances, and their susceptibilities are always ready to be outraged by the most trifling breach of the regulations.

In one way or another they insist upon our focussing attention on them throughout the day. " I can't get away from her for an instant. I must always be looking for her handkerchief or her keys which she has mislaid simply for the pleasure of making some one search for them. I have to tell her what she ought to do next, since she does not know herself ; and yet she does not do it when she has been told."—" When my daughter comes into the room, it seems to fill with sunshine ; I need her to come every five minutes at least."

They demand to be cared for both by day and by night in all possible and conceivable ways. A woman of forty has succeeded in persuading her husband, a man not otherwise lacking in intelligence, that he must spend hours holding her head in his hands. He has to exercise strong pressure on the back of her head, and while doing this he has to utter raucous cries that sound like belching. The gases confined in Madame's body have to pass out through Monsieur's hands, and must then be belched up by him. Monsieur goes on pressing his wife's head until his muscles are utterly exhausted, and belches until he makes himself sick.

These patients have again and again and yet again to be assured that their illness is not a serious one, " that their pupillary reflexes are active, and that they show no signs of general paralysis," that they are incapable of committing a crime. Sometimes these patients can only be reassured by some set form of words. For instance: " When I meet any one in the house, I ask : ' Does God really exist ? ' Then they must answer without fail : ' Of course he does, you little silly ; it would really be too wretched if God did not exist.' This is what they must answer, do you see ? It's absolutely neces-sary."—Mp. (m., 60) is able to live peacefully if he is con-stantly encouraged in a peculiar tone of voice ; he has to be chaffed about his countless ailments ; the current of his thoughts has to be changed by making him laugh ; and this process has to be repeated again and again.—No. (f., 50), who is afflicted with innumerable phobias and hypochondriacal algias, needs to be sympathised with, to be pitied because of her earaches, because of her heels which are sensitive to the hard floor, because of her breasts in which she fancies that tumours are growing ; all day long she has to be taken notice of, her veins must be examined, also her patellar tendons, her stools, her pupils, and so on. " My husband is so hard-hearted, he will never do any of these things ; he won't even join his lamentations to mine ! "

Nor does this suffice. They have to be everlastingly encouraged and stimulated ; and, since nothing produces the desired effect so well as praise and compliments, they demand a constant flow of flattery : their vanity is as colossal as their sensitiveness. Sometimes this vanity inspires them with boastfulness, and then they recount the glorious deeds of their own doing, and expect their hearers to be full of admiration for their prowess and never to show any scepticism as to their veracity. Others, again, display their vanity by the assumption of a whining personality of demeanour. Such persons are for ever repeating that they are " no good," that they are not intelligent, have no talents. In reality they do not believe a word of it ; on the contrary, they are persuaded that they have been especially well endowed by nature, and have wonderful talents, but that their gifts have been eclipsed by illness. They would be filled with despair if any one else were to depreciate them in the same terms, and they eagerly await the compliments for which they have been fishing.— Aj. (f., 37) says : " I count as less than nothing in my own home ; I have such dire need of being flattered ; my troubles would be greatly relieved, if only I could always have some one with me who knew how to flatter me."—" My mother is always demanding that people shall pay her compliments ; she only cares for people who flatter her or who help her to look as if she had achieved a success."—Lsx. needs to be pleased with himself, and in order to attain to this comfortable feeling he would like to be told that he is an extraordinary man ; he never has any visitors save those who are capable of proving this to his own satisfaction.—Ya. innocently remarks : " Of course I know at bottom that I am a very superior woman ; but I should like to feel my superiority. I am surrounded by idiots who don't understand a bit ; their real duty should be to show how superior they think I am."—Sophie, especially at the onset of her attacks of depressions, is so afraid that she may become insane that she needs constantly to be reassured as to her intelligence. It is sometimes surprising to find really intelligent women caught in the toils of a flatterer from whom it is no easy task to release them.

The Mania for being Loved.—The craving for obedience, for being tended and fussed over, and for flattery, may find expression in other ways. These tributes must be tokens of love, and not extorted. Here we encounter the famous need to love and to be loved which plays so important a part in the words and the deeds of neuropathic patients. " I do so need to adore and be adored. I have not got the husband (or the wife, as the case may be) that I had dreamed of having.

. . . I do so crave for caresses, for coaxing ways, for affection, for love ; I have never yet had as much as I could enjoy. . . . I can only be cured by affection, by love, " and so on. These are the plaints of hundreds of patients. I have already dealt at length [1] with this sentiment in all its variations. Here I wish merely to make certain points clearer by considering once again just what these patients mean by the expression : " I do so need to be loved."

A simple explanation which has been fashionable in Germany and Austria consists in interpreting the word " love " in the literal sense, and in considering the lament as an expression of ungratified sexual needs. Certain patients do seem to justify such an interpretation.—Céline (f., 32) is for ever awaiting the man who will marry her ; she listens with anguish in her heart for the sound of his footstep on the stair ; she cannot get up interest in anything, in religion, or art, or science ; she only feels interested in kisses.—" Love, alone is interesting," says Héloïse (f., 40). " If I had only had a husband to pet me, I should never have fallen ill."—Other patients amply justify the above interpretation. Bs. (m., 41), who was timid and never succeeded in what he undertook, found a mistress who initiated him into the sexual life ; she educated him, in fact. She was the first person through whom he was able to achieve a success. He was filled with despair when she left him. In his case it is not difficult to understand what he means when he sighs : " I want to be loved." His obvious yearning is for sexual satisfaction.

I fancy that even in such cases (as we shall see later) the satisfaction or gratification of sexual desire is more in the nature of a stimulant, and is resorted to instead of alcohol or morphine. Already in the cases quoted above, the issues become very quickly complicated ; and, side by side with the excitation caused by physical love, we find the gratification of all the other needs.—When Bs. mourns the loss of his mistress, he mourns the loss of one who was capable of guiding his life in all ways.—Aza. (m., 30) demands, not only a mistress, but " a woman who can guide me and buck me up."—Pepita (f., 42), when looking out for a lover, is gratifying her love of adventure ; and her need for moral excitation is satisfied by

[1] Cf. Les obsessions et la psychasthénie, 1903, vol. i, pp. 32, 40, and 388 ; vol. ii, pp. 11, 48, 92, 404, 410.

the danger she runs.   This is well proved in her latest adventure
of the sort.   Her lover was a ne'er-do-well who never gave
her any physical gratification ; but he fascinated her because
he was an etheromaniac and half crazed, and she had the
delight of running grave risks through her connexion with
him.—On the other hand, in a far greater number of cases,
there is absolutely no question of sexual gratification : here
we have to do with men and women who are incapable of
feeling sexual desires, who neglect the occasions when they
might gratify such desires if they had them, and who are
preoccupied with utterly different matters.

What these people mean by being loved is that no one shall
attack or molest them in any way.—" Isn't it horrid to feel
one is quarrelling with some one, or competing with some one ?
I simply cannot live if I fancy I am in any one's bad books." [1]
—More frequently, the person who loves the patient is the
person who renders innumerable services, who acts for the
patient on countless occasions, and who thus spares the sufferer
many efforts and many worries.—Fik. (f., 55) is always bemoan-
ing her loneliness, for every one has fled from her authoritarian
ways and her bad temper.   She is in despair because nobody
loves her.   " There's no one awaiting me at home ; and in
order to live happily I must know that some one is there,
expecting me.   I have got to make journeys all alone, and
nobody is there to take my ticket for me or to call a cab.
Surely a man is expected to call a cab for a lady at the
station ?   I have no home circle ; it is killing me ;   I am
terrified at having no one to love in the whole world."—
" When one is loved," says Pepita, " it's so easy to get out
of a carriage, his hand is always there to help. . . . Yes, an
ideal lover, wealthy and not too busy, a foreigner rather than
a Frenchman, they are more interesting, not so fed up with
things, exquisite natures, so considerate where women are
concerned, just a trifle loose, maybe, but so reasonable, liking
to have a good time but not to excess, knowing the place to
take me to and where I shall be best entertained.   That's
the sort of thing I need to cure me.   Have I not just as much
right as any one else to find him ?   Oh, to have a young page
like Cherubino in love with me !   A lad who could .be
affectionate and kindly, who would spoil me.   I do need it so

---

[1] Cf. Les obsessions et la psychasthénie, 1903, vol. i, p. 400.

much ! " In cases of this kind the craving for love belongs
to the class of impulses which are the expression of the search
for rest, and which secure an outlet along the line of least
resistance.

Another group is made up of persons who expect rather
more delicate service from the lover ; the services thus claimed
are hardly recognised as services at all ; the patient is inclined
to veil their nature by describing them vaguely as " love."
The one who loves is also the one who comforts, who revives,
who stimulates ; these ends may be attained by means of
sexual excitation, but more often the effect is produced by
social acts which are in themselves stimulating, not for the
performer, but for the person in whose interest they are
performed. A type of such acts is the giving of praise, and
flattery of every kind. Flattery is praise given with more or
less sincerity, but the aim of which is to raise the psychological
tension of the person to whom it is addressed. " Here is a
soldier who writes from the front to say I am his ' charming
godmother ' ; true, he has not seen me, but that doesn't
matter ; his letter did me good for a whole week. I do so
need a little tenderness ! "—Bm. (f., 52) has an amorous
obsession for a young man whose energy has impressed her.
Though she leads a regular life, she is romantically inclined,
dreams of adventures, feels a need for intimacy which she has
never been able to satisfy with any one, would like to be
guided and dominated by a person who all the time continued
to feel a great respect for her.—Aj. is perpetually repeating
that her husband does not love her enough. " I should like
him to be more tender and gentle, to give me advice and not
orders, to reanimate and stimulate me, to take a good deal
more trouble to incite me to action."—No. (f., 50), notwithstanding the expressions she uses, has no other wish than to
be incessantly reassured, condoled with, and tended. " If
any one will reassure me, I brighten up immediately, my
distress vanishes, I appreciate everything ; a suitable word
will fill me with beatitude, and my associates seem harsh to
me because they refuse to say this word."—When people of
this type are in search of some one to love them, they all
want the same thing, to find a person who will defend them,
help them, flatter them, reanimate them ; they want an
intelligent slave who will adroitly perform on their behalf

all the actions necessitating psychological tension, all the actions which they are unable to perform.

But there is another element in their conception of love. They must feel assured that the person whom they find to fulfil this role will go on playing it in perpetuity, will never change, will be always at their disposal to defend them, console them, stimulate them, etc.—" If she really loved me, she would not leave me for a whole day to look after myself." —" If my husband loved me, he would have continued to tend me as sedulously as he used to."—But the analysis of these persons' idea of love would be incomplete without the addition of another important notion. For them, to be loved means, not only that the innumerable services they look for shall be rendered for an indefinite period, but that they themselves are never to pay for these services in any way whatever. I need hardly say that material or monetary payment seems horrible to them.—" Your doctor and your nurse are giving you all the care you need. You can have a companion as well, an intelligent woman who will do all that you say you need."—" Perhaps, but that sort of thing would not satisfy me. She would be paid; she would not serve me out of love."—I told Fik. that several members of her family had been to see me, and that they were all eager to help her, to be companions to her, to distract her thoughts. She became quite angry. " Of course I know that, and I don't want to have anything to do with them. They are influenced by self-interest; they hope I shall give them presents, they are on the look out for legacies, they want me to give things to their children. People like that are of no use to me. I want some one who really loves me, who loves me for myself."— I have been surprised to come across the same feeling in a domain where there is no question of payment. I have told some of my patients at the hospital that they will receive all possible attention from doctors and students; that these spend hours in talking to the patients, in understanding them, in reanimating them.—" Oh, yes, but they are studying, are taking notes. They will use the observations they make on me. That is not love, that is not true affection. If only I could meet some one who loves me for myself ! "

Some of these patients are intelligent enough to understand that it is, after all, necessary to pay for services rendered. They will give little presents, freely, when it suits them; they will render little services, which are often imaginary. But, owing to their infirmity, they act awkwardly and without perseverance; and they expect their presents and their services to be greatly overvalued. " The most trifling thing that I do would seem of inestimable worth if I were really loved."— Lsx., who has such a craving to be loved, does not get to work in a way which is likely to bring him satisfaction. He blundcringly tries to make his wife jealous by courting another woman in her presence. " He shows a Teutonic kind of sentimentality, and yet is heartless; and he is indignant because he is never loved for himself."—A woman of forty says that when she was young she had plenty of girl friends. (At that time, she had no lack of psychological tension.) " Now I can't make any friends. I am ill, and people find me a bore. No one can love me for myself."

We may think in this connexion of the Freudian explanation of all psychological phenomena, of the explanation that they are universally dependent upon sexual phenomena. These patients, these women, do they simply mean that everything is to be given them provided only that they give themselves in return? Some of them would agree to the bargain. The sexual act costs them little, and is not distasteful to them. For many women, a lover or a husband is simply a cheap slave. But the majority will indignantly exclaim: " How selfish and brutal men are! I should still be paying, and how could you call that being loved for oneself?" Moreover, I sympathise with the protest. What they want is certitude, security in love; a guarantee that absolute devotion will be continued for an indefinite time, and whatever circumstances may arise. But if they are to pay for love monetarily, or by having their symptoms studied, or by rendering services, or by giving their bodies, they no longer have the absolute and unconditional certitude they desire. They may cease to be rich, to be interesting cases, to be vigorous and young and beautiful; then the conditional devotion will vanish. " It would be much better if I could be loved for myself." The payments, whatever form they take, involve activity on their part. They have to make an effort to give something, or to give themselves; they dread that they will not always be able to perform these actions, and they dislike the thought of having

to perform them in order to ensure others' devotion. " I
want to be loved for myself alone ! "

What do they mean by this phrase ? I think our talks
with our patients enable us to divine the meaning. A particularly instructive case in this respect is that of Ya. She is
a rather pretty woman of thirty-five. Her intelligence is by
no means profound, but she sparkles. She is incapable of
acting, or of rendering any service to others. Since she is
sexually frigid, sexual relationships have no lure for her.
She simply cannot understand their attraction ; and, like
frigid women in general, she is ostentatiously prudish in these
matters. She is continually railing against her husband, and
against men in general, for failing to appreciate her adequately.
" He is not worthy of such a wife as I am ; a handsome,
refined, and distinguished woman. . . . A woman such as
I am, ought to be loved for her own sake. . . . Do there no
longer exist any true lovers, chivalrous enough to love their
ladies without asking any return ? "—" But Madame," I reply,
thinking to put her in a quandary, " even the truest of lovers
are sometimes a little exacting. If you were to meet this
perfect lover, would you not make him a few concessions ? "
—" What are you talking about ? " she said. " You are
thinking, like all the rest, of love in the vulgar sense ; of
love which asks for payment. He would see me sometimes,
and would hear the sound of my voice. He could love me.
Am I not a charming woman, and is not that enough ? "
Substantially, what she means by being loved for herself alone
is that she is to secure perfect and unending devotion without
having to make any return, without having to do anything
herself ; she is to secure this devotion simply by the fact that
she is a pretty woman. She wants to pay for the devotion
by her natural qualities, which she believes she possesses
once for all, so that she need never make any effort now or
in the future. All these patients are animated by some such
idea. The natural qualities of which they are thinking will
vary from case to case, but they are regarded as a permanent
possession. An elderly woman will speak of her white hair ;
a girl of her youth and her maidenhood ; a man of his bodily
strength and his past exploits, or of his intelligence and his
straightforwardness. These natural qualities, the gift of birth
or acquired once for all, are what they have in mind when they

use the phrase " I want to be loved for my own sake " ; it is in the name of these qualities that they demand love.

Here we touch upon a very important notion, that of " rights," for a right only means that the holder of the right can demand of another or of others the performance of certain actions without having to make any return, himself, in the way of action. Those whom we speak of as " men of action " do not concern themselves about their rights but about their duties, about the actions which they themselves have to perform. Abulics, on the other hand, think only of the rights which entitle them to expect actions from others, and which dispense them from the need for acting themselves. That is why psychasthenics are continually talking of their rights, like the rights we were considering in the last paragraph, those of a pretty woman.—Gh. will tell us of a young man's rights in the field of love. " How artificial they are, these working-class girls who cannot give themselves simply for love. When they make fun of my proposals, they are really immoral and spiteful. I never have the luck to come across the Jenny of the novel, or Béranger's grisette. Nowhere can I find nature, for everywhere I encounter artifices and prejudices, innumerable obstacles to be overcome, things which ought not to exist in a really natural nature."—The great argument used by a mother who tries to impose an almost incredible slavery upon her married daughter and her son-in-law is the " right of motherhood." " How can my daughter go out in this way and leave me alone ? How can she go on talking without saying anything about me ? Am I not her mother ? No matter what she does, she can't get away from that."—Others speak of the rights of age, lineage, wealth, education. " Surely a man of family like myself ought to have plenty of friends for his own sake."—Or the talk will be of benefits forgot, of the rights possessed by the doer of services in the past. " I was so good to them twenty years ago. There is no gratitude in the modern world."—No less remarkable is the way in which the working of natural laws may be regarded as establishing rights. A young woman who has no children, and is obsessed with the thought of this, is never weary of complaining that she has been unjustly treated. " A married woman ought to have children ; it is her right. Why should I be deprived of my rights ? "—Many of those who have a mania for love use similar phrases. " Love prevails throughout the world ; the cow loves her calf ; when a house was on fire I once saw a bitch sacrifice herself for her pups. Love is natural, and I have a right to love."—Moral laws will initiate the idea of rights even more readily than natural laws. " My husband is behaving badly when he does not love me as he ought."—" Certainly my wife ought to love me. Religion ordains it, and if she does not love me with all her heart, she is wicked."—The " rights of man," finally, may be made the foundation of individual rights. " No one should try to injure me, or to humiliate me ; I have a right to justice ! No one should try to deceive me, to tell me a lie ; I have a right to the truth ! " All these feeble souls take refuge in the idea of rights and justice. When they boast of their own scrupulousness, what they really want is to make other people extremely scrupulous towards themselves. Moral notions, like philosophical notions, are not infrequently the outcome of disease.

The Mania for Devotion.—Some patients protest against such an interpretation of their mania for being loved. They declare that they do not merely wish to be loved, but wish to love. They want to protect others, to do services to others, to pay compliments, to overwhelm the objects of their affection with flattery and delicate attentions. In a word, they want to devote themselves to others.

I need not recapitulate the description of the neuropaths who try in every possible way to put themselves into the limelight, to attract attention. Glaring colours, eccentricities, are not peculiar to hysterics. Similar characteristics are met with in a great many neuropaths suffering from depression, who seek to obtain excitation through success and especially through love. What it behoves us to remember is that in a good many women " efforts to please, to charm others " may become a definite cause of overwork. Calls, parties, conversations, are for many such women serious operations demanding a great expenditure of energy and resulting in extreme exhaustion.

Some patients go further than this, being constantly agog for opportunities to perform minor services and to give unexpected presents.—" I have a strong desire to help, flatter,

and cajole those whom I love.   I like to overwhelm them with
attentions.   Why is not my loving kindness acceptable ? "
—" He is harsh to me, disagreeable.   No matter, I want to
be something in his life.   I am always giving him little
presents, even if I have to steal the money from my husband.
I want to devote myself to him.   I should be happy if I could
only be an inkstand on his desk."—Héloïse is continually
boasting of her love, her generosity, her devotion, the caresses
she can lavish.   She glories in having been called " a woman
who is an incarnate caress."   She says : " I am a lover quite
as much as a mother.   There are no limits to my love.   What
would I not give to those whom I love ? "

Such devotion, such generosity, have invariably some
strange and abnormal element.   The attentive observer can
usually detect a flaw somewhere.—An unhappy son-in-law
said to me : " You will do me an immense service if you can
deliver me from my mother-in-law's presents."—" That is
rather a strange request of yours ! "—" Nothing could be more
natural than my wish.   My mother-in-law is an odious woman,
and we know perfectly well that she does not care for us at
all.   Her dread is that her daughter's marriage will be a
success, and her one thought is to humiliate and degrade us.
But she has a mania for making us presents.   They are wretched
little things, but they enable her to boast everywhere of her
generosity, and to demand unending thanks."—The same
trait was to be seen in another lady who had a way of continually giving trifling presents to her grandchildren, simply
in order that her daughter and her son-in-law might have to
overwhelm her with thanks.   When they had gone away, she
would burst into tears, and exclaim : " Oh, dear, they only
thanked me three times to-day ! "—Again, I knew a mother
who made herself a perfect nuisance to her children.   She
would be continually giving one or other of them a present in
order to single that one out from the others and to have a
perpetual reiteration of thanks.

But, in most cases, this ostensible devotion is merely a
mask for other appetites.   Yd., a man of twenty-three, the
sexual invert who was always trying to find " an ideal friend "
among the young scamps with whom he associated, had a
strange way of depicting his enterprises as acts of devotion.
" If I am on the look-out for this young friend, it is that I may

be able to reform his life alike in the physical, the moral, and the religious respect. I want to have him properly dressed and housed ; to have him given music lessons and literature lessons ; to make a gentleman of him. That would be my mission in life, and would fill my days with interest." Imagining himself to be successful in his search, he will again and again pick up a young rascal who will flatter him ; will even, to please the patron, pretend to be jealous and make scenes ; and who will, in the end, run away with an abundance of plunder. But this does not deter our friend, and he makes a fresh start with some new object on whom to lavish devotion. —The mania for " raising fallen angels " played a considerable part in a dozen of my cases in which there was an impulse towards love affairs or adventures.

In other instances, the devotion may seem genuine, so that it is difficult to detect the element of self-seeking.—Sophie, when she relapses into depression, has a craving to tend her mother and to perform all sorts of services on behalf of other members of the family. In fact, when she becomes unduly charitable on her walks abroad and too anxious to please at home, when she is eager to fetch a footstool for this person and to put pillows under the head of another, it is time to watch out for a fresh crisis.—Byl. (f., 25) heralds her relapses by talking about leaving her parents' comfortable home and going to live among the poor ; and quite a dozen of my patients become aware at these times that their true vocation in life is to be a hospital nurse.—Ig. (m., 30) wanted to devote himself to some one, to help some one to success in life. " I should like to be able to make a change in some one's existence, to be the chief cause of his happiness."—If we analyse these urges to devotion, we shall find that, underlying them, is a wish to be rewarded by infinite gratitude, a desire to ensure protection and recognition and flattery for the remainder of the doer's life. There is, in fact, the same longing for love ; but there is also a desire to secure excitation by playing a great part, by performing a heroic action.

5. THE AGGRESSIVE IMPULSE.

Unfortunately, these efforts to dominate, to inspire love, are apt to be unsuccessful. More especially, they seldom succeed in freeing the patient from depression. In many instances, therefore, they become complicated by other forms of behaviour which tend, in turn, to degenerate into manias.

The Mania for Teasing and the Mania for Sulking.—The root of teasing lies in the desire to probe the power we really exercise over those about us.[1] The invalid makes an attack, inflicts a wound or a humiliation upon some one, not because of dislike, but under the spell of a wish to dominate, or to secure caresses, flatteries, and love. If the person who is attacked does not care for the attacker, he will defend himself and hit back ; but, in the other event, if he really loves the person who is making the onslaught, he will not defend himself ; he will accept the wound or the humiliation ; he will merely show his distress at the causeless aggression ; and perhaps (oh, joy !) will weep because of the wound. Then the teasing will have attained its end, and the success will bring a moment of infinite satisfaction.

Here is a letter from Héloïse which contains an excellent description of teasing. " The maximum of pride and satisfaction is to know oneself loved. But I want to be sure that the acts of devotion, the compliments, are sincere. I need a sincere, immutable, unvarying, steadfast affection ; I am not content to be fed upon comfits. . . . The real test of love is, not ability to give pleasure, for this is nothing ; the test is, ability to give pain. . . . No matter what form of pain it is. If the indifference, the absence, the neglect of one person extracts a cry of pain from another person, the former is loved by the latter. This is the most splendid victory, the most ideal happiness, when the indifference has only been a test, and when the neglect has merely been a mask in order that we may ascertain if we have really stirred those intimate and hidden fibres where true love vibrates ; if we learn that we are loved enough to be able to inflict pain."

The unfortunate thing is that the satisfaction is but transient, and that the doubt speedily recurs. Thereupon the successful experiment has to be repeated, the teasing has to be renewed.—Dl. (m., 55) cares for no one except his eldest daughter, and he is always teasing her, so that most evenings

[1] Cf. Les obsessions et la psychasthénie, second edition, 1908, p. 407.

he reduces her to tears at the dinner table. Then the mother takes the girl's part, and battle is joined night after night. —Héloïse does her teasing by letter, and there are no limits to the ill-natured things she will write to persons of whom she is fond and whose affections she wants to test.—This particular characteristic of teasing can be well verified when we note how it may undergo a marked development during periods of depression, and may disappear when the depression is over. It is during the week following menstruation that Noémi always feels the urge to make her husband weep ; and it is in the same phase that Héloïse begins anew to write spiteful letters to all her friends. When these two women are perfectly well, the impulses are in abeyance. Sometimes the mania for teasing may take extreme forms, and it must never be forgotten that in such patients the most signal manifestations of ill nature may be merely teasing.

The mania for sulking is closely akin. It, too, is a mania for verifying the existence of love, but in this case by a pretended indifference or a simulated rupture. If any one really loves us, nothing will distress him more than suddenly to break off relationships, than suddenly to replace affection by indifference. The victim will want to know the cause of the change, will offer excuses for an unwitting fault, will do all that can be done to bring about a reconciliation and to revive our affection. These signs of distress and these efforts may, for a brief space, tranquillise the mind of the doubter ; but soon the doubt recurs, and therewith a new fit of sulks begins.—Vkp.'s mother would sulk in this way for months, and Vkp. was ill advised enough to make a great to do about the matter.—In the case of Bkn.'s mother, sulkiness was a means for the extraction of money from the daughter.—Dl., in his relationships with his wife and his daughter, was a past master in the art of sulking as well as in that of teasing. " There are some people," said his wife, " towards whom he has been in the sulks for twenty years."

The Mania for making Scenes.—The before-mentioned types of behaviour are often supplemented by a kind of activity which is extremely characteristic of the mental condition of the neuropath. I refer to what is called " making a scene." The best way of defining this form of activity is to say that it

is a simulated battle, just as teasing is a simulated attack and
sulking a simulated rupture.

To begin a great battle with the person whom we love,
to volley abuse, reproaches, threats of death, as if we were
dealing with a real enemy ; to win an easy victory because the
opponent is not really an enemy, does not resist, allows himself
to be disarmed or even crushed ; then magnanimously to
offer pardon, to achieve a formal reconciliation, with embraces
and promises of eternal love—what excitation and what joy !
The enfeebled subject is stimulated by a battle and a triumph
which have cost him so little ; and he is confirmed in his
faith in the devotion which is able to endure such a test.
That is why the mania for making scenes is so common. I
have frequently had occasion to describe the cases of women
who took delight in making scenes with their husbands, saying :
" How jolly to be able to make it up afterwards ! " Here
I shall adduce a few additional examples.

Ek. (m., 30) admitted frankly enough that it did him good
to make a scene. To begin with there was obviously an
increase in his depression, with a feeling of despair and anxiety,
these being manifestations of psycholepsy. Then he would
utter vague recriminations against society, and, after a few
divagations, he would concentrate upon his father. " It
would seem," said the latter, " that his mind is at work in
order to discover satisfactory reasons for getting into a rage,
and ere long he succeeds in excogitating reasons which really
seem to him adequate. Then his anger is impetuous, sombre,
arrogant, savage, brutal ; he is incredibly rude ; nothing can
divert his attack. I, his father, become the central object of
all his hatred. He wants to make me suffer, longs to be
revenged on me. At the climax of the outburst, he flings out
of the house, tears across the country, collapses on to the
ground, and remains there for half an hour, panting, and
working off his emotions. Then he comes home again,
tranquillised and amiable, with his serenity restored for
several days."

Sometimes such scenes will assume a melodramatic form,
thanks to the working of the tendency towards symbolisation
and comedy to which I have frequently referred.—Fj. (f., 35),
when making a scene, will bring to her husband's bedside a
photograph of her mother. The husband then has to get up,

kneel down, and ask pardon of the photograph for the crime he has committed by not showing enough subserviency and love for the daughter of this revered lady.—Za. (f., 40), when going to bed with her husband, brings with her a paper-knife which is quite formidable enough to be used as a dagger. Then the scene begins. From time to time she picks up the dagger and brandishes it, threatening to use it now against herself and now against her husband, and declaring that it is time to put an end to this wretched existence. After the shrieks and threats have lasted for an hour or two, she gets up in her nightgown and goes out of the room, taking the dagger with her. Since she does not return, the husband rushes out, and in the passage he finds his wife prostrate. As soon as the husband comes, she gets up quietly, and goes to make a glass of orange-flower water for each of them. Inasmuch as the scene is reproduced every fortnight, the husband, having grown a trifle weary of the routine, sometimes stays comfortably in bed after she has left the room. In that case, the wife will lie for hours in the passage, until at length the husband, afraid that whe will get a serious chill, goes out to her. " We have lived in this way for years in the company of the paper-knife dagger."

Manias of Jealousy.—Another type of morbid affection is jealousy, which is a complex psychological phenomenon, and one whose precise anlaysis is by no means easy. We have not merely to do with a peculiar form of behaviour in relation to the object of affection, who is hunted and monopolised ; furthermore, there is, in the jealous, a special mode of behaviour towards other persons, who are excluded, repelled, annulled, in so far as they are real or possible rivals. Jealousy comprises both the monopolisation of the person or thing that is loved, and hostility towards other persons who may covet the same person or thing.

This exclusivism is in part dependent upon the desire to secure to the uttermost the person who is loved ; upon the very simple idea that we shall obtain less for ourselves if we have to share our ownership. In part it is dependent upon the dread of rivalry, upon the fear of having to compete with other individuals who may be more worthy of being loved than we are ourselves, so that we may be hard put to it if we want to maintain our ownership. Nothing clashes more violently with our tendency to dominate than the success of another individual who competes with us for the same object. Parents can no longer suppose that their daughter's love is theirs exclusively and for an indefinite term, when they perceive that another person has already secured an important place in her affections. The thwarting of so powerful a tendency gives rise to vigorous derivations, to intense distress, to formidable hatred.

Different varieties of jealousy may be distinguished in accordance with varieties in the fundamental monopolisation, in accordance with differences between the tendencies which give rise to this monopolisation. In persons whose primary thought is wealth and station, jealousy is directed against those who are well-to-do, and especially against those who are rising in means or position. Hh., a man of forty, suffers from several sub-varieties of this form of jealousy. He cannot endure " people born in the gutter who now actually drive about in carriages just like me—a pretty pass the country is coming to ! " He pushes this tendency so far that he hates whole villages " which for some years, now, have been so impudent as to grow, and which, if they are allowed, will soon regard themselves as the equals of the county town in which I live." Jealousy makes psychasthenics prone to associate by preference with persons who are beneath them in fortune and position. They are fond of the humble and the poor ; and, as we have seen, they have a special liking for their own employees and subordinates. Conversely, they have a natural detestation for their social superiors, and for persons who are wealthier than themselves ; but their special animosity is reserved for those who rise in the social scale, and thus become superiors when they have been inferiors. The success and the enrichment of others arouse their spleen, and they are enraged when they have to encounter the rivalry or opposition of those whom they have hitherto regarded as nothing better than menials.

Any kind of activity which may be conducive to success may arouse jealousy. Ya., a woman of forty, who has literary ambitions, is jealous of her son who is growing up and is doing well in his literary studies ; she has taken a dislike to him, and is always loading him with despiteful reproaches.

Here there is a factor of " monopolisation " at work, for she wants to be the only one in the family to exhibit an interest in literature ; but obviously this is not the exclusive factor. Her jealousy has another component, namely a peculiar way of conceiving and practising struggle and rivalry. This factor of jealousy is likewise extremely important.

We sometimes see a form of jealousy which is connected with the urge to dominate, and issues out of the authoritarian tendency. Here, in addition to the desire for a monopoly of despotism, we have hostility towards the person or persons who might also exercise dominion over the same subject, and a desire to drive these rivals out of range.—Gi., whom I class as a jealous tyrant rather than as a jealous lover, wants to reign alone in his wife's mind. He forbids her to see her parents, sequestrates her, locks her up when he leaves the house, hides her clothes, forbids her to look out of the window, watches her continually, and even goes with her to the water-closet. All these activities are inspired by the dread that she may speak to some one else, and thus become subject to an alien influence.—Jsa., a woman of thirty-eight, gives the following vivid description of the attitude towards her assumed by three of her customary associates, her husband, her sister, and an old friend of her own sex. " They always keep their eyes on me ; they tell me how I am to walk, and even how I am to do my hair. But they are terribly jealous of one another, and each of them is urgent with me to send the others away. They are all agreed in thinking that I can do nothing on my own initiative, with the result that when I resist the orders of any one of them I am immediately supposed to have been influenced by the others. . . . They are perpetu-ally intriguing to spy upon me, to find out where I am going, to make me take a side in their quarrels, to win over my little girl for the same purpose." As I have already said, this woman gives these authoritarian persons the idea that she will be a splendid prey, at once easy to win and well worth winning. Hence the perpetual hunting, and the everlasting jealous rivalry among those who want to dominate her.

As another embodiment of the commonest type of jealous affection, with monopolisation of the love of one person and the fending off of all those who may have a claim to love or be loved by this person, we may mention the case of Fv., a woman of seventy. Having for years tried to detach her daughter from her son-in-law, she is now trying to monopolise her grandson and to embroil him with his parents by making him believe that he is neglected by them and that they love his sister better than him. Such, indeed, is the traditional behaviour of mothers-in-law, who are so apt to pay court either to their daughter or to their son-in-law, and who are continually trying to sow discord in the young household. Divide and rule is a leading principle for authoritarian and jealous persons. That is why they have such a mania for setting people by the ears, for starting quarrels between husbands and wives, parents and children, friends. This seems to be almost the only occupation of many people.

" I want some one who will be my very own," says Héloïse. " I have such a craving for affection. I must have the first place, the only place ; must be preferred to everything and everybody ; must have all other things sacrificed to me. An ' omnibus ' does not suit me at all in matters of affection ; I like a private carriage, or if I am travelling by train I want the whole compartment to myself. . . . I used to be very religious. Shall I tell you why I am not religious now ? I'm out of humour with God because he loves everybody." —A girl of twelve, who is already very neuropathic, mono-polises her mother. The mother must never pay the least attention to any one else. The patient is jealous of every one who comes near her mother, of her girl cousins who visit the house, and even of the family cat.—A woman is jealous of her children, saying : " They have taken my husband away from me and have stolen my place as wife." She wants them to go away. " If they were not here, my husband would turn to me once more, would be gentle and tender, would let me share his life." Her moral sentiments lead her to offer a little resistance to the invasion of her mind by this hatred. " And yet my husband and my children are very happy together. The whole thing distresses me so. I don't want to make them unhappy, but what am I to do ? "—Ya. is jealous of her children. This jealousy is the source of her hatred for " these unwanted little creatures who demand so much care from us."—Zso. (m., 46) is jealous of every one who comes near his wife. He cannot bear that his wife should think of anything or any one but himself.—I could quote hundreds of similar cases. Perpetual jealousy is a character-istic trait in the mentality of these persons.

The types of jealousy may be classed from another outlook, in accordance with the varieties of the second main factor, the varieties in the hostility towards real or fancied rivals. But these varieties constitute very important types of mania, and deserve separate study. It will readily be understood that each distinct form of hatred can be combined with the manias for monopolisation we have just been studying, and may thus give rise to as many specific forms of jealousy.

The Mania for Disparagement.—In the competition which is an inevitable feature of life, a normal human being endeavours to triumph by rising above his rival. But one who feels him-self to be a weakling and has a terrible dread of effort, has a different idea of competition. His aim is to triumph, not by raising himself but by lowering his rival. Thus it is that the psychasthenic secures a partial and thrifty success by pre-venting others from acting. His opposition to all action on the part of his associates may arise out of a desire for immobility in his environment, out of a fear lest he himself should become involved in changes taking place in that environment ; but, in many instances, an additional factor is his dread of others' success. He does not wish his associates to rise, to increase their psychological tension by successful action. As we have seen, the persistent desire of the psych-asthenic is that others shall aid him in his work, and shall then efface themselves and leave him all the credit ; but the assistance he is thus continually claiming is what he is himself utterly incapable of rendering to others. Not only does he invariably refuse to collaborate in others' successes, but he does his utmost to impose obstacles in the way of those who are trying to act on their own account and to advance before him.

This characteristic is even a factor in a lover's jealousy, for the jealous person does not merely try to monopolise the affection of others ; furthermore, he cannot bear the thought that others may have more success in love than himself.—" I do not feel that I am loved enough, that I have sufficient experience of the joys of love. I feel that it would be shameful to me if my husband were to secure these joys elsewhere more fully than I can. In fact, I dread that he may be fortunate in love."—Héloïse says : " I cannot bear to see love flourishing everywhere. To see the loves of the insects and the flowers makes me jealous."

Although these efforts to lower a rival play a notable part in jealousy, they do not constitute the most important part of the neuropath's behaviour. The hindering of others' actions, the positive lowering of others, demand a struggle, necessitate efforts which are fairly difficult. The psychasthenic lacks courage for a frontal attack upon those of whom he is jealous ; he is not bold enough to hinder their actions and to lower them in the concrete world. In most cases he contents himself with trying to lower them in the estimation of the onlookers, and also in his own estimation, by fighting them with his tongue when they are absent. This is what we know as backbiting, which is the most characteristic activity of the jealous person.—Lox. (f., 40) has only one topic of conversation, carping criticism of all her associates, and especially of her daughter-in-law. As her husband remarks, criticism is the only thing that enlivens her attention. She is taciturn as long as there is no opportunity for talking about the disorderliness and misconduct of one of the women members of her family.—Such behaviour is distressingly common. I have a hundred or more well-marked instances of it in my records. Simple-minded folk will explain with a wealth of detail how Mrs. So-and-So dresses badly, cannot run her house properly, neglects her children, and plays her husband false. Persons who are somewhat more cultured will utter long tirades upon the artificiality and pretentiousness of this or that acquaintance, upon their conventional lies and self-interested behaviour. Both types are continually engaged in backbiting. We are apt to regard this tendency as an indication of a malicious temperament and an aggressive disposition. The judgment is not wholly accurate. The type of behaviour we are considering must be regarded as mainly the expression of an urge to lower others, to reduce others to one's own level, or, better still, to a lower level than one's own. Substantially, it is an important symptom of psychasthenic depression.

The Mania for Recrimination.—When the patient is a trifle more aggressive, he tends to explain all his failures, mortifications, and sufferings, as the outcome of others' clumsiness or malice. He tries to console himself, to raise his own spirits by blaming his associates. The very converse of the over-scrupulous person, who is continually lamenting his own sins of omission or commission, the recriminator can never forget what he regards as the misdeeds of others, and is never weary of blaming the offenders.—" If my aunt had not made me go out that Friday morning, three months ago, when I needed rest, I should soon have got well. . . . If my father had gone to fetch the doctor the instant I asked him to do so, I should have got well directly. My one chance was missed, and I shall never get over it. Everything that has happened is the fault of my aunt and my father."—" If that doctor had not told me that I had a nervous disorder, I should not have been ill. What made me ill was that my attention was drawn to my mental sluggishness."—A young man of twenty-four is continually uttering recriminations concerning the harm done him at school, concerning the tortures inflicted on him.—A woman who is always dissatisfied with herself and others, has for twenty years been declaiming against the injustice of society because it does not allow young women before marriage the same freedom as young men.—In the case of two girls, twins, who have both gradually passed from obsession to psychasthenic dementia, perpetual recrimination is the only remaining sign of mental energy. Although they have become incapable of action, and remain motionless in their chairs, they continue to recriminate, sometimes in loud tones, and sometimes in a half-whisper. The curious thing is that they use almost identical formulas. " This is the wrong place for me ; it was a terrible mistake to send me here. . . . My brother is a perfect idiot. All that has happened is the fault of this fool whose only idea is to please the crowd. . . . What a horrid sort of place this is, advertisement, puffery, like the wings of a theatre. . . . I am treated as an inferior, given no initiative, robbed, I am left to rot like a pig on a dung-heap, they have made of me the shutter of a confessional changed into the consecrated host. . . . This nurse ought never to be employed here ; she seizes me like a kidnapped child. . . . I am cut off from religion, from the sacraments ; everything is forbidden me. . . . Just the human beast at its worst. . . . How dreadful to be intelligent and to be herded with such beasts. . . . It's Mother's fault ; she sent me to the convent, she did not take me home again when I came back from my journey, she sent me to live with that gang. . . ." These tirades went on unceasingly all day, and sometimes all night. The patients could utter nothing but recriminations, which came easily, as the expression of the only mental operation which persisted amid the ruin of all the other activities of the mind.

The Mania for Spitefulness.—In patients of a more active type, the desire for domination and the desire for excitation are too often complicated by tendencies to cruelty. Some of these patients are really dangerous, but those who can be classed as psychasthenics in the strict sense of the term are active in word rather than in deed. A good many women, as I wrote some time ago, can never keep from saying disagreeable things to husband or daughter, especially when there are witnesses, so that what they say will be more wounding.[1] They want to degrade those whom they desire to subjugate ; they want to inflict a conspicuous humiliation. That is why they have recourse to contumelious expressions, to cruel and mocking phraseology.

Simone declaims against the taunts which she cannot bear when they are directed against herself. "I cannot endure people who take a delight in wounding others, who know what will give most pain and are not satisfied until they have touched the sore spot. They make me feel as if they were turning the dagger in the wound." But no one is more skilled than Simone in the discovery of phrases that will wound her unfortunate nurse, at whose poverty and domestic troubles she is continually jeering.—Zso.'s main desire is to torment and humiliate his wife. He looks at her with eyes full of hate, and grows spiteful directly he fancies that she is not submissive enough. He tries to make her uneasy by pretending to be ill. He refuses his food in public, and eats on the sly, in the hope that she will believe him to be starving.—Ew. likes " to give people a lesson " in public. She is continually humiliating her daughter before witnesses. She makes the girl stay in the drawing-room while she explains at great length how she has been able to secure for herself

[1] Les obsessions et la psychasthénie, second edition, 1908, p. 404.

the whole of her husband's fortune and that her daughter will have nothing. " I hope I shall live long enough to make her realise that a daughter must always be subordinate to her mother."—Md. plays the same comedy. She takes a delight in plaguing her daughter, who is a tall and handsome young woman of twenty-five. The daughter is sent for to the drawing-room to receive a stream of orders " to keep her on the go " before the visitors. The mother criticises her, tells her that she does not know how to behave and that she makes herself ridiculous, says sharp things to her until she blushes and bursts into tears. Thereupon the mother makes a parade of devotion, hastens to console her, says she must on no account go out, and brings her glasses of sugar-water. The same scene is repeated day after day. If the girl is steadfast and does not weep, the mother is very much upset, is extremely piqued, and sulks for a fortnight.

In all these cases, and in many others of the same kind, we must note an important psychological fact. We have not yet reached the domain of real hatred. Indeed, these authoritarian persons are continually vaunting their great love for the victim. Nor do I think that they are wrong. Love and hatred have always been defined in a very vague way, and I cannot agree with the general view that the essential characteristic of love is to do good, and of hatred to do harm, to the person who is loved or hated. These complicated tendencies are derivatives of the more fundamental tendencies towards approximation and withdrawal respectively. Pain is a tendency towards a simple movement of withdrawal ; hatred is a tendency towards complete removal, towards effecting the disappearance of an object regarded as a living creature. Love, which derives from the act of taking food, from sexuality, from the act of touching, is a tendency to approximate to oneself a living creature, to keep that creature near oneself. Now, it is quite true that authoritarian persons have an overwhelming desire to keep in close contact with themselves the individuals whom they torment. They would be most unhappy if their victims were to withdraw to a distance, and still more unhappy if their victims were to disappear. We have seen that Zso. adores his wife, and cannot bear that she should be out of his sight for a moment. We see the same thing in the other cases. Noémi, who plagues her husband for hours at a time until she succeeds in reducing him to tears, is in despair when he is called up for military service. Their cruelty is the form their love takes. The persons whom they love are for them a means of excitation, and as such these individuals must be kept close at hand.

The Mania of Hatred.—Unfortunately this pathological evolution may advance yet further, to culminate in the obsessions or delusions which are often subsumed under the name of delusion of persecution, but which could, I think, be more aptly described as a mania, an impulse, or a delusion of hate. Delusion of persecution, as I have frequently pointed out, has been too sharply distinguished from psychasthenic states. In many instances, it is no more than the final stage of these psychasthenic conditions.

When any one resists our will and fails to perform the action we order, he annoys us; he checks the development of a tendency which has been aroused in us; and, by compelling us to undertake the struggle on our own account, he imposes on us a certain expenditure of force. In a normal person, this expenditure is not of great importance, for it will not be ruinous. But for a depressed person, the expenditure is a very serious matter indeed. It brings about a further lowering of the psychological tension, thus giving rise to dread of death and to other anxieties. The subject therefore naturally tries to rid himself of this obstacle, of this person whose presence threatens him with mental death; and he consequently becomes inspired with hatred for the offender. The cruelty of the mother who tries to humiliate her daughter in order to raise her own spirits is not hatred, for the mother does not want to rid herself of the daughter; on the contrary, she wants to keep the daughter near herself. But if the young woman does not allow herself to be humiliated, if she does not comply with her mother's wishes by bursting into tears when her mother nags at her before witnesses, then the mother's feeling is accentuated to become true hatred. The same feeling of hatred arises against persons who will not give way, and whom the patient cannot succeed in moulding to his will.—" As far as I am concerned," says Ya., " every difference inspires hatred. I detest everything different from myself, and I want it to disappear. I am deep but narrow."—This hatred which tries to suppress people's existence, to make them disappear completely, finds its counterpart, where social tendencies are concerned, in the tendency to the liquidation of situations —a tendency to which we have referred when speaking of fatigue. When Ot. takes a dislike to his flat, saying " I want to destroy the place completely, never to see the house again, and never to hear any one speak of it," he resembles Yd. who wishes at all costs and without a moment's delay to dissolve his business partnership or to break off his betrothal. But in the case of hatred, the obstacle to be suppressed is usually a living creature, a human being. That fact is characteristic of this emotion.

When hatred undergoes its fullest development, which can only take place in an energetic mind, it arouses a tendency to the complete suppression of the enemy by his murder. This is what we see in some of the homicidal impulses of sufferers from delusion of persecution ; but it is rare in the patients I have been describing, for they lack energy. " I am seldom on sufficiently bad terms with any one to be moved to attack him openly ; I don't want to make a scandal." Usually these patients confine themselves to disparagement, recrimination, various manifestations of petty spite.

Even at a somewhat more advanced stage, the destructive attacks that issue from hatred will be confined to the realm of words. A great many of these patients breathe threatenings and slaughter. Gh. fills the letters he writes to me with abuse of the working-class girls who have repelled his advances. He fancies that they have taken possession of his mind, that they control his will, and compel him to adopt their voice and their gestures.[1] When alone in his room, he makes faces at himself in the mirror as if he were a little girl ; and he shrieks imprecations against " these girls who are worse than prostitutes, and who have taken possession of my mind." The invectives and insults which are so often mouthed by such patients are the climax of an evolution which begins with the feeling of weakness ; passes on to the desire for domination, associated with love ; and culminates in the desire for annihilation, associated with hatred.

In other cases, when the neuropath finds that life in

[1] Dépersonnalisation et possession chez un psychasthénique, " Journal de Psychologie Normale et Pathologique," 1904, p. 28.

contact with the enemy has become insupportable, he drives this enemy out of the house. Ew. finds from time to time that the presence of his daughter is intolerable, and he will make her live elsewhere for months at a time.—When the patient has not the power to drive away the person he hates, he will himself take refuge in flight, and this is the initiating cause of a variety of neuropathic fugue which is not always properly understood.—Oy. (f., 50) tried to live in her son's house and wanted to dominate him. Finding that she could not master him, she suddenly left without telling any one beforehand. " I can't bear to see them any longer ; I hate them so much that I know I should kill them if I were to stay." —Neb. runs away from home, and explains his flight by saying : " I could not bear, to be in my wife's company any longer. It agitates me too much."—Ya., too, ran away from home, to the great alarm of her husband, who was unable to discover her whereabouts for several days. She had conceived a hatred for her husband, her children, and all her neighbours. —A very typical case is that of Px. A woman of thirty-seven, she lived with her mother and her sister, and for a long time had held despotic sway over the household. At first she was obsessed with love for her sister, having a mania both for loving and for being loved ; then came an obsession to dominate and monopolise, accompanied by an intense jealousy of the sister. At length, since the sister offered some resistance to domination, and tried to retain a shadow of independence, she became more and more irritated until there ensued a sort of delusion of persecution which was in reality nothing more than an obsessive hatred of the sister. She came to feel that she must leave the house once for all. " I was no longer mistress of the others, and I should have had to do things which I could not do. I had begun to see red, and I realised that I had better clear out."—In twenty of my cases, delusion of persecution or the mania of hatred appeared, in like manner, as an outgrowth of obsessions of love and longing to dominate.

Interesting observations can be made as to the persons who become, by preference, the objects of such hatred. Ya., who has six children, detests the three older ones, but still retains some affection for the three younger ones. This is a very frequent phenomenon. Psychasthenics are fond of young children, and begin to dislike them after a while, usually towards the age of fifteen.   An old woman under my care had first adored and subsequently hated all her children, and then all her grandchildren.   Towards the end of her days, the only person she could bear to see was a little girl of eight, her great-granddaughter ;   and she died before this child's turn for being hated had come.   Our behaviour as adults towards very young children is comparatively simple, so that only a low psychological tension is requisite.   Besides, these little children are very much alike, are frankly recognised as inferiors, offer no disquieting resistance, and require very little effort on our part.   As they grow up, they become differentiated one from another and differentiated from ourselves.   The child forms a personality which is capable of independence and resistance ; hence the change of attitude towards the growing child exhibited by psychasthenic patients.   We have already noticed that neuropaths cannot endure people who enjoy an increase in wealth and station.   The dislike of children who grow up belongs to the same category of feelings.   Such patients are especially apt to hate persons who to begin with seemed especially docile and affectionate, and persons whom they have tried to monopolise.   As soon as a little resistance to monopolisation becomes manifest, love is transformed into hatred.

In most of the cases I have been describing, these different tendencies, though strange and abnormal, do not give rise to the gravest forms of mental disorder.   The resulting manias and impulses are not very serious, and the patient is more or less aware of their existence.   Though he gives his tendencies free rein, he will generally admit that they are absurd, or at any rate exaggerated.   Most of the foregoing descriptions are given in the patient's own words, or based upon their own statements, for, when they are talking to the doctor, they are usually quite ready to laugh at their own follies.   Obviously, the symptoms may develop, and may then give rise to dangerous delusions.   In that case, however, the nature of the illness is recognised, and the patient is subjected to treatment.   My aim here has been to describe the social behaviour of persons who are supposed to be suffering from nothing worse than infirmity of character, persons who are regarded as quite fitted for ordinary domestic life.   My desire has been to show the effect which the behaviour of these persons can have on the mental condition of their associates.

6. EXHAUSTING AND ANTIPATHETIC PERSONS.

It has frequently been pointed out that a neuropath's exactions do not always redound to his advantage. If he gets his way with his associates, he is apt to become more ill than before; undue compliance with a neuropath's wishes is not good for the patient. Playfair pointed out how pitiable was the association between the self-indulgent patient, on the one hand, and a person in good health who betrayed exaggerated devotion, on the other. " Does the patient complain of a pain in the spine ? She is urged to lie down at once. Is she unable to read ? Her self-appointed nurse reads to her. Does she say that the light hurts her eyes ? Her mother shuts herself up with the girl in a darkened room throughout the livelong day. Is the patient afraid of a draught ? All the doors and windows are closed."

Ac. (f., 22), suffering from muco-membranous enteritis, has gradually become affected with manias and fixed ideas concerning defaecation. She is well aware that her troubles have been aggravated by the sedulous care of her family. Her mother follows her about everywhere with a chamber-pot, watches her continually, looks to see if she is flushed, or examines the whites of her eyes, asks whether she wants to go to stool, and produces the chamber-pot from the folds of a cloak. " As soon as I turn my back, my father, my mother, and my grandmother begin to whisper about me ; they never let me forget my illness for a moment." When the tendencies to achieve domination and to seek love are excessive, and when they have given rise to manias and morbid impulses, they compel the patient to a perpetual struggle. He exhausts himself in his search for love, as others may weary themselves trying to remember a forgotten name or seeking for a proof of the existence of God. An interesting indication of the bad effect of such prolonged efforts is the transformation we have just been considering when a mania for love is changed into a mania for hatred. If we are to be able to detect this symptom whenever it is present, we must carefully distinguish between manias for domination, for teasing, for cruelty, on the one hand, and true tendencies to hatred, on the other, the latter being characterised by a longing for the removal or suppression of the object of hatred. It is also very important that we should be able to detect the moment when mental manias and obsessions are tending to be transformed into psychasthenic delusions. These various symptoms show that the resistance of the patient is becoming enfeebled, that his psychological tension is being more lowered than ever, and that he is growing exhausted in the contest with his environment.

In this connexion, we have to consider another field of psychological study, and one which has been very little examined. In view of the character of the subjects we have been describing, what effect does their presence induce in their associates ? Usually people are content to say that the subjects are extremely disagreeable, and that their presence is a nuisance for every one concerned. No doubt ; but we want to know a good deal more than this.

All the types of behaviour I have been describing have a reaction upon the patient's associates ; and the reaction is of course a complicated one, difficult to describe. The patient's abulia and indecision render him incapable of performing useful actions. Obviously, then, any work which the patient has been doing in the household will now have to be done by some one else. We remember the complaints of Aj.'s husband. " The matter is far more complicated than you might think. It is not easy to live for two people. I am overburdened by this necessity, and cannot bear it much longer." The worst of it is that the associates have to will for the patient, to decide everything for the patient, while keeping in mind the patient's interests and tastes. We have to accept full responsibility for these actions, while we are subject to the reproaches and protests of those for whom we do them. If we want to make them act (because this is essential, or because we wish to give them something to do which will distract them) we must carefully get things ready, must make all the efforts on their behalf, and then involve them in the movement. But the last step is the most difficult, for they are not interested in anything. They need to be guided and incited all the time if they are to be made to do anything ; it is frightfully hard work. If we want them to collaborate with us, we have to bear in mind how incredibly slow they are, and must set a very slow pace. " In the end, one gets so impatient that one would rather do the whole thing oneself."

Nor is it easy to hold converse with these patients, for they speak with difficulty, and their unfinished sentences demand sustained attention on the part of the listener if he is to grasp the meaning at all. They are afraid of conversation, and, above all, of discussion. " They rarely venture to express a personal opinion, and if they do so they will abandon it at once lest they be called upon to make an effort to sustain it, and so they leave you in the void. . . . Or they will purposely so confuse the issues as to make their meaning quite incomprehensible, and secure peace for themselves by this means." Subjects for conversation fail them, for they are not interested in anything and do not follow outside events. " Here we are in the thick of a war and in the midst of death, and all she can talk about is the misdeeds of the cook. . . . Besides, there are so many things we must not mention in her presence ; whole days are passed in her company without exchanging a word ; it's deadly. . . . You simply cannot imagine what it is like to have lunch with that family ! " If the matter seems urgent, we have to give ourselves no end of trouble to make them understand, for they are hopelessly inattentive, and have very little interest in what we are explaining. Lkd. is in despair because his wife, whom he finds too childish, does not respond to his endeavours to educate her. " Intellectually, we are misfits."

In the end, their inability to love, and to adapt themselves to their surroundings, makes living with them an intolerable burden. Though they are for ever demanding caresses and thanks, they are incapable of appreciating the love and the service bestowed on them ; on the contrary they pretend not to notice what is done for them, so as to avoid the feeling of humiliation, and the fatigue of having to manifest gratitude. The services rendered to these unfortunates have to be absolutely disinterested, and we must never look for a sign of real affection in return. " My husband is cold and unjust to me ; he is always in the sulks, and does not seem to have really accepted the idea that he has married me. I am so sad and troubled ; I feel, somehow, as if I were merely a provisional wife, as though I had no proper home ; it is so distressing, makes life so difficult." The unstable nature of such patients' feelings is an additional worry. "One never can tell how they are feeling towards one. Are they friendly? Or are they hostile? All the time one has to be on guard. . . . It is never possible to find out whether they are sincere; they look daggers at you, and call you 'darling' at the same time. . . . At bottom, they are so indifferent and so selfish that one is quite discouraged." The embarrassment they show in social relationships is catching; the shyness such patients display makes their associates feel awkward, for nothing is more fatiguing and more arduous than trying to hold converse with a shy person. It is no easy matter to understand their unfinished sentences, which are uttered hesitatingly, so that a very great effort of attention is demanded to follow them. No intimacy is possible: these patients pretend to want it, but they behave as if they dreaded it. They are always seeking to hide themselves. "They are for ever telling falsehoods, and never can they be brought to speak frankly, . . . neither are they able to understand frankness in others. They always behave as if they thought you were lying. It is a terrible worry." We must, however, do our utmost to understand these patients in order to give them all possible help.

They are sad and discontented. "They are always so splenetic, and there does not seem to be any reason for it. Their ill humour casts a gloom over the whole house." The members of Lox.'s family become tired and lethargic as soon as they set foot in the home, or have been there a few days. They dread these family gatherings, mealtimes are a veritable torture. "The gloomy atmosphere, without a spark of gaiety, more than we can bear; and the perpetual criticism of every one and everything, never a word of approval. We none of us dare breathe a syllable if she is about—too many forbidden topics—and we have to keep too rigid a watch on what we say; we can't do anything; misfortune seems to be brooding over the house."

Not only do these patients do nothing themselves, but they try to prevent their associates from doing anything likewise; they sometimes bring every particle of energy to bear on the prohibition. We must resist their objections, and for ever

keep our idea of action in the foreground, in spite of the fact
that their actions and their words tend to crush activity of
any sort. This will need additional effort on our part.—
" My father hinders us in carrying on the business ; he is an
obstacle. . . ."—" My daughter will not allow us to have any
cooking done. . . ."—" My word, it has been difficult to get
anything done in the house, . . . he wanted me to succumb
with him, he wanted to drag me into the swamp with him.
. . How I had to struggle to keep my own end up ; to
prevent myself from going downhill along with him. . . ."

Or, again, they will allow us to undertake certain activities,
but on condition that they may take part by issuing orders,
giving advice, and suggesting details which are absolutely
valueless but which give them a feeling of contributing something important to the undertaking ; our action is thereby
rendered considerably more complicated. They wish to help,
to collaborate, or simply to look on, while the other person
does all the work. Such collaboration demands the utmost
display of tact on our side, and we must learn to recognise
the precise moment when to step into the background ; for
these patients have a mania for freedom, and are always
complaining that people are trying to boss them, to bring
pressure to bear upon them ; they think that it is their role
in life to influence others, not that others should influence
them. Our intervention needs to be masked ; we must lead
them to believe that the decisions come from themselves,
must allow them to reap the full benefit of the work in hand.
Rv. knows that his wife, who usually refuses to accept any
proposal, will perform the required action in a few days' time
if she can be persuaded that the idea originated in her own
mind. But he regards such behaviour as absurd ; he thinks
that it panders to her selfishness ; and he finds it very difficult
to resign himself to these manoeuvres.—The patients say to
us : " Go ahead, don't mind me, work with me or work in
my presence, behave just as if I were not there, it gives me
real pleasure to see you busy and to give a few words of advice,
and it does not cost you anything."—" Don't you believe
that it does not cost me anything ; I can't ignore your presence,
for you are not invisible ; I have to do my work knowing all
the time that you are there, that you are watching me, judging
me ; my whole activity is transformed. It may seem to be

the same ; but, psychologically, it is rendered far more complex ; I have to substitute constant watchfulness for my customary free-and-easy way of performing the task. You do not sit motionless and silent ; you wish to increase the feeling of collaboration, for it invigorates you to take part in my work, be that part never so small ; and so you make remarks, such as : ' That's fine, what you're doing now. . . . But I'm not sure that I would have done it in quite the same way. . . . Look here, I think it ought to have been begun this end. . . .' Doubtless, I should not take any notice of what you say ; I have thought about the work more than you have, I realise that you really know nothing about it, I have already dealt with the solutions you propose. Unfortunately you awaken thoughts about the difficulty of the task, you make me hesitate, you force me to make once more the initial effort which I had already made ere I began the job ; what a terrible expenditure of supplementary energy ! "—A famous banker is staying in the country ; on medical advice he undertakes to do a little gardening. Friends rush to the rescue. " Just look at the great financial magnate who is handling a watering can and the pruners. . . . Cincinnatus, are you not afraid you will tire yourself ? . . . Doctors are such queer fish. . . . Please, allow me to help you." The amateur gardener is embarrassed, he tries to put a good face on the matter, he smiles at the ladies while continuing to clip the rose-trees but he becomes awkward and nips his finger ; in order to hide his clumsiness he pretends there is no pain. . . . What a lot of needless effort ! His attempt to do a little gardening has completely exhausted him.—In especial, it is very difficult to show one's real feelings in the presence of witnesses. A mother-in-law says to me : " I never leave the young people by themselves, for I do so like to see their pretty ways with one another ; I want to take part in their love. Unfortunately they are very cold to one another, and never exchange a word so long as I am there."—" I should like to show more affection to my father," says Mademoiselle Md., " but poor dear Mother is always there ; she does not exactly frighten me, but—well it's difficult to describe the effect she has upon me ; she seems to freeze me, and I can never utter a word at home."

The mania for issuing orders determines modifications

in the actions of the bystanders ; it transforms all their doings into acts of obedience. Real obedience, which consists of difficult actions for the performance of which genuinely helpful directives are given, as a rule lessens the work of deliberation and of decisions which such acts usually demand, and tends to make their performance easier. But in the case of simple actions for which no guidance is needed, or in the case of useless actions which would never be performed by a free agent, the performance of such actions is rendered more complicated by having to act under command. Instead of being performed automatically, the action is consciously performed ; instead of being personal, it becomes social ; it is no longer carried out for its own sake, but to give pleasure to some one ; it has to be executed in a spirit of submissiveness ; and the beneficent excitation caused by the performance of a personal action is absent. The result is that, though obedience may diminish the cost price of expensive actions, it increases the price of cheap actions. Among persons who are weak, and so poorly endowed with energy that they have to consider every outlay, the transformation of a commonplace action into an act of obedience is rendered so costly that the action is simply suppressed. A little child, all smiles and hunger, was just going to eat a plateful of soup, when the mother rushed in exclaiming : " Now then, eat your soup ! " The child immediately began to cry, and refused to eat the soup.—A girl with a kodak stops in her walk to take a snapshot. She has just got the picture nicely focussed, and is about to press the button, when her mother calls out : " I say, here is a lovely little corner. Do snap this." The girl folds her kodak and slings it over her arm again without taking any picture at all. She says that, on reflection, she did not consider the light good enough. But she is put out because she vaguely feels that she has been thwarted in the accomplishment of an action by an interference which has rendered it more difficult. It is no easy matter to live with a person suffering from a mania for ordering others about, for we are perpetually called upon to perform more complicated actions, actions which are more costly than they need be, and we have to renounce the benefits accruing from independence and initiative. It is well to remember that initiative and freedom are favourable stimulants of which we are deprived by the authoritarians in our midst.—

" They have got accustomed to leading me by the nose, and
are furious and amazed if I ever venture to do something on
my own ; . . . it robs me of my feeling of satisfaction, deprives
me of lightheartedness. . . . Not only are they always ordering
me about, but they do it in front of strangers ; even in the
tramcar one of them will place a hand on my shoulder and give
me my orders, just to show he is my owner . . . it is so
humiliating. . . . I never have the joy of doing something
which has not been commanded. . . . That is partly why we
are all of us so inert . . . we are led to think we are poor
creatures. . . . I should be doing things if only I were not
told at every turn to be doing so and so. . . ."

Manias for love are likewise difficult to bear with. Great
care is needed not to wound these patients, never to criticise
them, never to give them the impression " that they may be
in any one's bad books." Constantly we must dance attend-
ance upon them, with never a thought of reward : a very
complicated, very difficult task ; a painful servitude.

All these peculiarities have similar characteristics. They
all tend to trouble the healthy persons who have to come in
contact with such disorders ; and tend, likewise, to arouse in
the healthy sentiments of an analogous nature.—Vkx. (m., 29)
is unable to live with his grandmother and his father : " They
criticise everything, they are always harping upon ideas of
illness, ruin, disaster ; they say they are crucified ; they declare
that terrible things are impending ; and so on. And, all the
while, they assume melodramatic airs and speak big. . . .
They think out loud the things I am only too prone, myself,
to think in silence : their talk saddens me and fills me with
alarm."—Disquietudes thus suggested must be courageously
resisted ; we must constantly repeat that these poor things
are invalids, and need not be given credence to ; but such
resistance constitutes an effort, a struggle. Instead of allowing
ourselves the luxury of yielding to the anxiety which they
inspire us with, we have to work hard in order to reassure
them, to console them, to revivify them.—" I'm just back
from a journey with a neurotic aunt who is sad, disagreeable,
and jealous. All my time was spent in bucking her up. How
awfully complicated and difficult life is in her company !
What a rag she reduced me to ! "—Other patients are always
expecting thanks and flattery. We have to realise the need

there is to supply the demand, give up our own little vanities, and labour to provide the patients with the compliments they are in search of. And the labour is no small one, for these invalids are very suspicious, and require that the compliments shall sound sincere and spontaneous, so that they can be accepted without the slur of ridicule. The dispensing of such compliments becomes a veritable fine art, and demands a great deal of practice and close attention to detail.

While rendering all these services, we needs must reassure the patient as to the future, guarantee that our devotion will last a life time. We must be on our guard lest a thoughtless manifestation of self-interest should escape us, and must constantly assure them that we want nothing from them in return for what we do. We have to persuade them that we "love them for themselves alone," and that, by the very fact that they are alive, they have the right to be loved.

This "rights" mania exposes us to constant humiliations ; for it goes without saying that if the sufferer can claim such manifold services from us without ever doing anything in return, we must, inferentially, be inferior beings to the patient. This is how they understand the matter, and they are very fond of showing up our inferiority. Such behaviour naturally awakens in us a defensive reaction : the constant assertion of rights on the part of the patient rouses in us the thought that we, too, have rights which the invalid never respects. This thought has to be resisted, so that we may maintain a high moral attitude of mind—but, psychologically, the resistance is costly.

When the patient takes it into his head to love, to render services, or to make presents, far from simplifying our task, he considerably complicates matters for us. For he is, in actual fact, incapable of rendering a service ; what he wants is that, to all our other labours, the labour of giving thanks shall be superadded, and that his sense of obligation shall thus be lightened. He wants it to appear as though he were paying for the love he demands ; but he wishes to choose the method of his payment, or to make fictitious payment which we are expected to receive as if it were a genuine one. In reality, what he calls for is gratuitous devotion.

True, from the giver's point of view, such devotion is the finest, a devotion which is given as a duty and is therefore on a high moral plane. Madame X. is right when she says : " What I ask for is really a very simple thing ; all I want is that my associates shall behave towards me according to the rules imposed by morality. . . . If my husband and my children were really moral, I should always have had what I asked for. . . ." This is quite equitable, and I am loath to admit that such conduct is impossible : too often one has to witness the most admirable devotion lavished upon a perfectly odious psychasthenic; I would merely observe that normal humanity is not invariably in the habit of behaving like a saint, and that such conduct is extremely complex, on a very exalted plane, and, psychologically, altogether too costly. Nor need we be surprised at the complaints and protestations of those who make no claim to the saint's aureole. Héloïse's daughters are afraid of her when she has one of her passionate outbursts of love towards them ; they find her " exclusivist and in the way," and have no desire to live with her. The unhappy mother is all astonishment : " Is my need for bestowing love so alarming ? Am I an ogress when I love ? Those girls simply don't know how to love, they are afraid of becoming entangled."

In spite of every precaution and the most absolute devotion, these patients are devoured by doubts and jealousy. Then the mental labour on the part of the onlookers is enhanced, for they have to put up with attacks, recriminations, and scenes that beggar description. Such onslaughts, inspired as they sometimes are by hatred, are not without their dangers. Notwithstanding abulia and unskilfulness, the psychasthenic is momentarily carried along by an impulse which may deal an unmerciful blow. The patient is cunning in his knowledge of the best ways to wound, and his mania for disparagement is often amazing. Above all he excels in the art of setting the onlookers by the ears, for he always endeavours to rule by dividing. These onslaughts must be recognised as important ; they must be parried so that we do not have to suffer too acutely ; and yet, in parrying, we must be careful not to wound the patient. Even when we feel impelled to dread him and despise him, we must continue to show him unlimited affection and admiration.

Of course these attacks are not always inspired by genuine hatred ; for the most part they are resorted to in order that

the patient may rekindle his energies at our expense; they
are also very often the outcome of a mania to tease and a
mania to make scenes. But all too frequently there is real
hatred in the background. We therefore need to make a
diagnosis, and this demands a good deal of psychological
shrewdness and attention. Again, if we come to realise that
the attacks are only a form of teasing, we have to beware of
a natural tendency violently to repulse the attack; we must
arrest such a tendency by the thought that these patients
need our utmost affection and respect, even in their most
tiresome vagaries; and we must for ever buoy ourselves up
with the hope that some day they will change their behaviour
towards us. Thus, we have to adopt a special and quite
unnatural kind of behaviour; we have to counter an attack
with a smile, or with a look of wonder and distress. " At first
I was in despair, I wept fit to make myself ill, when she was in
one of her tantrums, when she hurled her wedding ring into
the baby's cradle; then I felt like laughing at all these tragic
airs. Now I know that I must do neither the one nor the
other; but it has taken me years to learn ! " The behaviour
needed may wellnigh be qualified with the name " scientific " ;
it resembles the behaviour of the practising psychotherapist
who does not allow the sufferings of his patients to afflict him,
seeing that he is absorbed in the study of an interesting case ;
it is akin to the attitude of the alienist, or to that of the nurse ;
but it is not the natural attitude of mind of a husband towards
his wife. " I don't want to be a nurse to my own grandmother ;
it is because I refuse to act in this capacity that I find visiting
her so exhausting."

Nothing is more painful or more depressing than to spend
all one's days with a jealous person. In order to avoid or to
reduce to a minimum the terrible scenes provoked by the
mania of jealousy, one is constrained to keep constant watch
on one's most trivial actions, or gestures ; and one has to
renounce almost all participation in social life. The only hope
of preserving a spark of naturalness in one's behaviour lies
in passively tolerating a perpetual succession of the most
appalling scenes.

The best way to bring home to ourselves the complexity
of behaviour incumbent upon the associates of a psychasthenic,

is to picture our attitude when in company with a liar and humbug. An individual whom we know to be capable of lying, one whom we suspect, requires from us a complicated method of procedure : we have to listen to him and at the same time to resist the natural tendency which impels us to believe what he is saying, must withstand being " suggestioned " by his words ; we have to believe something different from what he is saying. Hence our behaviour becomes extremely intricate. Well, not only does the neuropath constantly lie, but his whole conduct is really the embodiment of falsehood ; he seems to love, and does not love (any way, not in a normal fashion) ; he seems to hate, and yet, in reality, he does not hate ; he demands implicit obedience, and yet is incapable of ordering the performance of anything important which might justify his command. All the time he puts forward false statements in order to learn the truth, and when he declares that his illness is incurable, we have to understand that he does not think anything of the sort, and is awaiting our refutation. " The thing that makes life with my husband peculiarly hard is that I cannot take a word he says seriously ; I can never be spontaneous, cannot allow myself to be natural, for nothing he does is natural, and nothing he says has the ordinary meaning his words imply."—" My husband," says Madame Zso., " tells me he never eats, and certainly in my presence he refuses food with an expression of the utmost loathing, and says he hopes he will die of starvation. But directly my back is turned he eats plentifully. He howls with despair when he knows I have found him out, and that I am unhappy about his behaviour ; and yet I know that the minute I leave the house he calms down. When I enter the room he turns away from me, and pretends to hate me, pretends he is not in the least interested in me ; yet, if I take no notice, he tries every device to ascertain whether I am there, whether I am thinking about him, and so on. It is all so trying, and how can I sift the true from the false ? " The life of falsehood becomes so obvious sometimes that even the patient grows aware of it, and murmurs : " I seem to be feigning ; it would appear that I am acting a part." It is probably not quite correct to say that these are genuine lies. But such behaviour is certainly analogous to falsehood : the real motive underlying the action of the patient is to revivify himself at our expense ;

but this is not openly acknowledged, it could not be, for it is not clearly recognised ; it is masked under another sort of behaviour whose ordinary aim is something quite different, but which, incidentally; has the property of stimulating the sufferer. Thus the patient, by his endeavours at domination, by teasing, by sulking, by scenes, causes his associates to assume the same sort of attitude they would when dealing with a liar.

In spite of all, seeming, this complex behaviour provoked by the neuropath and forced upon all those who come in contact with him, leads invariably to the same results ; it is very exhausting to the patient's associates, and upon them likewise entails a great expenditure of energy. We constantly hear identical remarks from those who have to associate with a neuropathic individual.—" Grandmother is so terribly tiring."—" My sister wears me out and exhausts me."— " My wife is very fatiguing. My whole household is sad and wearisome."—" Goodness, how tiring my poor husband is ! He is clumsy, heavy, queer, anything you like ; but, above all he tires me out."—" Home life is impossible. Father is always bewailing his fate, and the process of comforting him is utterly exhausting."—" Mother is so fond of us, she never gives us a moment's privacy. She comes and turns our rooms topsy-turvy with the excuse that she is tidying them ; all day she is trying to render us services for which we have never asked, and she makes such a row if we don't seem to like what she does. It is absolutely wearing us out. As for me, I need a quiet life above all things, and I am at the end of my tether."—Such is the constant refrain sung by those who have to live with a neuropath.

A fatiguing individual forces us to make an excessive expenditure of moral energy, an expenditure we should not have to make were such a person not living with us. Let me try to show, by allegorical means, why it is that such beings are " costly." A man has a twenty-franc piece in his pocket. This amount of money should in the ordinary course be ample to meet his expenditure for several days. He thinks he is well enough off to indulge in a day in the country on the following Sunday ; he will go by train and take a third-class ticket ; he will lunch at a wayside inn and drink fresh water from the running brook ; and thus he plans an enjoyable excursion. He need not spend much money. . . . He meets a friend who is wealthier than himself, who wishes to go with him, and who promises to share expenses. The friend says that in this way the day in the country will work out cheaper. But he is making a big mistake ! The man will not have the courage to travel in a third-class carriage if his wealthy friend is with him, he will go to a more expensive restaurant, and will slake his thirst elsewhere than by the brookside. . . . When he gets home in the evening he will have spent eighteen francs and will, therefore, have no more than two for his expenses during the following days. He is disappointed with his excursion, out of humour with himself, and furious with his friend. Such a one has proved to be an expensive friend.

When we come to the study of antipathetic individuals we are faced with analogous phenomena from the mental outlook, and we find very definite instances of fatiguing and costly persons. In studying the phenomenon of antipathy, philosophers, such as Ribot, quite recently [1] have been inclined to relate antipathy to fear properly so called. Antipathetic individuals, they maintain, are a danger to us, but, still, the danger is not very obvious. First of all, it is not easy to find out precisely in what the danger consists ; and, secondly, we cannot determine the signs by which we shall be able to recognise that they are dangerous. The danger is not clearly perceived, rather is it intuitively or instinctively sensed.—My own conception of the matter is somewhat simpler. True, antipathetic persons are persons whom we fear, flee from ; but we flee because they threaten us with a very real danger, one which all mankind is alarmed at, but which the expert psychologists have not understood. These patients threaten us with exhaustion, and with mental depression as a sequel of exhaustion.

We are all of us thrifty in our outlay of mental activity, and we have a feeling of aversion for persons who wring from us, as soon as they approach us, a greater expenditure of energy. We have a desire to spirit such persons away, out of our vicinity ; consequently we experience an initial feeling of hatred towards them, and resent the fact that they should compel us to squander our mental energies. Monsieur X., the

[1] Cf. Ribot, Problèmes de psychologie affective, 1909 ; Bourdeau, La philosophie affective, Alcan, Paris, 1912, p. 104.

journalist, is nothing more than an inquisitive and loquacious man. He obviously wants to know my opinion on such and such a question, or my feelings towards such and such friends ; he will make use of whatever I may say in his articles or in subsequent conversations. Can he be said to be really a danger to me ? Not much of one. I need but be careful of what I say, and he will have nothing to repeat which can incriminate me. But he constrains me to carry on a more complicated conversation, during which my mind is occupied with avoiding certain subjects ; and, while thinking of these things, I have to utter words concerning quite different things. Such a conversation is an act performed at high tension, and is quite another sort of conversation from one carried on in a free-an-easy spirit. It exhausts me, it necessitates serious expenditure on my part, it is hateful to me.—The liar who constrains us to complex behaviour, the authoritarian, the touchy person, the boaster whom one has to tolerate and not humiliate, he who makes claims on account of whilom rights which have no value in the present, and so on, are costly individuals and may very easily become antipathetic individuals. The feeling of aversion will naturally vary according to individual powers of resistance : those who are strong and well-endowed with mental energy will hardly be aware of an increased expenditure when fate brings them into contact with certain persons ; such lucky people have few antipathies. But the poorly endowed feels the smallest outlay as a serious one ; and the feebler such a person is, the more speedily does he come to feel that he is being ruined, the more readily does he become inspired with sentiments of antipathy or aversion.

Neuropaths are, in the extremest sense of the term, " expensive " persons. Also, by the irony of fate, they are often surrounded by individuals whose psychological tension is easily lowered. Such persons soon suffer from the effects of the complex and exhausting behaviour demanded of them, and they soon harbour special kinds of sentiments towards the patient, these sentiments being the expression of a profound and subtle antipathy.

Alienists are fond of recording a remarkable phrase they often hear their patients use. " Some one is stealing my thoughts, some one is stealing my consciousness." Such words, and their variance, are constantly on the lips of neuropaths, doubters, and obsessed individuals, who are, nevertheless, not suffering from a mania of persecution. Px. (f. 37) observes, when speaking of her mother and her sister: " I no longer possess my thoughts when I am with my mother or my sister; these two women trouble me, they petrify me, they clip the wings of my fancy; they gnaw me and suck me dry, they aspirate my very being out of me; they steal my thoughts. Never shall I be owner of my thoughts so long as I live with them ! "—" The people who are around me," says Ec. (f., 34), " suddenly rob me of my thoughts, and that leaves me without consciousness."—" As soon as they come into the room they steal my thoughts, they rob me of my presence of mind, of my power to act on my own initiative."—Tt. (m., 30) remarks: " It is so difficult for me to live with nervy people, especially when I myself am tired. It tires me, empties me. My sister should certainly not be allowed to live with Mother. I am sure she will become ill as I have. It is too exhausting to be in the same room with Mother, she seems to empty you out; she steals your thoughts."—In more serious cases, the impression of being robbed of one's thoughts occurs at every turn, and in connexion with many different individuals. " At meal-times," says Agathe, " every one seems to fall upon me and take away my will to eat, as though the person opposite me were cutting off my arms and legs; I am at the mercy of a rout of people, who rob me of my thoughts." The patients who express fancies of this kind are very numerous.

Though this particular expression appears akin to many others, I feel we must draw a distinction. Emile, for instance, complains that some one is penetrating into his thoughts, or reading his thoughts, " just as though I were transparent."— " As soon as any one claps eyes on me," says Su., " he can seize hold of my thoughts, as though he could hear them."—In such cases we are faced with a mania for secretiveness, with a phobia of having our innermost thoughts read. Emile exclaims : " I can't stand any one knowing some idiotic thought which flits through my mind and finds expression on my face. It is hateful that such thoughts can be guessed by the coincidence of some circumstance or the other and the expression on my face."—Other patients complain that all the time their thoughts " are being repeated." This is merely the phenomenon of the echo of thought in response to the patient's automatic utterances.—Others fancy that their thoughts do not belong to them. " I have some thoughts which I know to be my very own, and other thoughts which I feel are not my own. These latter seem as though they walked apart, and had been foisted upon me." Here we have the sentiment of automatism (which occurs so often when we are dealing with the sentiment of incompleteness) superadded to the phenomenon of " thought theft."

For my part, I feel inclined to interpret the phenomenon of " thought theft " as follows. Individuals in whom psychological tension is unstable, suffer from sudden relaxations of this tension, succumb to psycholeptic crises which have been brought on by their relationships with certain persons in their immediate circle. At first this lowering of mental level takes place slowly during the execution of the depressing action (any of those I have been enumerating) ; then, as time goes on, the pace quickens. " I can't help it, but little by little the scenes my mother revels in have become for me increasingly exhausting. When they first began, I used to put up with them willingly, and I would quickly squeeze out a few tears in order to please her. But I simply can't weep now. I feel I want to go away ; I am becoming indifferent ; I cannot guide my thoughts any longer ; the world seems to be losing all reality. As soon as she begins one of her scenes, I have to rush away from the drawing-room if I am to keep my wits about me." Psycholeptic crises are of frequent occurrence in these circumstances, they are the essential constituent of timidity.

Persons suffering in this way wish to ascribe the modification of psychological tension to some exterior happening. (As a matter of fact they find this needful in the case of all the changes which take place within them.) Thus Simone (f., 26) says : " When I am not amiable, it means that some one is present who fidgets me, paralyses me, and makes me perform idiotic feats." It is quite natural that a sudden depression of this sort should be laid to the charge of the persons who happen to be present at the moment. Nor is this deduction altogether false, for it is certainly the fault of the persons who happen to be present, inasmuch as they demand the performance of actions which are too complex for the subject, and which occasion fatigue and depression. After a time, the theory that the thoughts are being stolen is apt to possess the patient's mind whenever some particular individual is present. We can verify this in an almost experimental way. Take Simone, for instance. It cost me no end of time and trouble to overcome her inveterate shyness. She is conversing with me and expresses herself quite shrewdly ; she is satisfied that she is proving herself intelligent, and is sufficiently stimulated not to be under the dominion of any delusions. The door is flung wide, and Simone's mother, rigged out in the latest fashion, bursts into the room, exclaiming : " How is the dear child ? Doctor, don't you think she is quite well again now ? Don't you think she is fit to put on her smartest frock and come to receive my guests ? " The " dear child " pulls a long face ; her mind works slowly, and she detests surprises. The sudden and noisy irruption of her mother has caused Simone a great emotion, and has already depressed her ; her mother's get-up shocks her, for she is jealous and knows that she herself is incapable of dressing so smartly ; the mother's talk disgusts Simone, for the words don't ring true. Simone feels sure that her authoritarian and jealous parent has come in thus precipitately in order to catch what might be said to the doctor, and she has to repress a violent desire to reproach her mother for unseemly behaviour. All this depresses the patient in many ways ; and, as always happens when her psychological tension is lowered, she becomes coarse and brutal, and begins once more to rave about the ownership others exercise over her. She turns to me, and whispers in my ear : " There, you see, Mother is angry with me, she has come once again to steal my thoughts."

The other phenomena concerned with " thought theft " have the same origin. The sentiment of automatism, and the sentiment of being possessed, are sentiments of incompleteness closely akin to psycholepsy itself. " These girls have great power over me," said Gh., " They steal my thoughts, then they pierce me through and through with their eyes ; they eclipse me to such a degree that I find myself acting, posturing, and speaking in a way that is quite foreign to me." Others fancy they have been suggestioned, hypnotised, decomposed, or dissected, through outside influence. " Under the spell of those who associate with me," says Simone, " I feel as if parts of my mind, my intelligence, my understanding, my judgment, were flying away. . . . It is as though they were carrying off sections of myself, cutting little beefsteaks from this part of me and from that. . . . When I see such stout women, I feel as if I had had a stroke ; it makes me ill as though their filthy hands had passed over me, and as though their bodies had taken the place of mine. . . . I try hard to find myself once more ; I rub myself so that the pieces of fat woman shall drop off me." The many varieties of sentiment and mania of persecution derive from these fundamental facts.

The depression caused by the presence of such fatiguing and costly individuals may even find expression in physiological symptoms. Muscular energy is lessened; troubles of circulation and respiration appear in certain cases simply because of the presence of fatiguing persons. Above all, the digestion goes wrong.—Tt. (m., 30) tells me that he cannot digest properly when he has a meal with his mother.—Another man, twenty-eight years of age, complains : " How can any one eat in my family circle ? There are perpetual quarrels in progress, and I always get indigestion in consequence."—This is a commonplace, and has been frequently observed by medical practitioners.[1] Many neuropaths suffer from enteritis if they take their meals in the family circle, whereas when they are away and staying in hotels, where the food is certainly not better in any way, they digest quite easily. The main factor in such disturbances is the depressing influence exercised by his associates, upon an individual endowed with low vitality, especially when the associates belong to the category of neuropaths who are exacting and costly.

7. THE NEUROPATHIC GROUP AND NEUROTIC CONTAGION.

The foregoing studies are confirmed, if I mistake not, by a clinical phenomenon which attracted attention long ago, but one to which, in my view, insufficient importance has been attached. I am referring to the existence, not of a neuropathic *family* but of a neuropathic *group*. All medical men who have

[1] Cf. A. Bliss, The Influence of Mind on Digestion, in Parker's Psychotherapy, IV, iii, 59.

had experience of this type of patient will agree with me when I say that in a given circle of persons a neuropath is rarely to be found as a solitary specimen. Almost invariably, one or more others will be suffering in various degrees and in various ways from the same sort of depression of psychological tension. It often happens that these others are far more seriously ill than the subject who is brought to us ; but, for one reason or another, their illness has not been recognised. Such persons may bring a patient, declaring him to be a neuropath, without ever dreaming of the far graver symptoms they themselves are afflicted with.

I might adduce, in this connexion, many hundreds of observations, but will be content to enumerate a few cases which have not been noted in any other of my books. When all the members of a family live together, the ailment may be met with in the father and in one or more of the children.— Cx. is an anxious man, authoritarian, exacting, who suffers from crises of depression ; his son is likewise depressed, abulic, and subject to phobias.—Lkc. is an authoritarian and an ascetic ; his daughter has sexual obsessions.—Ao., timid and inclined to phobias, with a mania for being loved, has a daughter who suffers from anorexia and hypochondria, and is authoritarian.—Similar facts are to be observed in fifteen additional cases. Frequently we meet with the same illness in the mother and in the daughter, or, maybe, in several of the children. I have noted this in twenty of my cases.—Lox. is abulic, jealous, and suffers from obsessions ; she has two sons who are both of them abulic, and suffer from anxiety and from doubts.—Emma is obsessed by love, she is photophobic and impulsive ; her mother was an authoritarian who was afflicted with delusions of persecution.—Anna, in whom we witness such remarkable manifestations of the sentiment of unreality and metaphysical obsessions, is the daughter of an authoritarian and jealous woman.—Vkp., a hypochondriac suffering from an obsession of fatigue, has a mother who is authoritarian, exacting, hypochondriacal, and has passed her whole life in frightening him.—Neb. (m., 32), who suffers from a most peculiar obsession connected with defaecation, has led a preposterous life with his mother, who is abulic, phobic, and authoritarian. " She never knows what she wants, and yet she always insists upon her associates doing what she wants, to the accompaniment of the most terrific scenes."—I have had occasion to refer to Ew.'s strange conduct more than once in these pages. She is authoritarian and jealous up to the point of delusions; is for ever bringing her daughter to be examined by brain specialists in the hope they will declare her mad; Ew.'s trouble arises from the fact that she suffers from anorexia and from obsessions.—I need not further emphasise the familiar fact that the children of neuropathic parents are often congenital neuropaths.

Side by side with the foregoing we may place other groups which are far more interesting. I refer to instances in which there is no blood relationship between the members of a neuropathic group, so that there can be no question of hereditary influence.—Bnb. (f., 22), hysterical, anorexic, with fixed ideas; lost her mother in childhood (the mother, who died of tuberculosis, had no neurotic taint). Bnb.'s father soon married again, and the young woman has thus lived practically all her life with a stepmother who suffers from obsessions accompanied by delusion of touch, and from a mania for domination.—Cmc. (m., 20), depressed, etheromaniac, and with an impulse to fugues, lives with a stepmother who suffers from hypochondria, from a mania for love, and is perpetually lamenting.—In the family Dld., the girl who is actually ill is the daughter of a man who was normal; he died, and the mother married a second time. The girl has lived for many years, therefore, with a stepfather who is suffering from what has been called neurasthenia, though he is really affected with psychasthenic obsessions.—More frequent still are the cases where a young woman, hitherto apparently quite normal, goes to live with her husband's family. Ere long she begins to present signs of a psychological depression analogous to that from which her parents-in-law have been suffering.—Here, then, we have examples of malady in the mother-in-law or the stepmother and the daughter-in-law or the stepdaughter, in five cases; and in the father-in-law or the stepfather and the daughter-in-law or the stepdaughter in two others. I fancy that many similar observations might be made.

It seems to me, however, that a more interesting study is that of groups to which I have devoted special attention. In this case the group consists of husband and wife, or of lovers who have lived together for many years. Both members of the group exhibit well-marked psychasthenic disorder. I have had thirty-two such cases through my hands. Unfortunately, I have not space enough to deal with all these cases in detail. In each case, however, we find that one of the partners, normal before the union, falls ill after some years of cohabitation with an individual suffering from psychasthenic disorders. In certain instances, of course, matters are more complicated, and we find that, in addition to the father and mother, one or more of the children become affected.—In the Bgl. family, for instance, we find the father, the mother, and two daughters all suffering from obsessions.—In the Lob. family, the father, the mother, and one daughter are invalids.—In the Wkx. family we have the maternal grandmother who suffers from agoraphobia, from manias of domination and of touch ; the mother is a doubter, who is afflicted by anxiety and manias ; the father is abulic, and hypochondriacal, has crises of reading mania, and refuses to leave his bed for months at a time ; the son is a doubter, has a mania for asking questions, and suffers from metaphysical obsessions.—In Sophie's family, the father, the mother, one daughter, and one son, are all afflicted. Such groups occur more frequently than might be imagined, and their study is peculiarly interesting.

The neuropathic family is usually accounted for by invoking the influence of heredity. This explanation is quite adequate in the case of the first groups I described. But even here, I am not absolutely convinced that heredity is the sole factor. I have noted in certain instances that when some of the children of the same family have for various reasons been brought up away from the rest of the family circle, these children escape the affliction. For example, in the Wkx. family, mentioned above, the girl is quite free from neurotic symptoms because she was lucky enough to marry very young, and thus avoided the morbific influence of the family circle.

The appeal to hereditary influence has no bearing where stepchildren are concerned, in the case of connexion by marriage, or in the relationship between a lover and his mistress. In these neurotic groups where there is no tie by blood, we must seek for some other explanation than direct or collateral inheritance. Nor do I think that we can be content to talk of coincidence. We are unscientific if we disregard the law of probability so flagrantly as to suppose that illnesses of the same character can chance to coincide among associates as frequently as, in actual experience, they do coincide. Such an explanation can only be a last resort. I am no better satisfied with the facile explanation that imitation or suggestion accounts for all the facts. The members of such groups are not all suggestible hysterics ; besides, they would have to be ill to begin with to be as suggestible as this theory implies ; the primary fact which demands explanation is the depression which might make them suggestible. At an earlier date, when I was dealing with a comparatively small number of such groups, it occurred to me as a possible explanation that psychasthenics have a taste for the society of their own kind ; that like draws to like ; that the patients seek out persons who share their fondness for reverie, their inclination to over-scrupulousness, their flight from reality. I still think that such a tendency may play its part sometimes, but I do not think that it is ever a notable factor. Although many of the patients are clever at self-analysis, they are apt to be incapable of understanding the character of any one else ; they have few active preferences ; and they are grouped by external causes, rather than as the outcome of spontaneous impulses. Besides, I have sometimes been able to ascertain that, prior to the association, one of the associates was free from psychasthenic traits, or at any rate did not exhibit them to a degree rendering their recognition and study an easy matter. Such explanations are, for the most part, inadmissible ; and I think that the study we have undertaken in the present work enables us to find a more satisfactory way of accounting for the facts.

We have learned in the foregoing chapter that circumstances which make life difficult, complicated types of behaviour, and the fatigue brought on by sustained effort, are frequent causes of mental depression. Our analysis of the characteristics displayed by the psychasthenic in social life, and our study of the complicated reactions demanded from such a person's associates, have taught us that those who have to live with these patients find life difficult, fatiguing, and costly. Are not we entitled to infer that a good many of the cases of depression observed among the associates of a psychasthenic are the direct outcome of this social fatigue ? Not infrequently, such patients give us definite information as to the origin of their depression, and what they tell us bears out the foregoing theory. They complain of having found it terribly fatiguing to live with a neurasthenic whose spirits they were continually trying to keep up.—For ten years, Eke. (f., 38) nursed her brother with great devotion. The brother was half-insane, abulic, and authoritarian. " I had to do everything for him. But that was not all, for he wanted to monopolise my feelings, my actions, and my thoughts. He was perpetually saying : ' I shall compel you to believe everything I believe, and if you don't I shall kill you.' He ended by sucking me dry, by living on my energies ; and whenever I went into his room I felt he was robbing me of my thoughts." At length she fell ill in her turn, manifesting a different form of depression.—" My father," says Cx., " deprives other people of their strength without knowing it."—Fjj. (f., 40) said of her lover : " He dominated me so as to completely absorb me. He would never let me go out, and prevented my doing the things which interested me and raised my spirits. He was constantly making me feel small, and dragging me down. . . . He did his work so well that now I no longer wish to occupy myself with anything ; I am good for nothing, I despise myself, and can only think of my own distresses."

When one of two associates is extremely jealous, this will often gravely affect the life of the other, and nervous symptoms are apt to arise in the latter. We see this again and again. Sometimes the resistance of a healthy subject will last a long time.—Monsieur Lox. bore his wife's jealousy valiantly for ten years before he succumbed ! " Now," he says, " I can't bear it any longer. All her energy seems to be devoted to watching my doings and my words. I never feel free. She works off all her troubles on to me. I am like a supersaturated liquid ; the most trifling allusion to the fixed ideas which I have never heard the last of during ten or twelve years, overwhelms me and makes me ill."—Gih. (m., 50) explains how he broke down at last. " For years and years my wife has suffered from agitations. She has been impulsive, incoherent, prone to exaggerations of thought and conduct. I have had to endure the scenes that were the outcome of her perpetual jealousy of myself, the children, and others. But the poor woman was kept in hand, to a great extent, by her mother, who sustained a considerable part of the burden. When my mother-in-law died, the entire load was placed upon my shoulders. At this time, too, I made the mistake of relinquishing an occupation which used to take me away from the house occasionally. Thus I was more persistently exposed to these troubles, and in the end I myself broke down."—I have several times referred to the household of Zso. Here the husband was authoritarian and jealous. He deprived his wife of all initiative. In the end, she became abulic, was affected by a sentiment of unreality, and suffered from various obsessions of over-scrupulousness. " I suppressed myself completely," she said. " I abdicated my own individuality. I renounced my own happiness, hoping that this would make my husband happy, and you see where it has led me. It seems to me that I took refuge in illness for the very reason that I had suppressed myself mentally and morally."

When the disease has extended to several members of the group, they themselves become aware that they have a bad influence on one another.—Rv. complains of his wife, saying : " She has nothing to talk about ; she won't go out ; she opposes everything I want to do ; she shuts herself off from life, and then suffers because she is not really living. All this has driven me crazy in the end." Madame Rv. complains of her husband's " abominable selfishness." She says : " He is afraid of everything ; he is always making me keep up his spirits ; and he has no sympathy with me now that I have become depressed in my turn."—Madame Dl. says of her husband : " He has a fine character, but he is so exhausting to live with ! " Monsieur Dl. puts the matter philosophically : " It is really impossible to say which of us is more domineering, which of us is more jealous, or which of us has a more exhausting effect upon the other."—" We all get on badly when we are together," said one of Byl.'s daughters. " Father is selfish and cold ; he is unfitted for any kind of activity, and cuts us off from the world. My sister, who is ashamed of herself and of her looks, is continually making scenes. I can't bear them any longer. I can't bear myself. I have become incapable of self-control, and cannot force myself to any effort. I am afraid of railway travelling, theatres, going to church, driving in a cab. I am afraid of everything, and the others find my dreads catching."

Should we use the word " contagion " to describe such an influence ? Should we speak of the contagion of the neuroses ? The question has been much discussed, and it may be contended that the connotations of the word contagion make it inapplicable here. As Georges Dumas has shown, the term implies that one patient exercises a direct action upon another, either by the transference of a poison or a specific microbe, or else by a directly suggestive influence. Now here we are not concerned either with the transmission of a microbe or with suggestion in the strict sense of the term. Even imitation plays a part in quite exceptional cases only. The influence of one patient upon another is indirect. One patient, by his presence, makes social life more difficult and more costly for another or for others. It is this increase of expenditure which leads in the others to exhaustion and to a lowering of psychological tension. Whether the word contagion be or be not used to describe the phenomenon, the point we have to keep clearly in mind is that those who live with certain neurotics become involved in a causal sequence which is apt, in them likewise, to induce and maintain neurosis.

I may be told that the foregoing considerations have no very important bearing upon the treatment of nervous disorders. Such cases, it will be said, are rare. We have to do with groups centring round some one who is definitely suffering from an illness of the type known as neuropathic or psychasthenic. Every one knows that a sick person, and especially a neuropath or a psychopath, has a disturbing influence upon his associates. Still, such patients are not met at every turn ; they are not to be found in many families ; they cannot have much influence in the causation of nervous disorders.

This criticism is based upon a misunderstanding which often affects the discussion of the problem of mental disorders. The general view would seem to be that " mental disorder " must signify " lunacy." There must either be complete lunacy or perfect sanity. " Since you say I am not mad, I must have all my wits about me." Let us first clear the ground of these terms which have a purely conventional significance.

The words "madness," "lunacy," "insanity," "mental alienation," are police terms and not medical terms. They mean no more than that, for various reasons, an individual has become dangerous to himself or others. Thus the term "insanity" has a purely relative sense, for mental disorder which may be dangerous in a man who is poor or neglected, may be free from danger in one who is carefully watched and is well-to-do. Leaving out of consideration madness in the legal sense of the term, people are apt to believe that mental disorders are terrible and incurable calamities which attack certain individuals in a very clear and definite way, but which, happily, are extremely rare. The general view of mental disorder resembles what used to be the general view of tuberculosis, which was only known under the comparatively infrequent but terrible form of "consumption." To-day, most people have come to realise that there are a vast number of cases of slight but curable tuberculosis. The same evolution will take place in our knowledge of mental disorders. Some day, people will come to recognise that they exist on all hands, in more or less attenuated forms, affecting large numbers of persons who are not ordinarily regarded as invalids at all.

All kinds of outward circumstances determine our decision that a particular individual is a "neuropath." A young person, one who is subject to parental control, and one who willy-nilly is brought to consult the doctor, will be regarded as a neuropath much sooner than one who is fully adult and master of his own actions, and who does not seek the advice of a neurologist. What brings people to the doctor is, in most cases, pain, suffering. But suffering has never been the true index of the gravity of a disease. Besides, in neuroses, suffering often assumes forms which make it difficult to recognise ; or it may be masked by peculiar kinds of excitation, as happens in the case of authoritarians. The result is that in a good many instances neuropathic disorders are not recognised as neuropathic. The general public overlooks these disorders entirely, or else classes them as peculiarities of disposition. The miser, the misanthrope, the hypocrite, were described by the imaginative writer long before they were claimed by the doctor as his patients. Many of the characteristics I have been enumerating have been popularly attributed to the mother-in-law. It will take some time to convince people that the type is not a monopoly of the woman whose daughter has been married, but that it is a type found in many depressed women approaching the fifties, who suffer from abulia, and are dissatisfied with themselves and their associates, who are authoritarian and jealous because they are afflicted with a mania for being loved and yet are incapable of attracting love. In a great number of the foregoing cases, the diagnosis made by a member of the family was far from being officially recognised as correct. Many of these women would be greatly astonished to find that I consider them to be as ailing as their daughters. Their own acquaintances look upon them as queer and malicious individuals, but never as invalids.

The result is that persons who are suffering from the various disorders I have just been enumerating, from a loss of will power, a lack of the power to believe, social abulias which occasion the many varieties of timidity, manias for being loved and for loving, and the countless forms of authoritarianism, are very numerous in present-day society. It matters little whether the laity does or does not recognise them as invalids. Their very presence and their behaviour cause profound modifications in the people who come in contact with them. The sufferers transform every simple act of their associates into a complex act, and constrain their associates to maintain a high degree of psychological tension which would not be necessary if such invalids were not present. Thus they are instrumental in leading their normal associates into a constant expenditure of energy; and if the associates are not plentifully endowed with the requisite psychological strength, they soon become exhausted and in the end are utterly ruined. We see that the presence of these neuropaths determines in those around them, not only mental depression, but similar neuropathic symptoms, which in turn foster the same complaint in yet other beings. This influence on the social environment, this kind of " mental contagion," must be taken into consideration in most cases when we are prescribing treatment for neuropathic patients.

I have used the fact of the presence of a neuropath in a given social environment, merely as an example in order to arrive at the concept of a social environment which is both fatiguing, and mentally unwholesome. We may now widen the concept. An individual need not necessarily be a neuropath in order that his presence should render the social environment more complex ; it will not be difficult to find other persons than neuropaths who will exercise the same disastrous effect. The introduction of a new comer, one who has not yet, as it were, been assimilated by the group of old friends among whom he is suddenly thrust, complicates matters very greatly, and easily becomes a source of exhaustion to the members of the original group. A woman, having been left a widow with two daughters, asks her sister, who also has just lost her husband, to come and live with her and the two girls. She is at a loss to understand why the presence of her sister should upset one of the girls.—Madame By., likewise, welcomed her brother into her home. He accepted her kindly offer and brought his son with him. In this case there is an extra cause for complication owing to the difference in financial position of the two families. This financial difference has rendered cohabitation more difficult, and has been contributory in causing the neurosis of the son of By.—It frequently happens that a widower living with his children will try to introduce his mistress into the family group. This will be a cause of depression and of neurosis among the children, especially among the daughters.

We often find that, from the outset, the group has been badly selected, is too complex. Twin sisters insisted that their respective households should always live together ; this led to inextricable difficulties, for they wished perfect equality to reign, and such an ideal is not for this world. The difficulties presented by the situation were largely responsible for the serious neuropathic illness of one of the twins.—In many other cases the young married couple insists upon one or more of the parents coming to live in the new home. This is always an imprudent step. I need not enumerate the hundreds of young married people's lives which have been ruined by the presence of the mother-in-law in the young couple's home. The fact is proverbial.—Wkw. (f., 30) from the first tried to attract her father-in-law ; she wished to be in his good books, and to behave in an exemplary way towards him. Thus she not only had to adapt herself to her husband, but likewise to her father-in-law. This meant a very great deal of work on her part. Soon she began to perceive that her father-in-law did not value her as highly as he ought, that he loved his own daughter better ; jealousy ensued, followed by an attempt at seduction, failure, and regret for all the sacrifices which the poor young woman thought she had made. In a word, adaptation was rendered more and more difficult ; the effort to achieve adaptation led to exhaustion and to depression; and the invalid was constantly asking herself whether she should desire the death of her father-in-law, or offer up prayers that he might live on indefinitely.

Great divergence in cultural acquirements or temperament among the members of a group may likewise engender serious troubles. If one partner in marriage is superior to the other (a thing which it is almost impossible to avoid), the more cultured partner has to adopt an attitude of condescension towards the other ; the less well endowed partner, on the other hand, has to make an effort to rise in order to bring about an equilibrium ; or else the difference has to be accepted by both, in which case a kind of hierarchy is established. This state of things may often be witnessed among perfectly healthy persons, and we know only too well how unfortunate the results are apt to be. If the member of the couple who is inferior in any respect is at the same time a sufferer from inadequacy of will power, this partner will exhaust himself or herself in fruitless efforts to keep level, will not accept the other's superiority, and will fall sick.—A converse type of disorder was that which arose in the case of Pz., who became obsessed with hatred for her husband because he was really less well educated and less refined than she was.—Lydia, a young woman, belonging to a rich, smart, and cultured family, married into a family of much lower degree and at a much lower level of education. She described herself as suffering because of all the happenings of her new life. " I cannot endure the meals, the speech, the manners, the way the men slam the doors, and their roughness when they are playing cards, the absurd sort of things they read, nothing but picture papers. They are so different in character from what I am accustomed to. Of course these things are not catastrophes, but they are the sort of pinpricks which wear one out. I have had to give up so much. Smart dresses, gay parties, presents, dances, all the pleasures of my youth—all vanished. People used to make so much of us ; we were always welcomed with flowers wherever we went ; young men used to vie with one another in paying court to us : that is all over now. None of these people behave themselves like my old friends ; I have had to adapt myself to quite a new sort of life. I have done my best, but I have not succeeded."

If, in any social group, there are two persons ill adapted to one another and who therefore carry on a perpetual contest, this will suffice to make life very difficult for other members of the group.—Vkf. (f., 21) is exhausted by the scenes between her father and her grandmother, and is " wearied by the everlasting reconciliations."—Quite a number of young people fall sick when there has been a divorce between the parents, so that the offspring of the marriage have been placed in a false situation.—I cannot go into these matters further, for this would involve a detailed study of the pathology of social groups, and of its relationship to individual pathology. Enough to remind the reader that in all these instances it would be possible to make the same sort of analysis that we have made concerning the presence of a neuropath in a family. Where an invalid is a member of a social group, the social behaviour within that group is complicated thereby, and will prove exhausting for those members of the group whose resources are inadequate. We must always bear the fact in mind when we have to treat a neuropath.

8. Social Rest by Isolation.

These studies of neuropathic groups are not merely instructive as concerns the pathogenesis of certain types of exhaustion, for they likewise furnish valuable indications as to the treatment of the same diseases. When we have studied those members of the group who have become ill, we shall do well to examine the others, the ones who have remained in good health, and to enquire how they have managed to escape.

Some of them, we may presume, had considerable powers of resistance, which enabled them to avoid being bankrupted by the claims of the environment. Sometimes, as we shall see later, they have been able to derive important resources from elsewhere. But some of these immune persons would appear to have availed themselves of other methods. It has often been pointed out that certain members of a neuropathic family escape the illness when, for one reason or another, they are brought up outside the family group, or are removed at an early age from the dangerous environment.—This is what happened in the case of Jean's brother, who was brought up away from the family and remained immune ; and I could quote a dozen similar instances.—I have already mentioned the case of Mademoiselle Wkx., the only normal and healthy member of her family, in which the grandmother, the father, the mother, and the brother are gravely affected with neuropathic disorder. Her escape seems to be due to the fact that she was a very short time in the family environment, and that her early marriage was successful.—I have notes of five other cases of the same kind.—The case of Ey. (f., 35) is rather different, for she was already gravely affected when she left the family environment, but was cured by the change. We have seen that in her family, the father, the mother, and one of the sisters were neuropaths of a marked type, and that her father in especial made the life of other members of the family a very difficult one. Ey., like her sister, manifested neuropathic symptoms quite early in life. She became affected with various digestive disorders, such as chronic enteritis ; her mental state was extremely characteristic, for she had hypochondriacal obsessions, was obsessed with the thought of death and with the desire for independence, made attempts to run away (fugues), etc. ; and no treatment did her any good. When she was twenty-six, she married, and her new home was far away from the old one. In six months her bodily and mental condition had greatly improved, and at the end of the year had become perfectly normal. Are we to suppose that this change for the better on marriage was the outcome of sexual experience ? I am sceptical of such an explanation, for I have known so many young women of the same type whose symptoms have been aggravated by marriage. A good many people who knew this young woman well, believed that the curative factor in her marriage was that she was removed from her family and was freed from the noxious influence of her father. This seems to me the most plausible explanation.—Similar considerations apply to the case of Neb. He was a young man of thirty-two, who had already had normal sexual experience before marriage, but was suffering from depression and phobias. Marriage cured these troubles because, as he said, it took him away from a gloomy household and from his mother.—Px. (f., 37), whose obsessions of persecution were becoming aggravated to the point of delusion, was cured through going to live by herself and thus getting away from her mother and her sister.—Cxc. (m., 30) had suffered from several crises of depression while living at home. One of these attacks was so severe that he had to be put under restraint for a time. Then he came to a rather remarkable decision. Not only did he make up his mind to leave the family circle, but he determined to go abroad. " My life will be more tranquil in a foreign land. I shall know hardly any one there, and shall not always be running up against acquaintances. I find social life exhausting, and it seems to me that I shall do well to avoid it as much as possible." In actual fact, he has for six years been living a somewhat eccentric and a very retired life, but he has lived sensibly enough, and has been free from serious relapses. It would be easy to multiply instances.

Even while living in a morbid family circle some persons are able to isolate themselves, and thus remain immune. Monsieur Ar., the husband of the hypochondriac who " for twenty years has stood dangling her arms and doing nothing but lament over her organs, one after the other," came to me in order to justify his conduct. " My wife has probably led you to believe that I am very selfish and cold-hearted. I know she is for ever complaining about me, and that she tells all and sundry that I only meet her on formal terms. At the beginning of our married life, I tried to take care of her, to lavish on her the consideration and tender compassion which she naturally expected. I soon realised that my efforts could do her nothing but harm ; and that before long, if I continued, I myself should become an invalid. We have three children, and I am the bread-winner. It would be a catastrophe for us all if I, too, went off my head ; and I should fatally succumb were I to yield to my poor wife's claims. So I came to change my way of living. I took to leaving the house early in the day, and not returning until late. When I get home at night I sternly refuse to discuss with my wife either her obsessions or her imaginary physical ailments ; for fifteen years I have not once asked her about the state of her health. Every year I go away for two months, in order to get a very necessary spell of mental rest. I do not believe that my behaviour has made my wife any worse, far from it ; and by this means I have succeeded in keeping healthy myself. Do you think I have acted badly ? " In several other families I know of a son or of a daughter who has adopted a similar line of conduct, and with good results.

Rx.'s children are calmer, cease having tics and manias, as soon as the father is away from home and they are living alone with the mother.—Sw. (f., 50) has had many crises of depression which had as their starting-point a few weeks' visit to her mother, a sufferer from hypochondriacal obsession. As soon as Sw. returned to her own home she was restored to health.—Tv. (f., 40) has to leave her husband every year for a couple of months, otherwise she falls ill. " My digestion only gets right if I no longer have to be caring for my husband all the time."—Sometimes the need to get away for a while leads to characteristic fugues. Ua. (f., 40) has lived for fifteen years with her husband, who is afflicted with obsessions of jealousy, and who converts her life into a veritable farce. She gets depressed in her turn, becomes alarmed, and takes refuge in hysterical flight ; her fugue lasts twelve days and is followed by complete amnesia.—Wkx. (m., 29), also, is impelled to quit the fatiguing circle in which he lives. " At a pinch, a man can live with my grandmother ; it is difficult, and needs a good deal of attention and suppleness. But my father never succeeded, he is not careful enough in what he says ; he does not thank her enough, or flatter her enough. For this reason they are constantly having scenes. Such a life is too wretched and too exhausting ; it has made both Father and Mother ill, and I cannot stand it any longer. I am a better hand at diplomacy than Father, but it wears me out ; and as soon as I begin to feel as though the world has no reality, as though I were in danger of falling over the edge of life, I have to go away for a time. "

In an earlier chapter we learned that the phobias of certain neuropaths could give us hints as to the precautions it would be wise to take in their cases. The timidities and phobias of many neuropaths are highly characteristic in this respect. As the depression increases they come more and more plainly to manifest a fear of living with their associates, and express a desire to be isolated; they may even go so far as to say they would like to live on a desert island. This is certainly a morbid manifestation, an exaggerated form of social abulia; at the same time, however, it is an indication that social life, and especially one particular form of social life, is exhausting to them.

Treatment by isolation endeavours to meet this demand. If the isolation could be made complete, if the invalid could live in the desert island he yearns for, a wonderful change would have been wrought in the tenor of his life, and more than three-quarters of his psychological expenditure would be docked at one stroke. The invalid, delivered from all his erstwhile associates, would no longer have to worry about the family, or the profession; no more demands would be made on his store of social politeness; he would be saved from business affairs, from engagements, from a thousand nothings which were wont to complicate his behaviour in the social environment. Social functions are the most important and also the most difficult and the most costly; life in a desert island would speedily bring about very great economies. This is a particularly important fact, and one we cannot afford to overlook when considering treatment by isolation. Isolation must therefore be envisaged as a rest cure, as a means for achieving psychological rest; and such rest is far more potent for good than any amount of staying in bed.

Isolation in a sanatorium does not fully achieve this. The invalid is still surrounded by human beings, even though these human beings are other invalids, or nurses, servants, and doctors. But he is under no obligations towards his fellow invalids, and he need not worry his head about their symptoms in the way he was wont to do where the members of his own family were concerned. The nurses and the doctors do not approach him in a normal spirit of equality and of combat but adapt themselves to his needs, and never demand that he should adapt himself to their requirements. The doctors are satisfied with their reward as scientific observers, and the salaried members of the staff are paid for their attentions; they do not expect any quid pro quo. They furnish the sufferer with social aid without expecting him to reciprocate, or asking him for affection and sympathy in exchange. If he can succeed in forgetting the sum paid for his residence in such an institution, he may come to feel that in the sanatorium he is loved for himself alone.

The change of environment, the installing of an invalid in a hospital or a sanatorium, where he lives away from the family and from his customary surroundings is certainly a method of treatment which acts beneficially upon the sufferer's neuropathic condition, especially when the morbid symptoms are not of very long standing. We may place in a first group all those patients in whom a cure has been effected, and in whom the healthy state has persisted for one year after quitting the institution. Many cases could be classed in this group, patients who have been cured after a few months' release from social obligations.

I have among my notes the record of a very large number of cures effected under such conditions ; the patients were hysterical neuropaths under twenty-five years of age. Forty-two such cases among young women included all kinds of disorders of movement, fixed ideas, refusal to take food, and, above all, attacks of hysterical delirium. In most of the cases, a cure was effected after two or three months' residence in the hospital ; in two cases the cure took five months. Many of these patients who, when at home, suffered from crises of delirium lasting twelve hours, and recurring at weekly intervals, had no further crises as soon as they were admitted to hospital. Lm. (f., 18), ever since her mother's death a year previously, had suffered from serious somnambulist crises almost every night ; I was unable to take any notes of this particular state, for the girl had not a single attack once she had entered the hospital. Seven additional cases presented similar phenomena. In other cases, the symptoms persisted for a time ; but very soon their gravity diminished, and they speedily disappeared in the new environment. The treatment which proved so beneficial was simple in the extreme ; it consisted merely in preventing the patients' going home and, for the most part, forbidding them to see anything of their friends and relations. The healing effects of such treatment are indisputable, and it is not difficult to understand why so many sanatoria have come into existence to deal with illnesses of this kind.

When we come to consider psychasthenic troubles, the benefits of isolation treatment are less obvious. Happy and decisive results are rare; most of my patients have had to stay very much longer at the hospital, and have had to undergo other treatments simultaneously; most of those who did repond to rest and isolation treatment, had a relapse before the year was out. Still, I have notes of a dozen young persons suffering from grave psychasthenic disorders, such as tics, mental manias, and paroxysmal obsessions, who were cured in a few months simply by isolation treatment, and who remained free from relapse for many years.—Kn. (f., 19), suffering from tics, screaming fits, a mania for asking questions, and various phobias, underwent isolation treatment, and left the hospital in excellent health at the end of four months. She had no relapse until she was twenty-two years of age, and this relapse was cured in the same manner in five months.—Jj. (f., 19), who was afflicted with the strange tic of pulling out her hairs one by one and eating them, and was suffering from other mental manias, was cured after a few months' isolation treatment, and had no relapse for eighteen months.—X. (f., 24) suffered from grave crises of over-scrupulousness, and from hand-washing mania, etc. She was cured after five months' treatment, and has had no serious relapse for many years.

Among more elderly patients the results of the treatment are far less definite, and I have not seen many successful instances. Emma, a typical psychasthenic, whom I have attended during several serious crises, developed, at twenty-six years of age, a fresh form of obsessional crisis accompanied by photophobia. Since she was more agitated and troubled in her family circle, I placed her in a sanatorium where, after six months' treatment by isolation, she regained her health. When she was leaving the establishment she said: "I feel so calm and so sedate that I hardly recognise myself." I might quote a dozen similar successes. If, among my notes, I have very few records of such cases, the reason is that I usually prefer to deal with these patients by other methods. If, however, isolation is used in conjunction with other methods, and a cure results, I regard the isolation as the chief factor of the cure.

When we have to do with more serious crises of psychasthenic delusion and delirium, wherein the patient loses all power of criticising his obsessions and gives vent to every impulse, treatment by isolation, even in a lunatic asylum, is definitely indicated; it is the necessary accompaniment to any other treatment. It is a needful precaution to protect the patient from himself, and to induce him to accept the other forms of treatment the doctor may deem requisite. We do well to remember that, in spite of their ostensible gravity, these attacks are more often cured than not. Even when the patient seems to be raving, we may notice that he will pull himself together from time to time; that he will have spells of complete intelligence during which he will realise how absurdly he is behaving, and will manifest the existence of the sentiments of incompleteness which are so characteristic of psychasthenics. These are important signs, which show that confusion of mind is not complete; they enable us to distinguish the condition from psychasthenic dementia, wherein the psychological tension falls very much lower and wherein the prognosis is much worse. I have seen grave cases of psychasthenic delusion and delirium cured by this treatment.— Pg. (f., 25) has always been timid, anxious, and scrupulous; she was seduced at the age of sixteen, and devoted herself to the upbringing and education of her child. She has already suffered several times from obsessions of scrupulousness on account of her child, and from foolish fears that he will be taken from her. After any strong emotional strain or physical fatigue, these fears, which she ordinarily laughs at, become exaggerated; she thinks she is being pursued by hooligans who want to rob her of her child; she wishes to become a martyr, and imposes tortures upon herself for her imagined neglect of her child; she refuses all food; etc. As soon as she had been isolated from her child and her family circle, she got rapidly better, and was able to leave the hospital in three months. It is true that the poor woman relapsed very gravely, but this did not happen until after many years.—Sophie was put under restraint on two occasions, for several months each time, since only in an asylum was it possible to tranquillise her, and to free her from the agitation and the delirium which had been superadded to her obsessions.—Fq. (m., 24) had likewise to be sent to an asylum. He had a very severe crisis of psychasthenic delirium. Thanks to being kept for eighteen months under restraint, he recovered sufficiently to play his part fairly well in ordinary social life.—Emile spent a year at the asylum, the isolation diminishing, though it did not completely cure, the social phobias and the psychasthenic delirium which had been superimposed upon his dread of being seen, and of having his thoughts read.—Cp. (f., 34) feels much calmer when she is in a sanatorium. " It seems horribly selfish, but I must admit that I find it extremely restful to be alone from morning till night, to have no responsibilities, no one to direct ; to live alone without having to account to any one for what I am doing."—Vkp. (f., 37) exhausted by living with her mother, who was an authoritarian person, and by a life which was too complicated for her powers, had to spend a year in a sanatorium. There, thanks to the isolation, her health was fully restored. Thence forward, she was able to organise her life more successfully, and to avoid suffering from depression serious enough to necessitate her being put under restraint.— We all know that attacks of mental confusion, mania, and melancholia, need asylum treatment in most cases, and that this treatment often cures.

But with these successful cases, we have to contrast those in which we cannot speak of a cure, for although the patient may improve greatly in the institution, he relapses as soon as he makes any attempt to return to ordinary social life, so that he has to spend year after year in the artificial social environment of a sanatorium or asylum. Still, even in these cases, the simplification of life does the patient good. Sufferers from more or less advanced dementia, when sent to an asylum, are not merely protected against themselves, but are enabled to behave better than when they are living a free life. Sufferers from what is termed dementia praecox (which is often nothing more than severe psychasthenic dementia) are subject to agitations and are apt to be violent when living in the complicated environment of the family, but are tranquillised by the simple environment of the asylum. As soon as they are secluded, we shall find in many cases that they are able to perform satisfactorily various actions which they had lost the power of performing before they were sent to the asylum.

Undeniable though these advantages are, we must not ignore the drawbacks of asylum or sanatorium life. In such institutions, social life is completely or almost completely suppressed, and this suppression exercises a terribly restrictive influence upon the mind. Such a sacrifice should not be made if it can possibly be avoided. Unquestionably there are patients whose mental energy is so greatly reduced that they can only live in a highly artificial and extremely narrow environment. But most of our patients, although psychologically speaking they must be classed as "poor" are not positively "destitute." Their stay in the asylum must be made as short as possible, just as patients suffering from fatigue must be kept in bed for as short a time as possible. As soon as we can, and as far as we can, we must provide them with an environment which has more social reality than that of the ordinary asylum.

This new environment, although it must be somewhat simplified, must be as little artificial as we can make it. At Gheel in Belgium, and at Dun-sur-Auron and Aunay-le-Château in France, interesting attempts have been made to board out patients with rural families. Unfortunately, such attempts have hitherto been made only in the case of dements and other lunatics of an incurable type, requiring simply to be watched and cared for. It would be well if the same sort of treatment could be organised for curable neuropaths. As Münsterberg writes : " The neurasthenic and all similar varieties are, sent away from the noise of the city, away from the rush of their busy life, away from telephones and street cars, away from the hustling business and politics." [1] I should add : " Send them away from their families, from their friends as well as from their enemies ! " In seven of my own cases, I have made attempts of the kind, either boarding out the invalid in a family, or sending the patient to a service flat organised specially for the purpose. In four of these cases, the results were markedly good. Nadia, in especial, was not sent to a sanatorium, but remained to a considerable extent her own mistress, living in a flat where she was completely separated from her family. She spent years in this artificial environment which I had organised for her. " I no longer have fits of temper," she said, " for there is no longer any reason for them. I don't see the people I used to see. There is no longer a bustle all round me. I am not worried by

[1] Psychotherapy, p. 192.

hearing people laugh, chatter, and amuse themselves when I am unable to do anything like others. It was a constant irritation to feel that I was despised, and to be teased by persons who did not understand me. I am not made to live with others. They harass and bore me because I am so different from them." After three years, the treatment had been so successful that the patient was able to resume a more complicated and freer life. Still, it has to be admitted that such an arrangement is costly and is difficult to organise.

In former days, the religious houses provided suitable retreats for such patients. It may well be that conventual life was sometimes a cause of mental disease, but there can be no doubt that in a good many instances it prevented the development of mental disorder which would have inevitably supervened in a free life. I quite agree with de Fleury [1] that for many people the disappearance of the religious houses in France has been a disaster. I know a number of persons (Sophie is one of them) who would be free from mental disorder if they could live in a convent. De Fleury believes " that during the next century there will come into existence a number of lay convents in which our descendants will find temporary refuge when they want to recruit their energies, tranquillise their nerves, fortify their will for the struggles of the ensuing year." Grasset advises that persons predisposed to neuropathic disorder should be sent into retreat for a time, just as those who propose to enter a religious order have to go into retreat.[2] Ossip Lourié makes the same demand in his work on the disorders of speech : " Isolation is the only effective treatment of verbomania. . . . In these days of generalised neurasthenia, every civilised country ought to have lay convents where the most efficient nervous motors of society can retire for intellectual rest, and for refreshment by devotion to manual work for a time." [3] Until such establishments have been organised, we must be content to advise our patients, in suitable cases, to take refuge in the quiet countryside whenever possible. Those who have to remain in town must seek social groups or pursue avocations in

[1] Op. cit., p. 473.
[2] Grasset, La défense sociale contre les maladies nerveuses, " Revue des Idées," 1906.   [3] Le language et la verbomanie, 1912, p. 256.

which they can lead a regular and simple life like that of convents.

For all such persons, and particularly for those who have to live with their families, I have found it well to advise the enjoyment of solitude from time to time. It is wrong to suppose that human beings must be continually under observation, cared for, worried by affectionate friends and relatives ; and this remark applies more especially to exhausted persons. Nothing is so restful as a few hours of solitude ; nothing can bring about so complete a release of tension ; nothing can ensure so true a distraction. " Solitudo alit ingenium."—Zoé (f., 30) has fully realised that she is freed from her " attachments " for a time by a spell of solitude ; that this enables her to get on with her journey through life. She knows that she must spend several hours quite alone every day if she is to behave normally to her associates for the rest of the time.—Tx. (m., 45), when he has been exhausted by a long walk or by conversation, can only recover, can only " get rid of the black dog," when he is alone. " My head is like a vessel that has been over-filled ; if any one pours a drop more into it, it will overflow ; I must stay quite alone in my room for a time."—Uw. (m., 47) finds that his ideas of persecution vanish and that a kindly feeling towards his associates is restored if only he can be left by himself for a time.—" When the sense of vacancy in the head comes on," says Nebo. (m., 40), " what I need is a day or two's solitude ; that is the best remedy for me."—The prescription of solitude is a simple one, and we must not forget to recommend it in suitable cases. It is more often applicable than people might think.

An even more important point, however, is that we should try to simplify the family life of these weaklings, to simplify the social life they have to lead day by day in their customary surroundings. My aim has been to show that neuropaths and those who are candidates for neurosis tend to get worn out in their everyday relationships with their associates, either because the associates, being more active than the invalids, tend to involve the latter in a life which is too complicated for their inadequate powers, or else because the characteristics of their associates are thorny and exact great expenditure from the weaklings. Morton Prince showed a good many years ago that the most essential feature of treatment by isolation was the withdrawal of the patient from home, the removal of the patient from contact with the other members of his family.[1] I think that we can put the matter somewhat more definitely, saying that it may not be necessary to separate the patient from *all* the members of his family. We have to discriminate, and to isolate our invalid from those individuals contact with whom is especially dangerous.

It is often of importance to simplify the group by advising certain persons to withdraw from it. Familiar experience has shown that difficulties and dangers arise when, after young people have married, their parents continue to live with them. This form of association becomes quite impracticable when the family contains any one suffering from psychasthenia.— Mt. (f., 41) was rendered crazy by the presence of her mother-in-law as a member of her household. Both the women were far happier when they lived apart.—The Wkx. family was greatly tranquillised by the departure of the grandmother, but here the neuropathic disorders were too severe for a complete cure to be achieved in this way.—Sz. (f., 48) had had in earlier years serious crises of depression. Notably, during several months, she had suffered from a remarkable phobia, a dread of the wind. However, for some years, she had been in good health. Then her daughter married, and the husband came to live in the house. Thereupon the elder woman had a serious relapse, was troubled with regrets for having agreed to the marriage, with doubts as to whether her daughter really loved her, and so on. She recovered within a few weeks after the departure of the young people to a separate establishment.—Cf. (f., 52), who had always lacked energy, found it impossible to live with her married children, for this imposed various activities upon her, such as attending parties, and luxurious living. She suffered from sleeplessness, persistent headache and hypochondriacal obsessions. All these symptoms were occasioned by her incapacity for participation in so complicated an existence. It was necessary to provide her with an establishment of her own, retired and extremely simple, accordant with the low level

---

[1] Prince, Educational Treatment of Neurasthenia, etc., 1898.

of her psychological tension.—I have seen the same sort of thing in nine other families.

But other separations have to be considered in this connexion, besides the removal of parents-in-law from young households.—Vv. had a sister-in-law living in the house, and ere long the sister-in-law became his mistress. This involved various complications and frequent emotional disturbances. The removal of the sister-in-law from the family environment was essential to his cure.—In Madame Rv.'s case, tranquillity was restored by the departure of a pupil of her husband's. This young man had been living in the house and had been making love to her.—In quite a number of cases, the dismissal of some particular servant or servants has simplified the life of the family group and has enabled nervous weaklings to lead a life which was healthier because it demanded less expenditure of energy.

Even when the members of the younger generation do not marry, but have simply grown up, it is sometimes impossible for them to remain with their parents if some member of the family should happen to be neuropathic and inclined to be abulic, authoritarian, or a tease.—Qc. recovered when he ceased to live with his father and his sister.—Sw. (f., 40) lived with her mother, and the two women were continually bickering. Sw. had a morbid dread of all kinds of little noises which her mother could not help making when blowing the nose, taking snuff, rustling a piece of paper, and so on. When the two women lived apart, they were both in much better health, and were fonder of one another.—A good many patients, acting on my advice, followed the example of Cxc., and went to live abroad in order to get out of reach of their families. In these instances, the measure seemed to prevent the onset of a serious neurosis.—Cdc., though she was only twenty years of age, had to have a separate establishment, so that she could get away from her mother. As soon as this had been arranged, she was freed from her nervous troubles.—I have seen a number of cases of this kind. Where we have to do with very young persons, we can get them away from their families by advising that they should be sent to boarding schools. When they grow up, marriage will often ensure their removal from the uncongenial family environment, as we have had occasion to note already in several cases. Even when that way out of the difficulty is not forthcoming, the doctor may find it necessary to insist upon a separate establishment, for this will be an advantage to all the members of the group.

In certain cases, which are commoner than is usually supposed, we may have to separate husband and wife, even at the risk of breaking up the marriage altogether. I have already had occasion to refer to the mental disorders which may be brought about by conjugal life in persons suffering from sexual phobias, or in persons who cannot endure the complications entailed by married life.—Lo. (f., 26) ran away from the house on her wedding night. She then suffered from serious depression and nothing could cure her but divorce. She would certainly have gone mad had she been compelled to return to her husband, but she had a fairly adequate mental life as a celibate.—I have recorded the sufferings of three women who had to be separated from their husbands, and who recovered mental balance to a considerable extent after the separation. In the treatment of mental disorders, we must sometimes have recourse to a sort of surgery, must be bold enough to make amputations when they are requisite. Besides, in a good many instances we shall not find it necessary to break up the household permanently.— From time to time it became necessary to separate Lox. from his wife, for only in that way could he be given the sense of freedom which for him was an absolute necessity. I used to send him away on a journey upon one pretext or another. After a few weeks he would come back in better health and "less supersaturated." He was now better able to endure complaints and recriminations, and had again become competent to exercise over all his words and deeds the strict supervision which was indispensable. Such separations, for a shorter or longer period, are useful in a great number of households, and reanimate affection.

When separation is out of the question, or when it is not essential, the psychiatrist may have to take other measures, and to reorganise the life of the group. R. C. Cabot writes interestingly anent the maladjustments of family life. "We all know how peculiarly and subtly members of the same family may wear upon each other—how the quality of an uncle's cough may be the one thing that his niece cannot abide, or how the habit of tapping or scratching with the foot which it is impossible for the patient's mother to stop, may be the very thing which the patient cannot stand. . . . We should take full cognisance of the facts in order to consider at least the possibility of their modification. . . . To diminish the number of hours spent at home each day is sometimes a more effective way of reducing home friction than to send the patient away altogether. Often the trouble is merely that members of the family pass too many hours at close quarters. . . . Now and then I have seen the best results follow the introduction of a new member into the family, as a sort of 'buffer' between its warring elements. . . . A family may behave quite angelically to each other in the presence of a comparative stranger, even after his first strangeness has worn off. . . . Exceptionally, it may be the physician's duty to take a hand in even more intimate domestic affairs—to help to reconcile a man to his wife, or to persuade a father to allow his daughter to get married when the objections to this step are not serious." [1]

In some cases, when the doctor has acquired authority over the group, he will not find much difficulty in reorganising their joint lives. But there is one thing which those who have to treat such cases should never forget, though it is often overlooked. When we have to prescribe for a neuropath in a family, it is almost always desirable to treat several other persons at the same time, to treat the patient's associates. Here we encounter a difficulty, for these individuals are not likely to be willing to regard themselves as invalids, and they may look upon some of the absurd things they do as legitimate actions based upon sacred rights, while they will tell us that other absurdities are acts of splendid devotion. Of course it is far easier to write a prescription for a soothing syrup than to contend with the authoritarian manias of some of the patient's associates and with the self-sacrificing manias of others ; but this regulation of the invalid's domesticities is an essential and fruitful part of psychotherapeutics. I shall not, at this stage, say anything more about the modifications which must be gradually induced in the bahaviour, for this concerns the education of particular kinds of action, and

[1] Cabot, The Analysis and Modification of Environment, in Parker's Psychotherapy, III, iii, 6–9.

excitations of special sorts. These are matters to be considered in subsequent chapters. It has been enough here to point out that the difficulties dependent upon social life in a particular group may be minimised by modifications in the social life of the group, and that by bringing about such modifications we shall sometimes be enabled to obviate the need for separations and isolations.

CHAPTER ELEVEN

TREATMENT BY MENTAL LIQUIDATION

WHEN a man, harassed by a sad memory, tries to rid his mind of it by journeying to a far country, " his trouble rides pillion with him." All the famous moralists of old days drew attention to the way in which certain happenings would leave indelible and distressing memories, memories to which the sufferer was continually returning, and by which he was tormented by day and by night. This inclination to brood over past troubles plays a notable part in causing the exhaustion from which neuropaths suffer, and for a long time it has been the aim of many psychiatrists to bring rest to their patient by tranquillising the mind and by freeing it from such exaggerated and persistent disquietudes. This attempt has been the starting-point of more than one therapeutic method in the development of which I have myself been to some extent concerned. But, in especial, it underlies a philosophical and medical system which has of late years undergone extensive development in Germany and the United States under the name of psychoanalysis.[1]

1. THE STUDY OF TRAUMATIC MEMORIES.

Again and again psychopathologists have pointed out that a good many neuropathic disorders are induced by an emotion, a disquietude, a grief resulting from some particular happening. Moreau de Tours, Baillarger, and, above all, Briquet, insisted upon the pathogenic importance of grief and similar emotions ; but in their day it had not been generally realised that such an exciting cause was a common antecedent of mental disorder, and might play an important part in its subsequent develop-

---

[1] The present chapter is based upon a report I made to the Seventeenth International Congress of Medicine held in London in the year 1913. This report was published in the " Journal of Abnormal Psychology," 1915, and in the " Journal de Psychologie Normale et Pathologique," 1917.

ment. Thus, the accepted ideas as to the working of such influences remained vague.

When lecturing in the years 1884 and 1885 upon the symptoms of hysteria, Charcot was able to give definite proof of the pathogenic influence of events that have made an impression on the mind. Describing certain cases of hysterical paralysis in which the trouble ensued after an accident, he showed that the emotion caused by the accident at the time was not the only cause of the illness. Nevertheless, he went on to say, we must ascribe considerable importance to the memories left by the accident, to the patient's "ideas and disquietudes" anent the untoward experience. Many observers, and especially Möbius, accepted Charcot's teaching in this respect, and agreed that certain hysterical symptoms were the expression of bodily modifications connected with ideas and memories.

In my earliest writings (1886 and 1892) I myself adhered to the same view, referring to various cases of paralysis and contracture that had arisen after an accident, and appeared to be due to the memory of the accident. Subsequently, I was led to enlarge the notion, and to show that neuropathic disorders of the same kind might arise in consequence of happenings which were not accidents in the colloquial sense of the term, which had not caused any obvious material injury, but had simply induced moral perturbation. The memory of what had happened persisted in the same way as the memory of a material accident. The traumatic memory, in this case likewise, had its attendant train of sentiments. Directly or indirectly, it was the cause of some of the symptoms of the disease.

I had noted this fact in connexion with a number of patients, but my book upon psychological automatism was philosophical rather than clinical, and it therefore contained an account of only a small number of cases of the kind. Here is one of the most characteristic.[1]—Marie, a girl of nineteen, suffered every month during menstruation from serious crises, attended by convulsions and delirium, which lasted for several days. Menstruation would begin in normal fashion, but after a few hours the patient would complain of feeling very cold and would have a characteristic shivering fit. Thereupon,

---

[1] Cf. L'automatisme psychologique, 1889, pp. 160 and 439.

the menstrual flow would cease and the delirium would begin. In the intervals between these crises, the patient was liable to attacks of terror in which she had a hallucination that there was a pool of blood before her eyes. She also had a number of stigmata of hysteria, among which may be mentioned anaesthesia of the left side of the face with amaurosis of the left eye.

Study of this patient's life history and an investigation of her memories concerning the various things that had happened to her disclosed some remarkable facts. At the age of thirteen, when menstruation first appeared, she had checked it by getting into a cold tub. This had brought on a shivering fit and delirium. Not only was the menstrual flow arrested then and there, but there was no recurrence of menstruation for several years. When, at length, a normal periodicity was resumed, menstruation was attended by the disorders I have just been describing. Subsequently, the girl had a terrible fright through seeing an old woman fall down stairs and cover the steps with blood. Much earlier, when she had been only nine years old, she had had on one occasion to sleep in the same bed with a child whose face on the left side was covered with the scabs of impetigo. All night she had been filled with loathing and alarm.

It was possible to ascertain that these incidents had produced in the patient's mind impressions of a kind closely akin to those represented by the symptoms from which she suffered when she came under observation. The symptoms did not appear until after these unfortunate happenings, and as a sequel of the memories they had left. Thus, when she was grown up, a symptom could be revived by the recall of the appropriate memory. Finally, it was found possible, by modifying the memory in various ways, to bring about the disappearance or the modification of the corresponding symptom. It was natural to draw the inference that the memory of these happenings had played, and continued to play, a part in causing the girl's hysterical symptoms and in deciding the form taken by these symptoms.

My book, *L'automatisme psychologique*, contained reports of other cases of the same kind.[1] Subsequently, I was able to detect like phenomena in connexion with a remarkable

_____
[1] Cf. pp. 208 and 211.

case of abulia,[1] and also in connexion with the amnesic disorders from which Madame D. suffered. She was thirty-four years of age, and had suddenly passed into a neuropathic state after a violent emotion induced by a " practical joker " who shouted in her ear that her husband was dead. I was able to ascertain that this patient's persistent amnesia, her delirious crises, and all her other symptoms were connected with the traumatic memory.[2] In my later writings, there are many more reports of such cases, and I think it would be easy to collect from these books about fifty instances in which a traumatic memory was described as one of the essential factors of the disease. In some, there was anorexia or a delusion of starvation brought about by the memory of a seduction and a concealed childbirth. In others, there were various forms of disaesthesia, one of the most notable being a terror of anything red (erythrophobia) connected with the memory of a funeral at which the coffin was covered with red everlastings. In some patients there was paraplegia, with contraction of the abductor muscles (" the guardians of virginity ") brought about by the memory of rape or by that of sexual relationships with a husband who had become odious. In other cases there were systematised choreas, occurring as a futile and persistent reproduction of occupational movements, the cause being a continual thought of the poverty of the parents and of the need that the patient should work.[3]

The following remarkable case is worthy of close consideration in this connexion.[4] Ky. (f., 22) had for six years suffered from various hysterical symptoms, such as cutaneous and visceral anaesthesias, attacks of meteorism, digestive disorders, intractable vomiting, contractures of the legs, extreme astasia-abasia which for four years had made it almost impossible for the patient to walk. In the course of a

[1] " Revue Philosophique," March 1891 ; Névroses et idées fixes, 1898, vol. i, p. 25.

[2] The International Congress of Experimental Psychology held in London, August 1892 ; " Revue Générale des Sciences," May, 1893 ; Névroses et idées fixes, 1898, vol. i, pp. 116 and 139.

[3] L'état mental des hystériques, 1893, vol. ii, pp. 100 et seq ; second edition, 1911, pp. 275 et seq.

[4] Traitement psychologique de l'hystérie, in Albert Robin's Traité de thérapeutique appliquée, 1898, vol. xv, p. 627 ; L'état mental des hystériques, second edition, 1911, pp. 625 et seq. ; Névroses et idées fixes, 1898, vol. ii, p. 519.

conversation with the young woman when she was in the somnambulist state, I learned that at the age of eighteen, when she was living alone with her father, incestuous relationships with him had begun and had lasted for a year. The hysterical symptoms had appeared soon after this. I ascertained that there was an intimated relationship between the symptoms and the memory of the incestuous intimacy with the dread of its consequences. By modifying the patient's ideas, I was able to relieve her of all her symptoms, and thus to confirm my theory as to their origin.

I may also recall the remarkable case of Achille, whose delusions were obviously the outcome of the memory of a transgression. A married man, while away from home on a journey, he had had a casual amour. Thenceforward he was haunted by the thought of diseases and other dreadful punishments, so that his mind, which was not strong at the best of times, became unhinged. Manifestly the remembrance of his transgression was the main cause of the mental disorder, for a modification of this memory was speedily followed by the disappearance of the delusions.[1]

Further studies of the same kind were published in my book *Les obsessions et la psychasthénie* (1903), and since then I have been able to collect the notes of a great many cases in which the memory of being raped, regret for a lost lover, emotional reminiscences connected with a fire, and the like, have played the chief part in causing various nervous and mental symptoms. My studies in this field have been confirmed by those of many other writers, and it may be regarded as proved that the memory of some particular happening can cause neuropathic symptoms. The *traumatic memory* must be regarded as an important factor of neurosis.

From the very first, as far as my own researches were concerned, these considerations led me to take special precautions in the study of traumatic memories and in the endeavour to discover their existence. Both for the explanation and for the treatment of certain neuroses, every effort must be made to discover such memories should they exist. On the other hand, seeing that traumatic memories might be absent in other cases of neurosis (which would then have to be explained and treated in a different way), great care

[1] Névroses et idées fixes, 1898, vol. i, pp. 379 et seq.

must be taken to avoid discovering traumatic memories when they do not really exist. It was necessary, therefore, to collect with the utmost care all the indications the patient could give concerning his thoughts and his memories. The doctor must not be repelled by the tediousness or puerility of the patient's chatter. Listening attentively to all the patient had to tell, he must consider which of the events thus recorded might have acted as pathogenic factors.

Now, great circumspection was needed when an attempt was made to establish a relationship between this or that memory and this or that morbid symptom. We had to ascertain whether the onset of the symptoms had been concurrent with the appearance of a tendency to dwell on a particular memory; whether the development of the symptoms had run a parallel course with the development of the memory; and whether, now that the patient had come under our observation, it was possible to modify the symptoms by modifying the memory. Not until I had made a great many verifications of this kind, did I feel justified in believing that in certain cases, a traumatic memory had been a factor of disease.

Unfortunately, it soon became apparent to me that many of the most important traumatic memories might be imperfectly known by the subject, who was unable to give a clear account of the matter even when he tried to do so. It was necessary, therefore, to institute a search for hidden memories, for memories which the patient preserved in his mind without being aware of them. The gestures, the attitudes, the intonations of the patient, would often lead us to suspect the existence of such submerged memories. Sometimes we had to look for them when the patient was in a special mental condition; sometimes, lost memories would crop up in the somnambulist state, in automatic writing, in dreams.[1] Madame D.'s traumatic memories were mainly brought to light, to begin with at any rate, by a study of her dreams.[2] In all these cases we were careful to write down the actual words used by the subject during the state of sleep, to record them without any modification. Madame D. was kept under

[1] Traitement psychologique de l'hystérie, 1898, p. 191 ; L'état mental des hystériques, second edition, 1911, p. 630.
[2] International Congress of Experimental Psychology, London, August 1892 ; Névroses et idées fixes, 1898, vol. i, p. 127.

observation while asleep, and a record was taken of whatever she murmured. In other cases I had the subject wakened up suddenly, in order that a note might be made of what he said the instant after being awakened. These words were only recorded if they had a definite meaning and related to some specific happening.

In other cases I found that these traumatic memories secured a very definite expression in abnormal states, in hysterical paroxysms, in attacks of delirium, and especially in somnambulist states. We are familiar with the peculiarity of the hysterical fugue ; the subject cannot tell us about the incidents of the fugue, or explain why he ran away, unless we put him into the somnambulist state. The same characteristic was manifest in the fixed ideas which had brought on hysterical paroxysms, paralysis, anorexia, etc. This is a commonplace in the study of hysteria. The doctor must be aware of it, not merely for his guidance in treatment, but even if he is to diagnose hysterical symptoms accurately. The traumatic memories of Marie, the young woman who suffered from delirium periodically in association with an arrest of the menstrual flow, were mainly discovered during her hysterical paroxysms and while she was in the somnambulist states. It was when she was in a condition of induced somnambulism that she told me how she had suppressed her first menstruation by getting into a cold bath, and how she had had to sleep one night in the same bed with a child whose face was covered with impetigo scabs. She could not have related these incidents to me when she was in the waking state, for then, to all appearance, they had been completely forgotten.

This is not a true oblivion, for tendencies that have been really forgotten are no longer active; whereas the latent tendencies we are now considering are still active, for they give rise to dreams, delusions, attacks of delirium, and many other disorders. We must not suppose, either, that the patient is feigning forgetfulness, from unwillingness to avow the tormenting thoughts. We have to do with a genuine inability to cognise what is going on in the mind, and to express it to oneself. There is a peculiar modification of consciousness in the hysterical subject, affecting the individual consciousness rather than the tendency. As long ago as 1889

I attempted to describe this modification as " subconscious-ness due to psychological disaggregation." Thus, the memories capable of causing symptoms took the form of subconscious memories. As soon as my attention had been drawn to these phenomena, I studied them with considerable interest, and I was able to describe a score of striking cases in which, as I then phrased it, there were subconscious fixed ideas, or fixed ideas taking a hysterical form.[1]

This peculiar characteristic of certain traumatic memories in hysterical patients would seem to be important, for fixed ideas of such a kind are apt to be very dangerous. Hypo-thetically we may say that such fixed ideas are dangerous because they are no longer under the control of the personality, because they belong to a group of phenomena which have passed beyond the dominion of the conscious will. Theory apart, modifications of memory during induced somnambulism, in automatic writing, and in various other subconscious states, have often enabled me to rediscover the thought of happenings the memory of which had determined or was maintaining mental disorder.

When we find that a patient has a memory of this kind, it is interesting to study the way in which it has become traumatic, to elucidate the mechanism by which it has affected the physical and mental health. Charcot, when he tried to explain the symptoms of traumatic neuroses, appealed to a psychological mechanism with which he and his contemporaries were beginning to become acquainted, the mechanism of suggestion. He supposed that the memory of the event gave rise to very natural reflections concerning its possible con-sequences, concerning the wounds, the losses of power, and the weaknesses which it might entail. Suggestion tended to realise such ideas of infirmity and impotence, and thus gave rise to paralysis. To begin with, I accepted this interpretation as the true one in certain cases in which it could be shown that the idea of illness antedated the symptoms of the illness, and could be proved to have influenced the development of these. For a long time I laid stress upon the mechanism of

[1] Cf. L'état mental des hystériques, 1892, pp. 67 et seq. ; Un cas de possession et l'exorcisme moderne, 1894 ; Névroses et idées fixes, vol. i, p. 375 ; Les idées fixes de forme hystérique, " Presse Médicale," 1895 ; Névroses et idées fixes, vol. i, p. 213.

suggestion, and I showed that in a restricted consciousness the idea of illness had an exaggerated power owing to the absence of antagonising phenomena. It is needless to recapitulate these notions, for their truth is now generally admitted, and this aspect of the matter has frequently been overstated.

In a great many cases, it became plain to me that the idea of loss of power, the idea which could set suggestion to work, had not come into existence during the period between the trauma and the first appearance of symptoms, or at most had had a trifling intensity. The symptoms were induced by a far simpler mechanism, which I have described under the name of " psychological automatism." The actual memory of the happening was constituted by a system of psychological and physiological phenomena, of images and movements, of a multiform character. This system, persistent in the mind, soon began to encroach. By association, it annexed a number of images and movements which had at first been independent of its influence. Thus enriched, prepotent in an environment of other thoughts that had been enfeebled by the general depression, it became able to realise itself automatically without passing through the intermediate stages of ideation and suggestion, and thus gave rise to actions, dispositions, sufferings, and delusions, of various kinds. In this connexion, I drew a distinction between primary fixed ideas and secondary fixed ideas, and a study of the cases I have recorded makes it easy to grasp the distinction. When, in Marie, the menstrual flow is arrested through the memory of a cold bath, or when, in the same patient, amaurosis of the left eye is induced by the memory of a child which had the left side of the face covered with impetigo scabs, we are able to distinguish in each instance between the primary phenomenon and the secondary phenomenon.

The following passage from my study of the psychological treatment of hysteria, which forms the latter part of *L'état mental des hystériques*, shows how these automatic developments of psychological systems combine with the phenomena of suggestion to induce various symptoms. " The young woman who had for a year lived in an incestuous relationship with her father, was at first terrified at the thought of pregnancy, and this was probably the cause of the meteorism, for such abdominal distension is frequently observed in women who are afraid they have become pregnant. It seems likely that the meteorism and the idea of pregnancy were jointly responsible for the disorders of respiration, the disorders of digestion, and the vomiting. Fear and remorse induced thoughts of suicide. These, in turn, led to a refusal of food, anorexia, and even to the difficulty in swallowing which one doctor whom the patient consulted regarded as due to a lesion in the medulla oblongata. Various causes contributed to make walking more and more difficult : the idea of pregnancy ; the stimulation of the sexual system ; a remarkable hallucination of the tactile and genital senses, which cannot be described here, but which came on whenever the patient moved her legs. The obsessive idea that the last-named remarkable symptom would lead to the discovery of all that had happened, was now superadded, with the result that the patient suffered from extreme astasia-abasia for five years. Another patient, a woman suffering from painful ovarian congestion, is, before all, an abulic who dares not and cannot come to any decision. She is too fond of her husband and child to leave them, and she is too fond of her lover to give him up. She therefore, procrastinates her decision until she has been thoroughly cured. But she puts off her cure. She does not really want to be cured, for then she will have to give a definite answer to her lover's proposal. For six months she has been bed-ridden, and suffering more and more. When we add a constructure of the adductor muscles of the thighs (a common symptom in women affected with sexual disquietudes), we shall have grasped some of the intermediate stages by way of which the symptoms from which these patients are now suffering have been attained. What we have to understand is that the hysteric seldom has in her mind a fixed idea of this or that symptom. She does not think about having a fit of hysterics, or about having her mouth drawn to one side, as those who try to explain everything by suggestion are apt to suppose. Such a theory can only apply to exceptionally simple cases. The fixed idea in the hysteric's mind has no obvious connexion with the symptom, and it only induces the symptom through the intermediation of a series of mental and physical consequences." I concluded this study by saying that the symptoms are linked to the traumatic memory by the totality of the psychological and physiological laws which regulate the development and the manipulation of the emotions.[1]

Many other writers were at this date expounding similar ideas.[2] In especial, I may recall Morton Prince's remarkable study of *Association Neuroses*.[3] Here he showed that " neurosis often consists of the unfortunate evocation of associated psychological systems." In another essay, *Fear Neurosis*,[4] he explained that certain stereotyped movements which seemed extremely strange might be associated with an indefinitely persistent tendency to fear. He compared this association to the one disclosed by Pavloff's experiments upon " conditioned reflexes," the association between the secretion of saliva in dogs and the sound of the ringing of a bell. Recently, Morton Prince has returned to the topic in his essay on *Recurrent Psychopathic States*,[5] and I am glad to note that he adheres to an opinion formerly expressed by myself, for he writes : " The tendency to preserve complexes that have been organised with a certain amount of automatic independence varies greatly from person to person, but it can only be manifested to a high degree when there is a fundamental condition of mental disaggregation."

Why do certain tendencies assume this subconscious character ? I have been inclined to associate the phenomenon with the general characteristics of the thought of hysterics, for we note that such patients are liable to many other dissociations of like kind, and we can see in them the effects of certain depressing emotions upon this or that mental condition. It is easy to note that these subconscious phenomena only make their appearance during the most serious phases of the illness, and that they vanish as soon as the cure begins. We frequently find that when they are being cured the patients will spontaneously recover the memory of happenings which, hitherto, they have only been able to recall in the somnambulist state. The depressing effects of emotion may show themselves in the case of some particular tendency which happened to be functioning at the time of a distressing occurrence. This exhausted tendency can no

---

[1] L'état mental des hystériques, second edition, 1911, p. 627.
[2] Cf. Forel, L'âme et le système nerveux, 1906, p. 211.
[3] " Journal of Nervous and Mental Diseases," May 1891.
[4] " Boston Medical and Surgical Journal," September 1898.
[5] " Journal of Abnormal Psychology," July 1911.

longer be activated to a sufficient degree to take on the characteristics appropriate to higher-grade psychological phenomena ; it can no longer give rise to actions accompanied by personal consciousness. We are here faced once more by the problem of depression, which may depend, as we have seen, upon various causes, and may be due, now to some particular happening, now to a series of troubles, and now to a fundamental disposition. The subconscious fixed idea is a special form of depression localised upon a particular tendency. But, however this may be, such fixed ideas may become dangerous because they have escaped from the control of the personality, because they belong to a new mental grouping over which the conscious will no longer has any power.[1] " The power of such ideas depends upon their isolation. They grow, they instal themselves in the field of thought like a parasite, and the subject cannot check their development by any effort on his part, because they are ignored, because they exist by themselves in a second field of thought detached from the first." [2]

2. FREUDIAN PSYCHOANALYSIS.

Charcot's lectures on the traumatic neuroses and my own studies summarised in the foregoing section were the starting-point of a remarkable theory of the neuroses and of a new method for the treatment of these diseases. I refer to the work of Sigmund Freud of Vienna and his pupils, to the system known as *psychoanalysis*. Of late years the psycho-analytical school has come to play a considerable part in Austria, Switzerland, and the United States. The writings of the psychoanalysts have bulked largely. Their books are not only concerned with questions of psychology and psychiatry. These authors also make a resolute attack upon all the problems of grammar, linguistic science, literature, art, and religion. Such has been the comprehensive outgrowth of that which began as a study of the part played by traumatic memories in the neuroses. These outgrowths have given to psycho-analysis an importance which is perhaps greater than it

[1] L'automatisme psychologique, 1889, pp. 430 and 436.
[2] L'état mental des hystériques, 1894, vol. ii, p. 267 ; second edition, 1911, p. 419.

deserves, but in any case I find it necessary to give a separate account of *mental disinfection by the dissociation of traumatic memories*, although such a separate treatment of this psychotherapeutic method had not been part of my original plan. I cannot attempt here to give a bibliography of Freudian writings, or to summarise this vast literature. Besides, an excellent account of Freudian doctrine has recently been published in French by Régis and Hesnard, and I am content to refer the reader to their work.[1] Psychoanalysis has often been presented as " a new point of view, a revolution in psychiatric science " ;[2] and it has been propounded as a method of study which should, in many respects, replace the old form of psychological analysis practised by psychologists and psychiatrists. Let us try, then, to understand what feature in psychoanalysis is essentially new.

Freud's earliest writings on this subject, published in 1893 and 1895, acknowledged as their starting-point the studies of which I have just been speaking anent happenings which have aroused emotion and which have left dangerous memories. He agreed with the view which I myself took as to the part these memories played in causing the actual symptoms of neurosis. I must admit that at first it did not seem to me that the studies of Breuer and Freud differed much from my own, and I was simple enough to regard them as an extremely interesting confirmation of my own researches. " I am delighted to learn," I wrote, " that Breuer and Freud have recently verified the explanation I gave some time ago of the fixed ideas of hysterics." [3] In fact, these authors showed by aptly chosen instances that certain hysterical symptoms were due to traumatic memories ; and I was very glad to find that their observations tallied so closely with mine. At most these authors changed a word here and there in their psychological descriptions. They spoke of " psychoanalysis " where I had spoken of " psychological analysis." They invented the name " complex," whereas I had used the

[1] Régis and Hesnard, La doctrine de Freud et de son école, " L'Encéphale," April 10, 1913, p. 356, May 10, 1913, p. 446 ; La psychoanalyse des névroses et des psychoses, ses applications médicales et extramédicales, Alcan, Paris, 1914.

[2] Cf. Maeder, Sur le mouvement psychoanalytique, un point de vue nouveau en psychologie, " L'Année Psychologique," 1912.

[3] L'état mental des hystériques, 1894, vol. ii, p. 68, second edition, 1911, p. 249.

term " psychological system " to denote the totality of psychological phenomena and the movements whether of the limbs or of the internal organs which were associated to constitute the traumatic memory. They spoke of " catharsis " where I had spoken of the " dissociation of fixed ideas " or of " moral disinfection." The names differed, but the essential ideas I had put forward, even those which were still subject to discussion (like that of the psychological system), were accepted without modification. Down to this very day, if we disregard hazardous speculations and confine our attention to the accounts of traumatic memories published by Freud's pupils, we shall find descriptions closely akin to those which I published long ago. When we consider these primary doctrines and these cases of traumatic memory, we find it difficult to understand how it is that psychoanalysis can be supposed to differ so much from psychological analysis, and difficult to discern the novelty of the psychoanalytical contribution to psychiatry.

Nevertheless it is certain that these initial studies concerning traumatic memories must already have contained a new trend, at least in the germ, seeing that the whole of psychoanalysis has issued from them. Various authors have endeavoured to show that the essential characteristic of psychoanalysis is its method. Jung enthusiastically declares that people have tried to refute Freud without having made use of his method, much as if a professed man of science were to ridicule astronomy while refusing to make use of a telescope. Brill,[1] Maeder,[2] and Ernest Jones [3] have described the characteristics of this method, and a great number of published works are the fruit of its application. Let us endeavour to ascertain what elements in the method are peculiar to psychoanalysis.

At first, readers of psychoanalytical books will be a trifle disappointed, for the methods advocated by psychoanalysts do not appear to be novel or unfamiliar. Psychoanalysts insist upon the need for a prolonged examination of the patient, hours being devoted to the same individual day after day for months and even for years. Alas, there is nothing very original here. Innumerable observers, myself included,

---

[1] Freud's Method of Psychoanalysis, in Parker's Psychotherapy, III, iv, 36.
[2] Op. cit.   [3] Papers on Psychoanalysis, 1913

have spent hour upon hour, by day and by night, watching their unfortunate patients, turning the object of examination over and over to study it from every possible point of view, and perhaps failing in the end to understand what they are looking at. We shall do well not to say too much about this, for the answer is an obvious one, the answer made by Molière's Misanthrope when he is listening to Oronte's sonnet :

Allez, Monsieur, le temps ne fait rien à l'affaire.

Freud lays stress upon excellent advice, which is worth reiterating, but which has no claim to originality. Like a great many clinicians before him, he shows that we cannot fully understand the illness unless we know the whole history of the patient's life. Psychoses must not be regarded as temporary and local manifestations which can be effectively studied and treated in isolation by one who disregards the patient's antecedent psychological history. The great physicians of earlier days were continually declaring that the doctor must make himself well acquainted with his patient's previous history, must collect data wherever he could, must compare the details reported by relatives and friends with those reported by the patient, and must, above all, know how to listen to the patient's own story. This last matter is of especial importance in order that the doctor may be properly informed as to the events which have made a strong impression on the patient, and may have left a dangerous memory. The doctor must not only note the tenor of the answers made to definite questions, but must also pay close attention to whatever the patient volunteers, must listen carefully to the flow of chatter which comes when the patient is speaking unguardedly. The psychoanalysts advise that when we wish to note chatter of this kind, the patient should be placed in an armchair, and that the doctor should sit behind him and should urge him to relax his mind and to give vent in speech to all the reveries which arise spontaneously in his thoughts. This is what they call the method of " free association." I do not think much of the method, and I regard those who advise it as somewhat simple-minded, for the patient still feels himself to be under observation, and will be more inclined than we are apt to suppose to arrange his words so as to produce a definite effect. I do not advise this method if a better one is available. The patient should be watched without his knowledge, when he believes he is alone, this being a method I have often employed myself. The doctor must note what the patient does, and what he says when he mutters to himself. We must take into account, not only what the patient actually says, but also what he avoids saying ; and we must note his gestures, his tics, his laughter, his blunders, his forced jokes, and so on. For instance, say the psychoanalysts, when a young woman displays a sudden desire to get married, or is extremely uneasy, we must be intelligent enough to guess that these symptoms arise " because she has had an intimacy with her cousin," and we must realise that when she talks of appendicitis, " it is because she is afraid she has become pregnant." Excellent advice in a lecture to junior students, but really I should never have ventured to say anything like that to my alienist colleagues.

A more interesting method has been advocated by Jung of Zurich.[1] This author has revived an old experiment of the psychological laboratory and has turned it to clinical account. Having drawn up a list of words, the operator pronounces these words seriatim in the subject's presence, and after hearing each word the subject must utter or write down the first word that comes into his mind. While this is being done, measurements are taken of the reaction time in each case, and any peculiarities in connexion with the associations are noted. In 1901, Mayer and Orth had observed that associations of this kind are speedy when accompanied by a pleasurable feeling, and comparatively slow when they arouse a disagreeable feeling.[2] In like manner, Jung notes that the associations are always retarded, or modified in one way or another, when the word uttered by the operator awakens in the subject's mind a painful feeling connected with traumatic memories— memories of which, in many cases, he has ceased to be aware. If, for instance, we are dealing with a person who is tormented by a fixed idea of drowning himself, the words " river," " lake," " swimming," which call up the idea of death by drowning, will evoke associations tardily, and there may be other manifestations of abnormality about these particular

[1] C. G. Jung, Ueber das Verhalten der Reaktionszeit beim Associations-experiment, Leipzig, 1905.
[2] Cf. Claparède, L'association des idées, 1903, p. 285.

associations. Such experiments may be utilised in order to reveal the memory of incidents which have had a strong influence upon the subject's emotions, and perhaps to reveal traumatic memories. Of late there has been superadded to these methods the use of the galvanometer for the study of changes in the electrical resistance of the body during the emotion aroused by the reading of a word which calls up, by association, the traumatic memory. We are indebted to Peterson of New York for an interesting summary of these studies, which he has supplemented by work of his own.[1]

Practitioners of psychological analysis, when trying to disclose traumatic memories, have had recourse to examination of the subject in various morbid or normal conditions distinct from the waking state. They have examined the subjects in delirious crises, in states of natural or induced somnambulism, during periods of distraction, in the mediumistic condition of the automatic writer, or simply during sleep and in dreams. The psychoanalysts, in especial, lay stress upon the importance of such phenomena, and incline, above all, to study their patients' dreams. We have to note, however, that their examination of dreams has been made in a very original fashion. Instead of being content to note the gestures and words of the subject while dreaming or immediately after waking, and instead of being satisfied with the direct sense of these words, the psychoanalysts have been able to turn their data to infinitely better account thanks to the fruitful method of "interpretation."

Freud has published a very remarkable book upon the psychology of dreams,[2] and his pupils have developed the master's ideas a good deal. These studies on dreams tell us nothing about special methods for recording dreams accurately at the time or very soon afterwards ; and they tell us nothing of methods for inducing dreams. Freud does not appear to concern himself, as do so many writers, about the disorders of memory whereby so many dreams are transformed, or about the way in which the subject systematises his dreams after waking. The founder of psychoanalysis is content to record and to accept the dream as related by the patient

---

[1] Peterson, The Effects of Emotions on the Body, Parker's Psychotherapy, I, iv, 5.

[2] Die Traumdeutung, 1900 ; English translation by A. A. Brill, The Interpretation of Dreams.

after the lapse of a few hours or days. He does not try to criticise these accounts, for he has a very different aim. He simply wants to explain all reports of dreams by the light of a general principle.

In 1861, Maury, and ten years earlier Charma, in his book *Le sommeil*, said that the passions and desires of human beings secured freer expression in dreams than in waking thoughts. " The soul, being in a state of profound repose and being perfectly tranquil, discerns, as if in a clear pool, its true affections and yearnings. Often enough, that which we do not dare either to do or say when we are awake, will present itself to us in a dream when we are asleep."[1] Alphonse Daudet wrote : " The dream is a safety valve." But for these authors, the principle to which they referred was merely a particular law applicable to certain dreams and not to all. It is but one among many laws of the dream. Freud has transformed this partial hypothesis into a general principle. For him, a dream is never anything else than the realisation of a wish which has been more or less masked during the waking state. In the daytime, the wish is repressed by the conscious mind, which exercises a strict censorship ; it secures expression during the night, when the censor is at rest and when his vigilance has been relaxed.

Only in exceptional cases, however, can the wish realise itself fully and simply, even in the dream. Such realisation would awaken the censor, who would be annoyed, and would stop the game—I should say, the sleep. Even during sleep, the wish must disguise itself in order to avoid awaking the censor ; it must transform itself in such a way as to become unrecognisable. These transformations occur in accordance with very simple laws. By condensation, displacement, dramatisation, and secondary elaboration, the primitive wish is so effectively masked that when we listen to the recital of a dream we can no longer recognise the repressed tendency which has secured expression in the dream.[2] If we were to leave the dream in this condition we should not understand it at all, and it would be of practically no use to us in the way of throwing light upon the hidden tendencies of the

[1] Charma, Le sommeil, 1851, p. 85.
[2] Cf. Brill, op. cit., in Parker's Psychotherapy, II, iv, 41 ; Jones, op. cit., 1913, p. 27.

subject. But let us make a little effort, let us suppress the effect of the superadded modifications. It will be quite easy to do so, since we know them well enough. We need only strip off the masks imposed by condensation, displacement, dramatisation, and secondary elaboration, and we shall lay bare the tendency which was hidden in the subject's account of his dream. This is the process of dream interpretation which is the best way of discovering old traumatic memories, of tracing the source of the tendencies which are seeking expression in dreams. A woman dreams that she looks on unmoved at the death of her sister's only son ; she cannot admit that this is a manifestation of a repressed wish, for she had absolutely no desire for her little nephew's death. How are we to interpret the dream. When we ferret into her memories we discover that once she went into a house where a child died, and that there she met a man who became her lover. Obviously, when her little nephew died in the dream, this was the expression of a wish to meet the lover once more.

Freud's disciples have perfected this method of dream interpretation in a very remarkable way. I may refer, in especial, to an article by Maeder in which we find an account of the most usual explanations of some of the common symbols occurring in dreams.[1] Thus, it is just as well to know, lest we should be misled, that in dreams a cave or a small house denotes the female sexual organ, the vulva, and that a snake or a stick represents the male organ, the penis. If a man dreams that he is walking in a forest, this signifies that he is wandering through the hair of the mons Veneris. If we dream of a railway station, we are obviously dreaming of love, for the coming and going at a railway station is extremely characteristic. In the next section I shall consider the sexual theories of the Freudians ; but for the present, I only wish to draw the reader's attention to this method of interpretation as a means for discovering the memories of happenings which have left an impression on the subject's mind.

There is already something peculiar in this persistent interpretation of dreams, but we shall make ourselves more closely acquainted with the essential characteristics of the Freudian

[1] Essai d'interprétation de quelques rêves, " Archives de Psychologie," Geneva, April 1907.

system if we study Freud's researches into the causes of the subconscious. He seems to have taken as his starting-point (without criticising them) my first researches concerning the existence and characters of subconscious phenomena in hysterical patients. I am rather sorry he did this, for the studies in question were in need of verification and criticism. His main desire was to discover the mechanism by which the subconscious came into existence, to ascertain the reason why this or that phenomenon was transferred from the domain of conscious psychological phenomena to that of subconscious phenomena. As he wrote a few years ago, commenting on a case of hysterical blindness,[1] he considers inadequate my whilom explanation that such phenomena were due to the weakness of mental synthesis. This criticism is probably sound. He believes he has discovered a more profound and more accurate explanation in his conception of " repression " (Verdrängung).

Traumatic memories, and the tendencies and ideas connected therewith, are extremely distressing to the subject's mind ; they jostle against his sensibilities or conflict with his moral ideas. The subject, displeased at entertaining such thoughts, makes manful efforts to rid himself of them, and carries on a vigorous struggle against these ideas. When the phenomena intrude into his consciousness, he will not allow them to develop, to realise themselves as actions or as definite thoughts. He checks them at the outset, and does his utmost to avoid apperceiving them, tries hard to forget them. " Repression," writes Maeder, " is part of the defensive system of the organism." A memory or an idea which has been persistently repressed, disappears from the conscious, and no longer tries to manifest itself there ; it becomes subconscious, and lives apart ; dissociation has resulted from repression. As an outcome of this process, consciousness is freed from conflict, but it is restricted and lessened. Thus, in the case of hysterical blindness to which I have just referred, Freud thinks that the patient has vigorously repressed a sexual wish. Now, sexual desire is intimately connected with the eyes, for it is obvious that the eyes can subserve the work of love. When repressing love, the subject has repressed from consciousness all that his eyes might disclose to him in the way

[1] Freud, " Aerztliche Standeszeitung," 1910, No. 9.

of temptation. He has repressed his visual sensations into the subconscious, and that is why he has become blind.

This mechanism of repression, conceived as an explanation of the subconscious character of certain traumatic memories, comes to play a very important part in the explanation of all psychopathological phenomena First of all, there is a modification ; a fear becomes attached to the repressed thought as soon as the thought begins to appear. What was at first a wish, becomes a dread. " Every morbid fear," writes Ernest Jones, " is the indirect manifestation of a checked and repressed wish." Here is an example. A man wants to marry the wife of his friend, who is seriously ill. In actual fact, he is impatiently awaiting his friend's death. He cannot acknowledge this immoral wish, and he represses it with all his strength. As a result, he suffers from exaggerated fears, morbid anxieties, whenever his friend's health is disturbed in any way.[1] The fear assumes a morbid type because it replaces a repressed desire. These authors also lay much stress upon the phenomenon they term " conversion," " transference," " displacement." To begin with, these expressions seem to denote some of the phenomena I have just been describing. The memory of a child the left side of whose face was covered with impetigo scabs, gives rise to anaesthesia of the left side of the face ; the memory of freshly shed blood upon the stairs, or of red flowers upon a coffin, gives rise to a painful horror of the colour red (erythrophobia). We call these phenomena, psychological associations, invading tendencies. Morton Prince made them the basis of his " association neuroses." Paulhan, in his admirable book *L'activité mentale et les éléments de l'esprit* (1889), gave a very good account of the struggle between psychological systems, describing how they would steal elements from one another, waxing and waning as the outcome of their rivalries. The conversion of a mental or moral phenomenon into a physical phenomenon, or rather into a phenomenon that appears to be physical, need only be regarded as a particular case of this competition among tendencies. But it is obvious that Freud sees something more in such phenomena. He is struck by their illusory, false, deceptive aspect. In reality, the subject's

---

[1] Ernest Jones, " Journal of Abnormal Psychology," April–May 1911, p. 13.

emotions have been stirred by a mental or moral phenomenon, and in place of it he manifests a paralysis or an anaesthesia which has only a remote connexion, and sometimes a purely metaphorical connexion, with the initial emotion. There has been, as it were, a dissimulation. We have just seen that neuropaths often have the aspect of persons who are lying, and that they sometimes regard themselves as liars. Freud, too, accepts this easy interpretation, for he considers that the most essential feature of nervous troubles is a transformation, a dissimulation, whereby one phenomenon is substituted for another. Repression gives rise to this metamorphosis. Our wish, which does not dare to disclose itself to us in its true form, undergoes exaggeration, assumes a physical aspect instead of a mental one, and becomes to all appearance a bodily disorder. This is what takes place in the dream, where the manifest images are only the masquerade of the "latent content." The same thing happens in the neuroses, which are phenomena of the same kind as dreams.

This conception of repression is undoubtedly one of the most interesting in the Freudian psychology. My own opinion is that the phenomenon must be explained in a different way, but it is none the less of great importance. The part which it plays in the Freudian system enables us, I think, to understand what is the core of psychoanalysis. Morbid symptoms, like dreams, are regarded as psychological phenomena which have been transformed and masked by the process of repression. They are appearances, and behind them we must discover, by subtle methods of interpretation, hidden realities. I have myself drawn attention to the subconscious character of some of the fixed ideas of hysterical patients. This characteristic of subconsciousness is ascribed by psychoanalysts to all the morbid manifestations of the neuroses.

Why is it that the Freudians have extended the conception in this way, which is, to say the least of it, strange ? The reason is that they want at all costs to discover a traumatic memory underlying every neuropathic symptom, to disinter a more or less modified memory of an event which has stirred the subject's emotions. Psychoanalysis is not an ordinary psychological analysis which is trying to discover any kind of phenomena and the laws which regulate the occurrence of these phenomena ; it is a criminal investigation which aims at the discovery of a culprit, at the unearthing of a past happening which is responsible for the extant troubles, an event which must be recognised and tracked through all its disguises. Indeed, in Freudian writings we shall often come aross this comparison of psychological study to a criminal investigation, and of the psychiatrist to a detective. The enthusiasts for psychoanalysis are, then, right when they claim that their system contains something entirely new, and implies a revolution in psychiatry. The systematic generalisation of the subconscious traumatic memory gives this doctrine an indisputable originality.

3. THE SEXUAL THEORY OF THE NEUROSES.

Another line of research has supplemented the investigations concerning traumatic memories. This has been the most widely trumpeted part of psychoanalysis, and the noise made about it has often distracted attention from the other elements of the doctrine. I refer to the investigations concerning the part played by sexual disturbances in the pathogenesis of the neuroses.

From early days, this problem has attracted the attention of physicians. Hippocrates declared that hysteria occurs in women who suffer from an insufficiency of sexual relationships. Many doctors who came after him were ready to echo his teaching : " Get the young woman married, and her troubles will vanish." For a long time, the neuroses were associated with disorders of the sexual functions, so much so that the very name of hysteria came to have a degrading connotation. Louyer-Villermay, writing in 1816,[1] pushed this theory to an extreme. It is true that Briquet in 1859, and Charcot subsequently, protested against the absurd exaggeration of the sexual theory of the neuroses ; but these authors, none the less, were fully aware of the importance of the sexual life in relation to nervous disorders. They were continually referring to the neuroses of puberty or the neuroses of the menopause, to the influence which diseases of the genital organs could exert upon the nervous and mental functions, to the pathogenic effects of excessive masturbation and sexual perversions ; and, among the causes of neuropathic symptoms, they gave an

[1] See Bibliography, Louyer-Villermay.

important place to the emotions induced by happenings in the sexual domain, such as rape, concealed pregnancy, jilting, and other disappointments in love.

Axenfeld and Huchard likewise referred to the effects of a lascivious temperament, to those of continence, to those of undue sexual excitation, and to those of thwarted love. In my own experience I have again and again had occasion to study neuroses that were a sequel of sexual assaults, the breaking off of engagements to marry, and similar causes. One of my first cases, the one to which I referred a few pages back, was that of a young woman of twenty-three who suffered from paraplegia for years as a consequence of prolonged incestuous relationships with her father, and fear of pregnancy. The remarkable delusion of possession which I described as an instance of subconscious fixed ideas, developed in a man who was a prey to remorse because he had been unfaithful to his wife. I do not think there is any warrant for saying that psychological analysts have ignored this problem, or that they have failed to study the relationships between sexual disorders and the neuroses.

It is, however, true that, in this respect likewise, psychoanalysts have adopted an original attitude. If we are to understand this outlook, we must not forget that when they speak of sexual disorders they attach to the term a meaning peculiar to themselves. They are not thinking of physical modifications, whether within or without the limits of normality, affecting the genital organs or the functions of these. Puberty regarded as a simple physiological modification, the menopause, the checking of menstruation, blenorrhoea, metritis, and the like, do not play a notable part in the theories of Freud. He knows perfectly well that these disorders are frequent in persons who remain free from neuropathic symptoms, and he does not regard them as important etiological factors of neurosis. The sexual disorders with which he is concerned are those which have moral repercussions, those which can give rise to the neuroses through the intermediation of psychological phenomena. Here, once more, precise definition is requisite. Freud has no special interest in the general modifications which may arise in the mental functions in consequence of sexual phenomena whose sexual character is not obvious to the subject. Authors who write of mental depressions at the age of puberty or during the menopause, and consider these depressions dependent upon some form of intoxication, cannot, for this reason, be regarded as psychoanalysts. Psychoanalysis takes cognisance of sexual happenings which the subject recognises as sexual, which he regards as important, and of which he retains a distressing and disturbing memory. In a word, the attention of psychoanalysts is concentrated upon traumatic memories that are the outcome of sexual experiences. A girl has given herself to her lover, and the latter has then refused to fulfil his promise to marry. This is a grave trouble, and, by one of the mechanisms we have already considered, it gives rise to a traumatic memory and to a neurosis. Here we have a typical instance of the sexual disorders studied by the psychoanalysts. Masturbation, incomplete coitus, and sexual abstinence, are only of interest to the psychoanalyst because of the emotions by which they are attended and because of the traumatic memories to which they give rise. We are concerned, then, with traumatic memories determined by sexual mishaps, or (if the phrasing be preferred) with traumatic memories that have a sexual content. These are the phenomena which psychoanalysts, following in the footsteps of psychological analysts of earlier schools, study in order to ascertain their frequency and to elucidate their importance as etiological factors of the neuroses.

As regards the first point, the frequency of memories of the kind, the Freudians hold definite views. Whereas previous observers have held that traumatic memories relating to sexual mishaps are to be found in *some* neuropaths, the psychoanalysts declare, and this is their innovation, that such memories are to be found in *all* neuropaths. The psychoanalyst contention is that in the absence of such a mishap metamorphosed into a traumatic memory, there is no neurosis. If it is not easy to detect the existence of such a traumatic memory of a sexual mishap in every neurotic patient, this is because the doctor has not succeeded in making the patient admit what has happened, has not been able to break down the patient's reticence.

In certain cases, indeed, no notable skill is requisite to discover that there has been a sexual mishap. The patient volunteers the information of rape, abandonment, adultery, etc. Or, if this frankness is lacking, still, our study of the patient's delirious utterances, or of what he says in the somnambulist state, leaves no possible doubt that his mind is troubled by the memory of a sexual mishap. In other cases, however, difficulties arise. The patient has a clear memory of the happenings of recent years, and cannot recall any sexual mishap bearing on the trouble. We must assist the patient to go further back, and to recall the impressions of early childhood. Then, often with considerable pains, we shall be able to revive memories of serious import which have been masked. When the patient was only five or six years old, he or she saw a woman advanced in pregnancy, or caught sight of a dog and a bitch in the act of intercourse, or listened to the rattling of the bed when the parents were engaged in coitus. This incident caused intense emotion, and could never be thought of without trembling. But sometimes the difficulty is still greater. With the best will in the world, the patient cannot recall anything of the kind. Then we must study and interpret his dreams. A young man dreams of three stars. This, Maeder assures us, is obviously an erotic dream. " We say of a noted actress that she is a star ; a lover calls his mistress his star ; Ruy Blas is ' a worm in love with a star ' ; in Switzerland, girls talking among themselves speak of their sexual organ as their star." Or a young woman has dreamed of a sailing boat on Lake Geneva. The sails of these boats have a very characteristic shape, recalling that of a dagger or some other pointed object directed skyward. The interpretation is obvious. Even easier is it to interpret a dream of a snake and especially of a snake-dog, or a dream of a garden : " I am in a large and shady garden where the gardener is watering the plants." No less easy is it to interpret a dream of a cave, a dream of a bird, and so on.[1] We are well on the track of the traumatic memories that have a sexual content.

If this does not suffice, we must know how to interpret the feelings which the patient has experienced in various circumstances. For instance, he tells us that he has sometimes wanted to be a person of great importance, to be a

[1] Cf. Maeder, Essai d'interprétation de quelques rêves, " Archives de Psychologie " Geneva, April 1917.

prince, perhaps, or the son of a noted financier, instead of being the son of a nobody. This is extremely characteristic. It proves that at the time of which he is speaking he wanted to thrust his father aside, to extrude his father from his own life. Why should he have entertained this wish ? Manifestly because he felt that his father was a rival, because he had a sexual love for his mother, and because his mind had formulated the famous " Oedipus concept " which plays so important a part in the peculiar psychology of the Freudians.[1] A young man is aware that when the tender passion began to dawn in him he fell in love with a woman much older than himself. The interpretation is simple. He was in love with his mother, and transferred this sentiment upon elderly women, who to him were supplementary mothers. Does another young man recall that on several occasions he was in love with women of easy virtue ? Here, again, there is no difficulty about the interpretation. Indubitably he must have had a passion for his mother, and must have been in despair when he learned the nature of the relationships between his mother and his father. The " Oedipus complex " became active, and he longed that his mother should be unfaithful to his father, presumably for his own benefit. It is owing to this romance of childhood that so many men have a weakness for women of easy virtue.[2]

Furthermore, we can, in case of need, interpret the simplest phenomena in the same way. Do we find that in childhood the subject used to make mud-pies, or that in infancy it was his habit to suck his thumb ? These practices were indications of precocious sexual perturbations. Somewhat later in youthful life, a taste for playing the piano is to be regarded as having a close connexion with masturbation.[3] We are told that, where little children are concerned, we must be very much on our guard in the matter of sensations and sentiments relating to the anus. " The anus is a partial erotic zone " and may undergo a development independent of that

---

[1] Max Graf, Richard Wagner im " Fliegenden Holländer," ein Beitrag zur Psychologie des künstlerischen Schaffens, Leipzig, 1911 ; Rudolph Acher, Recent Freudian Literature, " American Journal of Pyschology," vol. xxii (1911), p. 420.

[2] Freud, Beiträge zur Psychologie des Liebeslebens, " Jahrbuch für psychoanalytische Forschungen," 1910.

[3] Ernest Jones, The Pathology of Morbid Anxiety, " Journal of Abnormal Psychology," July 1911, p. 103.

of the other zones. " The attacks of enteritis which are so common in infancy lead to an excessive stimulation of this zone, and thus pave the way for the onset of the specialised neuroses." Kurt Mendel no doubt gives way to irony a little when he is explaining the fondness of psychoanalysts for interpreting this alleged interest of infants in anal sensations as being due to a search for sexual pleasure ; but there is ample justification for the way in which he phrases the matter. " Perhaps," says the Freudian to his little child, " when you are unwilling to go to stool before being put to bed, you were refusing to empty the bowel because you hoped that the retention of the faeces for a time would increase the voluptuous delight of defaecation." [1] Unfortunately, considerations of space make it impossible for me to dwell upon such interpretations, which are very ingenious, and which abound in Freudian literature. I must content myself with having given a few indications of the way in which, notwithstanding the subject's dissimulations, and despite his forgetfulness, it is possible to show that underlying every case of neuropathic disorder there is a traumatic memory with a sexual content.

Coming now to the second point, to the question of what part these sexual disorders and these memories can play as pathogenic factors, the Freudians have likewise developed a doctrine peculiar to themselves. Their contention is that in all cases of neurosis these sexual troubles and these memories are not merely one of the causes of the illness, but are the essential and, indeed, the only cause. Just as to-day syphilis is regarded as the specific cause of locomotor ataxia and of general paralysis of the insane, so these sexual disorders and these memories are to be regarded as the specific cause of the neuroses.

The thesis is seductive in its simplicity. There are several ways of demonstrating it. Sometimes the proof takes the form of a comparison of the symptoms of the disease with certain phenomena of the sexual life. Consider, for instance, anxiety, which is so common in neuropathic disorders, and is especially frequent in psychasthenics. In 1895, Freud began to describe anxiety as an independent disease, characterised by multiform symptoms, such as respiratory disorder,

---

[1] Cf. Ladame, Névroses et sexualité, " L'Encéphale," 1913, p. 163.

palpitation, changes in the colour of the face, sweating, dryness of the mouth, peristaltic contraction of certain muscles ; and he showed that these phenomena are characteristic of the sexual act. His explanation, therefore, is a simple one. Anxiety is an incomplete sexual enjoyment, a frustrate enjoyment, occurring in persons who have formed the bad habit of cutting the sexual act short before it attains its climax. When, for one reason or another, sexual desire cannot run its natural course, when the impulse is prevented from achieving its end, whether by moral restraint, by celibacy, by incomplete forms of coitus, or the like, it is repressed. It then continues to act subconsciously, and manifests itself in the form of the disturbances which comprise what is known as anxiety.

As a rule, the proof of the pathogenic importance of sexual disorders and of the memory of these is supplied by what I may call a symbolical construction, based upon the principles already considered in connexion with repression and transference. When we are confronted with a morbid symptom, we are to ask ourselves how it may have arisen if we suppose its starting-point to have been a sexual disturbance which has subsequently been modified by transference and repression. If our theory enables us to build up something which seems akin to the symptom we are considering, we shall decide that the symptom does really represent a transformation of the primary sexual disturbance.

This ingenious method cannot be properly understood without the study of specific examples. Do we find that a patient has disorders of sensation, anaesthesia, or disturbance of vision ? All we need do is, ascertain in what way a sexual disturbance, such as a sense of shame on account of a manifestation of sexual debility, *might* produce the disorder of vision. We know quite well that various sensations which are ostensibly distinct from the sexual functions can nevertheless be associated with these functions. Just as the mouth does not serve only for the intake of food, but is also the instrument with which we kiss, so likewise the eyes do not serve only to guide our steps, but can be used for the examination of the lineaments of one whom we love. When we are ashamed on account of some sexual happening, a repression of the sexual impulse occurs, and the sexual curiosity of the eyes is also and simultaneously repressed. This leads to a serious disturbance of the relationship between vision and consciousness. The repression is excessive, so that the ego loses its dominion over the eyes, with the result that the whole function of vision, which remains at the service of repressed sexuality, passes into the domain of the self-conscious. The legend of Lady Godiva explains, in a parable, the onset of hysterical amaurosis. The lady had to ride naked through the streets of Coventry. The inhabitants of the city made it a point of honour to close the shutters of their houses. They lowered their eyelids that they might not see ; they blinded themselves out of courtesy. Who can resist the charm of so poetical an explanation ? [1]

Here are a few more examples of the same method of proof. We find that a woman has little inclination for the sexual act, that she suffers from frigidity. The explanation is simple. When she was quite young she had a guilty passion for her father (see above, Oedipus concept), and she forcibly repressed these incestuous 'longings. The repression was excessive, with the result that she remains frigid throughout life.[2]—A man exhibits homosexual tendencies. The explanation is not far to seek. Very early in life, he was passionately in love with his mother. At first we may be a little puzzled by the theory that this childish passion for his mother should, now that he has grown up, be transformed into a love for boys. Little boys, we learn, always imagine that the mother has a male organ just like their own. The hermaphrodite deities of ancient days were feminine figures to which male organs had been superadded, and a little boy who, in imagination, endows his mother with a penis, is merely recapitulating the ancient creed of the race. If the explanation seems unsatisfactory, another is forthcoming. Many of the persons who had an undue fondness for their mothers, repressed this feeling. The undue repression has made them thenceforward incapable of loving a woman. By excess of virtue, they become perverts, become homosexuals. Are you not satisfied even yet ? Well, there is another explanation ready. (One of the great advantages of such symbolical proofs is that

---

[1] Freud, Die psychogene Sehstörung in psychoanalytischer Auffassung, 1910 ; Acher, op. cit., p. 426.

[2] Sadger, Aus dem Liebesleben Nicolaus Lenau, " Schriften zur angewandten Seelenkunde," 1909 ; Acher, op. cit., p. 432.

they are infinitely variable.) The little boy's sexual passion for his mother was so intense that he came to identify himself with his mother, to confound himself with her, to make her sentiments his own. Now, this mother loved her little boy. He was a boy, and therefore, when he adopts his mother's feelings, he, too, loves a boy. The boy for whom he has a passion now that he is grown up is simply a memory of his own infantile personality, and he loves this as his mother used to love him in his infancy. In loving the boy, he loves himself, by a sort of Narcissism. In this way, he remains faithful to his mother when he loves a boy, whereas he would be unfaithful were he to love a woman.[1] We may study all neuropathic symptoms in the same way, and may demonstrate by this method of symbolical construction that every one of them is, directly or indirectly, the outcome of a bygone sexual memory which has been unskilfully repressed.

Such studies may be rendered extremely precise. They can show us that particular incidents in the sexual life can induce particular morbid symptoms. The psychoanalysts tell us that the mishap usually occurred in very early childhood. Hysteria, they declare, will never result from a sexual trauma unless the mishap occurred before the subject reached the age of eight. For a time, this initial trauma has no obvious ill effects. Subsequently, at puberty, a conflict arises between the sexual instinct and conventional morality. This conflict leads to a repression into the subconscious, to the repression of the memory of various sexual scenes in which the lad or the lass has played a part. Thereupon, neurosis appears. This neurosis varies in form according to variations in the nature of the primary trauma. If, of course before the age of eight, the child was subjected to a sexual aggression, if, in the sexual mishap, the child's role was passive, the subsequent neurosis will take the form of hysteria. If, on the other hand, in these early sexual adventures, the child assumed an active and aggressive role, the subsequent neurosis will take the form of obsessions and phobias, will be psychasthenia rather than hysteria. Because of this difference in the respective results of the passive and the active roles, hysteria is comparatively common in women, and psychasthenia is

---

[1] Freud, Eine Kindheitserinnerung des Lionardo da Vinci, 1910 ; Acher, op. cit., p. 414.

comparatively common in men.[1] Writing in 1896 (*Zur Aetiologie der Hysterie*) Freud declared that these discoveries in pathogenesis were for the science of neuropathology what the discovery of the sources of the Nile had been for the science of geography, namely the most important discovery of the nineteenth century.—In like manner, the other neuroses have specific causes. The sole cause of neurasthenia is masturbation ; the anxiety neurosis is due to incomplete coitus or to excessive sexual abstinence ; and so on. Thus, the interpretations enable us to be extremely precise in our diagnosis.

It is proper to add that at a later date (1905) Freud admitted that he had been led astray in certain respects by the fallacious reminiscences of some of his patients. He was, therefore, no longer inclined to be quite so definite in his views as to the etiology of the various neuroses. As Ladame phrases it, it would seem that he no longer claims to have discovered the sources of the Nile.[2] But he still maintains as a fundamental principle that " in a normal sexual life a neurosis is impossible." He continues to believe that the neuroses, and even some of the psychoses, such as dementia praecox, have unique and specific causes. He still believes them to be due to a sexual disturbance consequent upon a mishap whose influence persists in the form of a traumatic memory.

Among the critics who have done their best to understand the evolution of the ideas which comprise the system known as psychoanalysis, a good many have been astonished by the sexual theory ; they have asked why Freud saw sex wherever he looked ; and some of them tried to explain this remarkable illusion. Aschaffenburg's idea is that Freud must question his patients regarding their sexual life in a peculiarly impressive manner ; that he must influence them by suggestion in one way or another, so that he gets from them the answers he wants ; that he must take very seriously the patient's most trivial words concerning sex, catch them on the wing, pin them down, put them into their places in the mental constellation he is manufacturing.[3] Friedländer and Ladame offer an

---

[1] Though at present I am expounding the Freudian theory, rather than commenting upon it, I cannot refrain from an interrogative challenge here !

[2] Ladame, op. cit., p. 71.

[3] Aschaffenburg, Die Beziehungen des Sexuellenlebens zur Entstehung von Nerven- und Geisteskrankheiten, " Münchener medizinische Wochenschrift," September 2, 1906.

even more remarkable explanation. Their theory is that there must be a peculiar kind of sexual atmosphere in Vienna. They suppose that there is a sort of local demon which, by epidemic as it were, takes possession of the population, so that in this environment the observer is foredoomed to overestimate the importance of sexual influences.[1]

I think that both these explanations contain elements of truth, but another reflection must be superadded if we wish to understand the evolution of Freudian doctrine. The importance ascribed to sexual happenings is, if I mistake not, a logical outcome of the nature of Freud's early studies. As we have seen, his aim was to modify in an original way, by an unlimited process of generalisation, the prevailing conceptions of psychological analysis in the matter of traumatic memories. If an investigator has made up his mind to discover in every neuropathic patient the memory of some incident which left a powerful impress on the emotions and was able to stagger consciousness ; if he holds a priori that this memory may be partially or wholly repressed and may be masked by symbols or metaphors, and if he believes that the patient will be so reticient about the matter that only through effort can it be brought back into the light of day, this investigator will almost inevitably be led to probe the mind for the discovery of sexual secrets. In contemporary civilisation, the events which are most apt to induce emotion, and the facts about which men and women are usually inclined to be reticient, and to veil their references in Latin words, are almost always happenings in the domain of the sexual life. Freud's way of regarding traumatic memories and subconscious fixed ideas led him to exaggerate the importance of the sexual experiences which people are inclined to refer to thus allusively. We must not be surprised to find that he has applied to this particular study his method of ingenious interpretation and bold generalisation. I think, therefore, that we must summarise this new department of our studies in the same way as those which have preceded it. Psychological analysis had, by way of observation and theory, recognised that sexuality must play an important part in the pathogenesis of the neuroses. Psychoanalysis adopted this notion, but trans-

[1] Ladame, op. cit., p. 160.

formed it, if I may borrow Ladame's quip, into the dogma of pansexualism.[1]

4. The Problem of sexual Disorders in the Neuroses.

Let us first devote our attention to the last-mentioned manifestation of Freudian theory, the sexual theory of the neuroses. The matter is one of considerable importance, for if this view should secure general acceptance the treatment of neuropaths would take an entirely new trend.

I need not dwell upon the first factor of the theory, upon the contention that traumatic memories having a sexual content are frequent. Psychological analysts always recognised that in neuropaths sexual disturbances were common, that these patients had in many instances had sexual adventures and mishaps concerning which they had retained distressing and dangerous memories. Every doctor must have heard neuropaths of both sexes complain of having been overwhelmed by a disappointment in love, of having suffered greatly from the memory of a sexual reverse or failure, of being impotent, and the like. In the writings of the analysts of the old school we find accounts of such phenomena, and Freud is only in their line of succession when he describes sexual perturbations.

The difference between Freud and the earlier analysts is merely one of degree, but this is one of the cases in which a difference of degree is fundamental. Whenever Freud says " all patients," ordinary psychological analysts says " some patients " or " a great many patients." The difference is that which exists between unrestricted generalisation and a precise statement of particulars. To grasp the nature of the restriction, we must come to an understanding as to the meaning of the term " sexual adventure or mishap." In a sense it is perfectly true that every one has had sexual adventures, especially if we accept symbolical interpretations. The birth of a younger brother or sister, the beginning of menstruation in a girl and the first ejaculation in a boy, a disappointment in love, the hearing of spiteful gossip concerning the infidelity of a husband or a wife, and so on, and so on—all these may be termed sexual adventures. Since every one has such sexual adventures, obviously neuropaths must have had their share of them. But this teaches the doctor nothing about the etiology of the neuroses, for no factor can have pathogenic importance which operates in equal measure among the sick and the well. We must, then, be concerned with a sexual adventure or mishap serious enough to have disturbed the subject to such a degree that it has left a distressing memory, one still able, at the time when the patient comes to consult us, to arouse emotion, fatigue, and psychological disturbances. If the term be understood in this sense, then psychological analysts, as contrasted with psychoanalysts, declare that in their experience such sexual adventures have not happened to every neuropath. They declare that only in a restricted number of their neuropathic patients can they find evidence of the existence of traumatic memories of this kind.

The proportion of neuropaths in whom sexual disorders can be detected is far from easy to ascertain, first of all because observers have not always given their attention to this particular point, and secondly because the proportion would seem to vary considerably as between one environment and another. Oppenheim, writing in 1910, declared that only a small proportion of his patients had suffered from a definite sexual disturbance. It is true that this author was mainly concerned with the problem we are going to consider next, the problem of the etiological importance of sexual disorders ; and that he recognised the existence of sexual disturbances only in those patients in whom, as he thought, the disturbances had actually caused the disease. Löwenfeld and Ladame take a more liberal view, recognising the existence of sexual disturbances in three-fourth of their cases. Dejerine and Gauckler found that sexual disquietudes were present in 22 per cent. of the cases of psychoneurosis.[1] I have no precise statistics on the point, but I incline rather to accept the figures of Löwenfeld and Ladame, for I believe that the existence of distressing memories with a sexual content, and of sexual disturbances, can be detected in three neuropaths out of four ; but for the moment I reserve my opinion as to the etiological importance of these phenomena. Besides, I think we waste our time in trying to establish a precise percentage, for, in my view, the percentage is extremely variable.

[1] Op. cit., 1911, p. 344.

If Freud had been content to say that his statistics show a specially high percentage; that, in the region where he practices, genital disquietudes and sexual disturbances are commoner than elsewhere, I should not feel moved to contradict him. I have always thought that in this matter the reputation of Paris was undeserved.

The essential point of the criticism is that such disturbances are not present in all neuropaths without exception, that in these patients a traumatic memory with a sexual content is not a constant and necessary pathogenic factor, as syphilis is a constant and necessary factor of locomotor ataxia. The simplest observation furnishes proof of this assertion. Psychological analysts insist that they frequently have occasion to observe sufferers from grave neuropathic disorder who make no complaint whatever of their sexual functions, and who, however carefully we examine them, give no sign of having a distressing memory relating to some definite sexual adventure or mishap. As a specific instance I shall refer to the case of the young woman whom I have described under the name of Irène.[1] She has been under my observation for more than ten years, exhibiting the symptoms of grave and persistent hysteria. Her father was an alcoholic, and died of delirium tremens; her mother, psychasthenic to a high degree, died of pulmonary tuberculosis. Irène herself, exhausted by poverty, overwork, and sleepless nights, disturbed by the terrible emotions occasioned by the dramatic circumstances of her mother's death, has suffered during these ten years from a succession of major neuropathic disorders. Throughout that period I have watched her closely; I am familiar with all her thoughts and all her mental states; and I can asseverate that she has never had any sexual disturbances in the strict sense of the term, or any sexual adventures or mishaps which have produced a strong impression on her mind. Brought up in an easy-going proletarian environment, she made an early acquaintance with all kinds of sexual phenomena without attaching much importance to them; she is capable of experiencing normal sexual sensations, without going out of her way in search of them, and without

---

[1] L'amnésie et la dissociation des souvenirs par l'émotion, " Journal de Psychologie Normale et Pathologique," September 1904 ; L'état mental des hystériques, second edition, 1911, p. 506.

trying to avoid them ; it is difficult to conceive of a more normal sexual life than hers—and yet I do not know a more typical case of major hysteria. The same remark applies to a great many hysterical patients, and also to psychasthenics, who may be obsessed or phobic as regards other phenomena while they are perfectly sane as regards their sexual life. Even if such patients are rare, I consider it indubitable that they exist. But their existence is flatly denied by the psychoanalysts, who hold that there can be no neurosis when the sexual life is normal. Here is a very sharp distinction between psychological analysis and psychoanalysis.

Another important point may serve to emphasise the contrast. Impartial psychological analysis discloses in neuropaths disturbances and traumatic memories which we have no right to confound with memories of sexual adventures and mishaps. Let me quote from my own earlier studies concerning the psychological treatment of hysteria : " Emotions of a sexual order obviously exist ; they must naturally exist, seeing that sexual feelings are so frequent, so powerful, so prone to induce all kinds of emotion. But, first of all, we have to point out that we are not always concerned with true genital excitations, for love is an extremely complex sentiment and it may assume manifold forms. Further, we have to recognise that hysterical symptoms are often the outcome of fixed ideas of a very different kind. This woman is inconsolable because she has lost her mother or her child ; that woman has been greatly distressed by an accusation of theft. Need we recall the innumerable cases of traumatic hysteria induced by the obsessive memory of a shock or accident of some kind ? In a word, every memory, every thought, competent to arouse strong and lasting emotions can play the part of a fixed idea, and may originate hysterical symptoms. It is merely necessary to point out that some fixed ideas are specially frequent in certain patients, the nature of these fixed ideas varying in accordance with the age, the education, and the social position of the patient." [1] We should have to begin by eliminating all these other emotions, we should have to show by rigorous proof and not by symbolical constructions that they are really

[1] Traitement psychologique de l'hystérie, in Albert Robin's Traité de thérapeutique appliqué, 1898, vol. xv, p. 149 ; L'état mental des hystériques, second edition, 1911, p. 629.

identical with sexual emotions, before we could accept the theory that sexual emotions are the only ones that count. Now, psychological analysts consider that no such proof can be given.

On the contrary, they think that certain non-sexual adventures and mishaps, certain non-sexual memories, may be of very great etiological importance, and must be taken into account quite as much as sexual emotions. I. H. Coriat of Boston, Mass., has shown that, in certain cases, psychological systems connected with the emotion of disgust may play an etiological role.[1] Boris Sidis attaches more importance to the tendencies connected with fear.[2] He begins his article with a fine quotation from Rudyard Kipling : " Fear walks up and down the jungle by day and by night." He recalls that in earlier days fear must have played a great part in the world, and tells us how William James drew attention to the fact that the transition from brute to man was characterised by the disappearance of a great many causes of fear. In Sidis' view, exaggerations of the instinct of fear are common determinants of psychopathic disorders. There is a good deal of truth in this suggestion, and it would not be difficult to build upon such a foundation a system akin to that which Freud has founded upon the sexual instincts. I should myself be inclined, to-day, to add phenomena connected with other tendencies which are less familiar, but which, in my opinion, play a notable part as determinants of human behaviour. I refer to the tendencies to flee from depression and to seek excitation. Disturbances of these tendencies are competent, as I have frequently shown, to induce many obsessive and impulsive ideas. One of the differentiae between psychological analysis and psychoanalysis is that, whereas the latter is solely interested in the study of sexual tendencies, the former is also interested in the study of these other tendencies which may give rise to adventures, mishaps, emotions and memories.

The writers who reason in this way, and who display these wider interests, have been sharply criticised by the

---

[1] Discussion of the Symposium, " Journal of Abnormal Psychology, " July 1911, p. 167.
[2] Fear, Anxiety, and psychopathic Maladies, " Journal of Abnormal Psychology," July 1911, p. 120.

convinced psychoanalysts. J. E. Donley [1] and I. H. Coriat had the audacity to note that their patients had other disquietudes than those of a sexual order. Coriat had a patient under observation for a year and a half analysing his behaviour throughout, and studying his dreams. To the doctor's astonishment, there were no signs of fixed ideas having a sexual content. This subversive observation was strongly censured, and Coriat was told that his studies were worthless. " You did not use the method, the true, the only one ; you did not look through Galileo's telescope ; if you had psychoanalysed the subject you would have found a multiplicity of sexual disturbances, genital mishaps, and traumatic memories." Let us understand what we are talking about. If the psychoanalytical method means, at any cost, and with the aid of the most improbable and most ridiculous interpretations, the discovery of sexual fixed ideas, it is clear that the authors I have quoted, and I myself, have not practised psychoanalysis. Are we to be blamed for that ? The very thing we are discussing is the justification for pushing this method of sexual interpretation to an extreme. Before insisting upon its application to all and sundry in season and out of season, it would be well to begin by proving that it is legitimate, by showing, without " interpretation," that traumatism of a sexual kind is a general factor of the neuroses. Unless we are to fall into a vicious circle, we must search for these sexual disturbances without psychoanalysis, by the ordinary means of psychological analysis, and in accordance with the ordinary rules of this method, for we have no right to invent new rules. Who is entitled to insist upon our using a method which seems to us to be discredited by our own observations ? In 1910, Oppenheim said that psychoanalysis is a modern method of torture. He goes too far, for the psychoanalysts only torture their own imagination. " We must not," says Coriat, " push analysis to the extreme at which reason and logic are replaced by the imagination of the analyst." [2] To me it seems that the psychoanalytic method is, before all, a method of symbolical and arbitrary construction ; it shows how the facts " might be " explained if the sexual causation of the neuroses

[1] Freud's Anxiety Neurosis, " Journal of Abnormal Psychology," 1911, p. 130.
[2] A Contribution to the Psychopathology of Hysteria, " Journal of Abnormal Psychology," 1911, p. 60.

had been definitively accepted ; but its application cannot be insisted upon so long as that theory is still unproved. The foregoing observations remain valid, and they illustrate the difference between the two doctrines as regards the frequency with which traumatic memories of a sexual character are met with in the neuroses.

This first discussion is not enough, for we have recognised that in three-fourths of the cases there really have been sexual disturbances, and the patients have suffered or do suffer from disquietudes connected with these disturbances. We now have to enquire what share psychological analysis ascribes to such disturbances and disquietudes as pathogenic factors.

In some cases the decision is easy. We learn that the disease began shortly after the sexual mishap, and that there had been no trace of this particular morbid disturbance before the patient's emotions had been thus troubled. We see that the cure of the illness begins with the cure of the sexual function, that the other disorders do not subside until the disorders of the sexual function have been relieved. The only way in which we can modify the morbid symptoms is by influencing the patient's sexual ideas and actions. In a word, the strictest application of the accepted rules of induction shows us that the sexual phenomena have been necessary antecedents of the neuropathic disorders. In these cases, therefore, we shall be satisfied that the sexual mishap gave rise, not merely to a memory, but also to intense emotion and to exhaustion with lowering of the psychological tension, and that beyond question it was the starting-point of the illness. We may feel it incumbent on us to add that the noxious influence of the happening was dependent rather upon the emotion and the exhaustion it induced than upon its sexual characteristics in the strict sense of the term. But this is a minor criticism, since we agree with Freud that the sexual happening initiated the illness. What we have to point out is that facts of the same kind have been noted long since by all who have written on the subject.

Have we to interpret in the same way the far more numerous cases in which sexual disturbances make their appearance during a particular phase of the disease, to disappear sooner or later while the disease persists, so that the determinism of the phenomena is by no means obvious ? Freud tells us that in all such cases we must regard the sexual disturbances as primordial and essential, his reason being that we can detect a certain analogy between the symptoms of the disease and various sexual phenomena. For instance, anxiety, in some of its outward manifestations, resembles the voluptuous ecstasy of coitus ; therefore anxiety must be a sexual disorder. Vague analogies of this kind have never been accepted as proofs of a causal relationship, and they can be interpreted in a very different way. Anxiety also resembles fear or surprise, or the disturbances attending diseases of the heart. If our only guide is to be analogy, to which of these are we to link up anxiety ? The important matter is that we should ascertain under what conditions anxiety occurs. I have tried to show that it occurs in depressed persons, who are incapable of accurately performing certain actions demanding a high psychological tension. That is why I have been led to suppose that anxiety is a discharge, a derivation which affects the mechanism of the organic functions, and that it ensues when the higher-grade activities cannot be properly performed. Numerous observations and experiments concerning the production and suppression of anxiety seem to confirm this simple hypothesis.[1] However this may be, of one thing I am confident, that anxiety arises in connexion with inadequacy of actions of any kind, and not solely as an outcome of sexual inadequacies. The vague analogy between the symptoms of anxiety and sexual phenomena is not a sufficient reason for giving a preponderance to sexual phenomena in the explanation of the illness.

I need hardly say that I cannot accept as proofs the apparent analogies secured by means of symbolical constructions. The recognition that a phenomenon might possibly be explained by one of these constructions, is a very different thing from the proof that the construction must be regarded as an exclusive explanation. In actual fact, there is no proof which justifies any such generalisation of the causative significance of sexual phenomena. We are simply concerned with imaginary constructions which we can regard with favour or disfavour according to our own predilections.

[1] Les obsessions et la psychasthénie, 1903, vol. i, pp. 224–233, 561–566, and 736.

Unfortunately, moreover, we are faced with a difficulty which was pointed out long ago by psychological analysts. We are not really free to be guided by our preferences in this matter. Taking up an idea which had been frequently put forward by the alienists of earlier generations, I tried to show in 1903, in my book on obsessions, that we have at least a partial acquaintance with the determinism of sexual disorders in certain neuropaths. In many cases we can prove that sexual disturbances are not the cause of the nervous disorder, but are its consequence and its expression.[1] I see that F. Lyman Wells has now adopted the same standpoint. He shows that in our civilisation the sexual life has become a difficult matter, so that it is a touchstone of our powers of mental adaptation. Thus disorders of sexual behaviour are among the commonest and most inevitable manifestations of nervous disease.[2] Ladame refers to various authors who take a similar view of this causal sequence.[3]

The point is of so much importance in this connexion that I shall not hesitate to reproduce here some of my earlier studies on the subject. Having shown that the sexual life of the psychasthenic is frequently disturbed, I added that, whereas some of these patients accept the fact with resignation, others are annoyed, and make desperate and ridiculous efforts to reenter the lost paradise, thus becoming subject to all kinds of obsessions taking a sexual form. " I therefore admit," I wrote, " the existence of the facts referred to by Freud, I admit that sexual disquietudes exist in patients suffering from obsessions, but I do not accept Freud's interpretation. Freud considers that a sexual disturbance, such as an inadequate sexual gratification, is a primary disorder, the outcome of external circumstances or of the patient's voluntary behaviour ; he believes that this accidental inadequacy of sexual gratification is the actual cause of the neurosis, the latter being secondary. Now, in my view, the inadequacies are far from being primary and from being dependent on circumstances. . . . Even in masturbation, even in coitus reservatus, and a fortiori in normal coitus, these individuals could secure adequate gratification if they were normal. But they are not

[1] Les obsessions et la psychasthénie, 1903, vol. i, p. 623.
[2] F. Lyman Wells, Critique of impure Reason, " Journal of Abnormal Psychology," June and July 1912.
[3] Ladame, Névroses et sexualité, " L'Encéphale," 1913, p. 65.

normal, and the inadequacies of sexual gratification are no more than a manifestation, a particular instance, of their psychological inadequacies. It is because they become more and more incapable of pushing any psychological phenomenon to its climax, that they stop short of the end in this action as in the others."

To-day, I am even more strongly convinced of the truth of the contentions than I was when I wrote the foregoing passage a few years ago. My opinion has been strengthened by a number of subsequent observations. In many patients we can detect veritable amorous obsessions, even accompanied by erotic gestures and sexual agitation, although the starting-point has not been a sexual disturbance properly so called. These patients are continually displaying their affectionate disposition, they are perpetually trying to attract attention to themselves, they are always dreaming of caresses, and they seem to be constantly aspiring towards something which they are impatiently awaiting, as if they were aspiring towards love. We must not fall into the mistake of supposing that all such manifestations are the expression of unappeased sexual urges. Fundamentally, they depend upon a terrible dread of isolation, upon an impulsive need to love and to be loved—these manifestations being connected with the need for guidance, the need for excitation, and the sentiments of incompleteness, which are themselves the accompaniments of the patient's depression. Such amorous obsessions are equivalents of authoritarian obsessions, obsessions of jealousy, or, simply, impulses to take alcohol or morphine. They alternate, in some of these patients, with impulses to consume toxic stimulants ; they appear when the crises of depression occur, and disappear as soon as the psychological tension has been restored. We should make a great mistake were we to regard them as primary, were we to link them up to some sexual trauma of old or recent date, for they are merely to be classed among the multiform manifestations of depression.

Other patients, conversely, suffer from sexual frigidity. They complain that they never secure complete gratification. Their sexual pleasure is always inadequate ; and their own theory, like that of the psychoanalysts, is apt to be that their frigidity and the incompleteness of their acts of sexual intercourse are the primary and essential cause of their nervous disorder. The following case is of interest in this connexion. Newy. (f., 30), recently married and already pregnant, has remained entirely indifferent to her husband's caresses. " My husband is not what he ought to be to me ; that is what makes me so ill. I feel nothing when I am with him ; there is a void between us. He does not succeed in making me love him. . . . I had such a longing to be married ; but marriage has brought me nothing, and I feel that I must get away from my husband. . . ? It is so exhausting to feel nothing, to be like a block of wood, that is what makes me ill."

Let us note, first of all, that the trouble is far more general than the patient imagines. All her feelings are disordered. Consider, for instance, the remarkable disturbance of her sense of ownership. " Nothing belongs to me in this flat. . . . I do not feel at home in any of the rooms ; to me they seem strange and dead. The dresses which have been bought for me since I first became engaged are not really mine. . . . If I dared, I would hunt up my old dresses and would wear them, for they are really mine. . . . If, nowadays, I buy something for the house, when I get home I cannot even undo the parcel, for the thing inside it is not mine, and I have no interest in it. . . . I should not care if people came and took away everything in the house. I should not want to keep anything, for I have no fondness for anything, just as I have no fondness for any person." Her actions are affected as well as her feelings ; she can do absolutely nothing. " I have no thought of settling in here, of running the little household. If I try to begin any action, I am exhausted before I start, and I burst into tears without having achieved anything. My actions are unreal, just like all my surroundings. . . . I cannot even make up my mind to go to sleep." These general disturbances existed prior to her sexual relationships with her husband ; they became serious as soon as the engagement was fixed ; they even existed before that, although they were less marked. The patient's will power is very weak. She has always lived with her mother and her sister, and has been guided by them in all her activities. " My mother and my sister settled everything for me, and I was lost if I was left alone for a moment ; without them, I did not know which way to turn." Newy., before her betrothal, had already had crises of over-scrupulousness when she went away for a holiday where she stayed with an aunt, far away from her mother and her sister. These crises were not so severe as the present crisis, but they were characteristic.

In these circumstances, I think we should make a grave mistake were we to regard the sexual disturbances as the cause of all the symptoms, and were we to urge the patient to confess having practised masturbation at an earlier date. She is, in fact, only too ready to accuse herself of this ancient offence. Her inability to perform the sexual act correctly is on the same footing as her inability to buy anything satisfactorily or to order dinner properly ; the sexual abulia from which she suffers is only a manifestation of her general abulia. She had suffered from depression for several years before her marriage, and there were several causes of this depression. Heredity was certainly one of them. Education was another, for her education had been absurd ; she had been subjected to a bad physical and moral hygiene. Already predisposed to such troubles, she had been exhausted by the difficulties attendant on her engagement ; she had been over-whelmed by having to leave her mother and her sister, by the novelty of conjugal life, of the life that was a duet for part of the day, while for long hours she was independent and alone ; by the mere change of domicile ; and, finally, by the onset of pregnancy. This exhaustion, this lowering of psychological tension, disturbed all her actions, and two actions in particular, which demanded a specially high psychological tension. She became unable to acquire new objects with a sense of ownership ; and she became incompetent to perform the sexual act with enjoyment.

What proves the soundness of this explanation is that the patient gradually improved, although nothing was done to modify her sexual relationships or to organise them in a better way. Some hygienic directions, a moral guidance which lessened the difficulty of coming to a decision, a gradual education of initiative ; these sufficed, and one day the patient was astonished to find that the equipments of her new home had become her own property. " The dining-room is really mine, but not the bedroom yet." When she succeeded, with a good deal of help, in organising a little dinner party, she was very proud of her achievement. This restored her tension to such an extent that she was able to love her husband, to have complete sexual gratification, and even (a thing which she had thought would be impossible) to sleep a whole night by his side. Subsequently, the sexual functions oscillated concomitantly with the general activity; they were at a high level, so that a complete sexual act was possible, whenever her will power had been stimulated, although there had been no treatment especially directed towards the sexual functions. We see the same sort of thing in many other patients. A number of observations collected without bias, and simple experiments guided by the ordinary rules of induction, have shown that sexual disorders which may appear extremely serious, and the traumatic memories connected with them, are secondary phenomena, the result of the disease and not its cause.

When I published reflections of this kind, declaring my opinion that the sexual disturbances spoken of by Freud are not primary but secondary, I exposed myself to the trenchant criticism from which J. E. Donley and I. H. Coriat had already suffered. In an essay entitled *The Pathology of Morbid Anxiety*,[1] Ernest Jones summarises my remarks and, without troubling to discuss my arguments, he sweeps them off the board. My contention, he implies, is the outcome of my not having practised psychoanalysis. He writes : " Psychoanalysis shows, however, that these defects, like all ' psychasthenic ' ones, are the result of specific disturbances in the early development of the psychosexual life." [2] Alas, Dr. Jones is right, I have not practised psychoanalysis. That is to say, I have not interpreted the utterances of my patients in accordance with a preconceived dogma. I could not bring myself to do anything of the kind, for I do not believe in dogma, and my aim is to establish the truth. My critic reasons like the faithful who will not allow any one to say a word against their religion. —" I have read the sacred books," says the sceptic, " and I find in them numerous contradictions and incoherencies."— " That is because you lack faith," replies the believer. " If you had read the books with the eyes of faith, you would not have seen any contradictions."—I am only too well aware that faith is requisite in order to understand to the full the symbolical interpretations of the psychoanalysts.

[1] " Journal of Abnormal Psychology," July 1911, p. 98.
[2] Op. cit., reprinted in Papers on Psychoanalysis, third edition, p. 504.

Have the writings of the psychoanalysts concerning sexual matters been fairly summarised in the foregoing analysis ? A good many of those who profess this doctrine will reproach me for having given too literal and crude a signification to the word " sexual."

I think an essay of Freud's may be regarded as an anticipatory statement of the criticisms I may expect in this regard. A few years ago, a woman separated from her husband was suffering from depression and anxiety, and she went to consult a young medical man, a disciple of Sigmund Freud. This doctor, being a faithful disciple, told the patient that all her troubles were due to unsatisfied sexual needs. His prescription was a simple one : " You must either go back to your husband without delay, or else you must find a lover." Shamefacedly I must confess that I am not sure whether my young colleague was altogether wrong in his advice, and at any rate he seems to me to have made a very sound application of his master's counsel. Unfortunately the patient declared that she could not carry out the prescription, and she complained that the advice had made her anxiety more intense. Freud sympathised with her in this new trouble, and wrote a vigorously worded article censuring his pupil, whose excess of docility was embarrassing to the teacher.[1] The young practitioner, said Freud, had understood the term " sexual life " in too restricted a sense, and had applied it only to the somatic functions, whereas for psychoanalysts it had a much wider and more moral significance. All the tender and affectionate emotions must be regarded as forming part of the sexual life, for the primitive sexual impulse was their source in every case. When speaking of such things we must know how to " sublimate " the word " sexual." In order to avoid being made responsible for faulty applications of psychoanalysis, the director of the school had promoted the foundation of an international organisation whose membership would be limited to practitioners competent to apply psychoanalytical principles.

I will not dwell upon the remarkable character of this decision, which recalls the major excommunication of heretics. We have studied something of the same kind in the school

---

[1] Sigmund Freud, Ueber wilde Psychoanalyse, " Zentralblatt für Psychoanalyse," 1910, vol. iii, p. 91 ; Acher, op. cit., p. 425.

of Christian Science directed by Mrs. Eddy. Enough to say that a good many other writers have told us that we must understand the term " sexual tendency " in a far more general and more poetical sense than has hitherto been customary. Jung insisted that the sexual instinct was the substratum of all our loves and all our desires ; the " libido " was the essential force of life. J. J. Putnam declared that if we wished to understand psychoanalytical doctrines we must interpret the word " sexual " in the most comprehensive way, including among its connotations all the affectionate and noble sentiments, inasmuch as civilisation was exclusively dependent upon the transformation and sublimation of the sexual instinct.[1] Maeder advises us to understand the word " sexual " in the sense in which it is used by the poets when they say that hunger and love make the world go round.[2] Ernest Jones, finally, speaks yet more clearly. He explains that the sense in which Freud uses the term " sexual instinct " differs little from that in which the term " will to power " is used by Schopenhauer and Nietzsche, the term " vital impetus " by Bergson, or the term " life force " by Shaw.[3] The writers wish us to understand that when the psychoanalysts talk of sexual instincts, sexual wishes, a desire for coitus, libido, etc., they mean nothing more than the " vital impetus " of the metaphysicians.

Various protests against this indefinite extension of the significance of the term " sexual tendency " have been voiced. Otto Hinrichsen points out that Freud is really becoming a mystic in his use of the word libido. The theory of sublimation enables him to give the term so vast an extension that libido, at length, has a quasi-universal application. Ladame joins in condemning this abuse of language, and quotes the witty phrase of André Beauquier : " We must have a respect for words, and must handle them carefully. We must be afraid lest we should injure them and pervert their meaning by cutting their roots. Words are not ours to do with as we please." [4]

---

[1] Putnam, Personal Impressions of S. Freud and his Work, " Journal of Abnormal Psychology," 1910, p. 375.
[2] Maeder, Sur le mouvement psychoanalytique, " L'Année Psychologique," 1912.
[3] Ernest Jones, Papers on Psychoanalysis, 1913, p. xi.
[4] Ladame, Névroses et sexualité, " L'Encéphale," 1913, p. 59.

I fully sympathise with these criticisms, and I have myself long been at war with kindred abuses of language. At the time when the epidemic of suggestion was raging in France (and it may be noted in passing that there are close analogies between this epidemic and the psychoanalytical movement), the enthusiasts for suggestion were ready to declare that all psychological and physiological phenomena were suggestions. Diseases were all suggestions ; so were cures ; education was suggestion ; so was religion ; etc., etc. Since these adepts carefully refrained from defining suggestion, and used the word to denote any sort of phenomenon entering the mind or the brain no matter how, they had an easy triumph with their declaration that suggestion explained everything. At that time, I made vigorous protests against this way of confusing the issues, which was, I considered, no less disastrous to philosophy than to the science of medicine. To-day, when the game is beginning once again with a term even more unsuitable, the term " sexual desire," I feel it incumbent on me to renew my protest.

Such oratorical exercises are easy. With a little interpretation, displacement, dramatisation, and elaboration, in conjunction with a lack of critical faculty, anything in the world can be generalised, and anything can be made into an element of everything. Yesterday, all the neuroses were suggestions ; to-day, they are all sexual disturbances ; to-morrow, they will all be disturbances of the moral or artistic sense. But why stop short at the neuroses ? It is not so very long since locomotor ataxia was considered to be due to sexual excess, and in the end the patients believed what they were told by their doctors. I am prepared to prove in like manner that tuberculosis and cancer are indirect and unexpected results of masturbation in early childhood. I really cannot see the use of playing with words in this way.

Such oratorical exercises are not merely futile, they are dangerous. They might be excused if they were confined to terms manufactured for the purpose, and devoid of antecedent meaning, as happens in the language of the metaphysicians. But the term " suggestion " and the term " sexual desire " already have a precise meaning. Any one who sublimates them, gives two senses to the same word, and this does not promote clarity of discussion. While employing the term in its sublimated sense, we shall simultaneously convey the images and significations which attach to it in the material sense. Thus the psychoanalysts, even while they are subliminating the word "love" in the most admirable way, are perpetually talking of the "Oedipus complex," of the masturbations of Narcissus, of little children watching a dog and a bitch in the act of intercourse, and of a railway station as representing the to and fro movements of coitus. Such confusions do not help us in the study of the "vital impetus," nor yet in the study of the sexual phenomena of human life. The result of the alleged sublimation is only to confound the loftiest tendencies of the human mind with the instincts that are common to all animals. Even if it could be historically proved that a higher tendency were derived from a lower tendency, the former would remain higher, with characters peculiar to itself, and there would be no justification for confounding it with the phenomenon out of which it originated.

Nevertheless, I shall be assured, the study of the relationships between the sexual instincts and the affectionate sentiments, the study of the relationships between love and the arts and poetry and religion, cannot fail to be of great interest. No doubt, but there is a serious misunderstanding here. The problems in question are interesting, but they are interesting from a specific outlook and in relation to a particular order of studies. Such problems, at any rate when discussed in the way we have just been considering, belong to general philosophy, and even to metaphysics. Of course we must not try to suppress metaphysics, and I hasten to repudiate the idea that I am uttering so dreadful a blasphemy. But we must leave metaphysics in its proper place ; we must discuss it in the templa serena, in the tranquil atmosphere of philosophical congresses. It is absolutely essential that we should avoid introducing these discussions to our patients' bedsides and into the precincts of the hospital, where the atmosphere will be uncongenial. For my own part, I am far from believing that our religious and moral ideas have been exclusively derived from our sexual instincts. I should have plenty to say upon the matter if I were discussing it from the outlook of general philosophy, but I have no intention of sandwiching such a discussion between a couple of reports to a medical congress, one report dealing with dementia praecox and another with typhoid fever. No doubt ideas and terms have to be reformed now and again by philosophical speculations, but we must leave the philosophers plenty of time to make these reforms, and we must wait until the philosophers have come to a satisfactory agreement before we initiate changes in scientific teminology. Actual science, practical science, must accept ideas and terms as they exist in the thought of the day. Unless we wish to go back to the Tower of Babel, we must avoid applying in medical observation and study any philosophical conceptions which are the product of our own imagination and which the philosophers themselves have no inclination to accept. Before all, psychoanalysis is a philosophy, which might be interesting if it were offered to philosophers ; but at the same time it claims to be a medical science, and the psychoanalysts insist on applying it to the diagnosis of disease and to the treatment of patients. This is the real origin of all the difficulties and misunderstandings that arise in connexion with the new doctrine.

Unless I am greatly mistaken, the studies requisite to-day in neurology and psychiatry are of a very different kind. I do not think that psychology should be presented to doctors in this philosophical form. Often enough, in the past, the psychological studies of medical men have influenced the great generalisations of metaphysics. Attempts have been made to explain in one breath history, morality, religions, and fits of hysterics. By degrees, however, doctors have found it necessary to abandon such literary excursions, for they have come to recognise the truth of Aristotle's dictum that " we must not mix the kinds," and they have realised that it was not good either for metaphysics or for medicine to confound the two disciplines. Psychology will only secure acceptance in medical studies if it renounces immoderate ambitions, is content to describe the behaviour and the dispositions of patients in accurate terminology, and is willing to link up the phenomena under observation by the strictest determinism that can be achieved.

That is why I have felt entitled to consider the sexual theories of psychoanalysis in the plain light of day, to discuss them as a scientific thesis, while interpreting the terms " sexual " and " sexual traumatic memory " in a precise and literal sense. It is when we understand these terms literally that we find ourselves unable to regard as proved the theory that all the neuroses arise out of emotions of a sexual kind. It may well be true that sexuality plays a very large part in the neuroses, and this may be proved in days to come. But it is not true that sexual adventures and mishaps, and traumatic memories of these, are the exclusive causes of neurosis.

5. THE EXAGGERATIONS OF PSYCHOANALYSIS.

The sexual theories of psychoanalysis are, we consider, an outcome of the psychoanalytical method and of the general psychoanalytical conception of the neuroses. The psycho-analysts, analysing the subconscious, to which in my opinion they have attached undue importance, have come to the conclusion that all the morbid phenomena exhibited in the neuroses are phenomena which have been misshapen and blurred by a reaction on the part of the subject, by " repres-sion " ; and they declare that we must always discover beneath these appearances a traumatic memory. The time has now come for a discussion of these two contentions.

By repression, Freud means, a conscious activity by which an individual checks the development of a tendency, usually a personal tendency, by opposing to it other tendencies, which in this case are social and moral. At all levels of mental activity, the tendencies are in conflict, but it is only in reflective assent that the struggle takes the form we are now considering. In this group of operations, the importance of which I have repeatedly emphasised, the tendencies which have been activated up to the stage of desire are verbally represented in the form of ideas ; and deliberation consists in awakening by special interrogations other ideas opposed to the first. When the first ideas represent powerful tendencies, the struggle against them may assume importance, and the other tendencies, the opposing moral tendencies, may be intensified to the grade of effort. Then we have " the conflict between reason and passion," in which repression plays a great part. This is the special phenomenon which Freud regards as the starting-point of all the symptoms of the dream and the neurosis.

Unquestionably, phenomena of repression can be observed

in the neuroses, and there is no doubt that in many cases these phenomena play an important part. Many patients declare that they are tormented by criminal impulses, impulses to kill, to steal, to perform obscene actions, " to touch the fly of men's trousers," to masturbate, and so on ; but since, in reality, they are virtuous persons, they are incensed by these temptations, and strive desperately against them. " I am continually praying to be delivered from temptation ; I set my teeth in persistent effort." We have already studied a good many instances of this kind.

It is likewise true that, in certain cases, this persistent repression changes the aspect of ideas and wishes. First of all, it is very probable that, now and again, excessive repression is the cause of the manifest exaggeration of the impulse. When we expend a great deal of energy in the struggle with an adversary, we are apt to overestimate his strength, to consider him more powerful than he really is ; and these patients believe that their passions are titanic because they make such immense efforts to overcome them. In cases of over-scrupulousness, the trouble is rather a mania of repression than a true impulse. The case of Hermine (f., 40) is demonstrative in this respect, for the patient herself shows us the repression and its origin. The poor woman has suffered from several crises of depression and scrupulousness, and she was worn out with nursing her son when he was dying of an intestinal complaint. During the later stages of the son's illness, and after his death, the mother, in her despair, sought consolation in religious and moral practices. " The time had come for me to be more moral, to behave better. . . . The joys of love, intimate relationships with a husband, are all right for happy people. . . . Always, in these things, there is a flavour of debauchery. Such matters are no longer suitable for persons of our age, or for persons in mourning. . . . We must renounce them, or must at any rate renounce the pleasure they might bring." She devotes a great deal of energy to the repression of frivolous pleasures. " It has always been my way to keep a strict hand over myself." These repressions soon showed their effect in the appearance of obsessions of immorality, imaginary impulses towards indecency, obscene sensations, etc. " I love what I loathe. Not only do I have incredible longings, but I seek them out. I am no longer mistress of

my eyes ; I have voluptuous sensations when I catch sight of
a carrot ; I impart an evil signification to everything." Does
not such a case seem to be a signal confirmation of Freud's
theory of repression ?

In other cases, repression, although masked, still exists.
I am thinking of horrible wishes and sacrilegious obsessions.
Da. (f., 27) laments her sad fate, which condemns her to love
in an improper way. " I appear to be incapable of a seemly
love, of one which I can avow. I fall in love with my confessor,
with some other priest, with a hotel porter who drinks and is
disgusting ; I have impulses to perform absurd and unclean
actions with an old lady for whom I have the utmost respect."
In such cases, the action is simultaneously seductive and
repulsive ; longing and repression exist side by side. In
sacrilegious obsessions, we always find this juxtaposition,
and underlying them there is often a memory of resistance to
temptation. The man who told us that when in the church
at Lourdes he had an impulse to defile an old priest or to rape
a descendant of Bernadette, had been ill for a long time,
and had been compelled to practise sexual abstinence on
grounds of health. Having repressed his sexual desires for a
considerable period, he now attributes to them a remarkable
impulsive energy. The sacrilegious obsession would appear
to have resulted from a combination of repression and the
impulse.

Can repression also exercise an influence in the subconscious
of hysterical patients ? Probably it can, in certain cases.
In my study of Irène, the young woman who, after her mother's
death, suffered for several months from retrograde amnesia,[1]
I showed that, from time to time, the patient resisted when
we wished to make her revive the lost memories, or when she
seemed on the point of reviving them spontaneously. I
wrote : "At the beginning and at the close of attacks of
hysterical amnesia, there are periods during which there is
a phobia of memory, as if a memory began by becoming terrible
before becoming subconscious."—But especially, in this
connexion, I have laid stress upon the remarkable case of
hysterical paralysis an account of which will be found in the

---

[1] L'amnésie et la dissociation des souvenirs par l'émotion, " Journal de
Psychologie Normale et Pathologique," September 1904, p. 417 ; L'état
mental des hystériques, second edition, 1911, p. 506.

report I presented to the Geneva Congress in 1909.[1] Sah. (f., 30) has for ten years suffered from a succession of neuropathic disorders which ensued upon a dreadful shock. Her father, who was lying down, had tried to rise to his feet with her aid, but he suddenly collapsed in an attack of angina pectoris, falling upon the daughter and dying instantaneously. She lay several hours beneath the corpse, which pressed upon her left side. In her terror she did not dare to move. Since then, she has been liable to the recurrence of a strange delusion. She complains that her left arm has undergone a sudden change, and that this change is intolerable. It seems to her that her arm no longer belongs to her. " It is not my hand, but some one else's ; it is no longer even a human hand, but seems to be like that of an animal or of a reptile. . . . I do wish I could get my own hand back." She will no longer use this left hand, and she has a horror of touching her other hand or her face with it. But the power of voluntary movement of the left hand is retained, and the sense of touch and the sense of pain (pin pricks) are unaffected. In a word, she has become just like the psychasthenics who keep on saying · " This is not my arm, but some one else's ; it is not I that speaks, walks, etc." But there is a very remarkable difference, in that the disturbance is strictly localised to one limb. We rarely see anything of the kind in psychasthenics.

This condition does not last long, for a few days after the onset of the delusion she has a severe hysterical crisis in which she makes as if she would tear off her left arm. She then resembles the patient described by Barrows in 1860, whose case was commented upon by William James[2] in 1889, the woman who would strike her arm and call it an " old stump." After the crisis, Sah. is merely affected with hemiplegia and anaesthesia of the whole of the left side. She no longer says anything about her arm. She does not complain of it, but she cannot move it, and she can feel nothing in it ; or rather, movement and sensation in this arm have become subconscious.

From the clinical outlook, the case is a remarkable one, for in my experience such an oscillation between the symptoms of psychasthenia and the symptoms of hysteria is extremely

[1] Rapport sur le problème de la subconscience, Comptes rendus du Congrès de Psychologie, Geneva, 1909, p. 68.
[2] Automatic Writing, Proceedings of the S.P.R., 1889, p. 550.

rare. But from the psychological point of view, no less, it may be regarded as interesting, inasmuch as it might be interpreted in the light of the Freudian doctrine of repression. Might we not say that in a woman obviously predisposed to hysterical disorders, the memory of her father's tragical death became associated with the left arm on which his dead body had lain, and that this association was the cause of the patient's strange horror of her left side. We may suppose that this was the reason why the patient had both a moral and a material repulsion for her left arm. Finally, it would seem that this repulsion, this repression, must have been the antecedent and the cause of the hysterical hemiplegia, of the lapsing into the subconscious of all the tendencies attaching to the left side of the body.

Does repression play an equally important part in dreams ? Here the evidence is less clear, but we can certainly agree that repression is sometimes at work. A dream is the behaviour of a sleeping man, and this behaviour consists of the low-grade activations of tendencies that have been aroused by various internal or external stimuli acting upon the sleeper. These tendencies are aroused in a very vague manner, because there has been no preparatory state, no erection of the tendencies. Their awakening occurs haphazard, according as this or that tendency has a disposition towards activation, that is to say, according to the variations in the energetic charge of the respective tendencies. Such charges vary much from tendency to tendency, and are affected by numerous influences ; but we may agree that one of these influences must sometimes be the extent to which the tendencies have been exercised during the waking state. Tendencies which are continually being awakened by clumsy repression, which are continually being inhibited so that they find no satisfactory outlet, may become overcharged, and may thus be inclined to undergo activation very readily during sleep. There is an element of truth in the old observation of Charma and Maury. As for the distortion of the dream, this is due to so many different influences, that it is far from easy to ascertain how much of the distortion is the outcome of repression of one kind or another.

However this may be, since we admit that, in the neuroses

at least, repression plays an important part, we have to ask ourselves how we are to understand this phenomenon ? Are we simply to connect repression, as just described, with normal deliberation ? Are we to regard it as an outcome of an exaggerated effort towards moral behaviour ? Are we to suppose that Hermine's illness is entirely due to her decision to be abstinent as a sign of mourning ? If she had not had this rather remarkable notion, if she had not made up her mind to " behave properly," would she not have been ill to-day, and would she have escaped the prolonged suffering that resulted from her obsession of sacrilege ? I think such a hypothesis most improbable. We rarely find that the patient's will, the patient's decisions, can exercise so much power over the development of mental disorders. Seldom does it happen that so thorough an upset is the outcome of the struggle with our longings, however vigorous the struggle may be. Is it easier to accept the view that a struggle with our wishes can induce hysterical subconsciousness ? The struggle with our tendencies inhibits their manifestation, checks their development, with the result that, by degrees, they are reduced and annihilated. If, on hygienic grounds, I make up my mind to resist the bad habit of smoking, I shall not thereupon take to smoking subconsciously in the somnambulist state, but shall merely bring about the disappearance of the tendency to smoke. What is characteristic of the subconscious is, not that a tendency diminishes or remains latent, but that a tendency develops and undergoes realisation without the other tendencies of the mind becoming aware of this realisation so that they may be able to counteract the development of the first-named tendency.

But I shall be told, we are talking of powerful tendencies, which resist repression and will not allow themselves to be annihilated. So be it, they will resist, they will continue to develop from time to time, and will overwhelm the counteracting moral tendencies. There will be struggles, and pangs of conscience, but here we have nothing to do with the subconscious. The wish to perform an action which has been forbidden by the doctor or by the father confessor will be attended, if you like, by a dread of death, or by the fear of the pains of hell, but it will not itself be transformed into fear. I want to smoke a cigar, but I am afraid that smoking will

make me ill. I cannot see why you should call this cigaro-
phobia, or how it can become the action of smoking
subconsciously. Such objections naturally occur to the mind,
and we find them in various writings—notably in an essay by
Morton Prince entitled *Discussion of the Symposium*.[1]

In actual fact, what goes on in deliberation, or (if you
like) in the normal repression of dangerous longings, is very
different. Such repression is not indefinitely prolonged, and
it does not induce all these disorders, for it is no more than
a transient stage in an operation which soon transcends it.
Hercules does not go on deliberating indefinitely, and he does
not pass his whole life in practising repression; he makes his
choice between vice and virtue. Decision, whether of will
or of belief, is not content with thwarting or controlling our
tendencies; it synthetises them, and gives them all a common
trend. Inhibition, as McDougall has shown very well in his
studies of vision,[2] invariably implies the canalisation and
utilisation of the energy of the inhibited tendency; and I
have found it easy in my lectures to adapt these studies concerning the elementary inhibitions to the struggles that occur
at a higher level when the tendencies have assumed a verbal
form. In normal life, repression leaves no traces; and we
do not find in normal life the mingling of allurement and
repulsion which is characteristic of the persistent repressions
of our patients.

Repression, as we have been describing it, is not a normal
phenomenon which, through clumsy handling, becomes the
cause of subsequent disturbances; it is itself already a morbid
disturbance. Let us reconsider some of our cases in this
light. Hermine does not merely suffer from her imaginary
obscene impulses. We can easily ascertain that she has a
great many other disorders. Quite apart from her impulses
and her scruples, her sexual functions are completely disorgan-
ised: menstruation is irregular and abnormal; the secretions
are modified; the wishes and the pleasure normally attaching
to the sexual act are not present, even when the patient con-
sents to perform this act. Moreover, there are many other

---

[1] "Journal of Abnormal Psychology," January 1911, p. 179.
[2] The Sensations excited by a single momentary Stimulation of the Eye,
"British Journal of Psychology," 1904, p. 78.

morbid symptoms. The patient cannot do any work ; her artistic tastes and her talent for composition have disappeared ; she can apply herself to nothing, and has become incapable of understanding what she reads. Serious reflection has become impossible to her, as she herself realises when she finds herself unable to examine her conscience. She can no longer guide her thoughts, and is greatly vexed with herself because she is unable to think about her son when she goes to visit his grave. Now, not merely are these symptoms independent of her special act of repression, but they existed long before that act.

For a considerable period, Hermine had been gradually depressed by a series of fatigues and emotions, and her working powers had diminished, but there were no symptoms of disorder of the sexual life. Three years ago, her son had his first severe abdominal crisis, and his mother, caring for him throughout the night, had suffered from intense anxiety and distress. She had just begun to menstruate when this happened, and, perhaps in consequence of her emotion, or perhaps (as she herself thinks) because she was handling ice all night, the flow was arrested. The menstrual irregularity dates from this instant. For some months, Hermine slept in her son's room, and regular sexual relationships with her husband were discontinued. When she wished to resume them, not being as yet troubled by any scruples in the matter, she became aware that " something had gone wrong." I may remind the reader that in connexion with the case of Pya. (m., 40) I have already described the disappearance of the higher grades of activation and of triumph (a disappearance which is characteristic of the depression of the sexual tendencies). In Hermine, these tendencies have never attained a notable intensity, and when, after her son's death, she made up her mind to sacrifice them, the sacrifice was an easy one, for she was renouncing that which she can hardly be said to have possessed. The renunciation and the repression, far from being the starting-point of the lowering of the function, were in fact the expression thereof. Her ideas anent mourning are no more than pretexts, for they are incompetent to exercise any influence upon this elementary function. When Hermine had recovered, when she had got rid of her horrible obsessions and her phobia of carrots, and when she had rediscovered the sexual triumph, she continued to hold the same opinion about mourning, and still said regretfully : " Such matters are no longer suitable." —But they happened all the same ! We must not endow delusions with more power than they actually possess ; we must not ascribe to delusion phenomena which are really the direct outcome of the depression.

Now let us reconsider the case of Sah. I agreed that the hemiplegia from which she suffered might be explicable as a phenomenon of repression, for sometimes the onset of paralysis of the left arm was preceded by a sort of delirium in which the subject repelled with horror the sensation of her own arm and seemed to repress it. But to say that an explanation is possible does not imply that we accept it as the only valid explanation, and I must point out a difficulty. In the complete report of the case which I presented to the Geneva Congress, we see that in the relapses the sequence of events was what I have just been considering. But to begin with, when Sah. was found lying under her father's body, she immediately suffered from a hysterical crisis, and from left hemiplegia which persisted, more or less, for several months. Then it passed off for a time, until, after emotion and fatigue, she had a relapse, in which the trouble began with a sense of horror of the left arm, which lasted several days and was followed by a new attack of hemiplegia. We see that the hemiplegia with subconsciousness appeared for the first time without having been preceded by the sense of horror and by the repression. Can we be sure that the second attack of hemiplegia, which was certainly preceded by the repression, was really caused by the repression ? May we not suppose that, in the relapse, the horror of the left arm was the first manifestation of the oncoming hemiplegia ? Under the influence of the original violent emotion, the exhaustion of the tendencies connected with the left arm was, we may imagine, sufficient from the first to bring about total subconsciousness, with anaesthesia and paralysis. When emotional disturbances led to a relapse, the exhaustion may at first have been incomplete, and may simply have led to a modification of the tendencies, with a sense of strangeness, and with phenomena of derivation taking the form of fear ; but, in the end, the increasing exhaustion may have gradually induced complete subconsciousness. According to this view of the matter, the repression was not a voluntary action on the part of the subject, and was not the direct cause of the paralysis; the repression was not a cause but a consequence, was itself an outcome of the exhaustion. Féré has published observations of the same kind, relating to the abnormal sentiments that were displayed in the early stages of functional paralyses. My own view is that such an explanation is far more satisfactory, for it does not only explain the paralysis, but also explains the repression, which is itself, on this theory, a morbid phenomenon.

The exaggerated repression characteristic of these patients is, then, to be regarded as a consequence of the depression. This puts an end, more or less completely, to the mental operations for which a high psychological tension is requisite; and, in especial, it puts an end to decision, the final result of reflection. Since no decision is arrived at, and since there is, therefore, no canalisation of the various conflicting tendencies, there results an indefinite prolongation of vacillation, with an exaggeration, now of the impulse and now of the repression. The mania for repression, thus understood, is still an interesting symptom; and it explains certain remarkable phenomena, such as monstrous and sacrilegious longings. It will continue to form a part of mental pathology under the name of " Freud's syndrome."

If this be so, if repression be no more than one of the symptoms of a particular form of psychasthenic depression, there is no reason for invoking repression everywhere and always, no reason for assuming that repression has been at work in the production of all the other symptoms. We must not explain every modification or every succession of symptoms as due to repression, however alluring the explanation may seem. Ten years ago I published an account of the remarkable case of Cb. (f., 39). When she married, this woman expected that she would inherit a little fortune upon the death of an elderly relative. But when the latter died, it transpired that he had spent all his money in the purchase of an annuity, and Cb.'s intense disappointment brought on an illness, with incapacity for work, indecision, etc. Some time after the illness began, she noticed that her hair was falling out, and she thereupon became obsessed with the dread of baldness, was ashamed to show herself in public, and suffered from severe agoraphobia. It would be very simple and pleasant to say that this woman was ashamed at having disappointed her husband, that she had repressed her shame in order to avoid having to admit to herself that she had made a rash promise, and that she had transformed this moral regret into shame concerning her physical appearance. This theorising would be strictly analogous to that of the psychoanalysts. Unfortunately, in spite of the most careful examination of the patient, I could not detect any sign of repression. She had made no secret of her disappointment, and had not attempted to conceal her regrets from her husband. She defended herself, naturally enough, by accusing her elderly relative of having deceived her. She transformed nothing, for she retained the feeling that she had been deceived, and the regret for having been deceived. As a result of this disappointment and of overwork, she suffered from depression, and from sentiments of incompleteness which are so common in these patients. Such sentiments of incompleteness are "attached," as in all other patients of the kind, upon a fact and a particular kind of behaviour ; there has been no conversion.

We must not assume the existence of repression when there is no trace of it, and we have even less warrant for the supposition that all the other symptoms have been distorted by fancied repressions. Such a method of explanation enables us to dispense with the need for clinical observation and to replace it by fantasy. It gives rise to dream interpretations or to explanations of sexual inversion which are too improbable to be worth serious discussion. I think that the general characteristics of these methods have been aptly summarised by Lyman Wells in his article *Critique of impure Reason*. What characterises this method, he says, is symbolism. When it suits the theory, any mental happening can be regarded as symbolic of any other. Condensation, displacement, secondary elaboration, and dramatisation, can effect such vast changes that any phenomenon can signify whatever you like. Lyman Wells adds that, in his view, this is a rather childlike conception of psychological determinism. I think that the psychoanalysts are led astray by their trust in a general principle postulated at the outset as indisputable ; a principle which does not need to be proved by the facts, but can simply be applied to the facts.

But this is not all. The theory of repression and its exaggerations arose out of the idea of the traumatic memory modified by the subconscious ; out of the need for discovering, beneath all the symptoms (and especially at the starting-point of the illness, of the depression), the traces of some event that caused strong emotion. Here we touch the core of the problem. No doubt there are certain symptoms which are related to certain of the happenings of life. Twenty years ago I described the case of a poor fellow who whenever his emotions were stirred would become affected by a strange tic which took the form of blowing vigorously through one of the nostrils. This was the reproduction of an action he had been accustomed to perform long before when he had had typhoid, and when there had been epistaxis followed by the formation of a crust in the nose. Are we to assume a priori that all neuropathic symptoms are constructed upon this model ? Must we hunt for transformed memories as explanations of the authoritarian manias or the love-manias which are so natural an outcome of a desire for self-defence or of self-elevation ? When Wkb. tells us that all the people he has just encountered in the street were corpses, and that suddenly after the act of coitus he found himself in bed with his mistress' dead body, are we to search his life history for some incident connected with a corpse ? We ought to be familiar with the phrase used by Wkb., for a good many patients use it. It is a special way of describing the feeling of automatism and the feeling of unreality in the instances in which these feelings relate to the perception of living beings. If a symptom astonishes us, and seems accidental, the usual reason is our own ignorance. It is far more likely that a symptom is caused by the laws of the disease than by accidental memories. We must not interpret symptoms historically unless clinical observation makes such an interpretation indispensable, and we should never indulge in risky hypotheses.

The same remarks apply if we come to consider, not now the pathogenesis of this or that symptom, but that of the illness itself, the pathogenesis of the depression. Are we entitled to assert that an actual neuropathic depression is always due to a traumatic memory ? Certainly not. Incontestably there are cases in which no particular event in the patient's life has been an important causative factor. Probably such cases form the great majority. The subject has often suffered from depression since childhood. It may be due to his hereditary. constitituon, to his age, to bodily disorders, to intoxications of one kind or another, to gradual exhaustion dependent upon a succession of minor fatigues or even to a number of petty emotions which were insignificant taken singly so that not one of them has left a distinct or dangerous memory. The patient's symptoms and fixed ideas are, therefore, determined by the intensity of the depression, by its localisation in this or that function which was primarily weak or has been debilitated by a number of forgotten petty shocks. In part, too, they are determined by reactions proper to the subject ; by his temperament, his intelligence, his education, etc. In cases of this kind no great importance must be attached to any particular happening in the patient's life, and probings into his past will be of little interest— from the therapeutic outlook, at any rate.

In other cases, which are also fairly common, special happenings have had a like causative influence, sometimes considerable. These events, giving rise to struggles and efforts which have lasted for a long time, have been a cause of marked exhaustion and of a depression which still persists. But I cannot agree that we are concerned here with a traumatic memory, for the memory no longer plays an active part. In Sophie, for instance, and in Lydia, the first crisis of depression occurred in youth, and was due to a sister's death. For a long time, the patient's mind was filled by this sorrow, but she consoled herself eventually, adapted herself to the new situation. In both these patients, in fact, the influence of the event was trifling. Still, it is obvious that neither of them ever regained the previous level, and that the result of the initial depression was to lower the psychological tension permanently and to leave the patient more liable to nervous disorders. But the mere fact that a happening played an important part long ago does not prove that it still plays an important part to-day, or that we have to-day to take its action into account. A microbic infection in the past may have weakened the sufferer irreparably, and yet have quite ceased to exist to-day. In the latter case, we shall not now do the patient any good by disinfective procedures.

The main defect of psychoanalysis is that it does not make

sufficient allowance for such cases, which form the great majority. The psychoanalysts invariably set to work in order to discover a traumatic memory, with the a priori conviction that it is there to be discovered—like a detective who has a fixed idea where the culprit is to be found. The worst of it is that such detectives will always run their culprit to earth in the end. So, too, will the psychoanalysts; owing to the nature of their methods, they can invariably find what they seek.

Let us consider for a moment Jung's interesting method for the study of delayed associations. No doubt by preparing a list of suitable words we can detect prolonged and abnormal associations in the case of words which are related in one way or another to the subject's fixed ideas. I have myself succeeded on several occasions in performing this little experimental demonstration. But I am by no means convinced that such an experiment would be successful if we did not know beforehand the subject's fixed ideas, or if the subject had no memory which could play the requisite part. I believe that we should make grave clinical errors if we should try to guide our diagnosis by this experiment alone. It has seemed to me that every word capable of arousing emotion of whatever kind, even mere surprise, will cause a more or less considerable delay and will modify the association. A strange or shocking word introduced into a list of ordinary words will arouse a surprise of this kind. I have secured delays of from six to nine seconds by suddenly pronouncing such improper words as " merde " or " votre cul " in the middle of a list of permissible words. Yet the subject, with whose mental condition I had long been acquainted, had no traumatic memory connected with either of these words.

The method is one for experimental work in the laboratory, and if we use it as a method of clinical examination we shall expose ourselves, I think, to serious risk. The method, as I have frequently seen in practice, will invariably succeed in furnishing evidence of certain ideas or memories, for in a long list of words there will always be some which will induce slow or irregular reactions. The observer will thus be enabled to discover traumatic memories in all their patients, even in those whose neurosis has no connexion whatever with such a memory. Those who use the method clinically do so with a prior conviction that the patient has a traumatic memory, and their only aim is to discover what the memory is.

This characteristic of psychoanalysis becomes still more obvious when we consider the psychoanalytical study of dreams and the psychoanalytical method of dream interpretation. At the first glance, this method of interpretation appears strange and hazardous, for one and the same dream can be interpreted in many different ways. Recently one of my patients, a young man of twenty-five with a strong inclination towards mystical ideas, told me a dream of his which he regarded as having an important bearing upon his future. " I dreamed that an invisible force compelled me to look at a part of the sky where my fate was written. In this part of the sky there was a star, and there were two doves."—" Two doves and a star," I exclaimed. " That's plain enough ; the masters of psychoanalysis have given us the key to such dreams. The two doves denote love ; you are evidently in love. The interpretation of the star is a more ticklish matter. I might tell you that you are in love with a music-hall star, and Monsieur Maeder has let us know that ' star ' is a name which young women in Switzerland apply to the female genital organs. But I do not want to be accused of ' wild psychoanalysis,' and I think it better to tell you that the star of your dream is the symbol of something marvellous and inaccessible. You will be unlucky in love."—" Not a bit of it," he answered. " You don't understand in the least. The star signifies the navy, for sailors guide their course by the stars. One of the doves is the soul of Joan of Arc, which rose out of the flames at Rouen in the form of a dove. The other dove is my own soul, which, as you see, is so like Joan's. It is my mission to do on the sea something like that which Joan of Arc did on land. My dream tells me to have no doubt that I shall command a great fleet which is to deliver Brittany from its oppression by the irreligious prefects." I did not argue the point, for there was just as much to be said for the young man's interpretation as for my own. An interpretation is only possible when we know beforehand how we are to interpret. When it is added that the theory of repression can transform all the phenomena, we see how easily the dream interpreter can discover in his patients whatever memories he wants.

Arbitrary enquiries and arbitrary interpretations of this sort have their drawbacks for the patient. First of all, while we are applying a tedious and unsuitable treatment, we are wasting time which might have been devoted to a treatment which would have done the patient good. We weary him by the prolonged discussion and detailed study of complicated psychological phenomena, and shall be very apt to develop in him what I have termed the " psychological mania," which is common in such patients. We shall upset him needlessly by making him see terrible dangers in all the actions of his past life. A good many patients I have known, constitutionally psychasthenic, persons with a low psychological tension and liable to be exhausted by the slightest efforts, began to suffer from scruples concerning the immorality of their lives, and first became affected with manias of effort and work, in connexion with investigations of this kind. Young Emile had for some time been under the care of one of Freud's disciples. Emile's dread of social life was easy enough to explain; but this doctor, on the look-out for a subconscious memory, had tried to apply Jung's method of associations. The patient took fright, imagining that an attempt was being made to read his thoughts, and he therefore did his utmost to defeat the experimenter's wiles by prolonging the association time in season and out of season ; and he conceived a horror of the doctor.—I had occasion to treat two young women whose sexual memories had been studied by psychoanalysts. —Ws. (f., 26), a sufferer from congenital depression, exhausted by scholastic work, bored to death by being kept too long in bed during a rest cure at a sanatorium, was then accused by her doctor of all kinds of sexual improprieties. She was in despair when she learned that the world was full of abominations whose existence she had never suspected, and was rendered crazy by the thought that any one could believe her to be capable of a thing of the kind. A sensible doctor had to intervene in order to put a stop to these unseemly investigations.—Slava. (f., 24) had not taken the matter quite so seriously. She gave me a very amusing account of the treatment, of the enquiries to which she had been subjected by one of Freud's disciples, who was obviously a simpleton. " The doctor pressed me with queries as to whether I was not hiding from him the story of some mishap in love which must have gravely affected my life, and he twisted every word I uttered, always endeavouring to get upon the trail of this incident. One day he discovered from a dream I had told him that every night I must be having unconscious intercourse with my grandfather, and that I had a strong sadistic tendency, though I hardly understood what he was talking about. . . . He ended by telling me that I was in love with him without being aware of the fact, and you can't imagine how hideous and stupid I thought him." Such are the puerilities that result from a theory which has been imperfectly understood and has been generalised in a ridiculous way.

A great many medical practitioners have adversely criticised these investigations as injudicious and often hazardous. " I consider," writes Forel, " that Freud, through his gross exaggeration in this matter of the traumatic memory as a cause of nervous disorder, and above all by the way in which he generalises the theory and applies it to cases in which the patient has no such memories, himself, as a rule, suggests to his patients all sorts of notions (sexual for the most part) which are far more likely to be hurtful than helpful." [1] Régis and Hesnard, in their essay on Freudism, insist that it is very dangerous to question the patient in this way, and to make him dwell upon his fixed ideas. Such is the opinion regarding psychoanalysis which has gained general acceptance in the French medical world.

For my part, I think the opinion is unjust. Although psychoanalysis is marred by many exaggerations and illusions, such as those which I have myself pointed out, we are indebted to the psychoanalysts for a number of valuable studies upon the neuroses, the development of thought in childhood, and the various types of the sexual sentiment. These studies have drawn attention to facts which were little known, and were indeed neglected owing to our traditional reserve concerning such matters. In due time, the overstrained generalisations and fanciful symbolism which to-day seem typical of psychoanalysis, and to separate the doctrine from other scientific studies, will be forgotten. Only one thing will be remembered, that psychoanalysis has rendered great service to psychological analysis.

---

[1] L'âme et le système nerveux, 1906, p. 214.

6. Unassimilated Happenings.

Exaggeration invariably leads to reaction. After suggestion had annexed the universe for a few years, it completely vanished ; and I myself, who had been trying to counteract its excesses, was compelled to take up the cudgels in its defence. It will be the same thing with the search for traumatic memories ; after the doctors have psychoanalysed all comers they will cease to analyse any one. We must foresee this reaction, and must save from it all that is of interest and value in my own earlier researches on the topic and in the additional studies made by various authors.

We have just seen that in most of the cases of neuropathic disorder, the trouble was not the outcome of any definite happening in the patient's life. But this being granted, it is none the less impossible to deny that there are other cases in which an event and its persistent effects continue to play an important part in the illness. Let me first give some further examples of this. I will recall a case published a few years ago, which is of considerable interest in this respect.[1] Irène, a young woman of twenty, who had displayed incredible devotion in nursing her mother when the latter was dying of tuberculosis, became seriously ill after the mother's death. At first, Irène's symptoms could best be described as negative. She did not behave like a young woman who had been passionately devoted to her mother, who had cared for the invalid night and day during many months, and who had just seen her mother die. Immediately after the death, she found herself unable to break the news to some relatives she was calling on ; she could not make the arrangements for the funeral, and could not even behave properly at the ceremony. She attended the burial, under pressure, but burst out laughing in the cemetery. When reproved for this, she said she did not believe that it was her mother's funeral at all ; her mother had gone away, but would soon be back. Thenceforward she gave no sign of sorrow, shed no tears, and refused to wear mourning. She made no attempt to take her mother's place in the little household, or to manage her father (who was a drunkard) as the mother had done. Moreover, it was plain

[1] L'amnésie et la dissociation des souvenirs par l'émotion, " Journal de Psychologie Normale et Pathologique," September 1904 ; L'état mental des hystériques, second edition. 1911, p. 506.

that she did not understand when any one spoke to her about her mother's illness and death, for she seemed to have completely forgotten the death and the three months that had preceded it. Were her other reactions to the extant situation more appropriate? By no means. She could no longer work ; she could not make up her mind to anything ; she had no normal feelings ; no interest in her associates.

On the other hand, she had grave symptoms of illness, being frequently affected by delirious crises which assumed a very dramatic form and lasted for several hours. In these crises she rehearsed with meticulous accuracy the chief scenes of her mother's last hours and death. She imagined herself to play a part, recapitulating her own words and gestures at the bedside when she had been trying " to prevent Mother coughing up her lungs," or when she had been doing her utmost to reawaken the dead woman. In the waking state she suffered from hallucinations, contractures, and a number of visceral disorders. These symptoms continued for a good many months without any change.

Let us turn to another example, one of a very different kind. Léa and Lydia, twin sisters, were inseparable. They dressed exactly alike, always did the same things and did them together, and shared the same feelings to an amazing extent. They would have been an excellent pair upon whom to study the psychology of the life of twins. When the young women had reached the age of twenty-four, the parents were so imprudent as to marry off Léa, who was thus separated from her sister. Lydia thereupon fell sick. She moped persistently, had no appetite, and spent her nights weeping. She was incapable of adopting the behaviour appropriate to the only daughter left at home ; she simply did nothing at all. At the same time, there was going on in her mind a strange discussion of an insoluble problem. Although she was good-looking, and was so like her sister that the two were often mistaken for one another, she was continually questioning herself about her face, her gait, her good looks or her bad looks. " Am I or am I not as pretty as Léa ? Is it because I am ugly that people like Léa better than me ? Did I make a failure of things because I was out of sorts at that time, as I was told ? Was I really ill then and did the others know that I was ill ; did they think that I failed because I was ill ? " This self-depreciation led her to seek retirement. She refused to see any one, and had a phobia of the street. She, in turn, was married, without herself paying much attention to what was going on ; and she derived no benefit from the change. Nor did it do the least good when it was arranged that she should once more be brought into contact with her sister, and that the two couples should form a joint household. Lydia continued to be wholly obsessed with the thought of her looks. She would not go out, would not dress, would not even leave her bed. Things went on like this for ten years or more.

I might quote a number of cases resembling that of Irène or that of Lydia. There is no occasion to describe the delirious crises identical with those of Irène which occur in women who are continually reliving violent quarrels or scenes of rape. I need mention only in passing the case of the young woman who, in her crises, would hasten to the cemetery intending to exhume the step-father who had formerly tried to violate her. As I have already shown, in a great many patients with paralyses and contractures, the mental condition resembles that of Irène.—A young woman of twenty-two has a spasmodic movement of the head and a contracture of the neck because she is constantly looking back over her shoulder to see if her father is rushing at her, as he had done when drunk a few months before.—A girl of seventeen has a contracture of the shoulder. This shoulder was touched (or she so thinks) in the street by an omnibus. Even when she is sitting quite safe in a room she spends her time trying to guard herself against vehicles in motion.—A good many obsessions recall that of Lydia. A married woman of forty-four has for years been tormenting herself with questionings as to whether a schoolmaster's profession is a good one, the reason being that long ago a schoolmaster had wanted to marry her, and she cannot make up her mind whether she did well to refuse him. —A young woman of twenty-two has a strange feeling towards all the little children she encounters ; she has a horror of any small child, wants to strike it, and runs away lest she should yield to an impulse to kill. This disturbance is the outcome of her having been seduced at the age of seventeen, with subsequent pregnancy and a clandestine confinement. Her feelings to-day are still determined by these distressing incidents which she vainly tries to forget.—A like horror of little children exists in a woman of forty who, after an imprudence, had suffered for more than a year from an obsession with the thought of pregnancy.—I shall not dwell upon these various symptoms. Suffice it to mention that all the patients were depressed persons, incapable of work, unable to make up their minds, practically unable to perform any actions except those connected with their crises, their tics, their obsessions bearing upon the event which produced so strong an impression.

The essential point in the foregoing cases is, I think, this particular event. All the patients seem to have had the evolution of their lives checked ; they are " attached " upon an obstacle which they cannot get beyond. The happening we describe as traumatic has brought about a situation to which the individual ought to react. Adaptation is requisite, an adaptation achieved by modifying the outer world and by modifying oneself. Now, what characterises these " attached " patients is that they have not succeeded in liquidating the difficult situation. Irène does not behave like a young woman who has lost her mother. Lydia does not behave like a girl who is left alone with her parents after her sister's marriage. A third patient does not behave as a person should behave who has escaped a danger in the street and has got safely home. A fourth does not behave like a reasonable woman who has refused one suitor and has married another. This lack of adaptation is characteristic of every one of the patients.

A very interesting detail in Irène's case is the amnesia. Not only is she incapable of realising her mother's death, of transforming it into real event, of believing in it ; she is also unable to remember the death and the events of the months that preceded it. I know, of course, that the psychoanalysts have a ready explanation of this forgetfulness. They will tell us that Irène has a horror of the memories, and that in her crises she represses them. I may even point out that in my description of the patient I have alluded to the accesses of terror that occurred in Irène when I tried to compel her to revive the lost memories. No doubt the accesses of terror, and the lapses of memory, may make us think of repression. But such an explanation is purely theoretical, and I cannot accept it. I could never discover, not even after Irène had been cured and after her memory had been fully restored, any evidence that there had been an effort at repression. Had I wished to believe it existed, I should have had to create it fictitiously. The phobias of memory were in Irène's case, as in those of the other patients, manifestations of a modification in the act of memory. If we find it difficult to understand this modification, that is because ordinarily we fail to understand the nature of the act of memory.

Memory, like belief, like all psychological phenomena, is an action ; essentially, it *is the action of telling a story.*[1] Almost always we are concerned here with a linguistic operation, quite independent of our attitude towards the happening. A sentinel outside the camp watches the coming of the enemy. When the enemy arrives, the first business of the sentinel is to perform particular actions related to this arrival ; he must defend himself or must hide, must lie flat, crawl in order to escape notice, and make his way back to the camp. These are actions of adaptation demanded by the event, and the perception of an event is nothing else than the totality of such acts of adaptation. But, simultaneously with these acts of adaptation, the sentinel must exhibit a reaction of a new kind; a kind which is characteristic of memory.; he must prepare a speech, must in accordance with certain conventions translate the event into words, so that he may be able ere long to tell his story to the commander. This second reaction has important peculiarities which differentiate it markedly from the first reaction. The actions which comprised this, the action of self-defence, that of lying flat, that of hiding in one way or another, are no doubt preserved like all the tendencies ; but they can only be reproduced, can only be activated anew, if the sentinel is again placed in the same circumstances, being faced by the same enemy and upon the same ground ; they will not be reproduced in different circumstances, as for instance when the sentinel has got back to camp, is among his comrades, and in the presence of the commander. On the other hand, the second reaction, his account of the matter, though it likewise is after a fashion adapted to the event, can readily be reproduced under the new conditions when the sentinel is among his comrades in the presence of the com-

---

[1] Concerning this explanation of memory, see the report of my lectures upon the elementary intellectual tendencies, " Annuaire du Collège de France," 1913, p. 37.

mander, and when there is no sign of the enemy. The stimulus which will arouse the activation of this tendency is a special form of social action, a *question*. Thus the essential characteristic of the sentinel's story is that it is independent of the event to which it relates, whereas the reactions which comprise his perception have no such independence. The upbuilding of this new tendency is what constitutes memorisation; and the activation of the new tendency in circumstances independent of its origin and as a result of a question is what we term rememoration. The action of telling a story is, moreover, capable of being perfected in various ways. The teller must not only know how to do it, but must also know how to associate the happening with the other events of his life, how to put it in its place in that life-history which each one of us is perpetually building up and which for each of us is an essential element of his personality. A situation has not been satisfactorily liquidated, has not been fully assimilated, until we have achieved, not merely an outward reaction through our movements, but also an inward reaction through the words we address to ourselves, through the organisation of the recital of the event to others and to ourselves, and through the putting of this recital in its place as one of the chapters in our personal history.

It is obvious that Irène has done nothing of the sort. She has not built up a recital concerning the event, a story capable of being reproduced independently of the event in response to a question. She is still incapable of associating the account of her mother's death with her own history. Her amnesia is but one aspect of her defective powers of adaptation, of her failure to assimilate the event.

In addition to such negative characteristics, we can detect symptoms which may be termed positive. These patients continue to make great efforts to react to the event, to assimilate the situation. Lydia persistently maintains the attitude of distressful questioning which she assumed at the time of her sister's marriage. This is not, as might be imagined, because she coveted her sister's fiancé in any way. Her trouble was that she could not understand how or why her sister could perform an independent action and leave her alone. She wearies herself out by searching for the responsibility in this matter, blaming herself, and becoming in the end incapable of feeling and acting. Such patients as the one who was perpetually trying to guard herself from being struck by the omnibus, or the one who was perpetually questioning herself about the worth of the schoolmaster's profession, are continuing the action, or rather the attempt at action, which began when the thing happened; and they exhaust themselves in these everlasting recommencements. Irène offers a remarkable instance of this, for in her crises she readopts the precise attitude which she had when caring for her mother in the death agony. This attitude is not that of a memory which enables a recital to be made independently of the event; it is that of hallucination, a reproduction of the action, directly linked to the event. We say that she is hallucinated because she goes on performing actions which from our point of view ought no longer to be performed, since for us the event has vanished and has been liquidated. Irène goes on performing these actions because, as far as she is concerned, the event has not been liquidated. The persistence of the attitudes, and therefore the persistence of the hallucinations, is invariably one of the consequences of inadequacy of the action at the time when the event took place.

Strictly speaking, then, one who retains a fixed idea of a happening cannot be said to have a "memory" of the happening. It is only for convenience that we speak of it as a "traumatic memory." The subject is often incapable of making with regard to the event the recital which we speak of as a memory; and yet he remains confronted by a difficult situation in which he has not been able to play a satisfactory part, one to which his adaptation had been imperfect, so that he continues to make efforts at adaptation. The repetition of this situation, these continual efforts, give rise to fatigue, produce an exhaustion which is a considerable factor in his emotions. As we have already seen, our patient resembles a man who persists in pushing up against a wall in the vague hope of overthrowing it. An example from normal or quasi-normal life will convey a better understanding of the mechanism of this exhaustion. I have just received an unpleasant letter, which must be answered although the writing of the answer will be difficult and distressing. I think about writing the answer, and I draft the answer in imagination, but I lack the courage to write it, and I leave the letter unanswered on my writing-table. Thenceforward, I cannot sit down at this writing-table, cannot walk past it, cannot even enter the room, without seeing the letter, without divining its presence, and without beginning again and again my effort to write an answer. At first, this answer could have been written in ten minutes. If I add up all the time spent in imaginary and sterile attempts to compose a reply, and increase the total by the sum of all the consequent emotions, I shall find that in the work of not writing an answer I shall have expended hours upon hours of arduous and distressing effort, and it will not be surprising if after the lapse of a few days I find myself utterly exhausted by this damnable letter which I have never written.

In reality, the illness caused by a traumatic memory is not a new thing in our experience. It is a phenomenon strictly analogous to the exhaustion we have studied in persons whose situation is too complicated and too difficult, so that they go on struggling for an indefinite time in their attempts to cope with it. Here are two illustrative examples.—Eq. (m., 40) continued after marriage to keep up a relationship with his mistress. The complications thus involved, and the need for perpetual dissimulation, induced exhaustion and depression. The case is identical with those we have been studying in connexion with fatigue.—Now consider the case of Bc. (m., 50), who broke with his mistress before marriage. In the world of concrete fact, the rupture was complete. His mistress left the town where he was living, and he had no further news of her. But he was tortured by regret for having cast off one who had been his companion for twenty years. He was continually turning the matter over in his mind, wondering how he could have maintained the relationship, how he could find her again, and so on. He, too, like Eq., suffers from exhaustion.—Materially speaking, and for the onlookers, the action is finished ; but it is not finished for the subject, inasmuch as the situation is not liquidated in his mind. Different though these two cases are when objectively considered, subjectively they are identical. In both instances we have to do with depression consequent upon a difficult action which has been indefinitely prolonged until exhaustion has supervened.

From the clinical point of view, however, there is a great difference. In the former case, there is still a concrete situation to deal with, one which really exists even for the onlookers, so that we can reduce the labours of the subject by modifying the situation. In such instances, we are able to facilitate the subject's adaptation; we can procure rest for him by breaking off an engagement to marry, by insisting upon a breach with a mistress, by simplifying the social environment through the removal of certain individuals. But in cases of the latter type there is no concrete situation to modify, inasmuch as the event no longer exists for the observer and cannot be acted upon objectively. This situation is subjective; it exists only in the patient's mind; it is one to which the patient has failed to adapt himself. Exhausting effort is being made, but this effort is of a different kind. If we want to put an end to the effort we must do so in some other way than by the modification of concrete relationships. These thoughts concerning the mechanism of the traumatic memory bring us face to face with a new and important clinical problem.

The study of these facts leads us to the consideration of a new element in adaptation, a final stage of action, and a whole new series of superior tendencies derived from this stage of action, just as the ergetic tendencies are derived from the stage of effort, and the reflective tendencies from the stage of desire. In my lectures I have denoted this final stage of action the *stage of triumph*, because it explains the important phenomenon of joy; but when I have considered it in the light of its effect upon adaptation, I have termed it the *stage of liquidation*.[1]

This final stage of action comprises a number of modifications of the personality and of the tendencies, for these have to be harmonised with the new behaviour. If a crude comparison be permissible, I may picture a barrel, which is filled with sand, pebbles, and scrap-iron, placed at the top of a slope, and adapting itself to the slope by rolling to the bottom. But the arrival of the barrel at the foot of the slope does not end the action. The various objects in the barrel have now to settle themselves into their places, the heavier objects falling to the bottom, and the sand filling up the interstices. In

[1] Cf. Cours sur les degrés de l'activation des tendances, " Annuaire du Collège de France," 1917, p. 69.

like manner, at the close of an action, an internal reorganisation must occur in the mind to liquidate all the
happenings. An important part of this reorganisation is the modification
of the old tendencies relating to the event which has just
happened and to the recent behaviour. One of the new tendencies to be organised is the tendency to repeat the recital
which constitutes memory, to make that recital independent
of the happening, and to settle it into its appropriate place
in our life-history. But more than this is requisite. In order
to finish the action we must put an end to all the movements
that have been connected with it. If the close of the action
is to be definitive, we must demobilise, must disperse, the
forces that participated in the action. It is this dispersal of
the recuperated energies which produces the temporary
excitation of joy (the joy " that is superadded to action, as
blossoming is superadded to youth "), and all the feelings of
triumph. This joy and this triumph are especially conspicuous
after the sexual act, but they are present after every action
that has been well completed. Finally, there is a last action
which is seldom recognised, and which I shall have to consider
subsequently ; I refer to the carrying to reserve, to the rein-
vestment of the unutilised energies. This totality of different
elements of behaviour, which I speak of as the triumph, is
extremely important. If I mistake not, it is the starting-point
of a series of tendencies, among which the most notable are
the aesthetic and artistic tendencies.

Like the higher tendencies of reflection and work, so likewise the higher tendencies we have just been considering are
liable to be disordered in the neuroses. Some very remarkable
cases that have come under my notice show how important
such disorders are, and prove that persons subject to depression
cannot endure without the appearance of morbid symptoms
the triumph which crowns action. I have recorded in psychasthenics the way in which feelings of ecstasy and of indescribable
happiness have been followed by a sudden fall of tension,
culminating in a psycholeptic crisis and even in an epileptic
fit.[1] Here are some additional examples.—Noémi (f., 26) had
a baby a few days since. She feels very well, is sitting with the
baby on her knee, and is receiving her friends' congratulations.

---

[1] Les obsessions et la psychasthénie, 1903, vol. i, p. 381.

" How gloriously happy I am," she thinks. " Everything I have longed for has come to me." Caressing the child, she is full of a strange enthusiasm. Then, suddenly, it all lapses. She is seized by the dreadful thought that this infinite happiness will not last for ever. It must come to an end some day, for she is mortal. She becomes obsessed with the thought of death, and the obsession lasts for two years.—Pby. (m., 29) is walking arm-in-arm with a woman whom he loves, and they are watching the sunset at the seaside. " My heart is flooded with a joy that is purer and more beautiful than I have ever known before. Life is suffused with splendour. Then something seems to go crack in my head, and all turns black and gloomy. I am seized once more by the obsession that I have to fight a man whom I used to know at college, a man I detested, but whom I have not seen for ten years. What rotten luck ! "

Pf. (m., 37) can perform coitus without any bad results when his partner is a woman in whom he has no interest and whom he does not passionately desire. But there is one woman whom he ardently loves. When he has sexual relations with her, the joy is intense, and immediately afterwards he has an epileptic fit.—Gf. (f., 29), who has long been psychasthenic, tries to resume her musical studies. If she goes on for some time playing a piece she loves, and into which she puts much feeling, she has an epileptic fit.—The most remarkable case of the kind is one to which I have already referred on several occasions, that of Paul, a man of thirty. An observant young man, he dreads the phenomena which he describes in the following terms: " If I let myself go in the way of enjoyment, and especially in the enthusiastic enjoyment of an artistic pleasure, I have to pay for it. . . . Recently I was induced to become one of a crowd of persons who had gone to see an airplane display. The sight of these marvels of human genius had a great effect upon us ; every one was full of a patriotic frenzy ; and I am sure that no one in the crowd was more strongly moved than I was by the wonderful beauty of the sight. . . . Suddenly, it seemed to me that I recognised the sight, I felt that I had seen it all before, seen the very persons who were now near me, had heard the same sounds. . . . All these people had flocked together for some sinister purpose. . . . It was against me that these preparations were directed ;

something terrible was to happen to me ; a fall into an absolute and infinite void. . . . What, then, was the use of life, what was the use of acting as we do, since the sun will not go on shining for ever ? . . . I don't know what happened after that." What happened, can easily be guessed. He turned pale, made a few steps to get away, and fell down in an epileptic fit.

I need not return here to the consideration of the kinship between the depression of psychasthenics and an epileptic fit. This is a matter which I have studied at considerable length,[1] although as yet the matter is very little understood. Suffice it to say that intense enthusiasm, fully conscious perceptions, actions performed in complete awareness, attentively, and accompanied by marked pleasure—enthusiasms, perceptions, and actions characterised by a very high degree of psychological tension—are, in these cases, suddenly followed by a marked fall of tension. It may be contended that the initial excitation has itself been morbid ; that it was the beginning of the depression, the last flicker of a lamp that was just going out ; and that, consequently, the depression is not caused by the initial excitation, and would have ensued in the absence of that excitation. I shall not argue the point now, and shall merely say that, while the explanation might apply to certain cases like that of Noémi, these are many cases which it does not explain. Such persons know how to prove this for themselves. They are able to recognise the enthusiasm in its initial stages, and can avoid it or check it in good time, as I shall show in a subsequent chapter when I shall discuss the precautions they have to take. The point is that, when the patient adopts these precautions soon enough, he escapes the depression which would otherwise have ensued. Paul can ward off an epileptic fit if, as soon as he becomes aware of the sentiment of pseudo-recognition, he shuns the sight of that which is stirring his emotions. It is obvious that in such patients excessive psychological tension induces exhaustion, which may have serious consequences. This confirms our previous remarks anent the danger of actions which are on too high a plane.

The majority of psychasthenics, however, do not behave in this way. They make no attempt to achieve the action of triumph. In them, action is checked at an earlier stage. They tell us that they never experience true joy or true sorrow ; that sexual intercourse gives no pleasure and is not followed by a relaxation of tension ; that if they pray, they have no religious emotion ; and so on. The lack of the actions and the sentiments of triumph is precisely what makes the neuropath feel, in most cases, that his action is unfinished, although objectively considered it may appear to have been adequately performed.

A woman may seem to have completed the sexual act, and yet she will continue to feel that the act is unfinished, for there has been no pleasure and no relaxation of tension. We see the same sort of thing in the persons who can never feel that a piece of work is finished. Vkp. has never finished her housework ; Emile (m., 16) has never finished his translation; Vol. (f., 27) has never completed her confession. No doubt Léa and Lydia were able to make their joint household work after a fashion, but they were not wholly satisfied. This sentiment of incompleteness is very dangerous in these patients, who are apt to succumb to manias, tics, and obsessions, who so readily become "attached." They make incredible and absurd efforts to attain to the joy which always flees before them. I have given instances enough of the persistent search for enjoyment in exhausting masturbation, in adventures which are equally dangerous and sterile.

The traumatic memory is merely one of these disorders of the triumph and the liquidation. The patients who are affected by such traumatic memories have not been able to perform any of the actions characteristic of the stage of triumph. They are continually seeking this joy in action, continually endeavouring to achieve this liquidation which flees before them as they follow. To recognise and understand such phenomena is to realise the importance of this peculiar morbid disturbance whose nature has by degrees been disclosed to us under the name of traumatic memory. The symptoms studied in the previous chapter were disorders in the activation of the superior tendencies, the reflective and ergetic tendencies. Traumatic memories connected with the superior tendencies of the triumph have now been added to the enumeration of the disorders due to psychological depression.

7. Treatment by the Redintegration of Conscious-ness; by the Dissociation, the Assimilation, and the Liquidation of Memories.

The traumatic memory, when thus understood, plays an important part in a certain number of neuroses and psychoses. Whereas some doctors never trouble their heads about traumatic memories, and do not even know that these exist, and whereas others fancy them everywhere, there is a place for persons who take a middle course, and who believe they are able to detect the existence of traumatic memories in specific cases. The doctors comprising the last group need diagnostic rules. Unfortunately, the psychological phenomena now in question are still imperfectly known, and it is far from easy to give precise indications.

By elimination, as it were, we can secure a primary indication. A depression which seems accidental, which is not related to the subject's condition from youth upwards, and which does not depend upon an obvious change in his health, may be related to a memory of this kind. I think, moreover, it is important to exclude the causes of exhaustion which may be supplied by the subject's situation, by his customary environment; and among these, as we have seen, social influences play the chief part. When we can find no explanation in the subject's extant life, we are certainly entitled to delve into his past.

Régis and Hesnard are afraid that if we do this we shall risk attracting the patient's attention to the details of his life and to his fixed idea. I cannot wholly agree with their critisism. Obviously, such a study of the patient's past history has been compromised by foolish exaggerations. But exaggeration in the other direction would be just as bad. We might as well say that a surgeon must never touch a wound for fear of infecting it. Every one knows that a surgeon must put his fingers and instruments into a wound, but that his fingers and instruments must be clean. If the doctor is careful not to make up his mind beforehand that he will find a memory responsible for the whole illness, and if he is not obstinately determined that the memory of which he is in search must relate to a sexual happening, he will be able to make his examination tactfully and without unduly troubling the patient's mind.

A study of the patient's history is indispensable, and we must make it with the patient's own aid, since we have to make ourselves acquainted with his memories concerning this or that period of his life, have to note the way in which he describes them, have to ascertain the extent to which he has assimilated them. The psychoanalysts have done well in that they have understood the worth of the researches made by French physicians into this matter, and have imitated their French colleagues. When we recall how light-heartedly a diagnosis is often based solely upon a few obvious and imperfectly understood symptoms, without any attempt to study the psychological evolution which has originated these symptoms, we cannot but admire the minute investigations made by these German doctors into the mental and moral history of their patients.

In many cases, the patient himself draws our attention to his disquietudes concerning this or that period of his life. Again, the moment at which the symptoms have appeared, their rapid or gradual development after this or that happening, the fact that certain symptoms are always related to some specific phenomenon—such indications as these may put us upon the right track. Our suspicions may be confirmed by the patient's more or less complete amnesia as regards certain epochs or certain groups of phenomena ; or by delusions, hallucinations, phobias, day-dreams ; or by emotions which arise when we draw the patient's attention to such points. If we discover the sort of memory of which we are in search, we have next to ascertain what part it may be playing to-day. A good many distressful things may have happened to the patient, may have left a memory which stirs his emotions more or less, and yet may play no notable part to-day. We are only entitled to regard as traumatic memories, those memories which recur again and again at the present time, and which lead the patient to make efforts which are frequent, obvious, and competent to induce exhaustion.

I cannot repeat too often that much caution is necessary in this diagnostic investigation. It is doubtless true that traumatic memories are not always perfectly definite, and that they may sometimes be masked in various ways ; but we must not therefore feel that we are entitled to accept all kinds of easy-going explanations. Beyond question, dangerous memories may, in certain forms of hysteria, manifest themselves in the patient's crises or somnambulisms outside the field of normal consciousness, may assume the form of the subconscious; but we must be on our guard against the subconscious. I was one of the first to describe this aspect which can be assumed by certain psychological phenomena, one of the first to bring forward this notion of the subconscious; and I have sometimes been rather rueful while watching the development of the idea, while watching its undue success. In the studies of the spiritualists and the occultists, the subconscious has become a wonder-working principle of knowledge and action at a far higher level than that of our poor ordinary thought; in the studies of the psychoanalysts it has become the principle of all the neuroses, the god from the machine invoked to explain everything. I do not think that the subconscious is worthy of so much honour, and I believe that a single precaution will enable us to confine it to its proper role. A psychological phenomenon, which is always in reality a particular form of the subject's behaviour, must invariably be something which an observer can detect. Phenomena detached from the subject's normal consciousness certainly manifest themselves in somnambulism, automatic writing, movements, and words. It is proper to take note of these phenomena whenever they appear, and to turn them to account. What we have to shun is the subconscious which we never see, and which we can only construct imaginatively. The exaggerations which have discredited admirable studies must put us upon our guard against the hasty interpretations of those who are too ready to base their conclusions upon psychological motions which are still extremely tenuous.

The Redintegration of Consciousness.—In my early studies concerning traumatic memories (1889–1892), I drew attention to a remarkable fact, namely that in many cases the searching out of past happenings, the giving an account by the subject of the difficulties he had met with and the sufferings he had endured in connexion with these happenings, would bring about a signal and speedy transformation in the morbid condition, and would cause a very surprising cure. Marie's case was typical. (Vide supra, pp. 590–591.) In the somnambulist state, this young woman told me what she had never dared to confess to any one. At puberty she had been disgusted by menstruation, and had dreaded its onset. When the flow began, wishing to check it, she got into a cold bath. This had made her ill, and she had questioned herself a great deal concerning the seriousness of what she had done. The questionings continued until the time when she became affected with hysterical attacks, shivering fits, and the arrest of menstruation. Thenceforward, she ceased to think of the origin of these troubles. After she had made this disclosure, her fits of hysterics ceased, and normal menstruation was restored.[1] Ky. (f., 22) disclosed in the somnambulist state that she had been her father's mistress for a year, that she had suffered terribly for months from a dread of pregnancy, that at this time she had been on the watch for the most trifling sensations and had believed she could feel something abnormal between her legs whenever she tried to walk; then she had ceased to think about these things, but had become quite unable to walk. While she was relating the distressing incidents, and in proportion as she regained consciousness of the whole story, she gradually recovered the power of walking, and was soon well again.—Achille's delusions soon passed away after he had been able to tell me how he had been unfaithful to his wife while on a journey, how he had fancied that he had contracted venereal disease, and how he had dreaded his wife's anger.—Another case, a quaint one, which I published in 1893, was that of Lie (f., 18), who for two years had been subject to frequent and severe hysterical attacks, in which she would cry " Thieves ! " and " Help, Lucien ! " In her normal condition she was unable to explain the significance of these two exclamations. In the hypnotic state she gave a detailed account of how the house where she had lived in the country had been burned down, and how a gardener named Lucien had rescued her from the flames. (I subsequently obtained independent confirmation of this story.) When her memory of the happenings had been fully restored to the waking consciousness, her hysterical attacks ceased.[2]

In these earlier writings, I drew the inference, though

[1] L'automatisme psychologique, 1889, p. 439; Les accidents mentaux des hystériques, 1894, p. 62, second edition, 1911, p. 244.
[2] Névroses et idées fixes, vol. ii, p. 234.

with some surprise, that the memory was morbific because it was dissociated. It existed in isolation, apart from the totality of the sensations and the ideas which comprised the subject's personality; it developed in isolation, without control and without counterpoise; the morbid symptoms disappeared when the memory again became part of the synthesis that makes up individuality. I was glad to find, some years later, that Breuer and Freud had repeated these experiments, and that they accepted my conclusions without modification. In their first work on hysteria, these authorities said that they had noticed how the hysterical symptoms disappeared one after another, disappeared for good, when it had been possible to bring the exciting cause into the full light of day, and to reawaken the affective state which had accompanied it. Subsequently, Freud came to hold the view that all the symptoms depended upon a sexual excitation which had been diverted from its original aim, his conclusion being that the morbid symptoms would be dispelled by redirecting the patient's attention to the primary sexual phenomenon. To-day, most of Freud's disciples seem still to regard this method of treatment as essential.

The Dissociation of Memories.—This happy effect of the redintegration of consciousness seemed plain enough in certain cases, but it was not manifest in all. It could not be said that in every case of nervous disorder the trouble ceased as soon as it had been brought back into consciousness. There came under my observation a good many instances of traumatic memory which were extremely dangerous although there was no apparent disorder of the individual consciousness. Morton Prince rightly points out that when memories become subconscious it is because they conflict with the subject's other ideas and feelings. If we drag them back into a consciousness which will not tolerate them, they will soon be driven out again, and we shall have to begin the whole process once more. Various other considerations might be adduced to show that we are not justified in applying this method of treatment invariably and as a matter of course. In most cases, the discovery of the fixed idea is no more than the first step, and there will still be a great deal to do before we can lead the patient back to health.

Moreover, I have myself often had to combat, in my patients, traumatic memories which were not cured by the redintegration of consciousness. During the years 1894 to 1896 I repeatedly drew attention to the case of Justine. She had nursed patients dying of cholera, and for twenty years had suffered from a fixed idea of cholera, the idea assuming an amazingly vivid form. She repeatedly suffered from crises in which she saw the dead bodies of cholera patients; felt the symptoms of cholera, and realised them as far as possible; heard the bell tolling for the burial of those who had died of the disease, herself among the number; and so on. Either during hypnotic sleep or in the waking state, this patient had full consciousness of her symptoms and their origin, but her crises continued none the less.

To cure her, I tried to put in practice a very simple notion, one which would naturally occur to any one dealing with such patients. It is natural to think that the patient will promptly get well if he can simply forget what has happened. This is what we all of us try to do in such circumstances. I have already referred to what happens when we have received an unpleasant letter, and lack courage to answer it at once. We leave the letter on our writing-table, where it is a persistent occasion of discontent and effort. One fine day, perhaps after the lapse of a considerable time, we seize it and tear it up, saying: " Hang it all, I can't answer the thing. Damn the consequences! " This action, which is itself a decision and an adaptation, is not achieved until after a certain time has elapsed. Time reduces the importance of past happenings. In this case it brings a season when the letter has lost much of its interest, so that to tear it up has become easy. Lazy people do not act at once, but they act after a time, when action has become easier. This is what happens in our patients when, as we sometimes see, they are cured by the influence of time— for time is a master craftsman, in psychotherapy as well as in other fields. There are plenty of memories which have been traumatic, but are no longer traumatic. They have ceased to be traumatic, either because the subject has renounced the attempt to make the appropriate adaptations; or because he has, at long last, succeeded in making the adaptations by " taking his time." It is not so simple as might be supposed to forget a happening immediately, without awaiting the effects of time. " To know how to forget," wrote Taine, " is a great thing, whether for nations or for individuals." It is knowledge which neuropaths lack, or at any rate it is knowledge which they are unable to apply. These patients who seem to have so little memory when it behoves them to acquire new knowledge, will retain for years the memory of some unhappiness, or of some unlucky adventure, and will think of it night and day. The faculty of voluntary oblivion would be a precious discovery in psychiatry. The importance of the subject gives considerable interest to these tentative experiments in treatment by the destruction of memories.

At first sight it may seem that we should try to suppress undesirable memories by suggestion. If suggestion can induce systematised anaesthesia and systematised amnesia, can it not rid us of a troublesome memory ? The results of such attempts are discouraging. A suggestion of the kind will succeed only in a few persons, only in those who are extremely suggestible ; and even in them the effect will be fugitive. The conditions are most unfavourable to suggestion. The essence of suggestion is the development of an isolated idea which does not encounter opposing ideas in the field of consciousness. But where an unpleasant memory is concerned, the suggestion of oblivion immediately awakens an antagonistic idea, and for this reason the requisite distraction is very difficult to secure. Still, in young and docile subjects, by the frequent repetition of the suggestion, we may succeed in annulling the memory.

In most cases I have had to abandon the attempt at simple negative suggestion, and have found it necessary to complicate the method a little. I regard a memory, and especially a fixed idea, as an artifact, as a system comprising a number of associated psychological phenomena.[1] Its factors are visual images, images attached to the other senses, a few motor tendencies, and, above all, words. In many cases, a fixed idea is incarnated in words, and the words call up all the rest. I have attempted to break up this system, to demolish it stone by stone; this is what I call the *dissociation of a fixed idea*. In my study of the dissociation of the fixed idea of cholera, I found it necessary to suppress in detail and by degrees the sound of the tolling bell, the sight of the corpses, the smell of these,

---

[1] Histoire d'une idée fixe, " Revue Philosophique," 1894, vol. i, p. 121 ; Névroses et idées fixes, 1898, vol. i, p. 167.

and then the very name of cholera—these being the various factors of the fixed idea. Sometimes I found it useful to effect a kind of substitution, to induce hallucinations whereby the scenes imagined by the subject were transformed. The task was long and difficult, but in the end I was able to dispel a hallucinatory fixed idea from which the patient had suffered for more than twenty years. In the same connexion I should like to refer to the good results achieved in two girls by the dissociation of dreams that were giving rise to intractable nocturnal incontinence. Jules Janet has given ample proof that nocturnal incontinence of urine is usually connected with dreams. These dreams may be of three kinds : sometimes they are strictly urinary ; sometimes they are sexual ; sometimes they are merely dreams which arouse strong emotion, such as terror. The dreams in my own two cases belonged to the third category. In one of the girls, the dreams always related to quarrels with her step-mother ; in the other, they reproduced the tragical end of her little dog, which had been run over before her very eyes by a tram. These dreams, reproduced in the hypnotic trance, were gradually dissociated, and the incontinence was completely cured.

I regard the method by which Zy. was cured as belonging to the same category. She was a woman of forty-five in whom awakening was intensely distressful, coming as it always did as a sequel of a persistently reproduced dream in which she was once again watching her son's death.—The contracture of the shoulder to which I referred a few pages back was persistent in its recurrence until I succeeded in dissociating the memory of the omnibus which had brushed the patient's shoulder. This dissociation was achieved in twelve sittings.—Identical was the method of cure in the cases of the young women who suffered from crises reproducing scenes of rape. In one of them, only four sittings were requisite.—In the case of Cam. (f., 26), the contractures from which she suffered reappeared again and again after having been dispelled, and she was not definitively cured until I had been able to modify her memory of the death of her two children. I had to deprive her of the little photographs which she had sewn into her dress, and I cured her by ridding her of her fixed ideas.

I may recall here a method of treatment already mentioned in the chapter on suggestion. In hysterical young women, when they are not very intelligent and not very well educated, it is amazingly easy, sometimes, to modify the love passion. All that is requisite is, by means of simple affirmations,' to transform the image of the well-beloved, so that a doubt arises in the mind whenever they think of him. In one of my earlier books I recorded the remarkable case of Vz. (f., 28), who was suffering from hysterical delirium after a disappointment in love, but was speedily cured when an irreverent suggestion had equipped her lover with a bestial face.

To sum up, I find in my notebooks the reports of twenty-six cases in which this method of treatment by the dissociation of memories gave good results.

But the method has grave drawbacks. It is unlikely to succeed except in very suggestible hysterics; it is tedious, as a rule, and its application is difficult. The destruction of the memory is imperfect. There will remain memories or fragments of memories dissociated from the personality, and these will be likely to cause symptoms at a later date. Even when the operation of psychological surgery seems to be completely successful, it will leave a gap in the mind, sometimes a large gap, and this may eventually prove serious. People are not sufficiently aware that those who have suffered from some form of mental trouble at an earlier date are apt, even though ostensibly cured, to retain undesirable traces in the form of a psychological scar. Dentists know that their patient was in childhood ill at some particular age when they detect a disturbance or malformation in a tooth which was developing at that particular age. Some day we shall be able to infer that a grown man is affected with disorders of this or that social sentiment, this or that sexual tendency, this or that religious or scientific idea, because he was ailing at the period of life when the tendencies in question are formed in normal individuals. Our treatment creates such mental scars; it is but a makeshift.

Assimilation and Liquidation.—The psychological study of traumatic memories enables us to devise a more rational method of treatment. The memory has only become traumatic because the reaction to the happening has been badly effected. Either because of a depression already induced by other causes, or else because of a depression induced then and there by the

¹ Névroses et idées fixes, 1898, vol. ii, p. 134.

emotion aroused by the incident, the subject has been unable to achieve, or has but partially achieved, the assimilation which is the internal adaptation of the individuality to the event. This process of adaptation he continues to attempt, but is unable to complete, and he therefore becomes exhausted ; but sometimes, unaided, he achieves complete adaptation after months or years, and then undergoes a spontaneous cure. Our business is to help him in the work of assimilation, so that he can effect it speedily. Just as, in another method of treatment, we dispel symptoms by helping the subject to perform the outwardly directed actions demanded by extant situations, so now we must help them to perform internal actions related to past happenings.

The latter process is much more difficult : first of all, because it is far less easy for us to perform the actions on behalf of the patient, as we can do when our business is to modify the extant objective situation ; and, secondly, because the science of psychology is still in its infancy, and cannot as yet furnish us with anything more than the vaguest notions concerning the actions which have to be performed to effect the complete assimilation of a past happening, so that the mind may cease to trouble itself about the matter.

" When we have made a mistake or done a foolish thing," says Forel, " we must hasten to put matters right, to repair everything that can be repaired, to take precautions against doing the thing again ; and then cry quits. We ought to do the same where we are concerned with the mistakes of others." [1] The familiar phrases " to get used to a thing," " to forget and forgive," " to give up," " to resign oneself," and the like, are ostensibly descriptions of simple phenomena of consciousness. But in reality these expressions denote a complicated totality of actions some of which have to be performed, and others of which have to be avoided ; together with new attitudes which have to be adopted—all being actions which liquidate the situation and enable us to resign ourselves to it.

Though this is very difficult of accomplishment, there are certain desirable actions which may be pointed out to the patient, and which the doctor may help the patient to perform. Emma has been seriously ill ever since the rupture of relations with her lover. You will say that she has not been able to

---

[1] L'âme et le système nerveux, 1906, p. 311.

resign herself to the separation. Maybe! But this lack of resignation consists in a series of actions which she continues to perform and which we have to help her to discontinue. She persists in trying to see the man again, she is always haunting his house, or paying him a visit, only to be met with a rebuff ; if ever she meets him, she adopts a beseeching or disconsolate attitude ; she is always thinking out ways and means of winning his affections once more ; in imagination she builds up the sort of life she might lead with him ; and so on. " I have always been very stubborn," says she, " I have always succeeded in doing what I set my heart on. . . . I never thought that if I had a lover, matters would take such a turn. . . . I simply cannot refrain from trying to arrange things as I think they should be. . . ." This obstinacy is frequently found among persons of feeble character ; they cannot change an action, cannot stop an action when once it is begun, even if the circumstances which led to its inception have completely changed. The doctor has to help such a woman as Emma to cease from performing these ridiculous actions ; he must help her to learn to perform others ; he must see to it that she adopts another attitude of mind. To forget the past is, in reality, to change one's behaviour in the present. As soon as Emma has been able to adopt this new kind of behaviour it matters little if she retains a verbal memory of her mishap, for she is cured of her neuropathic disorders.—Another woman is suffering from similar troubles though, perhaps, in a somewhat cruder form. She is for ever awaiting the advent of her lover, who never comes ; she gets ready to receive him ; she refuses to look at any one else. When I succeeded in making her burn his letters and his gifts, cease to keep her unending watch for his return, and consent to see other people, she announced that she had quite forgotten the scene during which the engagement had been broken off.

Irène's case is of special interest because her absurd behaviour was so out of place in the circumstances, and because of the lacunae in her interior assimilation which found expression in her amnesia. After much labour I was able to make her reconstruct the verbal memory of her mother's death. From the moment I succeeded in doing this, she could talk about the mother's death without succumbing to crises or being afflicted with hallucinations ; the assimilated happening had ceased to be traumatic. Doubtless so complex a phenomenon cannot be wholly explained by such an interpretation. Assimilation constitutes no more than one element in a whole series of modified varieties of behaviour which I shall deal with in the sequel under the name of " excitation." Irène, under the influence of the work which I made her do, threw off her depression, "stimulated" herself, and became capable of bringing about the necessary liquidation. The problems will crop up once more when we come to consider aesthesiogenism ; suffice it, here, to study the fact of the assimilation of an event, and the importance of such assimilation. Irène was cured because she succeeded in performing a number of actions of acceptation, of resignation, of rememorisation, of setting her memories in order, and so on ; in a word, she was able to complete the assimilation of the event.

The treatment of traumatic memories by the work of assimilation has only been applied to a limited number of cases ; I think I may say that it has been responsible for the cure of about a dozen of my patients. It sometimes entails many sittings, and is fraught with difficulties ; but it has the advantage of not necessitating the use of hypnotism, and it responds far better than the latter to the needs of the problem.

This is not the place for a detailed study of the matter, for it raises the problems of action, of education, and of excitation, and these I intend to study in a subsequent chapter.

8. TREATMENT BY DISCHARGE.

Local Discharge.—A phrase frequently used in the writings of Freud and his pupils implies, at times, a different outlook upon the treatment of traumatic memories. The complex which has come into existence in connexion with the event is, they say, " charged with affect," it has " an emotive charge." This charge must be expended, " abreaction " must be achieved, and the process is difficult owing to the repression into the subconscious. The aim of our treatment must be to facilitate the discharge. I regard the idea as a very interesting one, but I shall not try to expound it as understood in the Freudian system, for I think that Freud's exposition is vague, and I cannot attempt to discuss his terminology. All I propose is to summarise the way in which I myself understand the phenomena to which he refers, and the way in which I have set them forth for a good many years now in my teaching anent mental energy and psychological tension. These cursory reflections are not presented as explanations or even as hypotheses ; they are merely conventional expressions for the description of extremely intricate psychological phenomena of which we are only just beginning to catch a glimpse.

In this connexion, I shall rarely use such terms as " quantity of affect," " emotive charge " etc., for I do not understand them clearly, and in my own writings the word emotion is used in another sense.[1] I shall confine myself to the terms " mental energy," and " psychological tension," which have already been defined more than once. As I have said several times in this book, the various tendencies are not only endowed with a tension proportional to their hierarchic grade and to the degree of activation they can attain ; they are also equipped with psychological energy. By this I mean that by being activated they can give rise to movements which are more or less vigorous, rapid, and durable. The elementary and old tendencies have, as a rule, a great deal of energy ; the higher-grade and recently acquired tendencies have usually less energy. Thus pain (the tendency to rid oneself of things), fear (the tendency towards flight), anger (the tendency to attack), hunger, and the sexual tendency, usually have a great deal of energy ; but reflective beliefs and scientific ideas are, in most cases, scantily equipped with energy.

This energy may assume either of two forms. It may be latent energy ; energy in reserve, or capitalised energy, if the phrase be permitted. In that case, the energy is inconspicuous, and we do not know clearly in which psychological phenomena it plays a part ; but its part must, none the less, be important ; a latent tendency is far from being a tendency of no account. On the other hand, the energy is kinetic when the tendency has been awakened, and is undergoing more or less complete activation. The energy has been drawn from the reserve, has been mobilised ; it manifests itself in the form of a number of complete or incomplete actions which it tends to produce. Agitation is the expression of energy which has already been mobilised and is ready to act.

When an event occurs and necessitates a reaction, this

[1] Cf. La définition de l'émotion, " Revue Neurologique," December 30, 1909.

reaction is partly effected by the construction of a new tendency (not a very powerful one), this being the role of adaptation ; but it is mainly effected by the awakening of one of the latent tendencies which have been antecedently organised. According to circumstances, the event may awaken nothing more than recently acquired and feeble tendencies, or it may awaken long-established and powerful tendencies. If it arouses the tendencies towards pain, flight, anger, hunger, or love, the tendency to react will be promptly charged with a large measure of vital energy. The tendency thus charged will press for activation ; it will inhibit, or rather, canalise, other and weaker tendencies, especially those endowed with only a low tension ; if it be imperfectly adapted to the situation, it may induce a great deal of agitation and give rise to much disorder.

The tendency may lose its charge, may " discharge " itself, in various ways. One method of discharge is by the production of many vigorous, rapid, and long-continued movements ; but it would seem that this form of discharge is a slow one, especially in the case of strongly charged tendencies. It may be canalised by a tendency which has a higher tension ; nothing can discharge a tendency more effectively than a high-tension action effected at its expense. It is probable, as we are coming more and more to see, that the more highly a tendency is charged, the more essential is it that it shall be counterposed by a higher-grade tendency in order to effect canalisation. Finally, when studying the last degree of the activation of tendencies, we have been led to postulate the stage of triumph, to assume that in this stage there occurs a special canalisation of the energies that have been mobilised but unutilised, and a new carrying of energies to reserve in the latent form. I must apologise once more for the inadequacy of this summary statement. I hope, later, to present the ideas somewhat differently when I come to publish my lectures. As the exposition stands, its only value is that it has enabled me since I began my teaching career to expound somewhat more clearly a number of morbid phenomena.

Let us consider the individuals who are already depressed and in a state of hypotension, but who have not at the time of examination any crisis of obsession. They are comparatively calm, but they dread a crisis. " I have to be extremely careful," such a patient will say, " to dismiss the thoughts which enter my mind. I must not allow anything to stir me, for if I do, I shall have a most distressing crisis." What is it that they are afraid of ? What happens when some occurrence, or some chance word uttered in their presence, induces a crisis ? The occurrence or the word awakens in them a tendency which is vigorous, ready to be mobilised, in a state of erection ; it arouses the dread of a disease, the fear of hell, the tendency to over-scrupulousness, and so on. The awakening of this vigorous tendency endows the subject with activity competent to produce powerful, numerous, long-lasting movements ; gives the subject, if you like to phrase it thus, a strongly charged idea. A normal individual would be delighted, would turn the opportunity to good account, would canalise the energy usefully. The persons we are considering have too low a tension to be able to control, utilise, and recuperate this energy ; they do not know what to make of it, and they fall a prey to agitation. The vigorous tendency which has been awakened undergoes activation in the form of terror, remorse, interminable self-inquisition. The subject struggles desperately against it, and is exhausted by this distressing struggle.

One of my patients made an interesting remark in this connexion. " If at the very beginning of the impression which I dread so much, I pay careful attention to the matter, if I reflect about it, if I talk about it for a long time with some intelligent person who makes everything clear to me, I do not have a crisis. What is dangerous to me is the hearing of some chance word the significance of which does not instantly strike me, but which goes on working in the depths." We have already recorded a similar observation in connexion with the mechanism of suggestion by distraction. In other words, the energy which has been awakened and mobilised is not at first very large in quantity ; if it can be promptly expended or canalised, if it can be assimilated even by counterposing to it a high tension, there will be no crisis of obsession and no suggestion. But if the energies undergo mobilisation for a long time before the subject attends to them, they will accumulate, and the subject's tension will not be adequate to control them. A crisis will occur.

Let us consider the same patients when a crisis has ensued. How do they succeed in obtaining relief ? One of these patients said to me : " A little time after the onset of a crisis of obsession [this patient was obsessed with the thought of syphilis], when it had already become serious, it occurred to me that I would' go to see a relative of mine. The visit was extremely distressing to me, for I told him about all the follies I had committed, the follies which had exposed me to the risk of syphilis. I told him all kinds of things which did not concern him in the least, and which it cost me a great deal to tell him. From one point of view I regret very much having made a fool of myself in this way; but, from another point of view, I have no reason to complain, for this visit and this confession put an end to my crisis, and thus spared me a great deal of suffering." It is plain that, in his absurd and distressing confession, the patient must have expended the energetic charge of the morbid tendency, must have canalised the energy. This immediately relieved him of his distress.—Zob. (f., 50), intelligent, but extremely nervous, and liable to severe agitation after any emotion, knows that she can discharge her emotion, can rid herself of it, by drawing a picture or writing a poem. " I get up during the night and write a poem. Then I feel quite well again, and I can get to sleep." Unfortunately, this means is not at every one's disposal, but less talented persons can achieve similar results. In a great many of my patients I have been able to convince myself of the good effects of such canalisation.

It is probable that all the methods of treatment previously described as having an effect upon traumatic memories act in the same way. I am thinking of researches into the past life, avowals, efforts to express and to remember. These were, substantially, difficult, arduous, costly actions. In this connexion, I may refer to the remarkable case of Kl. (f., 45). She first came under my care fifteen years ago, when she was suffering from grave depression with obsessive crises which sometimes lasted for months. The crises were of a complicated and remarkable character, but I shall not here give a detailed account of them, since I have described them fully in an earlier work.[1] Their central feature was an anxious questioning anent a strange problem. " This birth-mark which my youngest child has upon his little behind—is it a proof that my husband is the child's father, seeing that he has a similar birth-mark upon his thigh ? " This question was, of course, connected with memories of a love affair that occurred before the child

---

[1] Les obsessions et la psychasthénie, first edition, 1903, vol. i, p. 441.

was born, and with moral situations which had been imperfectly liquidated in the subject's mind. By various methods, and in especial by assisting the patient to assimilate this story, I was able to promote a liquidation (though probably an imperfect one), and to check the crises for a time. But every two or three years, as a sequel of fatigue, the crisis returns. At first, on these occasions, Kl. is disinclined to regard the matter as serious. " It will soon pass off," she says to herself ; and though she is really aware that the malady is running its usual course, she takes no action for a few days, until she has relapsed into a condition of complete abulia attended by doubts and obsessive ideas. Then she writes to me, for she does not live in Paris, and she has to make a long journey in order to consult me. In her abulic condition, this journey is a very troublesome matter for her. Still, she comes to see me. When I ask her what she complains of, and why she has had to take so long a journey, she weeps, laments, and is unable to explain. She says : " You know quite well what the matter is. The same old trouble. I've told you a hundred times."—" I am afraid I have forgotten."—" But you must know ; you wrote it all down."—" I can't put my hand on my notes. Please be so good as to tell me once more."—Despite the utmost efforts on both sides, she cannot put into words what we both want her to tell me, and she goes away in despair. Two or three consultations are necessary before she can make a fresh avowal of her obsessive idea, concerning the birth of the child and concerning the birth-mark. While her phrases are being formed with great difficulty, the patient has laughing fits, twitchings, and contortions, and in the end she weeps copiously. She then feels bewildered and extremely tired, but is incredibly happy. " I am freed from my fixed ideas ; I no longer question myself about anything ; people's heads don't look funny any more ; I have ceased to be a mere machine." The transformation is a very rapid one, and (this being rare) it is durable. I can safely send her home, for I know by long experience that the crisis is finished. May we not say that the tendency created by the memory had been recharged, but that the journey, the arduous efforts to make a fresh avowal, and the labour requisite to express herself, have effected a discharge ?

This idea is an interesting one, and can be effectively associated with that dynamic psychology of energy and tension which seems to me to be the most fruitful to-day in clinical psychiatry. It is not completely satisfactory unless we link it on in some way to our previous studies. When the traumatic memory has been discharged by the avowal, why does it not promptly become recharged ? In their agitation, these patients have already performed, apropos of their fixed idea, a number of arduous and costly actions which have given them no more than a temporary relief and which have been rapidly followed by a recurrence of the agitation. If the avowal is nothing more than a costly action of the same kind, why should it bring about a definitive discharge ? My view is that there has not been simply a discharge. What has taken place is a discharge by a high-tension operation ; an assimilation which has liquidated the situation, has recuperated the energies, has carried them to reserve, and has checked their mobilisation. Kl., who is already familiar with the treatment, believes what we have made up our minds she is to believe regarding the birth of her child ; she accepts the decision, and this puts an end to her exhausting expenditure. We have always to get back to the high-tension action which restores the proper utilisation of energies.

Thus the notion of the discharge does not merely supplement the foregoing, but superadds interesting psychological conceptions, and, perhaps, valuable practical methods. It shows us that the danger does not only lie in the existence, the qualitative construction, of the tendency, but also in the energy of which the tendency can avail itself. It teaches us that the act of liquidation, the act of assimilation, is more difficult and demands a higher tension when we have to do with strongly charged tendencies. It shows that these delvings into the past, these distressing avowals, are not useless, for they serve to weaken the insurgent tendency and to facilitate the act of assimilation. Such conceptions are still extremely vague, but they will become more and more important as time goes on.

General Discharge.—These reflections anent the discharge of a particular tendency, anent a discharge which may be described as local, will be better understood if they are supplemented by a study of the general discharge and the part it plays in the neuroses.

It would be very instructive to consider what might be termed the paradoxes of agitation. In one of the foregoing chapters, when discussing treatment by rest, I pointed out that an increase of energy is not always advantageous to a neuropath, who may be worse after a good night or after a course of tonic treatment.

The converse phenomenon is even more interesting. I am thinking of the apparent improvement which a neuropath may exhibit, as far as the neurosis is concerned, when the organism is greatly enfeebled and when its energies are reduced. The very last case which has come under my notice is typical in this respect among a legion. Mba. (m., 35) had for several months been suffering from a severe crisis. He was incapable of action ; was tortured by doubts, feelings of unworthiness, a sense of shame, scruples of all kinds, obsession with the thought of death and madness ; in a word, his state was one of anxiety and intense agitation. Then he had a sharp attack of quinsy, the temperature ranging for several days between 102.5° and, 104°. For a fortnight he could take hardly any food, and had to endure an extremely painful local treatment. During this time, and after the acute stage was over, he was so debilitated that he could hardly stand ; but as far as his mental condition was concerned there was an amazing change for the better. His anxieties were dispelled. Although his life was really in danger, he was untroubled by thoughts of death or of madness. He had perfect confidence in his doctor, and was Spartan in his endurance of the painful local treatment. " This physical pain is a trifle when compared with my former moral sufferings." He found no difficulty in making up his mind about matters of importance. To cut a long story short, all the symptoms of the neurosis seemed to have disappeared. The mental disturbances did not manifest themselves again until three weeks after the throat trouble had been cured, and when the physical strength of the patient had been reestablished.

Here are some other instances of the kind.—On several occasions Madame Z. had severe attacks of broncho-pneumonia, so that her life was endangered for weeks at a time. Invariably, the serious organic disease was accompanied by a marked improvement in the neuropathic condition.—We often find that an attack of influenza, typhoid, or erysipelas will quiet nervous disorders in such patients. I need not give special instances to show how melancholics are temporarily cured by an attack of typhoid ; how patients suffering from obsessions and anxiety will remain perfectly tranquil during febrile disorders ; how epileptics will be free from fits during an attack of pneumonia or one of the infective fevers, and will still be untroubled during the phase of convalescence. When these facts forced themselves on my attention, and more especially when I had studied the case of Marceline, I was led to infer that in some instances the improvement was due to the fever, to an excitation connected with the febrile intoxication.[1] But this explanation will not apply to all cases, for the improvement is likewise manifest during convalescence, when the patients are free from fever and are no longer suffering from febrile intoxication, but when they are still debilitated. In all these cases, the enfeeblement would seem to be a determinant of the mental improvement.

During the few days before menstruation, most women pass through a period characterised by greater vitality. The phenomenon is probably connected with changes in the ovarian incretion. However this may be, as an actual fact there is a gain in weight at such times, as I myself (following up the investigations of others) have been able to show by remarkable graphs. At these times, too, most of the bodily functions are more active than usual. Conversely, just after menstruation, and especially when the flow has been profuse, we note a loss of weight and obvious debility. In certain neuropaths, the mental condition exhibits similar waves ; there is improvement before menstruation and increased debility afterwards. But the cycle does not always take this form. In a number of instances, neuropathic women pass through a bad period, when all their symptoms are aggravated, during the days just before menstruation, whereas their tranquillity is restored during the phase of enfeeblement which follows menstruation. Irène is subject to floodings when she menstruates, and some of these losses have been so abundant as to endanger her life. But after such severe menorrhagia, we note that she has been freed from distressing agitations, that she has recovered mental tranquillity, and that she can once more eat and sleep satisfactorily.

[1] L'état mental des hystériques, second edition, 1911, pp. 558 and 609.

A second group of phenomena may be compared with the foregoing. We shall see in the following chapters that convulsive seizures, weeping fits, attacks of migraine, etc., are usually bad signs. They are signs of a relaxation of tension, for they characterise the transition from a higher state of psychological tension to a lower. In all cases they are notable expenditures, they are exhaustions, reductions of energy. Why is it that in other cases, and sometimes in these same subjects, we are able to note a certain improvement after such critical phenomena ? Much further study is requisite concerning the varieties of these crises and the modifications of activity they induce. I have myself collected so much information bearing on the matter that I cannot consider it all here, and must reserve what I have to say for a systematic study of the oscillations of the mind. Enough, now, to summarise the general impression left on me by these cases. How frequently we notice that patients affected by various agitations, suffering from anxiety, and more or less delirious, will have convulsive crises in which they will howl and struggle for hours. Then the crisis will pass off, leaving the patient tired no doubt, but with a delicious sense of calm, so that he will be far more happy, and indeed more normal, than before the crisis.

Violent exercise, whether undertaken voluntarily or otherwise, may have effects similar to those of such crises. An instructive case is that of Gt. (m., 30). Physically, he is a very robust young man, but he is poorly equipped with moral energy, has a low psychological tension, and becomes affected with grave depression when there are any changes in the circumstances of his life, or when he is affected by any emotion. He then becomes gloomy, hesitant, and filled with doubts ; he suffers from sentiments of incompleteness, manias of interrogation, and anxieties ; he can neither eat nor sleep. He knows quite well the remedy he needs, for it is one he has found useful again and again. If circumstances permit, he goes for a tremendously long walk or a long bicycle ride ; or he takes a motor car to pieces and cleans it ; or he does some other hard manual work for several hours. When he is dropping with fatigue, he feels tranquillised, is freed from mental disturbance, eats a hearty dinner, digests his meal satisfactorily, and sleeps like a top.

Certain authorities, a very few, have turned their attention to these matters, and have tried to give a physiological explanation. Féré used to say that the nervous system cannot endure a high tension, and therefore discharged itself as soon as the tension rises. Deschamps says what amounts to the same thing. He writes : " The nerve centres cannot endure a tension exceeding a certain level, which is always the same for any particular state of the energies. . . . The subject must immediately expend the energy supplied by his motor. Failing this, excitation [agitation] ensues, for the nerve centres cannot bear too high a tension." [1] I think that we gain nothing and risk much by arbitrarily translating such psychological phenomena into physiological terms. For a good many years, therefore, I have tried to furnish them with an accurate psychological expression, setting out from clear definitions of psychological tension and mental energy. This was the foundation of my extensive studies concerning the hierarchy of the tendencies, and concerning the degrees of activation.

Mental or psychological energy, by which I mean the strength, number, and duration of movements, must not be confounded with psychological tension, which is characterised by the degree of activation of actions, and by the hierarchical gradation. It is probable that in normal behaviour, in well-balanced individuals, a definite proportion must be maintained between the available energy and the tension. If the tension is lowered when there is a great deal of energy at work, the result is agitation and disorder. Let me illustrate this imperfectly understood law by a comparison, Persons who are not trained to orderly and thrifty habits do not know how to behave when a large sum of money is suddenly placed at their disposal. The results are often disastrous. A poor woman said to me : " It was my employer's fault that I got so frightfully drunk. He gave me seventy francs all at once. Twenty-five francs all at once is as much as I can stand. What could you expect ? I did not know what to do with all that money, so I spent it on drink." When the psychological tension is high, it does not matter if there is an abundance of available energy, for this can be utilised in the performance of high-grade actions, which are advantageous and demand considerable expenditure, while in the last stages of activation, energy can be carried to reserve. But when the tension is low,

[1] Les maladies de l'énergie, 1908, p. 93.

it is better that only a small quantity of energy should be available. It is therefore a good thing, in many cases, that the superabundant energy should be dissipated in one way or another, so that a proper proportion between energy and tension shall be restored. No doubt, when the tension is low, and when the balance is restored thanks to the reduction of energy by a discharge, only low-grade activities will remain possible, but these will be better for the subjects, will be less dangerous. Such is the general notion of the discharge, and we shall find it helpful in the explanation of many morbid phenomena.

This explanation, given here in outline merely, enables us to understand some of the before-mentioned facts, such as the improvement which results in certain patients after violent activities, and the urge that some persons have towards activities of the kind. A discharge may be effected by a tremendously long walk, by fugues, dromomanias, quarrels, tantrums, excessive activity of various kinds. A discharge may also be effected by way of distressing actions, actions that arouse emotion, or by efforts to escape danger, or by acts of devotion. Many of these forms of behaviour are, from our present outlook, comparable to convulsive seizures. Consequently, the improvement that results from such actions—the disappearance of agitation, the onset of a sense of tranquillity, and the restoration of certain activities—may be regarded as due to a reduction of the amount of available energy, so that the energy becomes proportional to a low psychological tension. When, in the next volume, we come to consider the effect of actions, and to study the excitation they induce, we shall often be confronted by a difficult problem. We shall have to ask ourselves whether the advantages resulting from some particular action are the direct outcome of the stimulating effect of the action, or are simply due to the fact that the action has brought about a discharge. For the nonce, it is enough to indicate the importance and the mechanism of improvement due to discharge.

From the foregoing observations it would be possible to deduce the principles of a method of treatment by discharge, and I am surprised that no school of practitioners advocating such a method has come into existence. Charcot had already noticed that it was a good thing for certain patients to have convulsive crises, and he even went so far as to advise that in such cases a crisis should be induced. A good many authorities have pointed out that when we have to deal with a sufferer from agitation we must not be too ready to advise self-restraint, and that we shall often do well to let the patient expend his energies. I think that the rationale of certain forms of drug treatment, and especially of treatment with bromides, is to be found along these lines. Such substances would appear to induce a form of intoxication whereby the energies are lowered, so that the patient is tranquillised by a phenomenon akin to the discharge.

However this may be, the deliberate enfeeblement of the neuropath is not, as yet, a recognised curative procedure ; or, at any rate, a general expenditure of energy will only be recommended in very exceptional instances. Still, the possibility of employing such a method, and the recognition that it can certainly be useful in some cases, throw considerable light upon our recent study of local discharges in cases where traumatic memories are at work. We see that in some instances it will do the patient good to dissipate part of his energies, for he will then find less difficulty in controlling, utilising, canalising, and carrying over to reserve such energy as still remains at his disposal. Before the discharge, he exhausts himself in the continued effort to mobilise energies which were not doing him any good. It is actually an economy for him to let some of his energy run to waste, for when this expenditure has been made once for all, he will be saved from having to make additional and more serious expenditure in the future. The study of traumatic memories, and of treatment by liquidation, has thus led us to consider the more general problems connected with the discharge and the question of its importance in psychological therapeutics.

9. PSYCHOLOGICAL ECONOMIES.

From the psychological outlook, this chapter upon moral liquidation or treatment by moral disinfection, and the two foregoing chapters dealing respectively with treatment by rest and treatment by isolation, seem to me to present close analogies. I think, therefore, they can be classed under one head as treatment by economy.

Most neuropaths are depressed or exhausted persons, or

have been this at the outset of their illness, and the mental disturbances from which they suffer are the outcome of their depression. To recur to the comparison with pecuniary affairs, all these illnesses are, substantially, different forms of bankruptcy and ruin, but the causes of the bankruptcy are manifold. Some of the patients appear to have adequate resources, and their ruin has resulted from a persistent expenditure over ʾand above that required to meet the ordinary demands of life. It is the supplementary expenditure which has been disproportionate to the income. The reason for the supplementary expenditure has been the indefinite persistence of an unliquidated affair. The subject retains an interest in a concern which has got into difficulties, which demands very large and continuous expenditure, and will never return any profit. This is the way in which we have regarded traumatic memories, and a great many fixed ideas. The explanation will guide our treatment. We must stop the leak; the only aim of the methods of moral disinfection is to put an end to the fruitless expenditure. Since the patient cannot achieve this unaided, we must help him to liquidate the concern which is ruining him. When we have done so, his income will suffice for his current expenditure. Thus the methods of treatment which we have been considering under the name of methods of moral liquidation are nothing but methods of economising.

The importance of these methods is great, for a good many illnesses are the outcome of exhaustion dependent upon a persistent failure to achieve internal assimilation. In numerous cases a cure can be effected by one or other of the methods we have just been studying. When selecting from my own notebooks the cases I regarded as having been cured by liquidation, I was extremely critical, and I would not include in the list any patients in whom the depression was more or less completely independent of genuine traumatic memories. That is why I said that I had records of only fifty cases. Still, it would be easy to add a much larger number of instances in which patients suffering from various forms of illness have been relieved by moral liquidation, patients whose crises have been cut short in this way. When we have to do with young patients, when the liquidation is effected before the exhaustion has become profound and definitive, the cure and the restoration of energy may be complete. Some of these patients have remained free from crises for years and years.

But we must not delude ourselves as to the possibilities of this method ; we must avoid the exaggerations of the disciples of Sigmund Freud. Excessive expenditure is not the only cause of financial ruin, and expenditure outside the domain of normal budgeting is not the sole cause of psychological depression. When we come across some poor devil who has not a penny to his name and has never had one, we must not solemnly declare that he is destitute because he continues to lavish money upon a mistress, or because he is secretly keeping up a racing stable ; we must not insist that if he will only suppress these extravagances he will become well-to-do. There are, alas, many other causes of poverty besides unthriftiness. Even in the cases in which the illness was occasioned by a particular happening, the symptoms may, after a while, become completely independent of that happening. The mind has been exhausted by a fruitless struggle ; and, even if in the end the struggle be abandoned, the exhaustion may persist. To return to the financial simile, let us suppose that a person has been ruined by keeping up a second and irregular establishment secretly, quite apart from his regular household ; if the irregular expenditure be not cut off soon enough, his ruin will be complete, even though the leak be ultimately stopped. Such cases are, perhaps, exceptional. But in a great many instances the exhaustion from which the patient suffers is not due to any memory of a past happening ; it is the outcome of actual events which recur from day to day. The patient, though a poor man, has an income which would suffice to meet moderate demands, but circumstances compel him to keep up too costly an establishment.

If bankruptcy and poverty are to be avoided, we shall have to curtail the ordinary expenditure of everyday life. That is what the doctor tries to do when he forbids action of any kind and immobilises the patient in bed. Theoretically considered, the plan seems satisfactory, for thereby almost all expenditure would appear to be cut off. We have seen, however, that " rest in bed " does not always achieve this end. Moreover, it will often be enough to reduce expenditure ; it may not be necessary to cut off all expenditure. We need not invariably prohibit every kind of action. We must discriminate, must ascertain which actions are the most costly, which forms of expenditure most ruinous. It is these which must be prohibited; and the patient's activities must be restricted to such as are indispensable, simple, and inexpensive. But, even in this restricted form, treatment by rest is an economising method of treatment.

Furthermore, this simplification of life will also form a part of the treatment of traumatic memories. It is not enough to dispel the actual symptom. We have to think of possible relapses. We must be on our guard lest some new happening, causing emotional stresses and imperfectly liquidated, may not, ere long, establish a new traumatic memory. Remember the case of Paul, who has epileptic fits as a sequel of attempts to enjoy a triumph. The patient himself tells us of the precautions he finds requisite. He knows perfectly well that anything which stirs his emotions is dangerous to him; he avoids anything which can arouse a keen sense of joy or sorrow, can give him a strong feeling. He keeps away from public displays; he does not go to concerts, for he is " too fond of them." He does not travel, since the sight of new countries might stir his enthusiasm; he will not even allow his thoughts to dwell upon future pleasures or upon the possibility of making money. " It is essential to my health that my life should be colourless and unemotional, and I regulate my activities accordingly. No doubt he pushes these precautions too far, seeing that he never dares get into a train or pass beyond the suburbs of the little town in which he dwells. Nevertheless, he has good reason for this regulation of his activities, and thereby he has been able to make his epileptic attacks very infrequent, and has passed a whole year without a fit. He has reduced his infirmity to a minimum.

The precautions, I repeat, are excellent, and can be amply justified. Just as the patient must avoid circumstances that demand reflective assent and circumstances that necessitate prolonged labour, so he may have to avoid circumstances which will induce the sense of triumph, seeing that this likewise will involve difficulties and dangers. No doubt it is rather sad that we should have to cut off the patient from the joys of life, to forbid triumph and enthusiasm and excitement; but in many cases these prohibitions may do a great deal of good to the patient, and their enforcement is as a rule easy, for these patients are not cheerful folk. They are almost invariably in the first grade (at least) of depression, and they are accustomed to a dull life. Like our friend Paul, they must avoid festivals, ceremonies, places where crowds foregather. Only a few of our patients will be refractory, those who have a desperate longing, as it were by impulsive obsession, for joy and excitement. In these cases, we shall have to be continually pointing out the dangers, and insisting upon the need for caution. The reader may object that it is impossible to avoid occasions for sorrow, surprise, or regret, but the criticism is not altogether sound. We can avoid circumstances which would lead to partings or disillusionments ; we can be careful not to take things too much to heart ; we can shun circumstances which would lead to a triumph or necessitate a liquidation ; we can evade circumstances which might induce traumatic memories.

Finally, we learn from psychological analysis that the most complicated of all our actions are social actions ; that the expenditure necessitated by adaptation to our associates is the most lavish of all our expenditure. The inference is that it is especially this expenditure which we must avoid or curtail. In serious cases, the patient must be isolated as completely as possible, his social life must be reduced to artificial relationships, which demand very little expenditure. In less severe cases, absolute isolation will not be requisite : it will be enough to restrict social relationships ; to draw the important distinction between " expensive " and " inexpensive " persons ; to reduce social expenditure in conformity with a scanty income. Treatment by isolation and treatment by separation from costly individuals are the most perfect forms of mental economy. Here, then, we have an assemblage of kindred and extremely important methods of treatment. When we have to do with one in whom bankruptcy threatens, the most vital matter is to reduce expenditure and to insist upon strict economy.

The foregoing summary is rather metaphorical, but it has its uses, not only in demonstrating the value of these methods of treatment, but also in disclosing their inadequacies. First of all, we must not forget that the actions requisite for dispelling traumatic memories, the actions which will achieve liquidation, are often difficult and costly. We have just been studying their satisfactory outcome, but we have had occasion to note that they are difficult to bring about, and that they may entail a heavy expenditure. On the other hand, the restricted life characteristic of the foregoing methods entails serious inconveniences; it may be out of keeping with the patient's tastes or unsuitable to his position; in many cases, it is very disagreeable alike to the patient and his relatives. Finally, the future of which it affords prospects is by no means seductive, for it does not promise anything more than a very slow increase in psychological capital. We know only too well that thrift, however rigid, will rarely suffice to lead to fortune. That is why other methods of treatment have been advocated. These are, perhaps, somewhat more hazardous, but they offer more attractive prospects. I refer to the methods which I propose to consider in the fourth part of this work, under the title Psychological Acquisitions.

Classics in Psychiatry

An Arno Press Collection

American Psychiatrists Abroad. 1975

Arnold, Thomas. Observations On The Nature, Kinds, Causes, And Prevention Of Insanity. 1806. Two volumes in one

Austin, Thomas J. A Practical Account Of General Paralysis, Its Mental And Physical Symptoms, Statistics, Causes, Seat, And Treatment. 1859

Bayle, A[ntoine] L[aurent] J[esse]. Traité Des Maladies Du Cerveau Et De Ses Membranes. 1826

Binz, Carl. Doctor Johann Weyer. 1896

Blandford, G. Fielding. Insanity And Its Treatment. 1871

Bleuler, Eugen. Textbook Of Psychiatry. 1924

Braid, James. Neurypnology. 1843

Brierre de Boismont, A[lexandre-Jacques-François]. Hallucinations. 1853

Brown, Mabel Webster, compiler. Neuropsychiatry And The War: A Bibliography With Abstracts and Supplement I, October 1918. Two volumes in one

Browne, W. A. F. What Asylums Were, Are, And Ought To Be. 1837

Burrows, George Man. Commentaries On The Causes, Forms, Symptoms And Treatment, Moral And Medical, Of Insanity. 1828

Calmeil, L[ouis]-F[lorentin]. De La Folie: Considérée Sous Le Point De Vue Pathologique, Philosophique, Historique Et Judiciaire, Depuis La Renaissance Des Sciences En Europe Jusqu'au Dix-Neuvième Siècle. 1845. Two volumes in one

Calmeil, L[ouis] F[lorentin]. De La Paralysie Considérée Chez Les Aliénés. 1826

Dejerine, J[oseph Jules] and E. Gauckler. The Psychoneuroses And Their Treatment By Psychotherapy. [1913]

Dunbar, [Helen] Flanders. Emotions And Bodily Changes. 1954

Ellis, W[illiam] C[harles]. A Treatise On The Nature, Symptoms, Causes And Treatment Of Insanity. 1838

Emminghaus, H[ermann]. Die Psychischen Störungen Des Kindesalters. 1887

Esdaile, James. Mesmerism In India, And Its Practical Application In Surgery And Medicine. 1846

Esquirol, E[tienne]. Des Maladies Mentales. 1838. Three volumes in two

Feuchtersleben, Ernst [Freiherr] von. **The Principles Of Medical Psychology.** 1847

Georget, [Etienne-Jean]. **De La Folie:** Considérations Sur Cette Maladie. 1820

Haslam, John. **Observations On Madness And Melancholy.** 1809

Hill, Robert Gardiner. **Total Abolition Of Personal Restraint In The Treatment Of The Insane.** 1839

Janet, Pierre [Marie-Felix] and F. Raymond. **Les Obsessions Et La Psychasthénie.** 1903. Two volumes

Janet, Pierre [Marie-Felix]. **Psychological Healing.** 1925. Two volumes

Kempf, Edward J. **Psychopathology.** 1920

Kraepelin, Emil. **Manic-Depressive Insanity And Paranoia.** 1921

Kraepelin, Emil. **Psychiatrie:** Ein Lehrbuch Für Studirende Und Aerzte. 1896

Laycock, Thomas. **Mind And Brain.** 1860. Two volumes in one

Liébeault, A[mbroise]-A[uguste]. **Le Sommeil Provoqué Et Les États Analogues.** 1889

Mandeville, B[ernard] De. **A Treatise Of The Hypochondriack And Hysterick Passions.** 1711

Morel, B[enedict] A[ugustin]. **Traité Des Degénérescences Physiques, Intellectuelles Et Morales De L'Espèce Humaine.** 1857. Two volumes in one

Morison, Alexander. **The Physiognomy Of Mental Diseases.** 1843

Myerson, Abraham. **The Inheritance Of Mental Diseases.** 1925

Perfect, William. **Annals Of Insanity.** [1808]

Pinel, Ph[ilippe]. **Traité Médico-Philosophique Sur L'Aliénation Mentale.** 1809

Prince, Morton, et al. **Psychotherapeutics.** 1910

Psychiatry In Russia And Spain. 1975

Ray, I[saac]. **A Treatise On The Medical Jurisprudence Of Insanity.** 1871

Semelaigne, René. **Philippe Pinel Et Son Oeuvre Au Point De Vue De La Médecine Mentale.** 1888

Thurnam, John. **Observations And Essays On The Statistics Of Insanity.** 1845

Trotter, Thomas. **A View Of The Nervous Temperament.** 1807

Tuke, D[aniel] Hack, editor. **A Dictionary Of Psychological Medicine.** 1892. Two volumes

Wier, Jean. **Histoires, Disputes Et Discours Des Illusions Et Impostures Des Diables, Des Magiciens Infames, Sorcieres Et Empoisonneurs.** 1885. Two volumes

Winslow, Forbes. **On Obscure Diseases Of The Brain And Disorders Of The Mind.** 1860

Burdett, Henry C. **Hospitals And Asylums Of The World.** 1891-93. Five volumes. 2,740 pages on NMA standard 24x-98 page microfiche only